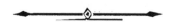

ISBN 978-0-260-85001-0
PIBN 10976361

ARCHIVES

OF

DERMATOLOGY AND SYPHILOLOGY

(Succeeding Vol. 38, 1919, the Journal of Cutaneous Diseases)

VOLUME 6

1922

PUBLISHERS
AMERICAN MEDICAL ASSOCIATION
CHICAGO, ILL.

CONTENTS OF VOLUME 6

Archives of Dermatology and Syphilology

VOLUME 6   JULY, 1922   NUMBER 1

ERYTHEMA MULTIFORME CONFINED TO THE MUCOUS MEMBRANES

WITH REPORT OF CASE

JOHN BUTLER, M.D.

Associate Professor of Dermatology and Syphilology, University of Minnesota Medical School

MINNEAPOLIS

Crocker [1] reported a case of erythema multiforme in which the mouth alone was affected, and which "showed attacks of bullous aphthae beginning on the buccal mucous membrane, and spreading over the tongue and mouth without any skin lesion. The affection occurred every two or three months. After being under observation for over a year, erythema iris lesions appeared on the back of the hands in one attack, and the patient then remembered that he had had a similar attack some years before."

So far as I can determine from a review of the literature and current textbooks, there are no other reports of cases of erythema multiforme confined to the mucous membranes.

Osler [2] reported eleven cases of erythema multiforme with visceral complications. In two of his cases in which the attacks were entirely visceral there were no skin manifestations. In none of them were the mucous membranes involved other than hemorrhage in five cases; but in the majority of these cases there were severe visceral complications. Two of the cases were fatal. The skin lesions were described as "polymorphic, ranging from simple purpura to extensive local edema, and from urticaria in all grades and forms to large infiltrating hemorrhages of the skin and subcutaneous tissues." Osler stated that "most of these cases would be described under the heading of purpura of peliosis, since hemorrhage was the most constant lesion; but the variable character of the eruption made a wider definition of exudative erythema multiforme more acceptable."

1. Crocker: Diseases of the Skin. Ed. 3. Philadelphia, P. Blakiston's So. & Co., p. 98.

2. Osler, William: Am. J. M. Sc., 1895, p. 629; Brit. J. Dermat., 1900, p. 227.

Pusey [3] says "these cases do not correspond to the accepted picture of erythema multiforme in which the systemic disturbance is practically of no importance.   They are, however, of interest as throwing light upon the toxic processes which underlie at least a great proportion of the cases."

In a western army camp, in 1918, I examined two patients suffering from severe stomatitis which the ward surgeon thought was syphilitic, but which I was unable to diagnose after a careful examination.   The

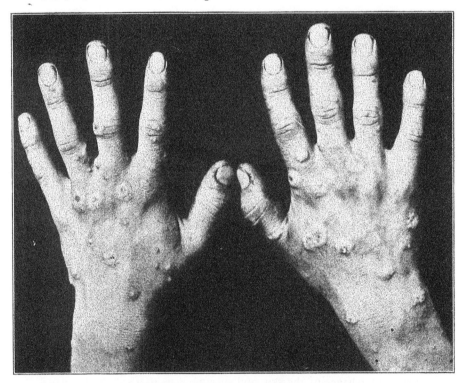

Fig. 1.—Bullous lesions on the dorsa of the hands.

mouth, tongue, and labial membranes were involved equally in both patients.   The skin was normal in every respect.   (A description of the lesions corresponds in every way to those in the detailed case report that follows.)

Syphilis was definitely excluded by the absence of clinical symptoms and by negative microscopic and serologic findings.   Vincent's angina was strongly suspected in one case; but the laboratory findings did not confirm the diagnosis.   Pemphigus confined to the membranes of the

3. Pusey, W. A.: Principles and Practice of Dermatology, Ed. 3, New York, D. Appleton & Co., 1917, p. 187.

mouth was considered, but it was dismissed on account of the fulminating development in two days of the lesions involving all of the membranes of the mouth, and the absence of skin lesions.

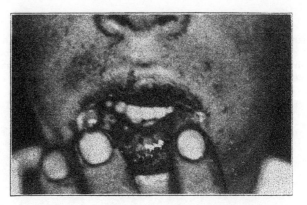

Fig. 2.—Involvement of lips and buccal and lingual membranes

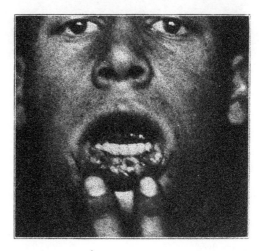

Fig. 3.—Involvement of lips and buccal and lingual membrane.

Two days following my examination one patient had beginning erythematosus patches on the dorsal aspect of the hands and feet that quickly developed into typical bullous lesions, and these made a correct diagnosis an easy matter. The other patient clarified the situation by saying that he, too, had suffered similar outbreaks on his hands and feet together with associated mouth lesions during the two preceding years, both attacks occurring in the Spring, and attributed by him to plowing in the fields during rainy weather. Careful observation of this patient throughout the course of his illness failed to reveal any skin manifestations of the disease.

REPORT OF CASE

A man, student, aged 16, had always been in excellent health. In October, 1918, he suffered an attack of erythema multiforme with bullous lesions on the dorsal surfaces of the hands (Fig. 1) and feet. The buccal and lingual mucous membranes were also involved, showing severe denuded areas. He had other

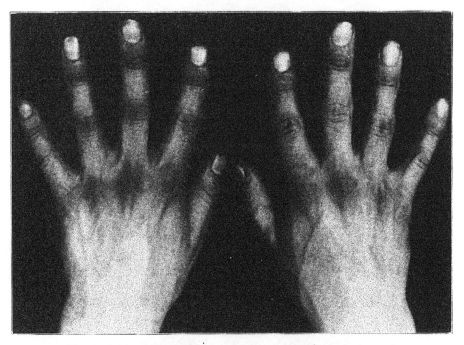

Fig. 4.—Lack of involvement of the skin during the second attack.

attacks in November, 1919, and in March and August, 1920. In all of these, the skin lesions were of the bullous and iris type, and the buccal, lingual, and labial membranes were involved.

I first saw this patient at the time of his fourth attack (Aug. 10, 1920), when he was admitted to the university medical school dispensary. On the palmar, plantar and dorsal surfaces of the hands and feet there were numerous bullous lesions. A few of those on the palmar and plantar surfaces corresponded more closely to the iris type. The buccal membranes were almost entirely involved, as were also the lingual, and inner surfaces of the lips (Figs. 2 and 3). The mouth lesions consisted of severe inflammatory, denuded areas covered with a grayish, viscid mucous secretion. There were numerous patches of the loosely attached grayish white shreds, the remains of the ruptured vesicle coverings.

There were similar lesions on the dorsum of the tongue and the inner borders of the lips. The patient experienced considerable difficulty in opening the mouth sufficiently wide to take nourishment. The ingestion of soft food, and especially of hot or cold liquids, was painful. There were no constitutional disturbances and the patient made an uneventful recovery in three weeks.

He was readmitted to the dispensary, Jan. 10, 1921, with erythema multiforme lesions of the buccal, lingual and labial membranes. No skin lesions were apparent throughout this attack . (Fig. 4). The mouth affection simulated and ran a course identical with that of the fourth attack. Esophagoscopy and proctoscopic examinations by Dr. R. I. Rizer revealed lesions similar to those of the mouth, reddened areas, covered with gray loosely adherent sloughs. The outline of the lesions was circular; some were confluent, gyrate patches. No other marked abnormalities were found. There were no constitutional disturbances other than a temperature of 101 F. on the first day, and a slightly dull, continuous pain in the right hypochondrium at the height of the attack. There were no hemorrhages. The teeth were negative. The tonsils did not appear diseased. The mucosa of the nose was turgid and congested, otherwise it was negative. There was some involvement of the anterior cervical and maxillary glands. The disease ran its usual course of three weeks. It was interesting to note that annular stains conforming to ringed lesions could be outlined in the regenerated buccal membranes.

The laboratory findings were: Blood culture was negative. In each hundred cubic centimeters of blood there was sugar, 0.80 mg.; creatinin, 2.30 mg.; urea. 15.9. Blood examination revealed: hemoglobin, 75 per cent.; erythrocytes. 4,920,000; leukocytes, 8,650; the differential count was normal. The urine was clear, straw colored and acid, and the specific gravity was 1.020. There was a trace of albumin. There was no sugar. The microscopic examination was negative.

COMMENT

Erythema multiforme of the mucous membranes without associated skin lesions is, no doubt, of rare occurrence. Naturally, such cases would gravitate to the oral specialist rather than to the dermatologist. so that it is little wonder that the dermatologist encounters this condition so seldom. A diagnosis of the affection naturally presents difficulties both to the oral specialist and to the dermatologist. The mouth affection might easily be, and no doubt often has been, mistaken for syphilitic mucous patches; and erythema multiforme being a self-limited disease, syphilitic treatment would apparently verify the mistaken diagnosis. Pemphigus confined to the mucous membranes would be equally confusing without sufficient time for observation. Stomatitis due to other diverse and unassignable causes would present diagnostic difficulties to the inexperienced.

CUTIS VERTICIS GYRATA (UNNA)

EDWARD A. OLIVER, M.D.

CHICAGO

It was recently my good fortune to see and study a case of this rare anomaly of the scalp. In looking over the literature on the subject, I found that in all about thirty cases have been reported. The majority have been recorded in the German literature, three in the French, and one in the American. Unna [1] and Jadassohn [2] termed the condition cutis verticis gyrata; Audry [3] and Lenormant [4] prefer the name la pachydermie vorticellie du cuir chevelu. Wise and Levin [5] reported the first American case in 1918.

REPORT OF AUTHOR'S CASE

My patient, E. B., aged 52 years, a lecturer, born in Central America, entered Cook County Hospital, Aug. 19, 1921, with a right-sided paralysis and aphasia, the result of cerebral hemorrhage on April 26, 1921. Up to that time he had been in fair health, but had had frequent attacks of vertigo, headache, and vomiting. I saw him through the courtesy of Dr. Lewis J. Pollock and Dr. Menke at the county infirmary.

He was middle aged, large, well built and well nourished. His skin was deeply tanned and his face wrinkled easily. The hair on the scalp was abundant, long and black. The scalp felt thick, was lax and easily movable. The forehead wrinkled easily, and one received the impression, on palpation, that the scalp was too large for the cranium. Pushing it back, it formed large gyri and furrows on his neck. When the hair was long nothing abnormal was seen, but when it was short a number of distinct gyri and furrows were seen on the top of the head. These simulated closely the gyri and furrows of the cerebrum. On top of the head was an oval area about 3 inches (7.62 cm.) wide, on either side of which, running symmetrically forward and arching toward one another, though not meeting, were three distinct furrows and two gyri. Running backward toward the occiput were five more furrows. These were not arranged symmetrically and pursued a rather jagged course. With the hair short the furrows and corresponding gyri were marked. Pushing up the scalp accentuated the condition. Down over the occipital region the scalp hung loosely. The gyri felt thicker than the other parts of the scalp and down in the furrows the hair grew abundantly. No scars were to be seen, and clinically there were no signs of a preceding inflammatory condition. There were no subjective symptoms.

The patient was unable to talk coherently or intelligently, and no history was obtainable. His wife knew nothing of this condition, although she had lived with him for twenty years, because he wore his hair long. The patient was well aware of the condition, but had never paid much attention to it.

1. Unna: Monatsh. f. prakt. Dermat. 45:227, 1907.
2. Jadassohn: Verhandl. d. deutsch. Gesellsch. Kong., Berne, 1907.
3. Audry: Ann. de dermat. et syph., 1909, p. 257.
4. Lenormant: Ann. de dermat. et syph. 5:225, 1920.
5. Wise and Levin: Interstate M. J. 25:380 (May) 1918.

CASES REPORTED IN THE LITERATURE

Jadassohn, at the ninth congress of the German Dermatological Society held at Berne, was the first to point out this peculiar anomaly. Unna, in 1907, published a report of three cases in men between the ages of 35 and 50. Von Veress,[6] in 1908, reviewed the previous cases, and reported eleven more of his own. Cases have also been reported by Pospelow,[7] Audry,[3] Bogrow,[8] Vignolo Lutati,[9] Vorner,[10] Oppenheim [11] Malartic and Opin,[12] Ronviere, Lenormant, and Wise and Levin. In a very complete paper published in 1920, Lenormant reviewed the previously reported cases and reported one of his own.

Wise and Levin reviewed the literature in 1918, and reported the first American case. Their patient was an Austrian Jew, a furniture upholsterer, aged 36, who had syphilitic periostitis. His attention was first called to his scalp at the age of 13. His mother was certain the condition was not present at birth. There were no subjective symptoms except that when his hair was allowed to grow for more than two weeks the scalp became tender and there was pain on pressure. There was no history of trauma or infection of the scalp, and the condition did not respond to antisyphilitic treatment.

Running transversely across the occipital region were three gyrus-like elevations, separated by two furrows. The gyri were parallel, most prominent in the central portion of the scalp, and tended to disappear at the lateral hair lines. The lower folds were more marked. The furrows were also parallel, and the lower was the deeper one. On palpation it was found there were five gyri; the upper two were perceptible to touch only; the others were elevated, from one-fourth to one inch (0.6 to 2.54 cm.) thick. The skin in the folds was thick, inelastic and freely movable on the skull. It felt more firmly attached in the furrows. There was no tenderness on pulling or pressing the hair on the scalp. The hair was dark brown and apparently normal. A Wassermann reaction was positive.

Lenormant believes that there are two varieties of this condition, one of inflammatory origin generally limited to a palm sized area on the superior portion of the scalp, and encountered in men; the other is always congenital, and anatomically resembles a giant nevus. The

6. Von Veress: Ztschr. **15**:675, 1908.

7. Pospelow: Russ. Ztschr. **18**:7, 1909.

8. Bogrow: Monatsh. f. prakt. Dermat. **1**:16, 1910.

9. Vignolo Lutani: Arch. f. Dermat. u. Syph. **104**:422, 1910.

10. Vorner: Dermat. Wchnschr. **54**:300, 1912.

11. Oppenheim: Arch. f. Dermat. u. Syph. **98**:100, 1909.

12. Malartic and Opin: Bull. et mém. Soc. de chir. de Paris. June, 1917. p. 84

cases described by him and Malartic and Opin differ essentially from other reported cases of which mine is a fair example, in that they are not characterized by furrows and gyri but are really giant nevi. The microscopic structure also differs materially in that it resembles closely the structure of nevi.

Lenormant's case was that of a woman, aged 30. Signs of the growth were apparent in childhood, but it was not until she was 13 years old that it began to attain any size. From that time until she was 30 it grew rapidly. The condition resembled a nevus lipomatosus; it looked

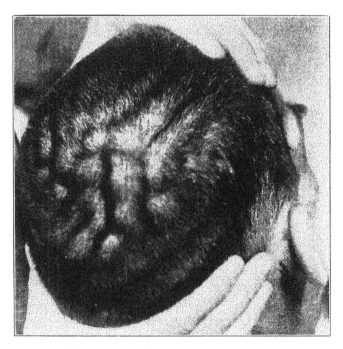

View of scalp showing gyri and furrows.

like a bonnet perched on one side of the head, covering almost the entire scalp except the right temporal and frontal regions. It had about the consistency of brain tissue, and the convolutions of the brain were closely simulated. There were a series of deep, irregular furrows which could be pulled or pushed apart. It was a heavy mass and was the seat of extensive ulcerations. Down in the furrows sebaceous secretions accumulated, and the odor of the decomposing secretions finally became so intolerable that the patient could no longer endure it. The mass was removed surgically. Malartic and Opin's case was of the same type.

The majority of these cases have occurred in men of middle age. In sixteen of the cases, the ages ranged between 35 and 50. In eight cases the ages were from 25 to 30, and in six the age was less than 25. The location was practically the same in all cases, a space the size of the palm on the uppermost part of the head. The condition in Oppenheim's case occupied one side of the head. In most of the cases the furrows ran perpendicularly. In a few they ran transversely. The history in nearly all of them was that the condition was discovered accidentally.

Jadassohn believed the condition was a congenital defect of the scalp which developed in later life. Unna, Pospelow and Vorner believed the same. Veress, Audry and Vignolo Lutati, however, assert that preceding inflammations and infections of the scalp are a prominent factor in its production. In three cases reported by Veress eczema, impetigo and psoriasis existed prior to its development. Audry's patient had an impetigo; one of Pospelow's patients had had an eczema, and another had had a syphilitic eruption on the scalp.

Welch made a thorough microscopic study of Jadassohn's case, and found nothing pathologic. Veress reported that in his first case he found a disappearance of the sebaceous glands and an atrophy of the sweat glands, whose glomeruli instead of having from ten to twelve convolutions had only two or three. There was an infiltration of plasma, lymph and mast cells in the papillary and reticular layers, and a complete disappearance of the elastic fibers. In his second case, however, he did not find any of the preceding lesions except a slight atrophy of the sebaceous glands.

Vignolo Lutati, after a microscopic study of sections from his case, concluded that the pathologic process started at the base of the lesion and that the furrows were secondary. He found no appreciable changes in the epidermis. In the deeper parts he recognized an infiltration of mononuclear, plasma, giant and epithelioid cells, localized about the deeper follicles. The superficial hair follicles remained unaffected. This infiltration was present at the top of the furrows and absent at the sides and bottom. He noted also a shrinkage of the papillae, swelling of the hair follicles, and atrophy of the sebaceous and sweat glands. In time fibrous tissue is produced and by contracting gives rise to furrowing of the scalp. Lutati believes that the hairs of the occipital region, when thick and short, acquire sufficient rigidity to exercise pressure on the bottom of the follicle when the patient is lying in the prone position and in this way provoke enough irritation to cause the condition. Its absence in women and children can thus be explained.

25 East Washington Street.

HEMANGIOSARCOMA OF THE SKIN

ARTHUR M. GREENWOOD, M.D.

Assistant Dermatologist, Massachusetts General Hospital

BOSTON

AND

THEODORE K. LAWLESS, M.D.

CHICAGO

The case which we report was presented at the clinical meeting of the American Dermatological Association, at the Massachusetts General Hospital in Boston, in 1921, and as there was no general agreement as to diagnosis and there had not then been opportunity for careful study, the following report is presented. We are indebted to Dr. Frederick S. Burns, who presented the case, and to Dr. Harvey P. Towle, in whose service it occurred, for the opportunity to study it. The report of the discussion of the case at its presentation may be found in the October, 1921, number of the ARCHIVES OF DERMATOLOGY AND SYPHILOLOGY, page 556.

REPORT OF CASES

J. C., a man, aged 62, born in Nova Scotia, married, a wood polisher, whose mother died of cancer, and whose father died of kidney disease, had five brothers, three dead; three sisters, all living; and one grandchild, who was well. There has been no condition similar to that of the patient in other members of the family, or any other skin disease. The patient was operated on at the Massachusetts General Hospital in 1920, and epididymectomy and vasectomy were performed for tuberculosis. As far as he knew, his skin was normal up to the time of the appearance of the present condition, and he thought there had been no birthmarks on his body.

The present condition began eighteen years previously, when he was 44 years of age, appearing on the face. The first thing he noticed was that the face was redder than normal, and he described the condition as a uniform redness which gradually covered the whole face and neck. From the onset, it had gradually spread over the neck, chest, abdomen, back, arms and buttocks. The patient thought that the spread had not been by direct extension from the original area but that it had appeared in new spots at some distance from the old ones. He was positive that the forearms were affected before the upper arms. He was of the opinion that there had been no extension for some months and our observation bore this out. There had been no subjective symptoms. The patient said that the eruption stood out much more distinctly after a bath or when he was cold.

Physical Examination. — The patient was well developed and fairly well nourished. The heart and lungs were normal. There was a right inguinal hernia, and the right testicle only was present. The urine showed a small amount of pus. The blood was normal; the blood pressure: systolic. 195. diastolic, 120; the blood Wassermann reaction was negative. The eruption or its sequelae involved the face. neck, chest, abdomen, back, buttocks, both folds of the axillae and the extensor surfaces of both arms and forearms. The skin of the active areas involved, seen from a distance, gave the appearance of a diffused, superficial, vascular nevus with varying shades of color, from a crimson red in the newer areas to a distinctly purplish-red in the older ones. There were seen on closer observation:

1. Areas of diffuse, fairly uniform purplish-red, in places a dusky blue, as is seen in asphyxia. These were on the chest and part of the abdomen and back. The color did not entirely disappear on pressure with the diascope.

2. Crimson red papules, slightly raised above the skin level. These were seen in or near the advancing borders. They varied from pinhead to pea size. Diascopic pressure did not efface them.

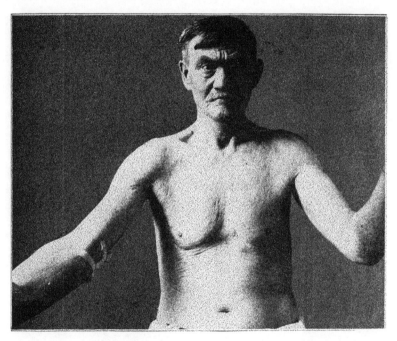

Fig. 1.—Front view, showing wrinkled, atrophic appearance of the chest over which the process has passed. The color is a dusky blue.

3. Many ringlike lesions in, and in advance of, the advancing border. The edges of these rings were elevated slightly above the skin level (approximately 1 mm.) and were about 1 mm. wide. The centers were lower than the edges but not depressed below the skin level. The process evidently consisted of a disappearance of the redness from the centers of the vascular papules leaving a pronounced red border with a rather paler than normal skin color in the center. There was no primary grouping of vascular papules in circles, but the rings were evidently all formed as described.

4. Pigmented lesions. These were circular, approximately pea-sized, brownish-yellow macules in, or just behind, the advancing borders. They were not marked and required fairly careful observation to be seen. They seemed much lighter in shade than those ordinarily made by blood pigmen

There were no distinctly atrophic spots. The centers of many of the vascular rings appeared whiter than normal and somewhat shrunken, but this seemed to us to be more from contrast with the red, raised periphery than from actual atrophy. On the other hand, the extended purplish areas appeared distinctly atrophic and wrinkled and crossed with a fine network of lines, considerably more so than in the normal skin of that age.

There were no telangiectases on the parts of the body affected by the growth. The general advance of the process apparently was by the appearance of the red papules in the normal skin beyond the areas of uniform redness, so that a schematic picture of the whole eruption, going from the normal skin to the oldest areas, would show: (1) normal skin; (2) vascular papules and rings

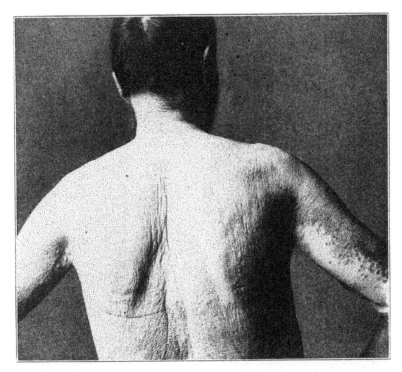

Fig. 2.—Back view, showing older area on the back and the active border on the upper arm. In this border are seen the outlying vascular papules and rings. The color is almost crimson, with a slight bluish tinge.

with normal skin between; (3) pigmented spots on a more or less uniform redness; (4) rather mottled, purplish redness on a wrinkled, atrophic appearing skin. There was no desquamation in any place. The most recent lesions occurred on the extensor surfaces of the arms and forearms and on the buttocks just external to the fold on either side. There was nothing to suggest "cayenne pepper grains" in any part of the lesion.

Below the buttocks, the skin presented a network of dilated capillaries and small veins on both thighs, legs and feet. This condition did not resemble the condition on the upper part of the body and, while perhaps more pronounced than is ordinarily seen, was not uncommon in a lesser degree.

Histology.— The tissues, from which the microscopic description was made, were obtained from biopsies, 1 per cent. cocain being used for local anesthesia, with immediate fixation in 4 per cent. formaldehyd solution for twenty-four hours. The tissue was taken from the advancing borders. the areas of uniform redness, and the oldest, atrophic appearing areas.

From these tissues, both frozen and paraffin sections were made. The staining was eosin and hematoxylin, Weigert's elastic tissue stain, and van Gieson's and Mallory's connective tissue stains. Each of the foregoing methods of staining, aside from specifically stressing the tissues for which the characteristic reactions were obtained, emphasized the same general structure throughout.

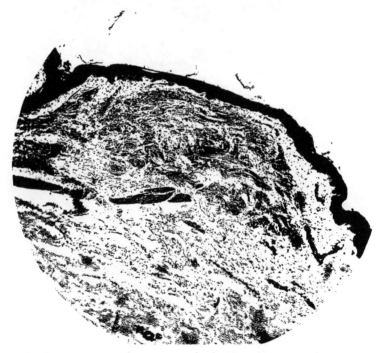

Fig. 3.—Low power photomicrograph showing location of the growth, its nevoid arrangement, flattening of the rete and keratosis of a follicular opening.

The epidermis gave no evidence of playing an active rôle in this condition or of being unduly affected by the activity of the process. with the exception of a slight increase in scale formation. a moderate degree of rete peg flattening over those areas of the corium where there was a proliferation of the neoplastic tissue. and plugging and keratosis of the follicular orifices.

The chief pathologic change was in the superficial corium. but occasionally the deep corium had also been invaded. Here we found. scattered at various levels, larger and smaller cell-rich areas. These cellular groups appeared mostly in an arrangement which was parallel with the epidermis. and were made up of islands and various sized cords and strands. in which were many vascular channels.

The character of the cells of this new formed tissue was constant throughout. A characteristic area presented fields of large ovoid to oval and, in places, flattened cells lining definite channels, and, in other instances, grouped and whorled and showing marked tendencies to line spaces in the tissue. The most striking component of these cellular masses was the presence of many large cells containing from one to five nuclei. These cells, as to nuclei and cytoplasm, resembled the definite endothelial cells but contained a larger amount of cytoplasm. This cytoplasm was finely granular and had a definitely reticulated appearance, and, like the cytoplasm of the cells lining the definite channels, was moderately basophilic in character. In many places, these multi-

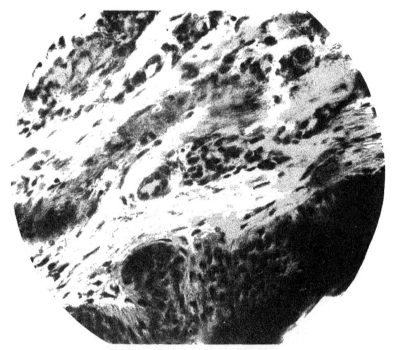

Fig. 4.—High power photomicrograph showing the newly formed vessels cut in cross section and longitudinally.

nucleated cells were sending out protoplasmic processes which apparently marked the first step in the formation of vascular channels. There were areas in which we found groups of these multinucleated cells apparently fused, or in the act of fusing, and a definite channel being formed by this act.

Within these proliferating areas, we found, here and there, either singly or in groups, cells of the lymphocyte series with a well formed, round to oval, deeply staining nucleus, and a small rim of acidophilic protoplasm. These cells were in the lymph spaces. Here and there were seen various sized, finely granular areas, with a reticulated appearance and without nuclear structures.

The connective tissue bundles were normal in appearance, but the spaces between them were increased. In those areas in which the number of new cells was large, the connective tissue fibers were diminished. The elastic tissue was apparently normal in quality although there was noted an increase in the amount of elacin. This, however, might easily have been a senile change.

The glandular structures were apparently normal, with an occasional invasion of the contiguous tissues by the neoplastic cells and with some follicular keratosis at the epidermal portions. There was nowhere to be seen the slightest evidence of an inflammatory reaction. The entire process impressed one as a postembryonal proliferation of endothelial cells, noninflammatory in nature, and the condition may be denominated hemangiosarcoma, or hemangio-endothelioma, with a distinctly nevoid arrangement.

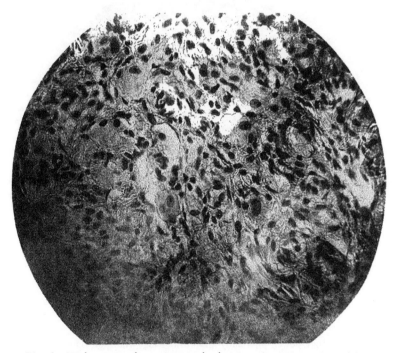

Fig. 5.—High power photomicrograph showing the large endothelial tumor cells, one of them with two nuclei and sending out a protoplasmic process.

In 1894, Dr. James C. White [1] reported a case of "so-called angioma serpiginosum," an abstract of which, with the histologic report, follows:

A boy, aged 12 years, had at birth, a "purplish-red mark" below the right shoulder blade. It increased slowly in size in an upward direction until he was 4 years old, when another spot no larger than the head of a pin appeared near the original one, which gradually became larger. Since then others had continued to appear and grow, up to the time of examination. The process began in the form of minute elevated points, of a bright red, which slowly increased in size until they were from one-eighth to one-sixth of an inch (3 to 4 mm.) in diameter. At this stage, they were elevated from one-twelfth to one-eighth of an inch (2 to 3 mm.) above the general surface. They were bright red, varying from scarlet to carmin, which could be made to disappear only partially by long pressure, and were of firm consistence. Having attained this size, they underwent involution at the center, which slowly sank down as the growth spread peripherally. In this way, rings were formed, and the disease progressed as an annular elevated margin, about one-eighth of an inch (3 mm.) in breadth, slowly creeping outward, until, by confluence with other lesions, the regular circular shape was lost. Within the ring, the skin had apparently returned to its natural condition except in

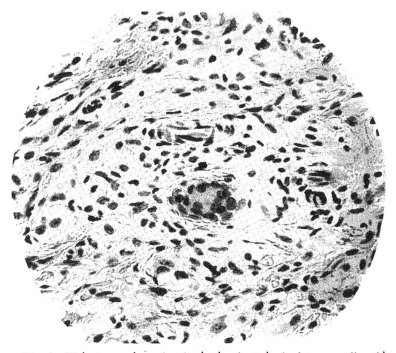

Fig. 6.—High power photomicrograph showing whorl of tumor cells with imperfect attempt at vessel formation.

color, which remained of a dull purplish or dusky hue. New foci, in the shape of minute points, appeared at some distance from the older areas, and assumed the same annular mode of progression, with central involution. The elevated margin or ring preserved a uniform breadth about its whole circumference. New foci were continually developing some distance, from one eighth to one third of an inch (3 to 8 mm.), beyond these older areas, which in turn were converted by central involution into the annular forms. The tissue in all stages of activity, the small papules and the rings in all their parts, presented the same character—a firm, smooth, elevated structure, varying in color from bright red to claret. The central areas after involution sank down to the normal level but remained stained, of a dull purplish-brown tint.

Histologic Report (Dr. Darier).—The epidermis was composed of its ordinary layers unaltered, and not infiltrated by the numerous migratory cells, as occurs in inflammations.

Examination by low power revealed a lesion occupying the whole extent of the derma, and consisting of a mass of cells deeply colored by the reagents. These masses were more or less sharply defined at their borders, and presented diverse outlines, circular or ovoid, with margins, festooned or angular, or drawn out into trails, which, in sufficiently thick sections. seemed to form, by ramification or anastomosis, a coarse network. In the deeper layer of the corium, on the border of the hypoderm, where the sweat glands lie. the masses of cells were abundant and large and were often seen in immediate contact with the glomerulas. The tubes of the gland were never invaded or destroyed.

With the high power lens, the cells composing these masses were seen to be fusiform, aplastic or angular in shape. Their protoplasm was abundant, and the nucleus was generally oval in form. This was manifestly no question of epithelial cells, but of cells having a mesodermic origin. There was persistence of elastic tissue. In all the masses, the flattened cells had a tendency to group themselves concentrically about a certain number of centers. Such a center was often made up of two or three cells of the same nature attached at their edges and thus forming a canal. At two or three points, the center was occupied by a cell much larger than the others with several nuclei (a vasoformative cell!?).

It appears, then, that we are dealing with a new formation of capillaries at the expense of the elements of the neoplastic tissue. How, then. is this lesion to be classed, and what name shall be given it? A neoformation. noninflammatory. composed of cells of the type of young connective tissue cells. should necessarily bear the name of sarcoma. But it will be observed that we are in the presence of an unusual form of sarcoma, not massed in a single tumor. but reticulated and infiltrated as a network. There is. moreover, to be noticed the tendency which the cells of this sarcoma have to form networks and clusters of more or less dilated capillaries, that is to say, to transform themselves into a true angioma. The title of this new formation might well be sarcome angioplastique réticulé. The information received. that this tumor started on the surface of a nevus, leads one to think that this is a nevus à structure de sarcome angioplastique devenu envahissant.

Comment.—Professor Councilman and Dr. Bowen, who examined sections from this case, found the epidermis and the hair follicles and sweat glands normal. The special pathologic condition consisted of groups of cells distributed in the corium, fairly well circumscribed and. in general. arranged parallel to the surface. The cells making up these groups were large. their nuclei oval in form and having something of the appearance of the nuclei of epithelioid cells. Various changes in the vessels could be made out. These consisted in swelling and proliferation of the endothelial cells of the vessels. frequently combined with proliferation of the cells on the outside. These vascular changes apparently affected small veins and capillaries. There was no evidence of anything corresponding to inflammation.

They noted. as a peculiarity in the process. the presence of small granular masses here and there in the cell groups. In the centers of some of the cell groups. a number of cells could be seen which were more granular and did not stain as brightly as the surrounding cells. and every gradation between this and total necrosis was found. Regarding the process as a whole. they said that it was one affecting the vessels of the skin; that it seemed to begin by a proliferation of the endothelium accompanied by a corresponding proliferation of the perithelium and that the degeneration in the older areas seemed to show that, with the advance of the cell proliferation, there was a corresponding degenerative process going on. They state: "From a purely histological consideration of the growth it may be compared to an angiosarcoma, it being understood that with this name only the histological appearance is taken into consideration."

It seems probable that the degenerative process which the last investigators found corresponds to the areas of involution which were so evident in both these cases. Similar granular areas were found in our sections.

At the discussion of this case at the meeting of the American Dermatological Association, two conditions were chiefly considered: angioma serpiginosum and poikiloderma atrophicans vasculare. This case differs from those included by Wise [2] under angioma serpiginosum, in the following points: (a) the absence of minute puncta; (b) the absence of telangiectases; (c) the fact that the outlying lesions were raised; (d) in the method of formation of the vascular rings; (e) in the histology, angioma serpiginosum being, to quote Wise, "a low grade inflammation . . . with secondary effects on the epidermis . . . in no sense an angioma."

The second condition considered was poikiloderma atrophicans vasculare, an excellent description of which, with the literature, is presented in Lane's article.[3] Our case differs from this condition in that there are: (a) no petechiae; (b) no telangiectases; (c) no reticular pigmentation; (d) no itching nor ulceration. There is nothing in this case at all suggestive of roentgen-ray dermatitis, which is marked in poikiloderma atrophicans vasculare, and, as Dr. Lane pointed out in the discussion, the eruption in this case is most intense at the borders, while in poikiloderma atrophicans vasculare it is most intense at the center and fades toward the borders.

As to the pathologic classification, Ewing [4] says:

Hemangioma hypertrophicum (Ziegler) is a cellular form of capillary angioma occurring chiefly in the skin. It consists of a large number of small vessels lined by hypertrophic and neoplastic endothelium. The vessels usually maintain a scanty lumen but the proliferation of endothelium may obliterate the lumen and yield compact groups of cells. In this form, the tumor is virtually an endothelioma and in this and the transitional forms, it may be designated as hemangio-endothelioma. Pure tumors of this type are usually progressive and if very cellular may exhibit local malignancy.

2. Wise: J. Cutan. Dis., 1913, p. 725.

3. Lane, J. E.: Poikiloderma Atrophicans Vasculare, with Report of a Case by Oliver S. Ormsby, M.D., Chicago, Arch. Dermat. & Syph. **4**:563 (Nov.) 1921.

4. Ewing, James: Neoplastic Diseases, Philadelphia, W. B. Saunders Company, 1919, p. 221.

Mallory [5] defines endothelioblastoma as "a tumor of mesenchymal origin of which the cells tend to differentiate into flat endothelial cells and to line vessels, cavities and surfaces." He says:

The endothelial cells of a hemangio-endothelioma tend to form blood vessels as they do under normal conditions. The vessels of the tumor may be capillary in type or cavernous, or of any gradation between these two extremes. The capillary hemangio-endothelioblastoma is relatively common, often congenital and frequently grows with considerable rapidity. It is always infiltrative in growth.

(a) In the large vessels the endothelial cells sometimes thicken up into two or more layers.

(b) Rarely the endothelial cells grow out into the lumina of the vessels in the form of papillary projections in which the endothelial cells sometimes accumulate in concentrically arranged masses or whorls. One tumor of this type started from a vascular nevus of the eyelid, invaded the orbit and destroyed the eyeball. Another, reported by Borrmann, recurred repeatedly at its site of origin beneath the breast after excision, and finally gave rise to multiple metastases in the lungs.

(c) If the capillary vessels are occluded or injured in any way so that the blood ceases to circulate in them, the endothelial cells continue to proliferate, but as they are no longer connected with the blood stream they do not form vessels. Instead, the cells collect in rows, groups, and especially on concentric masses or whorls.

The hemangio-endothelioblastomas are often congenital and frequently, perhaps always, arise from abnormalities of the blood vessels, especially from vascular nevi. They occur most often in the skin and subcutaneous tissue but may originate also in the muscles, nerves, liver, spleen, brain, bone marrow, etc. They are to be regarded on the whole as benign growths, although locally destructive, because their manner of extension is by infiltration of the surrounding tissues and by growth within and along blood vessels. Apparently but one case of metastasis is on record.

Dr. J. Homer Wright considers that conditions similar to this case are distinguished from the vascular nevi by the fact that in vascular nevi each nevus cell forms part of the wall of a blood vessel. When the endothelial cells form masses and are not confined to vessels, this fact takes the growth out of the class of vascular nevi and places it among the sarcomas, or the endotheliomas.

Oertel [6] says of angiosarcoma:

When the endothelial cells of angiomata assume greater activity (than in hemangiomata) and newly formed vessels remain incomplete, aborted, or when these cells only attempt to unite to vessels and grow more or less diffusely and undifferentiated, we speak of them as angiosarcomata.

5. Mallory: Pathologic Histology, Philadelphia: W. B. Saunders Company. 1914, p. 379.

6. Oertel, Horst: General Pathology. New York. Paul B. Hoeber, 1921. p. 285.

It has seemed to us that the outlying vascular papules in this case and the appearance of the growth in new areas at some distance from the old ones should be considered as metastases. Such a superficial process could hardly extend by continuity without showing some external change in the skin.

We must conclude, then, that Dr. James C. White's case and this one are similar, both being due to the manifestations in the skin of a tumor process, the tumor cells arising from mesoblastic tissue and showing a tendency to form vascular channels and to metastasize in the skin. Whether one calls it an hemangiosarcoma or an hemangio-endothelioma is a matter of nomenclature. The nevoid arrangement of the growth in this case would suggest its originating in a nevus, and Darier evidently considered Dr. White's case as of that origin. The patient's observation as to the absence of any nevi might easily be inaccurate. It is evident that the cases of angioma serpiginosum, so-called, and these two cases do not belong in the same category; and, if this condition is to have a dermatologic name, it would seem to be more in keeping with the findings to confine the name angioma serpiginosum to cases of this class, since it is both an angioma and serpiginous; while the cases included at present under that name are neither.

ADENOMA SEBACEUM AND TUBEROSE SCLEROSIS OF THE BRAIN *

GEORGE MANGHILL OLSON, M.D.

MINNEAPOLIS

Adenoma sebaceum is a germ plasm developmental defect of the skin, involving especially the sebaceous glands. Other elements of the skin, however, may be affected, as noted by Balzer,[1] Crocker,[2] and others, and confirmed by a study of the case herein reported. In the Balzer type of adenoma sebaceum, changes in the sebaceous glands may be slight. The Pringle type is characterized by an enormous hyperplasia of the sebaceous glands. The Hallopeau-Leredde type shows a predominance of the fibroma element; the surface may be verrucose. Mixed types, in which one lesion shows great hyperplasia of the sebaceous glands and a neighboring lesion may show only nonsebaceous changes, are not uncommon.

The germ plasm defect affects not only the skin, but also a number of other organs: the brain, kidney, heart, intestine and liver, and probably other organs. The changes in these organs are analogous to those in the skin, and consist in the formation of embryonal heart muscle tumors in the heart, the formation of a variety of tumors in the kidneys, and the condition in the brain known as tuberose sclerosis. These visceral changes, in their origin as germ plasm defects, in their microscopic structure, and in their clinical course, show a close relation to adenoma sebaceum and the nevus group of skin affections. They are often termed nevoid or organ nevi, in order to distinguish them from the ordinary birthmark.

Adenoma sebaceum is thus a part of a widely distributed disorder. The signs and symptoms of this disorder are largely dependent on the localization of the lesions. Marked involvement of the heart or kidneys often leads to a fatal result. Slight lesions in the skin with pronounced involvement of the brain or tuberose sclerosis give idiocy or epilepsy. Extensive lesions in the skin with slight or no involvement of the brain give a normal or nearly normal mentality.

In the heart and kidney, the study of this condition has been limited for the most part to a description of the predominating tumor. In the heart, this is a rhabdomyoma, which may cause death, often during the first few years of life. In the kidney, the predominating tumor has

---

* From the University of Minnesota Medical School.

1. Balzer: Arch. de Physiol. **6**:564, 1885; ibid. **7**:93, 1886.

2. Crocker: Diseases of Skin, Ed. 3, Philadelphia. P. Blakiston's Son & Co., p. 986.

been either a mixed tumor or a teratoma, or the tumors have been described as fibromas, fibrolipomas, leiomyomas, fibrolipomyomas, angiofibromas, angiosarcomas, and liposarcomas. In the brain, the condition has received more exact study under the term tuberose sclerosis of the brain.

TUBEROSE SCLEROSIS OF THE BRAIN

Tuberose sclerosis of the brain consists essentially of an overgrowth or hyperplasia of the neurologia, forming tumors or tumor-like growths

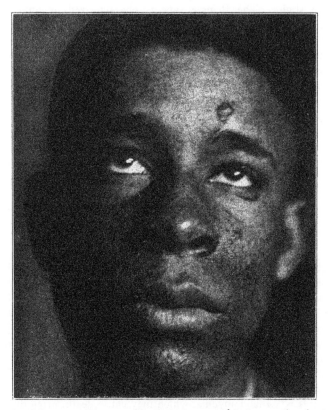

Fig. 1.—Adenoma sebaceum: The Pringle type of lesion on the cheeks and chin in the case reported. The larger Balzer type of lesions were removed by fulguration before this photograph was taken. Two padlike nevi are present on the left lower eyelid and forehead.

in the brain cortex and about the ventricles. The growths about the ventricles vary in size from a grain of wheat to a pea. Considerably larger growths are found in the cortex, and may be raised or sunken. Histologically, the findings are characteristic. There is great overgrowth of neuroglia, disorientation or dislocation of nerve cells, and very large cells which may resemble either neuroglia or ganglion cells. The process is analogous to, and genetically identical with, the adenoma sebaceum lesions of the skin. Depending on the size and location of the tumors or growths, the neurologic and mental symptoms may be absent, or there may be slight mental impairment, idiocy, epilepsy or symptoms of brain tumor.

REPORT OF A CASE

A. C., a man, colored, aged 18, had first shown symptoms of epilepsy when 5 years old. About one month later, numerous small tumors or growths appeared on the face, involving especially the cheeks and nasolabial folds.

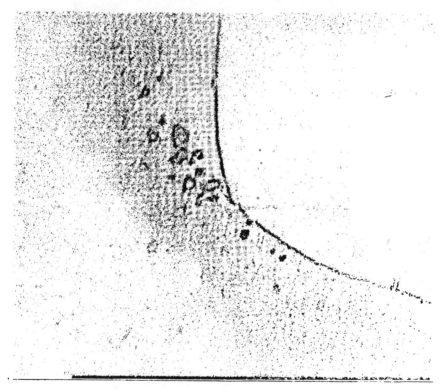

Fig. 2.—Back of the neck and shoulders; same case as Figure 1. The extremely numerous, closely set pigmented nevi are not well shown. Many tablike nevi are shown, one over the right shoulder projecting at right angles to the skin.

Epileptic attacks and new lesions on the skin had continued to appear since that time. He had four brothers and four sisters. No one in his family was similarly affected.

The numerous small tumors or growths on the cheeks, chin and forehead were red or yellowish-red in color. About the nasolabial sulci, the tumors

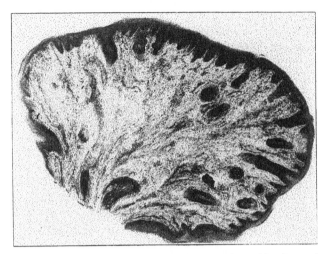

Fig. 3.—Balzer type of lesion: Photomicrograph × 25; from the right nasolabial fold. Alterations in the hair follicles in the case reported are shown.

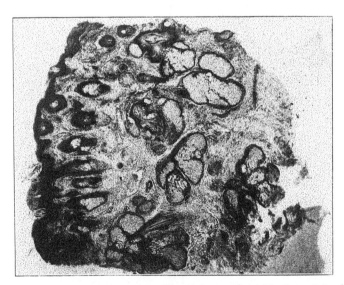

Fig. 4.—Pringle type of lesion: Photomicrograph × 25; from left cheek. Changes in the sebaceous glands in the case reported are shown.

included some that were larger and pale, showing no tinge of red. Most of the lesions were discrete, although some were confluent, forming patches like those seen in lichen planus. Over the face, there were many unusually large comedones. On the left lower eyelid and on the forehead, there were two soft pigmented, padlike nevi. Over the back of the neck and shoulders, there were hundreds of closely set, small pigmented nevi, with many projecting tablike nevi—nevus pendulum. On the right arm, there was a large patch of vitiligo, which was thought by the father to be due to a maternal prenatal craving for ice cream. Two quite large pigmented nevi were present on the abdomen. There were no subjective symptoms from the skin lesions. The mental condition was fair. He had been unable to continue in school beyond the sixth grade. The epileptic attacks had been moderately severe. Many of the larger lesions on the face were removed by fulguration, with excellent results.

MICROSCOPIC STUDY

One of the pale, rather large lesions, at the right nasolabial sulcus, was removed with the scissors, and found to conform to the Balzer type of lesion. The hair follicles were altered as regards size and shape, some were rudimentary, and some showed a high grade of degeneration. Changes in the sebaceous glands were slight. The hair follicles were surrounded by connective tissue, resembling a rather richly cellular fibroma.

One of the red lesions from the middle of the cheek was removed by the cutaneous punch. This was a typical Pringle type of lesion. There was massive hyperplasia of the sebaceous glands. Most of the sebaceous glands appeared to be simply hypertrophied or enlarged, the structure resembling normal sebaceous glands. At some points, the sebaceous cells were arranged in short bands or ribbons, did not resemble normal sebaceous glands, and were apparently true adenomas.

SUMMARY

1. Adenoma sebaceum is a germ plasm developmental defect of the skin, involving especially the sebaceous glands.

2. There are three types of adenoma sebaceum. The Pringle type consists of red lesions showing an enormous hyperplasia of the sebaceous glands. In the Balzer type, the lesions are pale, and show alterations mainly in the hair follicles. In the Hallopeau-Leredde type, the surface may be verrucose, and, microscopically, it shows a predominance of the fibroma element. Mixed types are not uncommon.

3. Adenoma sebaceum belongs to the nevus, nevoid or organ nevi group of disorders.

4. The brain and visceral organs, such as the heart and kidney, are often involved in a genetically identical and histologically similar process.

5. Adenoma sebaceum is thus part of a widely distributed disorder, nevoid in character, which may involve the brain and important visceral organs, and is characterized by an overgrowth of certain tissues, the formation of true tumors, and, in the visceral organs, may end in malignant tumor formation.

6. The involvement of the brain or tuberose sclerosis consists essentially of overgrowth of neuroglia, disorientation or dislocation of nerve cells and the presence of characteristic large cells. The tumors are found in the brain cortex and about the ventricles.[3]

---

3. In addition to the references given, the following will be of interest:

Freund: Berl. klin. Wchnschr. **12**:274, 1918.

Schuster: Dermat. Centralbl. **17**:2, 1914.

Fischer: Arch. f. Dermat. u. Syph. **134**:93, 1921.

Hauser: Berl. klin. Wchnschr. **12**:278, 1918.

Shelmire, J. B.: Adenoma Sebaceum, J. A. M. A. **71**:963 (Sept. 21) 1918.

Crutchfield, E. D.: Adenoma Sebaceum Associated with Teratoma of Kidney, Arch. Dermat. & Syph. **2**:368 (Sept.) 1920.

MORPHEA ASSOCIATED WITH HEMIATROPHY OF THE FACE

EARL D. OSBORNE, M.D.

Fellow in Dermatology and Syphilology, the Mayo Foundation, and First
Assistant in Section on Dermatology and Syphilology, Mayo Clinic

ROCHESTER, MINN.

Linear morphea or circumscribed scleroderma following closely a nerve distribution is of relatively common occurrence, but morphea associated with facial hemiatrophy is distinctly a rarity, if one may judge from the literature. Recently, two such cases have been observed in the Section on Dermatology and Syphilology of the Mayo Clinic. Barrs,[1] in 1891, reported a case of this type. Since then, three other cases have been recorded, all from the British Isles. Barrs' patient was a woman, aged 27, whose face was markedly asymmetrical, and the skin and subcutaneous tissue on the right side, from the upper border of the orbit to the level of the teeth in the lower jaw, were atrophied. The eyeball was noticeably sunken. Definite diminution in sensation over the area supplied by the superior maxillary nerve was detectable. Alopecia was not present. The patient had had neuralgia of the right side of the face for many years. In the right inguinal region was a typical patch of morphea.

In 1903, Savill[2] presented a case of morphea with well marked facial hemiatrophy and called attention to the relation between morphea and hemiatrophy, which he believed to be identical. The patient, a man aged 50, had struck the top of his head while running upstairs twenty years before. Two or three years later, he had noticed that he was losing his hair and eyebrows, and that the left side of his face was becoming sunken and painful. The atrophy was progressive and involved the subcutaneous tissue as well as the skin. Scattered patches of morphea were noted on other parts of the body. A depressed scar was found at the point of injury. At the time of presentation, an affection of the eye had supervened which Savill's colleague, Dodd, declared to be trophic in character.

In 1904, Galloway[3] reported the case of a woman, aged 37, with a typical patch of morphea involving the distribution of the first two divisions of the right fifth cranial nerve. The lesion commenced above the orbit and spread back approximately to the lambdoidal suture. There

1. Barrs, A. G.: Cases of Atrophia Cutis and Morphoea. Brit. J. Dermat. **3**:152-155, 1891.

2. Savill, T. D.: Brit. J. Dermat. **15**:106-107, 1903.

3. Galloway, J.: Brit. J. Dermat. **16**:20-21, 1904.

was also a small round patch on the upper portion of the right nasolabial fold. Distinct shrinking of the right nostril and ala nasi had occurred, with general atrophy of tissues of the right side of the face, especially around the orbit. The nasal mucous membrane on the right side was dry and atrophied. The eyeball had retreated within the orbit so that the eyes were noticeably asymmetric. The eyelids were unaffected. Bilateral deafness due to otosclerosis was also present.

In 1886, Steven [4] observed a remarkable case of scleroderma in a girl, aged 14 years, with pronounced hemiatrophy of the face, body, and extremities of the right side. When the patient was first examined, she complained of a moderately well advanced scleroderma of the right side of the body, of about two months' duration. The condition was first noticed as a hard patch of skin in the right groin; shortly afterward, the right hand became swollen. These lesions gradually extended, and new lesions were noticed on the upper right arm, extending over the shoulder and scapula. Seven months later, the condition was found to be much worse. The whole of the right arm was involved except for a small patch at the lower end of the radius. The right hand could neither be opened nor closed perfectly, and the arm could not be straightened at the elbow. The affected skin was more or less deeply pigmented, being brownish. On the abdomen, the condition had extended from the level of the umbilicus to Poupart's ligament, and was sharply demarcated at the middle line. The whole of the skin on the anterior surface of the right leg, from the groin to the toe, was extensively involved and presented all the characteristics of typical scleroderma. Besides this, there were a few small patches developing on the left arm, around the wrist, between the thumb and forefinger, around a vaccination scar, and in the axilla. There were also several small patches on the left side of the abdomen. The patient was in excellent general health. Sensation over the affected areas was normal. A month later, a patch was observed on the right temple and a very small cicatrix on the left. In 1897, Steven [5] made an extensive report on this case, the chief characteristic at that time being marked atrophy of the right side of the body, more particularly affecting the face, arm and leg, and very extensive and advanced scleroderma, which was not so strictly limited to the right side of the body. Atrophy of the

4. Steven, J. L.: Case of Scleroderma Adultorum, Glasgow M. J. **26**:280-283, 1886.

5. Steven, J. L.: A Case of Scleroderma, Leading to Pronounced Hemiatrophy of the Face, Body and Extremities, with Deformity and Fibrous Ankylosis of the Joints, After a Lengthened Period of Superficial Ulceration, Internat. Clin., S. 7, **2**:195-202, 1897; Case of Scleroderma with Pronounced Hemiatrophy of the Face, Body and Extremities, Death from Ovarian Tumor; Account of the Postmortem Examination; a Sequel, Glasgow M. J. **1**:401-408, 1898.

right side of the face was pronounced, being most marked on the chin and forehead. The right side of the lower jaw was markedly diminished in length, and a depression of the surface over the right temple and side of the frontal bone was distinctly visible. The depression of the forehead, however, began a little to the right of the middle line. The cutaneous sensibility and the hair were unaffected. The right arm and leg were practically universally involved in the sclerodermatous process associated with pronounced atrophy of the subcutaneous tissues of the fingers and toes. There were, besides, several old patches of scleroderma on the left side, evidently the patches seen at the time of the first examination eleven years before. No new patches were observed on this side.

The histories of both the parents and the patient were essentially negative, except that three years before the onset the patient had accidently drunk vitriol, with resulting difficulty in swallowing any but soft foods.

Twelve years after the first examination, the patient died, following an operation for ovarian tumor. When the brain was removed at necropsy, the cortex of the motor area was found to be slightly thinner in the left hemisphere (opposite the affected side), than in the right.[6] Sections from various levels of the cord were examined. The findings were as follows:

In each, there was a slight, though undoubted, diminution in size of the right anterior cornu (the affected side). The ganglion cells in this horn, besides being fewer in number than normal, presented signs of degeneration, in that their nuclei and plasma granules were not nearly so well defined as in the ganglion cells of the left horn. The neuroglia, too, in the right horn seemed denser than in the left. Changes corresponding to those just mentioned could not be made out with any certainty in either the medulla or the pons. Throughout the cord, medulla and pons, the arteries, especially those in the gray matter, were surrounded by certain spaces, sometimes containing a homogeneous structureless material, and in some cases free from any such contents. On transverse section, these spaces were round or oval in shape and most of them had sharply defined margins. The appearance they presented suggested dilated lymph spaces rather than a softening of the gray matter. They were best seen around the anastomotic arteries and, on the whole, were larger and more apparent on the right side of the cord than on the left. The nerve fibers from the cervical and lumbar plexuses showed a well marked parenchymatous degeneration. This change was evidently recent, and almost certainly had no connection with the more chronic changes in the cord.

Steven, in summarizing his observations on this case, concludes:

1. Scleroderma with hemiatrophy, as regards its essential pathology, is a trophoneurosis due to changes occurring in the trophic cells of the central nervous system, certainly in those of the spinal cord, and probably also in those

---

6. Unfortunately, a histologic study of the cortex was not made.

of the brain. As a result of this change in the nerve cells, the blood vessels, both of the cord and of the periphery controlled by the diseased nerve cells, are first of all affected.

2. Following upon the derangement of the blood supply caused by the central nervous disease, the atrophic changes in the skin and subjacent tissues are slowly developed.

REPORT OF CASES

CASE 1 (A347956).—A schoolboy, aged 9, was brought to the Mayo Clinic because of a depression over the left eye (Fig. 1). At birth, he was delivered by forceps; and he developed a large hematoma over the vertex which it was necessary to open. Measles and pertussis were his only illnesses until three years before, when a small whitish scar with a blue border was noticed below the left eye. The father referred to it as a "black eye." No history of trauma.

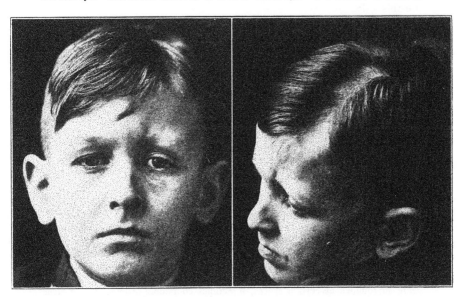

Fig. 1 (Case 1).—Morphea and hemiatrophy of the face of a boy, aged 9 years.

other than at birth, was obtainable. Four months after the appearance of the white scar, the left eyebrow began to thin and a depression which appeared over the eye gradually extended onto the forehead.

Examination revealed a typical patch of morphea on the cheek below the left eye and extending around the inner canthus onto the supra-orbital ridge. The skin was smooth, firm, and slightly elevated, with a definite violaceous border, especially marked below the eyes. There were no other patches on the face or body. The skin and subcutaneous tissue of the left side of the face were atrophied and the left ala nasi was retracted. The left eyeball was considerably sunken in the orbit. A partial alopecia involved the left side of the scalp anteriorly. The whole picture was one of definite asymmetry of the face. No changes were seen in the mucous membrane of the nose or throat. A careful neurologic examination did not reveal sensory changes in the area involved. There was, however, a suggestion of an extensor type of reflex in the left foot;

that is, an occasional Babinski, Oppenheim and Gordon reflex. Because of these findings, the consulting neurologist suggested a possible old inflammatory process in the brain._

Case 2 (A321327).—A girl, aged 7 years, was brought to the Mayo Clinic on account of an old fracture of the left humerus with limitation of motion of the elbow on that side (Fig. 2). Ten months before, she had fallen down a short flight of stairs, with consequent injury to the left elbow, and had since been unable to move her left hand. Sense of touch was absent. For some weeks, the arm was kept in a cast and later in a sling. Six months before examination, her parents had noticed slight thickening of the skin over the left side of the face and neck; this had gradually extended, but had not caused symptoms, except slight stiffness on movement of the head.

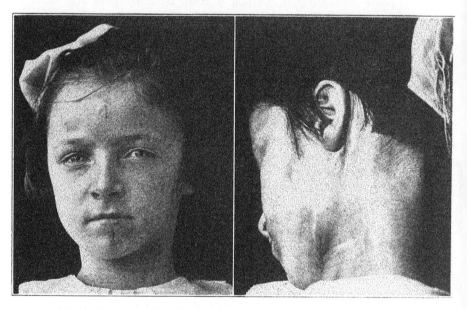

Fig. 2 (Case 2).—Morphea and hemiatrophy of the face in a girl, aged 7 years.

Examination revealed that the child was healthy and of normal weight and height. A diagnosis of ischemic paralysis of the left forearm and wrist had been made in the orthopedic section of the Clinic. A roentgenogram of the left elbow was negative. There were several discrete, firm, smooth, irregular patches of morphea on the skin behind and in front of the left ear and on the skin of the neck on that side. These patches were slightly elevated and had a very faint violaceous border. The hair was thin in front of the left ear. The chin was definitely asymmetric, and there was early atrophy of the skin and subcutaneous tissue of the entire left side of the face; but change could not be demonstrated in the bones of the skull. The mucous membranes of the nose and throat were normal. The cutaneous sensibility appeared normal. The basal metabolic rate was + 6 per cent. The Wassermann reaction on the blood was negative.

Because in these two cases morphea began definitely at the same time or shortly before hemiatrophy and the conditions existed together, it was thought that a review of the literature might reveal a common pathologic background and throw some light on the hitherto unknown etiology of both conditions. The cases of Barrs, Savill, Galloway, and Steven are the only ones in which a positive diagnosis could be made from the authors' descriptions. There are numerous cases reported of facial morphea, especially of the frontonasal type, in which coexisting hemiatrophy may be suspected from the description, but in which a positive diagnosis is not made by the reporter.

Some dermatologists question whether facial morphea and facial hemiatrophy are distinct entities. Sequeira,[7] who believes in a ganglionic neurotrophic origin of morphea says that progressive hemiatrophy of the face, involving bone, muscles and skin, sometimes occurs in conjunction with morphea. Hyde[8] classifies hemiatrophy of the face under scleroderma, but does not commit himself as to the etiology. Highman writes[9]: "Hemiatrophy facialis is scleroderma of one side of the face, which involves the deeper tissues. It is rare and usually accompanied by other evidences of scleroderma." On the other hand, neurologists are in accord in considering the two conditions as separate entities. Practically every textbook on neurology describes skin changes as one of the first symptoms of facial hemiatrophy. A white spot appears on the side of the face and gradually becomes larger, or, if there is more than one, they coalesce and become yellow or yellowish-white. The skin over these patches sinks and forms pits or trough-like depressions, owing to the disappearance of the subcutaneous fat. Pigmentation may occur not only in the areas where atrophy is marked, but on other parts of the face. This pigmentation is in small spots or patches, and varies in color from a grayish-yellow to brown or blue. The hair of the head, the beard, and the eyelashes may lose color and fall out in patches. The sebaceous glands are atrophied, and their secretion diminished and eventually checked. The secretion of perspiration is often increased.

The foregoing description of the skin changes in facial hemiatrophy is taken from one of the well recognized reference books on neurology.[10] The close similarity between the skin changes of facial hemiatrophy and morphea is apparent. It seems highly probable that the skin changes in patients who later develop hemiatrophy are of the morpheic variety.

---

7. Sequeira, J. H.: Diseases of the Skin, London, Churchill, 1915, 658 pp.

8. Hyde, J. N.: A Practical Treatise on Diseases of the Skin for the Use of Students and Practitioners, Philadelphia, Lea & Febiger, 1909, 1126 pp.

9. Highman, W. J.: Dermatology. The Essentials of Cutaneous Medicine, New York, The Macmillan Company, 1921, 482 pp.

10. Dercum, F. X., Ed.: A Text-Book on Nervous Diseases by American Authors, Philadelphia, Lea Brothers, 1895, 1056 pp.

In this connection, attention is directed to a case recently observed of typical hemiatrophy of the face of twelve years' duration (Fig. 3, Case A298444). The skin changes could very well have been the remains of an old involuted patch of morphea. The only diagnostic point lacking was the violaceous border typical in active cases. This patient also had had frequent typical epileptic attacks for eight years. The two other patients (Figs. 1 and 2) were observed in childhood, during the early years of the disease. In both cases, the morphea was typical and well advanced, whereas the hemiatrophy was just beginning. There are on record between 200 and 300 cases of hemiatrophy of the

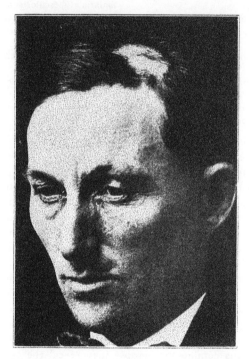

Fig. 3.—Hemiatrophy of the face in a man, aged 27. The scar of scalp and forehead is indistinguishable from that of an involuted patch of morphea.

face. It is impossible to estimate how many of these cases presented patches of morphea at some time. It is probable, however, that many of them would have been diagnosed by an experienced dermatologist as morphea associated with hemiatrophy of the face. Besides the similarity in symptoms between the two conditions, the recorded etiologic factors are practically the same, although the exact cause of each is unknown. The accompanying tabulation presents the supposed etiologic factors of both conditions according to standard works in dermatology and n u   · ·,

SUPPOSED ETIOLOGIC FACTORS IN MORPHEA AND HEMIATROPHY FACIALIS

Morphea	Hemiatrophy Facialis
1. Both sexes, females predominating.	1. Both sexes, females predominating.
2. Occurs at all ages, especially from 15 to 45 years.	2. Occurs at all ages, especially from 10 to 40 years.
3. Exposure to cold and wet and prolonged exposure to the sun are predisposing causes.	3. Exposure to cold and extreme temperatures are predisposing causes.
4. Often follows infectious diseases, such as rheumatism and erysipelas.	4. Often follows infections, such as erysipelas, scarlatina, pneumonia, malaria, tuberculosis and rheumatism.
5. Often accompanies emotional and nervous states.	5. Often accompanied with psychic disturbances, such as grief, anxiety and worry.
6. Often follows exhaustion from any source.	6. Often follows anemias and scrofulosis.
7. Local irritation or injury is supposed to play a part.	7. Traumatism sometimes precedes.
8. Thyroid diseases are as yet factors little understood.	

The etiologic factors are practically the same in both conditions except for the possible rôle of the thyroid in the production of morphea.

In summarizing the six cases reviewed, the evidence points strongly to involvement of the central nervous system. The history of trauma from four months to six years preceding the onset of symptoms in four of the cases, the necropsy findings of Steven, and the neurologic findings suggesting an old inflammatory process in the brain of one of the patients in the Mayo Clinic, are all incriminating evidence. The close relationship between facial hemiatrophy and morphea is emphasized by the common etiologic factors involved and in the similarity of skin changes seen in the two conditions. That the early skin changes seen in cases of facial hemiatrophy are always of the morphea variety seems unlikely, but that they may often be morpheic seems highly probable Further pathologic studies of the nervous system in cases of morphea and scleroderma coming to necropsy may reveal the essential etiology of these obscure conditions.

ACNITIS

REPORT OF A CASE

H. E. ALDERSON, M.D.

Clinical Professor of Medicine (Skin Diseases) Stanford University Medical School

SAN FRANCISCO

The subject of this report (private history No. 5971)—referred by Dr. W. W. Boardman—a man 20 years of age, employed as a clerk, presented many small follicular pustules on his cheeks, chin, forehead and in the parietofrontal regions of the scalp. These lesions, which healed slowly, leaving tiny depressed scars, had been appearing steadily for two years. The patient had lupus pernio of the lobes of his ears and typical papulonecrotic tuberculids on several fingers. There were also cervical tuberculous glands. These various cutaneous and glandular conditions had existed for about two years.

The skin lesions were typical. It would have been better, of course, had a biopsy and histopathologic study been possible, but it can be said that the evidence necessary to establish a positive clinical diagnosis was present.

REPORT OF A CASE *

History.—Seven years ago, after an attack of scarlatina, swelling of the glands, without pain, occurred on the right side of the neck. These gradually enlarged to the size of a walnut, and after about two years they broke down and were removed surgically. Healing occurred readily, but the right shoulder dropped and has remained lower; there has been no disturbance of function, however. There was no other trouble until two years ago, when glands on the left side of the neck began to swell, without pain or tenderness, gradually enlarging. A pustular eruption also developed on the face and scalp and vasomotor disturbances occurred in the fingers and ears, becoming aggravated by cold weather.

The family history was negative.

Two years before the cervical glands became swollen, the patient had a severe sore throat, after which his tonsils and adenoids were removed. There was nothing else of significance in his past history.

Physical Examination.—The patient was a fairly well nourished young man. His nose, throat and eyes were normal. His teeth were in poor condition. (The roentgen ray showed abscesses in the roots of several broken off molars). On the right side of the neck was a normal linear scar from an old operation. The right shoulder was low. On the left side of the neck there was a chain of glands rather closely adherent to each other but not to the skin or underlying tissues.

---

* The history of the case and report of the examination and general treatment were furnished by the patient's physician, Dr. W. W. Boardman.

Physical and roentgen-ray examinations of the chest revealed an old (healed) apical tuberculosis and diffuse peribronchial thickening with no active lesions. There was some evidence of the presence of mediastinal glands. No other abnormalities were noted. The blood Wassermann test was negative.

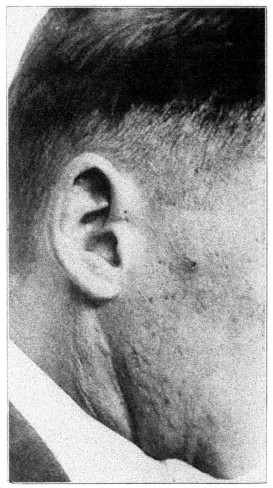

Fig. 1.—Acnitis of the cheek and scalp and lupus pernio of the rim of the ear. The scar resulting from an operation for cervical tuberculous glands is also shown.

The blood pressure was: systolic 120, diastolic 75. In the left axilla there was a small gland. The fingers showed passive congestion, and there was an occasional stinging, burning sensation. On the fingers were also indolent pustules and scars from former lesions. With the exception of a few enlarged glands in the left groin, nothing pathologic was found in the abdomen or pelvis.

The various reflexes were normal.

Treatment.—Under roentgen-ray treatment of the glands and fingers by Dr. Monica Donovan, and mercury-quartz lamp treatment of the skin lesions on the face (the latter steadily for six months), the glandular and cutaneous lesions subsided completely. Dr. Donovan reported that, from Jan. 18, 1921, to Jan. 24, 1922, the patient was treated at intervals of from three to six weeks, receiving in all thirteen treatments. The average dose was 23 milliampere minutes at 8 inches distance with a 9 inch gap (Coolidge tube) filtered through 3 mm. of aluminum and leather.

Mercury quartz lamp treatments were given by me twice weekly at first and then weekly—the intervals being regulated according to the persistence of the reaction each time. An effort was made to produce erythema without vesiculation followed by exfoliation. This was accomplished, and the skin became fairly brown.

A badly infected tooth was removed and the teeth generally put in good condition.

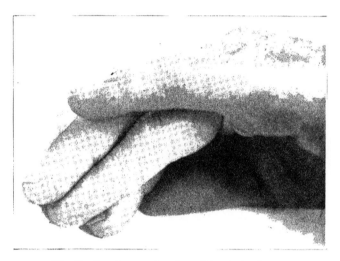

Fig. 2.—Papulonecrotic tuberculids of the fingers

Over a period of nine months semiweekly injections of tuberculin (B. F.) and iron arsenate were given by Dr. Boardman, the latter three times weekly.

Two series of tuberculin injections (B. F.) were given, ranging in dosage from 0.000001 to 10 mg. There were no constitutional reactions, but on two occasions slight local reactions occurred with the 10 mg. dosage. The patient's weight increased 10 pounds in eight months.

As for the skin lesions, the acnitis on the face, lupus pernio on the ears and papulonecrotic tuberculids on the fingers have all subsided, and the patient has developed no new lesions. Only numerous tiny scars remain on the scalp, face and fingers.

This association of three varieties of skin lesions, each one of which has been reported in tuberculous patients and one of which (papulonecrotic tuberculids) is very definitely caused by the tubercle bacillus, is most interesting. I feel safe in assuming that these skin lesions resulted from local destructive reactions brought about by the presence there of tubercle bacilli. These bacilli may have originated in cervical tuberculous glands. Metastatic deposits of tubercle bacilli in peripheral parts may be expected to produce such reactions, varying in degree with the virulence of the organism and the resistance of the host.

STUDIES ON BLOOD CHOLESTEROL IN SYPHILIS *

ALBERT R. McFARLAND, M.D.

Assistant in Section on Dermatology and Syphilology and Fellow
in The Mayo Foundation

ROCHESTER, MINN.

This study was undertaken with the idea of determining, if possible, any relation between the blood cholesterol and the serologic and clinical manifestations of syphilitic infections.

Cholesterol, according to Hawk,[1] is a monatomic alcohol containing at least one double bond and possessing the formula of $C_{27}H_{45}OH$ or $C_{27}H_{43}OH$. The exact formula is somewhat in dispute. It is soluble in ether, chloroform and benzene, and may be crystallized in thin transparent plates. Just as glycerol and the fatty acids unite to form glycerol fats, so cholesterol and fatty acids may form cholesterol fats. The cholesterol fats are more resistant to enzymic and bacterial action than the glycerol fats, and are thus found in the sebum of the skin and in the structural elements of red blood cells and tissue cells (Macleod[2]).

SOURCE

Cholesterol probably has two origins, exogenous and endogenous; some writers maintain that it is entirely exogenous. It seems to be the consensus of opinion that most, but not all, of the body cholesterol is exogenous, as shown by Luden[3] and others. Macleod has pointed out two factors that point toward its endogenous origin, namely, that the cholesterol in the feces of herbivorous animals is of the same variety as that in the feces of carnivorous animals and not phytosterol, which is present in plants, and that the universal presence of cholesterol in cells indicates that it must be manufactured there. Luden has studied extensively the effect of the ingestion of foods of high cholesterol value on the blood cholesterol. She has called attention to the fact that. since variations occur which depend on many factors, great care must

---

* From the Section on Dermatology and Syphilology. Mayo Clinic and The Mayo Foundation.

1. Hawk, P. B.: Practical Physiological Chemistry. Ed. 5. Philadelphia. P. Blakiston's Son & Co., 1916, p. 638.

2. Macleod, J. J. R.: Physiology and Biochemistry in Modern Medicine. Ed. 3, St. Louis, C. V. Mosby Co., 1920, p. 99.

3. Luden, Georgine: Studies on Cholesterol. IV. Experiments Concerning the Relation of the Diet, the Blood Cholesterol, and the "Lymphoid Defense." J. Lab. & Clin. Med. 3:141 (Dec.) 1917.

be exercised in choosing foods of presumably high cholesterol content. For instance, milk from cows may be different at calving time from that at other periods. The cholesterol content of cheese may vary according to the time consumed in ripening, and so forth. Luden has, however, apparently demonstrated the fact that certain foods, such as eggs, cream and butter, are fairly high in cholesterol content. Through the ingestion of an exclusive meat diet, a definite rise in the blood cholesterol may be observed. On the other hand, by feeding foods poor in cholesterol, such as fruit, vegetables and milk, the blood cholesterol can be definitely lowered. Hawk is of the opinion that most of the cholesterol is exogenous, but that under special stress the body may be able to produce endogenous cholesterol.

OCCURRENCE

Cholesterol is perhaps an almost universal constituent of the body tissues. It enters into the structural makeup of the cells. It is found most abundantly in the nervous tissue, liver and bile. It is found in the red blood cells, in the plasma and in the cerebrospinal fluid. It seems to be excreted largely in the bile, perhaps owing to the fact that the bile salts are a powerful solvent of cholesterol. It has been estimated that the bile itself contains about 1.6 parts of cholesterol for each 1,000 parts of fluid. This is probably an important factor in the production of gallstones.

FUNCTION

As has been stated, the cholesterol fats are resistant to the action of enzymes and bacteria. Hence, it is found in the sebum of the sebaceous glands and probably serves to protect the cutaneous glandular structures from the constant assault of these invaders. According to Macleod, it probably is an important element in the formation of the skeletal structure of blood and tissue cells. Kipp,[4] Denis[5] and others have shown that a definite relation exists between the blood cholesterol and the clinical course of such diseases as pneumonia and certain other acute infections. They have also called attention to the relationship of blood cholesterol to leukocytosis. The inference to be deducted is that the cholesterol plays an important part in the antitoxic and bactericidal powers of the body and probably is a factor in antibody formation. Luden, in a study of blood cholesterol in neoplasms, apparently has shown that there is a relation between the two. Whether cholesterol is utilized directly for the formation of cells or acts merely

---

4. Kipp, H. A.: Variation in the Cholesterol Content of the Serum in Pneumonia, J. Biol. Chem. **44**:215 (Nov.) 1920.

5. Denis, W.: Cholesterol in Human Blood Under Pathological Conditions, J. Biol. Chem. **29**:93 (Feb.) 1917.

as a catalyst (as suggested by Robertson) is not definitely known, but in malignancy there is evidence of disturbances of cholesterol metabolism.

CHOLESTEROL VARIATIONS IN VARIOUS DISEASES

During the past few years, numerous cholesterol studies have been made in specific diseases and syndromes in an endeavor to throw additional light on the real nature and function of the blood cholesterol. It is only natural to surmise that a substance so widely distributed in the human economy may be intimately involved in the process of immunity and that quantitative estimations may prove to be of diagnostic if not of therapeutic importance in combating disease.

Wilensky and Rothschild [6] have made a study of blood cholesterol in gallbladder diseases. As a result of a study of about seventy cases, they conclude: "It must be conceded that in any given case the diagnostic value of any determination of the cholesterol content of the blood is a variable and dubious one." They further conclude that when cholesteremia is found in a case of jaundice in which it is a question of whether the jaundice is obstructive or cirrhotic, the probabilities are that it is obstructive, provided no other conditions are present which may cause a cholesteremia, such as pregnancy, diabetes or nephritis.

Kipp, in 1920, in a rather extensive study of thirty-five cases of pneumonia and empyema, has found that during the period of invasion by organisms the blood cholesterol is low. As convalescence takes place, there is a gradual increase until cholesteremia obtains, the degree of which apparently depends on the virulence of the infection and the extent of pulmonary involvement. Several cases are cited in which the cholesterol values previous to death were very low. Henes,[7] in a series of twelve cases of chronic nephritis, has obtained almost uniformly high blood cholesterol values, and expresses the opinion that a cholesteremia in such cases is of considerable diagnostic value. He has also found, in cases of typhoid fever, that during the acute stage the blood cholesterol is low; later it becomes normal, and during convalescence a cholesteremia results. This observation seems to agree with that of Kipp concerning his cases of pneumonia.

Schnabel [8] studied a series of sixty cases of gastro-enterologic disorders. These included cases of pernicious anemia with gastric hyper-

6. Wilensky, A. O., and Rothschild, M. A.: Studies in Cholelithiasis. II. The Clinical Relationships of the Cholesteremia to the Pathologic Process. Am. J. M. Sc. **156**:404 (Sept.) 1918.

7. Henes, E.: The Prognostic Value of Cholesteremia in Chronic Nephritis. Arch. Int. Med. **25**:411-419, 1920.

8. Schnabel, T. G.: Blood Cholesterol in Gastro-Enterologic Cases. Am. J. M. Sc. **160**:423 (Sept.) 1920.

acidity, catarrhal and obstructive jaundice, duodenal ulcer, intestinal stasis, chronic constipation, gastric neurosis, and chronic appendicitis. He concludes that when a number of cases are studied, the results are too variable to be of any practical value in gastro-enterologic diagnosis.

From these observations, it may be seen that in certain diseases there seems to be a definite relation between the blood cholesterol and the pathologic conditions, while in others no definite relation can be shown.

Certain phenomena concerning the pathology of syphilis suggested that blood cholesterol determinations might be of clinical significance. The Wassermann test, founded on the conception of the formation of specific antibodies, supported the assumption that *Spirochaeta pallida,* or more strictly speaking its chemical composition, produced a specific antibody, which in the presence of the complement, formed a stable combination; and thus the test was applied in the diagnosis of syphilis. It was not until it was demonstrated by Landsteiner, Levaditi, Noguchi and others, that substances beside spirochete-containing tissue could serve as an antigen in the complement-fixation test that the specificity of the Wassermann reaction came to be questioned. Among the various antigens which have been devised, one of the most delicate is the cholesterol treated alcoholic extract of heart tissue. This would seem to indicate that the Wassermann reaction of syphilis might possibly be due in part to the cholesterol content of the blood.

Going back a step, it may be noted that cholesterol is present to the greatest degree in nerve and liver tissue. These tissues are often attacked by *Spirochaeta pallida,* and hence we might believe that cholesterol would be liberated, resulting in cholesteremia, and therefore would have some bearing on the positive Wassermann reaction. On the other hand, I had an opportunity to verify the well-known relative insolubility of cholesterol while working on Wassermann technic in the clinical laboratories. The antigens were prepared by adding 0.04 per cent. of commercial cholesterol to an alcoholic extract of human, beef or guinea-pig heart. It was noted that, at room temperature, even this small amount formed a saturation so that free cholesterol settled to the bottom of the flask. Heating was necessary in order completely to dissolve it. Even with this apparently saturated solution, many specimens still were found to lack antigenic power and others proved to be only equal or slightly stronger than the ordinary acetone-insoluble alcoholic extract fraction which was used for routine work in the laboratory.

In spite of the fairly well standardized methods of determining blood cholesterol, writers have reported widely varied data. Widal,

Weill and Laudat [9] consider from 175 to 195 mg. for each 100 c.c. to be about normal. Luden places normal values at from 70 to 100 mg. for each 100 c.c., with the Bloor [10] technic as used by her. Other investigators have reported data showing values from 50 to 450 in various conditions. The determinations in this series have all been made under the direction of Dr. Luden of the Mayo Clinic, with a uniformly standard technic, and by the Bloor I and Bloor II methods. While the data taken may not agree with those of other investigators, they should have a fair degree of uniformity for the cases studied.

TECHNIC

Two determinations were made on each specimen, one designated Bloor I and the other Bloor II. The chief difference between the two is that in the Bloor I method, sodium ethylate is added to the ether-alcohol extract in order to obtain the proper color for colorimetric determinations. In the Bloor II method, sodium ethylate is not used and the proper colorimetric qualities are maintained by the use of more care in heating the extract. The Bloor II values are as a rule higher than the Bloor I.

Five cubic centimeters of blood are withdrawn from the cubital vein by a large needle and syringe and immediately injected into 75 c.c. of an alcohol-ether mixture (3:1) which is then agitated for thorough mixing and heated just to boiling; the amount is then made up to 100 c.c. In the Bloor I method, 2 c.c. of sodium ethylate is added to each 10 c.c. of the extract. Evaporation to dryness is carried out on a water-bath and the residue is extracted three times with dry chloroform. To each 6 c.c. of the chloroform extract, 2 c.c. of acetic acid and 0.2 c.c. of concentrated sulphuric acid are added, in order to produce a green color. The test tubes are then exposed to the daylight for five minutes at a temperature of 20 C., in order to secure a color comparable to the standard. Calorimetric readings are made against a standard solution; each reading is checked repeatedly. A more detailed description of the technic may be obtained by referring to Luden's original article. By this method, it has been found that the normal Bloor I value is between 70 and 100 mg. for each 100 c.c.: values from 100 to 140 are increased; from 140 to 200 are high, and 200 or more are unusually high. The normal difference between the Bloor I and Bloor II values is from 17 to 34 mg. for each 100 c.c.

9. Widal, F.; Weill, A., and Laudat, M.: Comparative Study of the Contents of Free Cholesterol and Its Esters in Blood Serum. Compt. rend. Soc. de biol. **74**:882, 1913.

10. Bloor, W. R.: Studies on Blood Fat. II. Fat Absorption and the Blood Lipoids, J. Biol. Chem. **23**:317, 1915; Determination of Cholesterol in Blood, J. Biol. Chem. **24**:227 (March) 1916; Bloor, W. R., and Knudson, A.: Separate Determination of Cholesterol and Cholesterol Esters in Small Amounts of

The Bloor I value represents the unchanged cholesterol in the blood stream. The Bloor II value indicates the free cholesterol plus the combined cholesterol; the difference between the two represents roughly the rate at which cholesterol is being metabolized.

In this study, the cholesterol values are placed in three groups. Anything above 140 is classified high, from 100 to 140 medium, and below 100 low. The difference between the Bloor I and Bloor II values has been divided into three groups; namely, values above 34 high, below 17 low, and the remainder normal.

WASSERMANN DETERMINATIONS

The Wassermann tests were made by Sanford. A few salient points in the technic may be mentioned. The raw serum is employed without heating. The antigen used is the acetone-insoluble alcoholic extract of beef heart. Mixed guinea-pig serum furnishes the complement. Human cells and antihuman dog amboceptor are used in the second incubation series.

CONDITIONS OF THE EXPERIMENT

The tests were made on syphilitic patients taken at random from the section on dermatology and syphilology. The original diagnosis of syphilis in each case had been determined by the Wassermann test, examination of the cerebrospinal fluid, dermatologic examination, and the general examination, including neurologic, cardiovascular, and roentgen-ray examinations if indicated. The tests were all made under conditions as nearly uniform as possible. Each patient had been at rest for from six to eight hours and had not had food for the same length of time. Most of the Wassermann tests were made on the same day as the cholesterol test. Some were made the week before or the week after, which for practical diagnostic purposes may be considered within reasonable limits; a few made several months before were discounted. Problems as follows were considered:

1. The relation, if any, between the Wassermann reaction and the blood cholesterol.

2. The usual cholesterol value in cases of syphilis in general.

3. The relation between the cholesterol values and the progress of treatment; that is, the amount of arsphenamin already received.

4. The relation of the nearness of the last arsphenamin injection to the cholesterol values.

5. The constancy, if any, of difference between the Bloor I and Bloor II values in syphilitic patients.

6. The relation between the Wassermann reaction and the difference between Bloor I and Bloor II values.

7. The relation between the clinical and serologic response of patients and the cholesterol findings.

8. The relation of the clinical type of the syphilitic infection to the cholesterol findings.

9. The constant change, if any, in cholesterol values of a patient during a course of treatment.

Among the high cholesterol values (above 140, Bloor I), there were two positive and nineteen negative Wassermann reactions (9.5 per cent. were positive). In the medium values (from 100 to 140, Bloor I), there were twenty-two positive and forty negative reactions (25.4 per cent. were positive). In the low cholesterol values (below 100, Bloor I), there were five positive and fifteen negative Wassermann reactions (33.33 per cent. positive). In other words, of the twenty-nine patients with positive Wassermann reactions on the blood, 6.8 per cent. had high cholesterol values, 75.9 per cent. had medium cholesterol values, and 17.2 per cent. had low cholesterol values.

Thus it appears that the bulk of the positive Wassermann reactions are among the medium and low values, although in some cases high values occur. In general, it was found that of the 103 patients with syphilis, twenty-one (20.3 per cent.) had high cholesterol values, sixty-two (60.3 per cent.) had medium values, and twenty (19.4 per cent.) had low values. Here again the bulk of the patients seem to fall into the low and medium groups, which might be expected in any chronic infective process. The recent work of Craig[11] on injection of animals with cholesterol also corroborates these findings.

The patients with high cholesterol values had received an average of 8.9 injections of arsphenamin; those with medium values, 8.2 injections; and those with low values, 7.25 injections. The patients with high values had received from none to nineteen injections of arsphenamin; those with medium values, from none to twenty-eight injections; and those with low values, from one to seventeen injections. Examples of all stages of treatment were therefore included. There seems to be no relation between the amount of treatment and the cholesterol values.

A recent article by Strickler[12] contained the observation that a large percentage of nonsyphilitic patients give positive Wassermann reactions after receiving arsphenamin. To explain this, it was suggested that perhaps the arsphenamin acted on the liver, increasing the formation of

11. Craig. C. F., and Williams, W. C.: Experimental Observations upon the Effect of Cholesteremia on the Results of the Wassermann Tests. Am. J. Syph. **5**:392 (July 21) 1921.

12. Strickler, A.; Munson, H. G., and Sidlick. D. M.: Positive Wassermann Test in Nonsyphilitic Patients After Intravenous Therapy. Preliminary Report of a Study of Its Significance. J. A. M. A. **75**:1488 (Nov. 27) 1920.

lipoid, and thereby produced a positive Wassermann reaction. According to our observations and those of Kilduffe,[13] arsphenamin does not produce positive Wassermann reactions, and it seems evident that cholesterol is not one of the substances which are increased as the result of the administration of arsphenamin.

In considering the time relations between arsphenamin treatment and the cholesterol tests, it was found that the nearest previous injection varied from one week to ten months in the high values, from one week to eighteen months in the medium values, and from one week to four months in the low values. The proximity of the last arsphenamin injection, therefore, would seem to have no relation to the cholesterol values, although it must be stated that determinations were not made if the arsphenamin injection was nearer than one week to the cholesterol determination.

Fifty and seven-tenths per cent. of the entire series of patients had a high difference (above 34) between the Bloor I and Bloor II values; 34.6 per cent. had a normal difference (between 17 and 34), and 14.7 per cent. had a low difference (below 17). Twenty-seven and seven-tenths per cent. of the patients with high differences had positive Wassermann reactions; 53 per cent. with normal differences had positive Wassermann reactions, and 37.5 per cent. with low differences had positive Wassermann reactions. The bulk of the cases of syphilis, therefore, fall into the groups showing high and normal differences between Bloor I and Bloor II values. It is difficult to determine whether the positive Wassermann reactions tend to predominate in the groups with high or low differences, but certainly the majority seem to be within normal limits (17 to 34).

Cholesterol has been proposed as an element in the nonspecific mechanism of defense of the body. This mechanism is seldom recognized, but is a significant factor in the course of many chronic infections, and it seemed, therefore, that the possible influence of cholesterol as a defensive agent or index of nonspecific defense should be particularly conspicuous in a chronic infection such as syphilis. In recent studies by Tokuda, and by Bircher and myself, the globulin-albumin ratio, perhaps also to be included among the nonspecific defense indexes, was found to be considerably affected by syphilitic infection and by treatment. It was with the hope of detecting a similar rôle for cholesterol that the present study was begun.

Next, comparisons were made between the cholesterol values and the clinical and serologic responses of the patient. The cases were divided into three arbitrary groups. In Group 1, good response, were

---

13. Kilduffe, R. A.: Effect of Intravenous Administration of Arsphenamin, Neo-Arsphenamin and Mercury on the Wassermann Test in Normal Serums, J. A. M. A. **76**:1489-1490 (May 28) 1921.

placed patients who improved quite rapidly clinically and those whose blood easily became negative. In Group 2 were placed patients showing a fair response, who eventually obtained a fairly satisfactory result with regard both to their clinical symptoms and to their serologic findings, but who were rather resistant to treatment. Group 3 included the clinical "wrecks" and patients whose blood remained persistently positive in spite of apparently adequate treatment. The results of this classification can best be shown in tabulated form (Table 1).

TABLE 1.—Relation Between Clinical Response and Cholesterol Findings

Clinical and Serologic Response	Percentage of Patients				
	Cholesterol Values			Difference Between Bloor I and Bloor II Values	
	High*	Medium†	Low‡	High	Low
Good....................	15.9	68.2	15.9	36.3	63.7
Fair.....................	12.5	75.0	12.5	41.6	58.4
Poor...................	25.0	50.0	25.0	56.2	43.8

* High cholesterol, above 140.
† Medium cholesterol, 100 to 140
‡ Low cholesterol, below 100.

While there is some variation in the percentages for the different groups, this is perhaps no more than might be expected from a percentage classification in a comparatively small series of cases. It might be concluded that a small difference between Bloor I and Bloor II values means a good prognosis, but this would need further confirmation before it could be accepted as a fact. As a whole, the cholesterol values do not furnish definite information regarding the probable prognosis in a given case. In Table 2 the basis for classifica-

TABLE 2.—Relation Between Type of Syphilis and Cholesterol Findings

Type of Syphilis	Percentage of Patients				
	Cholesterol Values			Difference Between Bloor I and Bloor II Values	
	High	Medium	Low	High	Normal and Low
Latent (positive Wassermann only)	11.7	64.9	23.4	52.9	47.1
Primary and secondary.............	0	77.7	22.3	55.5	44.5
Tertiary (osseous, visceral, cutaneous, etc.)........................	0	82.3	17.7	47.0	53.0
Cerebrospinal......................	33.3	50.1	16.6	38.9	61.1

tion is the type of syphilis instead of the clinical and serologic results. The noteworthy feature of this tabulation is the high percentage of syphilis of the central nervous system which is associated 'with high cholesterol values, namely, 33.3 per cent. as compared to 0.0 and 11.7 per cent. in the other types.

Most of the data obtained for this study are from single tests, taken on patients at random. However, in a series of twenty cases, determinations were made at weekly intervals during a course or part of a course of treatment, with the idea of detecting any possible constant variation from week to week (Table 3). This was suggested by the behavior of the globulin content of the serum in syphilitic patients under treatment, as observed by Bircher and myself. It may be seen that it is possible for a wide variation in the determinations to take place from week to week. This may be explained on the basis of some inter-current infection of a nonspecific nature, although with few exceptions we were unable to locate such a factor. Certainly the variation cannot be explained on a basis of syphilis. This series of twenty cases included

TABLE 3.—CLASSIFICATION OF PATIENTS ON WHOM DETERMINATIONS WERE MADE WEEKLY DURING A COURSE OF TREATMENT

| | | Cholesterol Values Mg. for Each 100 C.c. Blood | | | | | | Bloor I Value Varied Enough to Change | | Difference Between Bloor I and Bloor II Values Varied Enough to Change | |
| | | Highest | | | Lowest | | | | | | |
No.	Type of Syphilis	Bloor I	Bloor II	Difference	Bloor I	Bloor II	Difference	Its Group	General Trend	Its Group	General Trend
1	Cerebrospinal	138	159	21	125	135	10	—	Down	+	Down
2	Tertiary	104	140	36	95	144	49	+	Down	—	Up
3	Cerebrospinal	208	230	22	102	114	12	+	Up	+	Up
4	Cerebrospinal	117	144	27	93	121	28	+	Up	—	Down
5	Cerebrospinal	133	171	38	120	163	43	—	Up	—	Down
6	Cerebrospinal	127	159	32	112	145	33	—	Down	—	Up
7	Cerebrospinal	171	249	78	145	200	55	—	Up	—	Down
8	Cerebrospinal	194	251	57	127	164	37	+	Down	—	Down
9	Latent	136	202	66	107	167	60	—	Up	—	Up
10	Cerebrospinal	144	167	23	117	133	16	+	Up	+	Up
11	Cerebrospinal	148	230	82	106	142	36	+	Up	—	Up
12	Tertiary	135	152	17	83	111	28	+	Down	—	Up
13	Cerebrospinal	103	155	52	95	117	22	+	Up	+	Up
14	Cerebrospinal	144	154	10	95	123	28	+	Down	+	Up
15	Tertiary	125	142	17	117	136	19	—	Down	—	Up
16	Latent	98	127	34	72	116	44	—	Up	—	Down
17	Latent	148	180	32	117	113	56	+	Down	+	Up
18	Tertiary	106	127	21	95	104	9	+	Up	+	Up
19	Tertiary	127	146	19	91	115	16	+	Up	—	Up
20	Tertiary	114	140	26	107	157	50	—	Down	+	Up

various types of syphilis. In twelve of the cases, the variation in Bloor I values was great enough from week to week to throw the result into a different group; that is, high, medium, or low. In eight of the twenty cases, the difference between the Bloor I and Bloor II values varied enough to change it from high to medium or to low. The general trend of the difference was up in fourteen instances and down in six instances. The general trend of the Bloor I values was down in nine instances and up in eleven. Treatment, therefore, in an individual case does not seem to result in any constant effect on the cholesterol values.

CONCLUSIONS

1. The positive Wassermann reaction on the blood apparently does not depend on high cholesterol value. While it is interesting to corrob-

orate this fact, it is not surprising in view of the probable complexity of the Wassermann reaction.

2. Blood cholesterol values in syphilitic patients, in general, tend to be medium and low rather than high. The occasional high values might possibly be explained on some other basis, but no attempt was made to determine this, since the study was confined to syphilis. This may mean that cholesterol as an agent of defense is low in a chronic disease like syphilis, just as leukocytosis is low in chronic infections; but from a practical standpoint it cannot be said that the cholesterol determinations, with the possible exception of findings in the cases of involvement of the central nervous system, have afforded results much different from those to be expected from a similar series of non-syphilitic patients.

3. The amount of arsphenamin given and the time between injections do not obviously affect the blood cholesterol values. If cholesterol is an agent of defense in syphilis, it has not been detected in most cases in greater amount than might be expected in a series of average nonsyphilitic persons, and hence it is not affected materially by treatment for syphilis.

4. The majority of syphilitic patients have high or normal differences between the Bloor I and Bloor II values, while only a few have low differences; the significance of this has not been determined.

5. There is, apparently, no relation between the cholesterol values and the clinical and serologic response of the patient.

6. The only recognizable relation between the clinical type of syphilis and blood cholesterol values is the large proportion of high cholesterol estimations in syphilis of the central nervous system.

XXVI.—RESULTS IN THE TREATMENT OF WASSER-MANN-FAST SYPHILIS BY INTRAVENOUS MERCURIC CHLORID *

A. H. CONRAD, M.D., AND C. H. McCANN

ST. LOUIS

The intravenous administration of mercuric chlorid is a comparatively recent method of treatment. Osler gives it passing mention in the eighth edition of "Principles and Practice of Medicine" (1914) under the subject "Treatment of Syphilis." Bavellie [1] of Rome began using it in 1917 and claimed to have had excellent results. Within more recent years mercurial salts have been advocated for intravenous injections by Spittel [2] of England, Sanz [3] of Spain, Bastron [4] of Lincoln, Neb., and Brocq. [5] J. C. Klecan [6] states that mercury can and should be given intravenously, his mode of administration being perfectly painless and safe. The results are prompt, from both the symptomatic and the serologic point of view. The patient is saved time and money, and the period of mental anguish is decidedly shortened.

By intravenous treatment Gutmann obtained 74 per cent. negative results; Zimmermann, 68 per cent.; Linser, 70 per cent., and Micheli and Quarelli, 86 per cent. Spiethoff states that he obtained negative results in a majority of his cases.

In these articles, none of the writers specifies whether his cases were routine or Wassermann-fast. The cases reported in this article are all Wassermann-fast.

The treatment was instituted on Wassermann-fast cases at the Washington University Clinic. A total of 1,679 patients were treated during the year 1920-1921, of which sixty-two did not respond to the usual routine treatment, their Wassermann reactions remaining positive in one or both antigens after receiving from one to thirteen courses of routine treatment as carried out in this clinic.

The standard course of treatment for early syphilis consisted of three arsphenamin injections one week apart, and twenty intramuscular

---

Studies, observations and reports from the dermatological departments of the Barnard Free Skin and Cancer Hospital and the Washington University School of Medicine, St. Louis, Mo., U. S. A., service of Drs. M. F. Engman and W. H. Mook.

1. Bavellie: Riforma med. **34**:893, 1918.
2. Spittel: Practitioner **21**:212 (Oct.) 1918.
3. Sanz: Medicana Ibera, August, 1920, p. 187.
4. Bastron: Am. J. M. Sc. **159**:118, 1920.
5. Brocq: Bull. méd., Paris **73**:574, 1914.
6. Klecan, J. C.: Northwest J. M. **22**:266, 1920.

injections of mercuric chlorid at two to three day intervals, between and following the arsphenamin injections. The course in late syphilis consisted of twenty intramuscular injections of mercuric chlorid followed by four weeks of mixed treatment. Patients were then given one injection of arsphenamin and returned in four weeks for a Wassermann test.

The intravenous treatment was carried out as follows:

1. A Wassermann test was made on all patients before the intravenous treatment was started.

2. All patients were started on 10 minims (0.6 c.c.) of a 1 per cent. solution of mercuric chlorid in physiologic sodium chlorid solution. This dosage was increased by 2 minims (0.1 c.c.) at each treatment until the patients were receiving 2 c.c. at a dose. They were then kept on this amount, if no signs of mercurial intoxication appeared. The injections were given twice a week. If at any time signs of toxicity appeared either by gastro-intestinal symptoms, or albumin or casts in the urine, the dosage was immediately reduced by one-half and then slowly increased to the maximum dose. A few of the patients received 2.5 c.c. of 1 per cent. mercuric chlorid solution, but as they showed no greater improvement than the other patients, the dose was decreased to 2 c.c. During the entire course no arsphenamin or other antisyphilitic therapy was employed.

The technic of injecting mercuric chlorid intravenously is very simple:

1. A 10 c.c. all-glass syringe and a fine platinum needle of twenty-one or twenty-two gage and 1½ inches (3.7 cm.) long is used.

2. The mercury is drawn into the syringe, a tourniquet applied above the elbow, the skin over a prominent vein is cleansed, the needle is carefully introduced so that the point rests free in the lumen of the vein, and from 8 to 10 c.c. (2 to 3 fluidrams) of blood withdrawn. The tourniquet is now removed and about half of this amount is injected. Blood is then withdrawn again up to 8 c.c., and the full amount slowly injected. In some cases the mercury fails to mix with the blood; this is overcome by slowly revolving the syringe with the needle in the vein.

The patients in this series received twenty intravenous injections, and were then given a four weeks' rest. At the end of that time a Wassermann test was made and the treatment resumed. We encountered no trouble from embolus, and in only a few cases was there thrombosis. This was not caused by the injection of mercuric chlorid, but was the result of faulty technic.

The intravenous method used by us differs from that of the other writers on this subject in that the mercuric albuminate is formed in the syringe without withdrawing the needle from the vein, whereas they either injected the mercuric chlorid directly into the blood or withdrew blood and separated the cells from the serum, mixing the latter with the mercury, heating it to 37 C., and then injecting it as mercuric albuminate. Some of the writers who injected the mercury direct report that they could use a vein only once, owing to thrombosis.

The intravenous injection of mercuric chlorid is a comparatively safe procedure, practically painless and free from alarming reactions, immediate or late—provided certain simple precautions are observed.

1. Be certain that the needle is free in the vein, and not in the walls of it.

2. Form the mercuric albuminate in the syringe before injection.

Violations of these simple precautions will cause considerable pain to the patient and thrombosis of the vein and possibly embolus.

The table shows the results of this treatment in the sixty-two cases referred to.

Our results show that forty of the sixty-two patients treated, or 64 per cent., had negative Wassermann reactions at the end of the treatment.

The minimum number of injections required to obtain a negative Wassermann reaction in this series was six, and the maximum was twenty-two.

In fourteen additional cases there was a decrease in the Wassermann reactions in one or both antigens; eight remained the same throughout the courses of treatment.

Distinct clinical improvement was noted in a number of cases in which the Wassermann reaction remained the same throughout the courses of treatment. Similar clinical improvement was also noted in a number of cases in which the Wassermann test did not become negative, but remained slightly positive in one or both antigens.

Case 12, for example, was one of tabes dorsalis. While the Wassermann reaction remained practically the same, the patient showed clinical improvement. Before intravenous treatment, he was unable to do any work; after receiving the injections, he was able to carry on his trade and walk very much better than he could before he was put on this treatment.

Case 36 is a fair example of the efficiency of the intravenous treatment in our series. This patient received six arsphenamin and 104 intramuscular injections of mercuric chlorid. At the end of the course, the Wassermann reaction was $+ + + +$ in the cholesterin and $+$ in the alcoholic antigen. She then received sixteen intravenous injections of mercury with an average of 1.7 c.c. to the dose, and was given a four weeks' rest—after which a Wassermann test proved to be negative.

Case 23 was that of a patient with late syphilis who had been unable to do any work for three years. After receiving twenty intravenous injections, he was able to return to his work. He is con-

Results of Injections of Mercuric Chlorid

Case Number	First Wassermann Test*		Type†	Number of Intramuscular Injections	Number of Arsphenamin Injections	Wassermann Reaction at End of Intra-Muscular Injections		Number of Intravenous Injections	Average Dose, C.c.	Present Wassermann Test"	
1	4	4	Late............	49	4	3	1	4	1.6	3	1
2	4	4	Late............	0	0	4	4	10	2.4	4	4
3	4	4	Latent..........	4	0	4	0	8	1.7	0	0
4	4	4	Latent..........	11	0	4	4	14	1.7	0	0
5	4	4	Latent..........	259	13	3	0	27	2.2	3	0
6	4	4	Late............	10	3	4	0	21	2.4	0	0
7‡											
8	4	4	Latent..........	132	10	4	0	40	0.8	2	0
9	4	4	Late............	0	0	4	4	27	2.3	4	4
10	4	4	Early...........	2	0	4	4	13	1.8	4	0
11	4	4	Late............	1	0	4	4	13	1.6	0	0
12	4	4	Late............	2	0	4	4	5	1.5	4	4
13	4	4	Cerebral neuro-syphilis, tabes	17	2	4	4	35	1.7	2	0
14	4	4	Cerebral neuro-syphilis	0	3	4	0	24	1.6	1	0
15	4	4	Late............	3	0	4	4	4	1.9	4	2
16	4	4	Late............	20	8	4	4	12	1.1	0	0
17	4	4	Late............	20	2	4	4	13	2.5	0	0
18	4	4	Late............	16	4	3	3	20	1.8	0	0
19	4	4	Late............	81	5	4	4	16	1.9	0	0
20	0	0	Tabes...........	15	6	0	0	22	2.6	0	0
21	0	0	Tabes...........	2	3	0	0	6	1.4	0	0
22	4	4	Late............	30	3	4	4	14	2.0	4	4
23	4	4	Late............	70	6	4	4	44	1.4	3	0
24	4	4	Late............	20	2	4	4	57	2.0	2	0
25	4	4	Late............	0	0	4	4	33	1.5	4	4
26	4	4	Late............	49	4	4	1	14	1.06	0	0
27	4	4	Late............	0	0	4	4	20	2.0	0	0
28	4	4	Late visceral....	33	3	4	3	29	1.7	0	0
29	4	4	Cerebral neuro-syphilis	52	3	4	0	22	1.6	3	0
30	4	4	Latent..........	22	3	4	0	18	1.9	0	0
31	4	4	Latent..........	10	1	4	0	6	1.02	0	0
32	4	4	Late............	145	8	4	4	23	2.0	4	4
33	4	4	Late............	150	6	4	4	22	1.6	0	0
34	4	4	Late............	41	6	4	4	16	2.0	0	0
35	4	4	Late............	71	6	4	4	11	1.7	0	0
36	4	4	Late............	104	·6	4	1	16	1.7	0	0
37	4	4	Late............	50	6	4	0	39	1.5	0	0
38	4	4	Late............	47	6	4	4	16	2.1	4	4
39	4	4	Latent..........	181	13	4	3	62	1.8	2	0
40	4	4	Late............	74	7	4	0	24	2.0	0	0
41	4	4	Latent..........	13	0	4	4	13	2.0	4	4
42	4	4	Latent..........	32	4	4	4	20	1.6	0	0
43	4	4	Late............	48	5	4	4	17	1.4	0	0
44	4	4	Late............	49	6	4	4	18	1.6	0	0
45	4	4	Latent..........	0	0	4	4	22	1.7	0	0
46	4	4	Late............	132	10	4	4	22	1.8	0	0
47	4	4	Syphilis (latent?)	16	2	4	4	10	1.4	0	0
48	4	4	Late............	50	3	4	0	18	1.5	0	0
49	4	4	Late............	20	2	4	4	17	1.6	4	
50	4	4	Early...........	40	3	4	4	10	1.2	3	0
51	4	4	Late............	141	12	4	0	10	1.7	4	0§
52	4	4	Late visceral....	4	0	4	4	30	2.0	0	0
53	4	4	Latent..........	4	0	4	0	8	1.7	0	0
54	4	4	Latent..........	11	0	4	4	14	1.7	0	0
55	4	4	Late............	15	3	4	0	21	2.1	0	
56	4	4	Late............	10	4	4	0	22	0.83	0	
57	4	4	Late............	1	0	4	4	13	1.6	0	0
58	4	4	Latent..........	20	8	4	4	12	1.1	0	
59	4	4	Late visceral....	20	2	4	4	57	2.0	2	0
60	....		Tabes dorsalis...	15	6	0	0	22	2.0	0	
61	4	4	Late............	20	2	4	4	13	1.8	0	0
62	4	4	Latent..........	16	4	3	3	20	1.6	0	

* The figures at the left in these columns represent the Wassermann test, using the cholesterin antigen; the figures at the right represent the result, using the alcoholic antigen; 0 = negative.

† Classification of syphilis according to Engman and described by Weiss and Cerrac. Am. J. Syphilis 4 : No. 2 (April) 1920.

‡ Incomplete record; hospital case.

§ Irregular treatment.

 ¶ Dose low owing to albumin.

tinuing the treatment and says that he feels better now than he has at any time during the past ten years.

In Case 48, at the time intravenous treatment was started, the patient could hardly walk; after the sixth injection he showed marked clinical improvement, and is now able to walk without any trouble. After the tenth injection, his Wassermann reaction was negative.

Case 47 was that of a woman who had practically lost her eyesight and showed other clinical signs of syphilis. Both her serum and spinal fluid Wassermann reaction were negative. At the time of her first visit, she was unable to see the letters on a signboard at a distance of 8 feet; the largest letters were about 2 feet high, and the smallest about 6 inches. After she received six intravenous injections of mercury, she was able to read the entire sign from across the width of the street.

Results obtained in the patients whom we have treated, although the number is at present small, lead us to believe that in those cases in which the routine treatment has failed to reduce the Wassermann reaction or improve the clinical symptoms, mercury administered intravenously should be given a fair trial.

Advantages claimed for this method over other modes of mercuric injections are that quicker results in treatment are obtained, a more accurate grading of dosage is made possible; the course of the disease can be more carefully observed, and a practically painless injection is assured the patient. As to the permanence of the serologic result:, we are, of course, not able to report.

SALOL IN SMALLPOX *

J. A. K. BIRCHETT, Jr., M.D.
AND
SAM R. LUSTBERG, M.D.
VICKSBURG, MISS.

The recent epidemic of smallpox in this section of the country gave us an opportunity to make some interesting observations as to the action of phenyl salicylate in this disease. This synthetic drug was suggested for use by one of our colleagues (J. A. K. Birchett, M. D.) to whom we are greatly indebted for cooperation.

The prevention of scarring covers an interesting chapter in the literature. Various measures have been pursued with varying success. Among the most popular are exclusion of light, local use of iodin, mercuric chlorid, boric acid, oils, glycerin, potassium permanganate or phenol.

It so happened that a member of our nursing staff who had been vaccinated was unfortunate enough to autoinoculate herself on a previous herpes about the lip, thus developing vaccinia of the lip. She was given 10 grains of salol four times a day, and the end result in four weeks was that no scar could be noted on the lip, while the original vaccination on the arm was evidenced by only a small scar.

A study was then made of the discrete and confluent forms of the disease. Salol, 10 grains four times a day was the sole medicament used, and careful observations were made of results. It was noted that the patients who began the medication in the preeruptive stage were left with only a few scars, and even those receiving the medicament during the eruptive stages showed less scarring than those who received no therapy. The severe confluent forms left a surprising aftermath. Some scarring, of course, remained as a remnant of the disease. but far less disfigurement than is usually seen in such cases.

In view of the epidemic, we were on the lookout for cases to develop in the institution. When a patient had a sudden rise of temperature. headache, lumbar pains and rapid pulse. and yet appeared well. salol was administered. After several doses the patient began to sweat. and as the drug was continued, the sweating became more profuse and continued so until the eruptive period. During this period there was some sweating. but considerably less than in the preeruptive stage. It was also observed that the temperature of patients treated with salol was lower than in those not treated with this drug.

---

* From the isolation wards of the Mississippi State Charity Hospital.

STUDY OF THE DRUG

Salol or phenyl salicylate is ordinarily used to disinfect the intestines. It is insoluble, but is decomposed in the intestine by the fat-splitting ferment of the pancreatic juice into salicylic acid and phenol. It is known that the salicylates have some antiseptic action, especially salicylic acid because of the acid ion. The drugs are eliminated in small amounts in the perspiration, and as perspiratioin is increased following the administration of phenyl salicylate in smallpox, it is fair to assume that greater amounts are being eliminated through the skin channels.

Salicylates prevent the breaking down of protein material, and preserve parts exposed to the air for a long period.[1] Phenol has a similar action, but is less stable. Cushny [1] remarks that the movements of plant protoplasm, protozoa and leukocytes are prevented by salicylic acid. It also retards digestion of the proteins by the gastric and pancreatic juices.

In smallpox, and more especially during the preeruptive stage, we have an increased elimination of two antiseptics whose action influences the disease. They both prevent protein decomposition, and when coming into relation with the lesions or with their oncoming location exert this special influence. The skin proteins are saved from destruction and little scarring occurs. Added to this factor, salicylic acid prevents the movements of leukocytes, and in this way accounts for the small pustule noted when salol therapy is used.

CONCLUSION

Salol (phenyl salicylate) as an internal medicament in smallpox diminished the degree of scarring. The best results were obtained when the drug was commenced in the preeruptive stage.

---

1. Cushny: A Text-Book of Pharmacology and Therapeutics, Philadelphia: Lea and Febiger, 1915.

SYPHILIS OF THE SALIVARY GLANDS *

JAROLD E. KEMP, M.D.

AND

JOSEPH EARLE MOORE, M.D.

BALTIMORE

The salivary glands, especially the parotid, may share in the general glandular involvement of the early stages of syphilis, or more frequently, may be the seat of tertiary lesions of the disease. Of about 5,600 cases of syphilis in all stages seen in the Syphilis Department of the Johns Hopkins Hospital, four, or less than 0.07 per cent., presented involvement of this glandular group, and so far as we have been able to determine, the literature contains the report of only sixty-one cases. The rarity of the condition, the paucity of reports in English and the differential diagnostic problem raised by these lesions warrants a report of our own cases.

REPORT OF CASES

CASE 1 (G39522).—*Chancre of the upper lip; enlargement of submaxillary glands.*

A white man, aged 36, was first seen Dec. 17, 1920, complaining of a lump under the right side of the jaw. He had been married two months before admission. His wife had acquired syphilis from her first husband. Otherwise the family and personal history were unessential.

About the middle of November, a painless sore appeared on his upper lip. It reached its maximum size rapidly, and had not grown during the month before admission. A week or so after its appearance, he noticed a swelling under the right side of his jaw, which had continued to enlarge, and which at present caused him some local discomfort.

Except for the local findings, the physical examination revealed nothing of interest. On the mucocutaneous border of the upper lip in the midline was an indurated, round, tumor-like erosion, measuring about 2 cm. in diameter. This was a typical chancre. Unfortunately, a dark-field examination was not made. The submaxillary glands on the right side were markedly enlarged, measuring 3 by 5 cm. The swelling was hard, indurated and slightly tender. The overlying skin was not involved. The left submaxillary gland was also enlarged, but not to such an extent. The other salivary glands were not involved. With the exception of polyadenitis, there were no signs of secondary syphilis. The blood Wassermann test was positive.

After six intravenous injections of arsphenamin, of 0.4 gm. each, the lesion on the lip had completely healed, and the tumor in the neck had practically disappeared.

CASE 2 (F51439).—*Gummas of the parotid, nasal septum and turbinates. Improvement under treatment.*

---

* From the Syphilis Department of the Medical Clinic, Johns Hopkins Hospital.

A colored man, aged 24, entered the clinic on May 3, 1916, complaining of a sore nose. The family history was negative. He denied syphilis by name and symptom, and stated that with the exception of mumps as a child he had always been perfectly healthy.

The present illness began in March, 1916, when he first noticed a sore in his left nostril. This was painless and was accompanied by little discharge. He made no mention of the other findings which were later noted, since they apparently caused no subjective discomfort.

Examination revealed these positive points: In both parotid regions were found large, firm, well circumscribed swellings about 5 by 3 cm. in size. The mass on the left was a little larger than that on the right. There was marked enlargement of the glands of the neck, the largest being about 2.5 cm. in diameter. The left nasal septum and the anterior portion of the left turbinates were ulcerated. The blood Wassermann test was positive. A roentgenogram of the skull was negative.

The patient was very irregular in his attendance at the clinic, but after one intravenous injection of arsphenamin, 0.3 gm., the nasal lesion had healed completely, and the parotid swellings had reduced greatly in size. A short time later he disappeared from observation.

CASE 3 (G22973).—*Gumma of the right parotid with sinus formation; paralysis of the terminal branches of the right seventh nerve; periostitis of the right tibia.*

A colored man, aged 35, was admitted to the hospital, Dec. 5, 1919, complaining of swelling of the face and a sore leg. He had been married ten years. His wife had had two pregnancies, both children dying about one month after birth. He admitted many Neisser infections and eighteen years previously had a genital sore which was later followed by a rash.

The swelling of his face began two and a half months before admission. It was painless and had gradually grown larger. Within a short time after its appearance, it softened and broke down exteriorly, with a resulting discharging sinus. This had closed spontaneously before his entrance to the clinic. About six weeks later, following a local injury, his right leg became swollen, painful and tender to pressure.

Physical examination revealed weakness of the right upper lid and the muscles around the mouth. There was complete paralysis of the frontalis on the right. There was also excessive lacrimation of the right eye, though no enlargement of the lacrymal gland on that side could be discovered. In the right parotid region was a tumor mass, extending from the level of the upper attachment of the auricle down to the lower attachment. The mass was firm and painless, and the surface temperature was not raised. The scar of the healed sinus was present. The overlying skin was freely movable, and the mass was not attached to the bone. A probe could not be passed into Stenson's duct, although the flow of saliva was not impeded. Over the lower third of the right leg and ankle there was swelling and tenderness, more marked over the tibia. The blood Wassermann reaction was positive. Roentgen-ray examination of the right leg showed periostitis of the tibia and fibula. The patient was treated for a short while only and showed definite improvement. He disappeared from observation before complete resolution of his lesions.

CASE 4 (G58197).—*Gumma of the parotid gland; nodular syphilid of the cheek; gumma of the right quadriceps femoris muscle.*

A colored girl, aged 23, came into the dispensary Dec. 14, 1921, complaining of swelling of the jaw. Her family history was negative. She admitted frequent sexual exposure since the age of 14. When she was 16, she had a miscarriage at one and one half months. On close questioning she denied any signs or symptoms of early syphilis.

Her present trouble began two years before admission, when a lump appeared above the right knee, and gradually increased in size. It was painful only at night, but was not especially tender to pressure, and the main subjective discomfort was slight stiffness of the right leg on walking. About eight months ago a swelling appeared on the right side of the face, which at first grew rapidly, and for a short time was painful, especially at night. The size of this mass remained constant, without any noticeable variation. About the time of the appearance of this lump, she noticed a "pimple" inside the left nostril, which gradually grew larger and opened exteriorly. After several roentgen-ray treatments, given by an outside physician, the nasal condition cleared up, but the mass on the right side of the face remained unchanged.

Examination revealed a diffuse swelling of the right side of the face. At the angle of the mouth on the right, deep beneath the skin were three cherry sized nodules, over one of which the skin was dusky red. Otherwise the skin was not involved. Beginning just below and behind the angle of the jaw, and extending up the right side of the face to the level of the zygoma, was an irregularly shaped, firm, elastic, painless mass about 8 by 8 cm. It occupied the position of the parotid gland, was not attached to the skin and apparently not to the bone. Stenson's duct was not obliterated. Inside the left nostril a large destructive scar was seen. On the outer aspect of the right leg, about 4 cm. above the patella, was found a hard firm mass about 2 by 4 cm. It was situated deep below the quadriceps fascia, moved with the muscle and was apparently not attached to the bone. There was slight tenderness on deep pressure. The blood Wassermann reaction was positive. A roentgenogram of the right leg showed only soft tissue swelling on the outer side of the femur.

After the intravenous injection of three weekly doses of arsphenamin, 0.3 gm. each, the parotid swelling and the other lesions had completely disappeared. No abnormalities could be detected at the site of the old lesions.

DISCUSSION

Richter,[1] in 1800, reported a case in which the parotid on one side was enlarged as a result of a chancre on the lip; and a few similar reports of involvement of the salivary glands when in the drainage area of the head or face chancres have since appeared. Our own Case 1 falls into this category. In secondary syphilis also, it has occasionally been noted, especially by Flandin and Aubin[2] that the parotid, submaxillary, or other salivary glands were enlarged, usually bilaterally, as a part of the general glandular involvement of this stage of the disease. In such cases, the enlargement is symmetrical, variable in size, usually painless, and it subsides as the other secondary lesions recede.

1. Richter, A. G., quoted by Gerber: Syphilis der Speicheldrüsen. Handbuch der Geschlechtskrankheiten **3**:109, 1913.

2. Flandin, C., and Aubin: Syndrome de mickulicz fruste à localization biparotidienne chez un syphilitique secondaire. Soc. franc. de dermat. et syph. 1920, p. 510.

In 1864, Virchow[3] reported the first case of tertiary involvement of the parotid gland. Important contributions to the subject were made by Lancereaux[4] in 1874, Bull[5] in 1878, and Lang[6] in 1880. In 1913, Gerber[7] compiled the cases reported up to that date, and the additional literature up to 1916 has been reviewed by Vuillet (1913)[8] and Haslund.[9] Cases have also been reported by Simard,[10] Guibaud[11] DeMassy and Tochman,[12] Letulle and Vuillet,[13] Lemierre,[14] Kjellberg[15] and Packard.[16] Including the four cases which we report, the literature affords the details of sixty-five cases of syphilis of the salivary glands, of which thirty-eight occurred in tertiary syphilis. We have not included in this total a few additional references which are not accessible to us.[17]

More than half of the total recorded cases of syphilitic involvement of the salivary glands have occurred in late syphilis, as is shown in Table 1. Six cases have been reported as late lesions in congenital syphilis. It also appears that in the majority of cases, as in our own, the parotid only is involved. Two or more glands may, however, share

---

3. Virchow, R.: Geschwülste **2**:439, 1864.

4. Lancereaux: Traité de la Syphilis, Paris, 1873, p. 253.

5. Bull, S.: Syphilis of the Conjunctiva, Am. J. M. Sc. **76**:405, 1878.

6. Lang, E.: Ueber Mastitis und Parotitis Syphilitica, Wein. med. Wchnschr. **30**: No. 9, 1880.

7. Gerber, P.: Syphilis der Speicheldrüsen, Handbuch der Geschlechtskrankheiten.

8. Vuillet: Syphilis des Glandes Salivaires, Thèse de Paris, 1913.

9. Haslund, O.: Ueber Parotitis Syphilitica, Dermat. Wchnschr. **62**:63, 1916.

10. Simard, A.: Gumma de la Parotide, Bull. méd. de Québec **8**:67, 1906.

11. Guibaud, M.: Un cas de syphilis de la parotide, Arch. de med. et pharm. Navales **105**:66, 1918.

12. De Massy and Tochman: Syndrome de mickulicz à début rapide simulant les orcillons chez un syphilitique, Bull. et mém. Soc. méd. d. hôp de Paris **42**:627 and 987, 1918.

13. Letulle, M., and Vuillet, M.: Syphilome de la parotide, Bull. et mém. Soc. méd. d. hôp. de Paris **35**:1149, 1913.

14. Lemierre, A.: Parotidite syphilitique bilaterale avec paralysis de la faciale gauche, Bull. et mém. Soc. méd. d. hôp. de Paris **43**:510, 1920.

15. Kjellberg, G.: Deux cas de parotide syphilitique, Acta dermat. venér. **1**:263, 1920.

16. Packard, F. R.: Two Cases of Suppuration of the Parotid Gland with Pus in the External Auditory Canal, J. A. M. A. **37**:450 (Aug. 17) 1901.

17. Felman, I.: Gumma a parotisban bujokoros gegeszükület; izomgummak, Orvosi betil, Budapest **45**:406, 1901.

Ito, T.: A Case of Gumma of the Submaxillary Glands, Hifubyog kiu Hiniokibyog, Tokyo **4**:126, 1904.

Kjellberg, G.: Om ett fall af Parotitis syphilitica med epikris, Hygiea, Stockholm **6**:1307, 1906.

in the disease process; and in rare instances other acinous glands of the body, notably the breast or the lacrimal glands, may be affected.

The local lesion may be, as tertiary lesions are elsewhere, either a diffuse fibrosis or a gumma. The latter apparently is the common form of lesion in acquired syphilis, while fibrosis is the usual accompaniment of the congenital cases.

TABLE 1.—INCIDENCE OF INVOLVEMENT OF THE SALIVARY AND ACINOUS GLANDS IN ACQUIRED AND CONGENITAL SYPHILIS: A COMPILATION FROM THE LITERATURE

Glands Involved	Acquired Syphilis Early	Tertiary	Congenital Syphilis
Parotid	17	28	6
Submaxillary	1	2	
Sublingual	1	3	
Parotid and submaxillary	1	3	
Parotid and sublingual	—	1	
Parotid and breast	1	—	
Parotid and lacrimal	1	—	
Blandin-Nuhn's gland (tongue)	—	1	

When the lesion is located in the parotid or submaxillary gland, subjective complaints are often absent. The patient notices only a gradually increasing swelling which may be only slightly painful. There is usually increased salivation. Mastication may be interfered with if the growth becomes large enough. The size of the swelling is not, as in the case of stone in the salivary duct, subject to marked fluctuation. When the sublingual gland is involved, there is often mechanical interference with mastication, deglutition and speech. If the gumma softens and breaks down, a salivary fistula results. In the case of involvement

TABLE 2.—SEX AND AGE OF PATIENTS WITH SYPHILIS OF THE SALIVARY GLANDS

Male 25 Age at Time of Appearance of Lesion	Female 22 Number of Cases
0-10	3
11-20	1
21-30	16
31-40	11
41-50	6
51-75	4

of the parotid gland, a pressure paralysis of the terminal branches of the seventh nerve sometimes occurs. Neumann[18] and Lemiere[14] each report one such case, and one of our own cases presented the same picture.

Lesions of the salivary glands are equally frequent in men and women, as shown in Table 2. The age at which the lesions appeared

18. Neumann: Ueber Syphilis der Parotis und der Glandula Sublingualis. Arch. f. dermat. u. syph. **29**:1, 1894.

could be determined in forty-one cases. More than half the cases occurred during the third and fourth decade.

The diagnosis is sometimes obscure. In the parotid, for example, one must consider stone in Stenson's duct, mixed tumor, ordinary infections, tuberculosis and actinomycosis. It is, however, rarely necessary to resort to surgical procedures to arrive at the diagnosis. In early syphilis the concomitant existence of other lesions of a secondary type should remove all doubt. In our three cases of tertiary syphilis, other syphilitic lesions were present, in one instance a gumma of the nasal bone, in another periostitis of the tibia and in the third typical nodular syphilids and a gumma of the muscle. Many of the reported cases also presented other lesions of syphilis, so that this factor is an important diagnostic aid. The blood Wassermann test is usually positive, as in our cases. The results of therapy are the final conclusive evidence of the syphilitic nature of the disease.

The results of treatment in the gummatous type are brilliant. Complete resolution occurs, and at the end of a few weeks it is usually impossible to find any residual of the lesion. In fibrotic lesions of these glands, on the other hand, it may be impossible to effect a complete disappearance of the tumor mass. After a partial resolution, the size of the mass may remain stationary in spite of the intensive use of anti-syphilitic treatment.

The pathologic condition of these lesions has been studied in only a few instances, and the reports available to us indicate that it does not differ markedly from that of fibrotic or gummatous syphilis in other organs.

SUMMARY

The literature on syphilis of the salivary glands has been reviewed and four additional cases reported.

Abstracts from Current Literature

A CASE OF SCLERODERMA FOLLOWING A PSYCHOGENOUS FUNCTIONAL DISORDER. BENEDEK, Deutsch. Ztschr. f. Nervenh. **72**: 5, 1921.

Benedek reports a case which supports the opinion that scleroderma is an angiotropho neurosis.

A NOTE ON THE ROENTGEN-RAY TREATMENT OF SCLERODERMA. DONATH, München. med. Wchnschr. **68**:41, 1921.

The author refers to two of his cases in which scleroderma was combined with aplasia of the thyroid gland. Stimulation of the thyroid gland had a beneficial influence on the scleroderma.

EXPERIMENTAL TAR CARCINOMAS. BIERICH and MOELLER, München. med. Wchnschr. **68**:42, 1921.

There are pronounced alterations of the cutis, that is, deposits of hemosiderin in the epithelial cells and of free tar in the meshes of the tissue. The frequent presence of arsenic in tar is not the effective ingredient. Prolonged painting with tar generally causes grave nephrosis.

COMBINED NEO-ARSPHENAMIN AND LUETIN ORGANOTHERAPY IN A CASE OF MALIGNANT SYPHILIS. MUELLER and PLANNER. München. med. Wchnschr. **68**:43, 1921.

This is a report of a case which not only resisted 5.1 gm. of neo-arsphenamin and ten injections of mercury but even became worse. Not until three injections of luetin (1 gm. each) were given followed by 0.6 gm. of neo-arsphenamin was there improvement. The author believes that luetin "prepared the ground" for the arsphenamin.

ETIOLOGY OF ACNE. SEIBOLD. München. med. Wchnschr. **68**:44, 1921.

This is a report of several cases of scabies in two families which after treatment developed obstinate acne. The question arises whether the scabies formed the disposition for the acne or whether the latter was a consequence of the therapy.

ARSPHENAMIN RESISTANT SYPHILIS. SIEMENS. München. med. Wchnschr. **68**:44, 1921.

This is the report of a case in a male patient who in the course of eighteen months had received six thorough courses of combined mercury and arsphenamin treatment. Both during the courses and after them *Spirochaeta pallida* were found in the lesions. There is no explanation for this case.

A NOTE ON TWO METHODS FOR PRESERVING THE COMPLE-
MENT IN THE WASSERMANN REACTION. KLEIN, München. med.
Wchnschr. **68**:45, 1921.

Sodium acetate added to fresh guinea-pig serum in the proportion 6:4 preserves the complement effect as long as seven days. However, this is not reliable,
as acetate complement even two days old tends to cause a negative reaction.
Nor is the other preserving method (freezing of guinea-pig complement in
carbon dioxid snow) reliable. The author advises heart puncture of the
guinea-pig for obtaining the complement quantity required on the day it is
to be used.

THE DIAGNOSTIC VALUE OF THE WASSERMANN, SACHS-GEORGI
AND MEINICKE REACTIONS IN MALARIAL COUNTRIES.
HEINEMANN, München. med. Wchnschr. **68**:48, 1921.

Nonspecific Wassermann reactions in malaria are frequent. In the flocculation reactions this "malaria error" is smaller than in the complement reactions. A nonspecific positive Wassermann reaction in malaria is always
transitory and disappears under quinin medication.

THE COMBINED SACHS-GEORGI AND MEINICKE REACTIONS.
STERN, München. med. Wchnschr. **68**:49, 1921.

The author tried both reactions synchronously in one test tube. In 500
cases the results attained were more exact than with the individual reactions.

EXPERIENCES WITH MORO'S DIAGNOSTIC TUBERCULIN.
PRAUSNITZ, München. med. Wchnschr. **68**:1015 (Aug. 12) 1921.

Moro's tuberculin and old tuberculin are practically equivalent. Moro's
has the advantage of revealing bovine infections also.

REGULAR ALTERATIONS IN LIPOID CONTENT OF THE BLOOD
UNDER SHOCK THERAPY (REIZTHERAPIE). GABBE, München.
med. Wchnschr. **68**:1377, 1921.

Small doses of the substances which cause only a slight rise of temperature effect an increase of the blood lipoids during some hours; larger doses,
causing pronounced fever, effect a transitory diminution of the lipoid quantity.

HOW TO SIMPLIFY THE CUTANEOUS TUBERCULIN TEST.
BRANDES, München. med. Wchnschr. **68**:1392, 1921.

The author recommends rubbing the skin with terra silicea, peeling it off
and then rubbing a little old tuberculin into this part with the finger.

AHLSWEDE, Hamburg, Germany.

ROENTGEN-RAY TREATMENT OF ADIPOSOGENITALIS. RANSCHBURG,
Deutsch. med. Wchnschr. **47**:43, 1921.

Frequent prolonged irradiation of the sella turcica region had a distinctly
beneficial influence on the brain symptoms. No damaging influence whatever
was observed. Two cases of adipose dystrophy with tumor in the sella were
successfully treated this way.

A NOTE ON THE PRECIPITIN REACTION IN THE DARK FIELD FOR FORENSIC PURPOSES, WITH A REMARK ON THE SACHS-GEORGI REACTION. OELZE, Deutsch. med. Wchnschr. **47**:45, 1921.

The Zeiss dark field condensor for suspended drops was used for examining a mixture of blood extract and specific antiserum. Soon after the mixing flocculation could be observed. The typical picture of a floccula is described. The Sachs-Georgi reaction is particularly suitable for examination in this way.

A NOTE ON THE RELATION BETWEEN DERMATOSES AND ENDO-CRINE GLANDS. BROCK, Deutsch. med. Wchnschr. **47**:47, 1921.

Dermatoses based on constitutional disposition are beneficially influenced both by injections of thymus organ extract and by irradiation of the thymus gland.

A NOTE ON THE ETIOLOGY OF THE NEVUS FLAMMEUS. POPPER, Med. Klin. **17**:22, 1921.

Popper assumes for the development of a nevus a primary damage to the nerve.

A NOTE ON THE PATHOGENESIS OF PRURIGO AND STROPHULUS INFANTUM. PULAY, Med. Klin. **17**:39, 1921.

Pulay holds that prurigo, strophulus and urticaria belong to one group of diseases, pruritus being the cardinal symptom of the three. The author proposes to call this group the "pruritus of childhood" (des Kindesalters).

EOSINOPHILIA IN QUINCKE'S EDEMA. GAENSSLEN, Med. Klin. **17**:40, 1921.

Eosinophilia is an anaphylactic reaction to the attacks and is caused by absorption of the serum.

TREATMENT OF VARICES WITH INJECTIONS OF MERCURIC CHLORID. LINSER, Med. Klin. **17**:48, 1921.

Linser injects 1 c.c. of a 0.5 to 1 per cent. solution into the varices. thus causing a necrosis of the vein intima. Thrombosis generally occurs within twelve hours after injection. Embolism was never seen. Up to ten injections are made on successive days. The kidneys require attention.

DIAGNOSIS OF TYPHUS. KLIENEBERGER. Berl. klin. Wchnschr. **58**:40, 1921.

A positive Weil-Felix reaction easily decides the diagnosis ($1:40 +$ is generally sufficient). Simultaneous typhoid agglutination and morphologic blood examination should serve as a control. There is generally a slight polynucleosis.

PRIMARY SYPHILIS IN THOROUGHBRED RABBITS. SCHERESCHEWSKY and WORMS, Berl. klin. Wchnschr. **58**:44, 1921.

The authors do not agree with the difference Kolle found between the spirochetes in rabbits and those in pallida with a fuchsin stain. They hold that it is impossible to differentiate between the two species.

FEVER DERMATITIS AFTER COMBINED MERCURY AND ARS-PHENAMIN MEDICATION. Peters, Berl. klin. Wchnschr. **58**:44, 1921.

This is a report of two serious cases of skin eruptions. The author discusses the differential diagnosis with regard to the literature on similar cases and sees the cause of the disturbance in mercury alone.

FREQUENCY OF SPIROCHAETA PALLIDA IN THE MALE URETHRA IN PRIMARY AND SECONDARY SYPHILIS. Friedländer, Berl. klin. Wchnschr. **58**:48, 1921.

Syphilitic patients with postgonorrheal catarrh or urethritis nongonorrhoica in eight cases out of thirty-two had *Spirochaeta pallida* in the urethral discharge. These were primary seropositive cases. Of forty cases of secondary syphilis there were *Spirochaetae pallida* in twelve. Endoscopically, lesions resembling plaques opalines were found in the urethra. From one of these lesions pallida were obtained not mixed with other spirochetes. The possibility of transmitting syphilis via the sperm is mentioned.

A CONTRIBUTION TO THE RELATION BETWEEN PEMPHIGUS NEONATORUM AND IMPETIGO CONTAGIOSA. Feilchenfeld. Berl. klin. Wchnschr. **58**:49, 1921.

The author reports three cases which point to a possible etiologic identity of the two disorders.

SPIROCHAETA PALLIDA IN THE CERVICAL CANAL IN PRIMARY AND SECONDARY SYPHILIS. Fuchs, Berl. klin. Wchnschr. **58**:51, 1921.

In eleven cases of Wassermann negative syphilis in women *Spirochaeta pallida* was found in the cervical canal.

A NOTE ON APLASIA CUTIS CONGENITA. Loenne, Zentralbl. f. Gynäk. **45**:46, 1921.

This is a report of three cases which are remarkable in that the lesions were not located on the scalp, which is the usual site.

THE LIPASE CONTENTS OF THE SPINAL FLUID. Resch, Ztschr. f. klin. Med. **92**:1, 1921.

There is no genetic relation between lymphocytes and lipase. In thirty-four patients suffering from cerebral and spinal disorders there was no coincidence in the spinal fluid between the lymphocytes and lipase. Though the lymphocytes were enormously increased in some cases, the lipase (Fettahspaltung) was not.

THE TREATMENT OF MENINGEAL SYPHILIS. Gennerich, Therap. Halbmonatsh. **35**:22, 1921.

The author advises lumbar puncture and examination of the spinal fluid as early as possible in all cases of latent syphilis whether the Wassermann reaction is positive or not. The chief indications for endolumbar arsphenamin administration are latent meningeal inflammation and cerebral syphilis with a high percentage of globulin and a strong positive Wassermann reaction. In many cases of tabes the endolumbar injection in his experience quickly removed pains while the other symptoms were more energetically influenced than by intravenous administration. In some cases of progressive paralysis, particularly during the initial stages, satisfactory results were obtained. In tabetic optic atrophy endolumbar injections must be made as soon as possible.

THE ROENTGEN-RAY TREATMENT OF RINGWORM OF THE SCALP IN CHILDREN. C. GUTMANN, Dermat. Wchnschr. **73**:1123 (Oct. 29) 1921.

Buschke and Klemm (*Dermat. Wchnschr.*, 1921, No. 22, p. 453), without defining their technic, described frequent syncope, headache and vomiting, and later roentgen-ray dermatitis, ulceration and permanent alopecia in a large percentage of the cases treated by them. Kleinschmidt (*Dermat. Wchnschr.*, 1921, No. 32, p. 855), on the other hand, was satisfied with the results he obtained in 231 cases, although headache and faintness were rarely manifest.

The author reports favorably on the treatment of forty patients, in spite of frequent headache, swooning and vomiting. Rays filtered through 0.5 mm. aluminum were used in doses measuring 9 X to 10 X with the tube at five placements. It was found that on scalps containing only single patches the entire hair had to be epilated in order to avoid recurrences.

Cultures revealed *Trichophyton cerebriforme* in twenty-six children, and *Trichophyton rosaceum, gypseum* and *violaceum,* each in two cases. Each gypseum case was a typical kerion, whereas the other scalps presented scattered, scaly, dry patches. No instances of trichophitid were noted.

THE DIGESTION OF CARCINOMA BY TRYPSIN. K. HUEBSCHMANN, Dermat. Wchnschr. **73**:1145 (Nov. 5) 1921.

The method of pepsin-hydrochloric acid digestion of pathologic material, as suggested by Unna, has been applied by the author to carcinomas of the stomach and intestines. Microscopic sections fixed in alcohol, after thorough washing, were incubated at body temperature in a 1 per cent. solution of pepsin in 0.5 per cent. hydrochloric acid, at twenty-four, forty-eight and seventy-two hours. After digestion, these sections were stained with hematoxylin-eosin and polychrome methylene blue. The nuclei of the carcinomas were preserved and the chromatin picture did not exhibit change until several days had elapsed. Then the nuclei manifested simple disintegration, rather than a transformation suggesting pepsin digestion. A similar procedure with a substitution of trypsin and soda solution for the pepsin-hydrochloric acid, soon exhibited loosening and elevation of the nuclei from the sections, succeeded by chromatolysis and falling out of the nuclei into the supernatant fluid. After centrifuging the sediment, they were found decidedly damaged and, in a short time, disappeared entirely. In thick sections, in which nuclei, if preserved, would have been noted, there was only the débris of disintegration.

LIVEDO RACEMOSA NONSYPHILITICA. S. PELLER, Dermat. Wchnschr. **73**:1157 (Nov. 25) 1921.

Syphilis is not always responsible for livedo racemosa, and there is not always demonstrable histologically an endarteritis of the deep cutaneous vessels. Two cases illustrating this point are described. Experiments on them with epinephrin and amyl nitrite revealed a paresis of the venous capillaries of the skin. It is concluded that there are two types of the affection: livedo racemosa as a venous disease without visible organic changes in the small arteries, in which there is a raised contraction threshold for the entire peripheral vascular system, and livedo racemosa as a secondary venous disease following local organic obstruction of the arterial flow in the skin, as in syphilis.

PROVOCATIVE EXPERIMENTS WITH MILK INJECTIONS IN THE LATENT STAGES OF SYPHILIS. J. Guszman, Dermat. Wchnschr. **73**:1172 (Nov. 12) 1921.

At the beginning of the arsphenamin era, it was discovered that apparently cured syphilitic patients with negative Wassermann reactions showed positive reactions after a single arsphenamin injection, demonstrating that although completely healed, to all appearances, a syphilitic process still remained.

The author gave, intragluteally, 10 c.c. of milk, in three classes of persons with negative Wassermann reactions. The first group consisted of known syphilitic patients who had become symptom free, seronegative and apparently cured. Provocative arsphenamin injections had failed to produce positive Wassermann reactions. Of seventy-three cases, from four to six days following the milk injection, 15 per cent. showed positive Wassermann reactions. The second group consisted of known, latent syphilitic patients with negative Wassermann reactions. Twenty-five per cent. of these showed positive tests after the milk injections. The third group consisted of patients who were not syphilitic, but who suffered from other venereal diseases. In these the milk injections caused no positive Wassermann reactions.

A COMPARISON OF THE VALUES OF THE SERUM REACTIONS OF SACHS-GEORGI AND OF WASSERMANN. F. Weise, Dermat. Wchnschr. **73**:1193 (Nov. 19) 1921.

For the Sachs-Georgi reactions, alcoholic cholesterinized beef heart extract was used; whereas, for the Wassermann reaction, alcoholic cholesterinized human heart extract was employed. After comparative tests on several hundred cases of primary, secondary and tertiary syphilis, it was concluded that the Wassermann reaction is superior to the Sachs-Georgi reaction in determining the syphilitic basis of disease and that the often made assertion that the Sachs-Georgi reaction becomes positive earlier in primary syphilis and remains positive longer in secondary syphilis is erroneous.

METABOLISM IN SKIN DISEASES. E. Pulay, Dermat. Wchnschr. **73**: 1217 (Nov. 26) 1921.

Analytic metabolic studies of a case of lupus erythematosus in which the history suggested an interrelation between the eruption and exposure to sunlight, demonstrated an abnormally high blood uric acid, as well as other minor changes in the blood chemistry. The theory is advanced that certain endogenous metabolic products become strongly catalytic in the presence of light and that proteins are photosensitive.

ARSPHENAMIN ERYTHEMA AND THE HERXHEIMER REACTION. M. Hesse, Dermat. Wchnschr. **73**:1241 (Dec. 3) 1921.

A dentist, with psoriasis of the palms and soles, presented a very painful paronychia with a marked lymphangitis of the forearm, swelling of the cubital lymph node and fever. After surgical treatment, the local symptoms subsided, but the fever persisted, ranging from 100 to 103 F. Internists made the diagnosis of pulmonary catarrh; whereas surgeons suggested the possibility of a metastatic abscess. Roentgenograms seemed to support the opinion of the internists, as there was a bilateral inflammatory process of the apexes and an infiltration of the hilus nodes. The tuberculin reaction was negative.

The rise in temperature persisted for more than a month, until Professor Matzenauer made the diagnosis of syphilis. After one arsphenamin injection, the temperature fell to normal. After the fourth injection, it again rose sharply to 104 F., and on the following day a typical scarlatiniform arsphenamin erythema appeared, most pronounced in the areas in which the lymphangitis had been. The author believes that the vasotoxin theory of the Herxheimer reaction also accounts for the subsequent toxic erythema.

A CASE OF EXTENSIVE OIDIOMYCOSIS RESEMBLING MILIARIA RUBRA (MILIARIA RUBRA OIDIOMYCETICA). G. Miescher, Dermat. Wchnschr. **73**:1265 (Dec. 10) 1921.

The patient, aged 28, during convalescence from a mastoid operation. developed an extensive erythema with numerous pinhead sized pustules in the genitocrural region, and on the back, chest, arms and legs. The appearance was typical of miliaria rubra. There was a predilection for the folds of the joints. The buccal mucosa was free.

Bacteriologically, there were a few staphylococci, but an oïdium was found more regularly and this seemed to play the main causative rôle. In cultures. the oïdium grew regularly in a manner different from that in which it grew in the skin. Workers are cautioned concerning the importance of this discrepancy in mycology.

THE MORE RECENT REMEDIES FOR THE PROMOTION OF HAIR GROWTH. H. Friedenthal, Dermat. Wchnschr. **73**:1281 (Dec. 17) 1921.

During the last year, the internal administration and the external application of the split products of horny substances have been advocated by various authors. It is improbable that the lack in the blood stream of prodncts necessary chemically for the formation of hair is the cause of alopecia. One frequently observes a profuse growth of body hair and the beard in bald persons. The primitive Europeans showed this characteristic.

Weidner has demonstrated that the internal use of digested horny substances is frequently harmful. The horny substances in the hair cells may be divided into those free of sulphur and those containing sulphur. Attention has been called to the administration of sulphur-containing keratin. Cystin plays an important rôle among the sulphur-containing split products of albumin. In animal experimentation, this has proved a dangerous poison. It may. however, be used externally on the scalp. Unna has advocated softening the horny layer of the scalp with a mixture of pepsin and hydrochloric acid in order to facilitate rubbing remedies into the deeply situated hair roots.

A satisfactory hair tonic should contain the primary split products of human hair. It should be of an alkalinity estimated to soften horny and albuminous substances in order to make the scalp penetrable to chemical molecules: it should have strongly bactericidal properties; and should contain drugs which. when introduced into the tissues. will cause an enhanced circulation of the entire scalp.

GLANDLIKE PICTURES IN BASAL CELL EPITHELIOMAS. W. KRAINZ, Dermat. Wchnschr. **73**:1297 (Dec. 24) 1921.

Two tumors are described. The first in its structure suggests a derivation from a sweat gland; the second, from a sebaceous gland.

The former, microscopically, showed round, hollow, club-shaped projections from the basal cell layer into the deeper cutis, hemmed in by bands of connective tissue. The projections were formed mainly of cylindrical cells, but on their inner sides the cells were oval and polygonal. Some of these cells were large with nucleoli. Within these epithelial nests were cavities containing a fine, fibrin-like network, staining heavily with eosin, and therefore considered hyalinized cellular elements. Some of the larger epithelial cells showed vacuoles containing fluid which caused the enclosing cell to be cylindrical. These were arranged in a radial manner, resulting in the formation of a small central lumen. The latter, microscopically, sprung from the side of a rete peg, with large projections and canals formed by long, oval and polygonal cells with large nuclei, rich in nucleoli. Frequently, the canals were enclosed by a zone of long, spindle-like cells and connective tissue, and contained cellular elements and homogeneous material which stained with eosin and gave a strong fat reaction. This gave the impression of a mature, gland-like growth, of already highly differentiated epithelial cells, secreting sebaceous material.

HIGH FREQUENCY CURRENTS. M. J. MARTIN, Gaz. d. hôp. **101**:1609 (Dec. 24) 1921.

These are employed in two methods to eradicate lesions. In the first method, the electrode is placed at a certain distance from the tissues to be destroyed. Sparks are produced which cause the destruction by mechanical action. This is fulguration. In the second, the electrode is in direct contact with the tissues to be destroyed. The action, therefore, results solely from generated heat, called thermoelectrocoagulation.

Fulguration employs currents of high tension furnished by the Ondin resonator. These are unipolar. Their action is not penetrating and it is employed only superficially. It produces a slightly retractile crust which, after being shed, leaves a wound which cicatrizes rapidly.

Doyen utilizes solely the thermic effect, and he shows that this action is infinitely more powerful and penetrating when currents of great intensity and low voltage are used, especially if the bipolar method is employed.

PRIMARY SYPHILITIC INFECTION OF THE TOES. RILLE, Dermat. Wchnschr. **73**:1313 (Dec. 31) 1921.

Primary syphilitic infection of the lower extremities, excluding perigenital localization, is much rarer than that of the upper extremities, in which the fingers are notably the sites of inoculation. The author has collected from the literature 557 instances of chancre of the fingers. Chancres are uncommon below the knees. Seven cases in the vicinity of the knees, are reported; twenty on the lower legs and fourteen on the feet. A primary infection of the right great toe is described. The patient, a girl, aged 19, had cut her toe on a piece of tin in a bathroom two weeks before the onset of a painful swelling of the digit. When observed the foot and leg were swollen and there was a circumscribed ulcer on the right great toe near the nail. The free margin of the latter was raised and covered with a greenish crust. The Wassermann reaction was negative. The lesion was not recognized as syphilitic until there was a secondary roseola and a positive Wassermann test.

LICHEN PLANUS AND LICHENOID ARSPHENAMIN DERMATITIS. P. KELLER, Dermat. Wchnschr. **74**:9 (Jan. 7) 1922.

Cases have been reported by Jadassohn, Buschke, Freymann and others, of eruptions resembling lichen planus in patients receiving arsphenamin. A similar case is reported by the author. The eruption appeared after two arsphenamin injections in a patient who had previously had a full course of antisyphilitic treatment, which had resulted in a negative Wassermann reaction. There was an itching exanthem of brownish-red, bean-sized, in places confluent, lesions on the buttocks, extremities and face, with lamellated, dry scaling. The buccal mucosae was negative. Biopsy revealed noncharacteristic, lymphocytic infiltration, with thickening of the horny layer.

These peculiar lichenoid arsenical eruptions may be regarded as precursors of arsenic pigmentation.

SUBACUTE AND UNIVERSAL LEUKODERMA IN SYPHILIS. W. FREYMANN, Dermat. Wchnschr. **74**:33 (Jan. 14) 1922.

Universal leukoderma seems to have increased in frequency. It occurs mostly in patients not previously treated. It is questionable whether therapy favorably influences the condition. The majority of cases show that lenkoderma does not originate from the soil of previously existing exanthems; but it apparently reveals, secondarily, a prior disease of a central nervous organ simultaneously regulating pigment distribution.

A CONTRIBUTION TO THE KNOWLEDGE OF ICHTHYOSIS HYSTRIX. W. BLOTEVOGEL, Dermat. Wchnschr. **74**:41 (Jan. 14) 1922

The histologic aspect of the keratomas of ichthyosis hystrix corresponds to that described by Unna. A transition between the keratomas and the diffuse body ichthyosis exists only so far as both forms of hyperkeratosis occur side by side in one person. However, in accordance with the dissimilarity in their histologic pictures, these two forms should be fundamentally differentiated.

THE USE OF A PARTIAL ANTIGEN IN THE PROGNOSIS OF SKIN TUBERCULOSIS. E. BERGMANN, Dermat. Wchnschr. **74**:57 (Jan. 21) 1922.

In the years 1919 and 1920, fifteen cases of lupus vulgaris were tested intracutaneously, according to the method advocated by Devcke and Much, both before and during the course of treatment. It was concluded that the titration afforded no indication of the prognosis.

TWO CASES OF KERATODERMA SYMMETRICA. R. WAGNER. Dermat. Wchnschr. **74**:81 (Jan. 28) 1922.

The symmetrical hyperkeratoses of the palms and soles, the so-called keratodermas, are separated into essential forms (malformations) and symptomatic forms. The latter arise through trauma, intoxication or localized disease of the skin.

The first patient, a woman, aged 32, first noted a thickening of the palms and soles ten years previously. There was a family history of mental disease, but no keratoderma. At the time of onset. her hands were exposed to chemicals. The horny layer of the palms and soles was about 3 mm. thick, yellowish, semitransparent, without scaling. The affected areas were sharply limited to the palmar aspects, and surrounded by a narrow, pale red margin.

The second case. that of a girl, aged 18, had for the last four years a similar symmetrical hyperkeratosis. Its onset was preceded for four years by erythema of the affected areas at each menstrual period. At these times, the patient was mentally depressed and subject to frequent spells of crying.

The late onset in both instances distinguished the disease from keratoma palmaris et plantaris hereditaria. These cases belonged to the symptomatic hyperkeratoses, resembling somewhat the keratoderma erythematosa symmetrica of Besnier.

EXPERIMENTAL RESEARCHES ON THE DURATION OF LIFE OF SPIROCHAETA PALLIDA IN CASES UNDER DIFFERENT FORMS OF ANTISYPHILITIC TREATMENT. E. Rubin and S. Szentkiralyi, Dermat. Wchnschr. **74**:84 (Jan. 28) 1922.

The duration of life of spirochetes was observed in twenty cases of syphilis under treatment with 1 c.c. of 10 per . cent. mercury salicylate given intragluteally every five days. The observations were made on lesions on the external genitals. These were cleansed with sterile gauze and a drop of the serum produced by this irritation was transferred to a slide, protected by a cover-glass, the rim of which to prevent drying, had been painted with a thick solution of shellac in alcohol. This preparation was observed at room temperature and not kept in the light and warmth of the dark-field reflector for a longer time than was necessary.

The duration of life was proportionate to the amount of treatment the patients had received. In untreated cases, it varied from twenty to fifty hours; but, in treated cases, the organisms lost motility in a much shorter space of time.

EXPERIMENTAL RESEARCHES ON THE DURATION OF LIFE OF SPIROCHAETA PALLIDA UNDER DIFFERENT FORMS OF TREATMENT (*Concluded*). E. Rubin and S. Szentkiralyi, Dermat. Wchnschr. **74**:107 (Feb. 4) 1922.

In patients treated exclusively with mercury the clinical symptoms slowly vanished, and the spirochetes disappeared from the lesions in a measure proportionate to the healing, their duration of life at the same time being shortened. The researches substantiated the old time observation that mercury causes principally a resorption of the syphilitic infiltration with doubtful spirocheticidal action. In many cases the spirochetes were as numerous in papules of patients treated with mercury as in spontaneously healing papules of untreated patients.

In patients treated exclusively with arsphenamin it was impossible to find spirochetes in the lesions a few hours after the injection; whereas, prior to the injection, the duration of life of the spirochetes under the cover glass was twenty or thirty hours, after the injection the duration of life was markedly curtailed.

Andrews. New York.

A STUDY OF RENAL FUNCTION IN ROENTGEN-RAY INTOXICATION. I. McQuarrie and G. H. Whipple, J. Exper. M. **35**:225 (Feb.) 1922.

The writers believe that renal tissue is much more resistant to roentgen-ray dosage than the small intestine epithelium, as strong roentgen rays, repeated moderate doses and lethal doses, with the kidneys shielded, produced no disturbance, but a transitory lowered function followed large doses directly over the kidney.

STUDIES UPON EXPERIMENTAL MEASLES. I. THE EFFECTS OF THE VIRUS OF MEASLES UPON THE GUINEA-PIG. C. W. Duval and R. D'Aunoy, J. Exper. M. **35**:257 (Feb.) 1922.

Characteristic reactions following a definite incubation period after the inoculation of guinea-pigs indicated that the measles virus could be propagated in these animals even though the symptoms and lesions were not entirely analogous to the symptoms and lesions of measles in man.

ROENTGEN-RAY INTOXICATION. S. L. Warren and G. H. Whipple. J. Exper. M. **35**: No. 2, February, 1922. I. Unit dose over thorax negative, over abdomen lethal. Epithelium of small intestine sensitive to X-rays, p. 187. II. A study of the sequence of clinical, anatomical and histological changes following a unit dose of X-rays, p. 203. III. Speed of autolysis of various body tissues after lethal X-ray exposures. The remarkable disturbance in the epithelium of the small intestine, p. 213.

In this series of experiments, it was found that dogs treated over the thorax with large doses of roentgen rays, up to 512 milliampere minutes, showed no clinical sign of intoxication, while those treated over the abdomen only with 350 milliampere minutes almost invariably died on the fourth day. Necropsy revealed that the epithelium of the small intestine had almost completely disappeared, which is held to account for the reactions and lethal intoxication following large doses of the roentgen ray, as the epithelium of the small intestine is very sensitive to this treatment. During the first twenty-four hours after such exposure, there is no change except histologically; the second period shows beginning clinical disturbance, which is increased during the third twenty-four hour period, while the fourth period is usually accompanied by coma and death. Histologically, the secretory crypt epithelium of the small intestine autolyzes first and the epithelium of the villi last, but the significance of this has not been determined.

VENEREAL SPIROCHETOSIS IN AMERICAN RABBITS. Hydeo Noguchi, J. Exper. M. **35**:301 (March) 1922.

A spirochete resembling *Spirochaeta pallida* has been found in papulosquamous and ulcerating lesions of the genitoperineal region of a number of rabbits otherwise normal. These lesions run a chronic course and are transmissible to normal rabbits; but no lesions were reproduced in monkeys after four months. The Wassermann reaction was uniformly negative and arsphenamin had the same effect as on syphilitic lesions. Noguchi calls this organism *Treponema cuniculi.*

STUDIES ON X-RAY EFFECTS. IX. THE ACTION OF SERUM FROM X-RAYED ANIMALS ON LYMPHOID CELLS IN VITRO. J. B. Murphy, J. Heng Liu, E. Sturm, J. Exper. M. **35**:373 (March) 1922.

Lymphoid cells from the rat thymus and lymph glands increased when incubated in the serum from animals which had been exposed to roentgen rays, but the serum must be obtained within an hour or two after exposure. If normal serum is used, the cells rapidly disintegrate.

Jamieson, Detroit.

NOTES ON ULCERATIVE GRANULOMA. P. A. Maplestone, Ann. Trop. M. & Parasitol. **15**:413 (Dec.) 1921.

A report of four cases among the Australian aborigines. All cases were treated with tartar emetic, intravenously, with uniformly good results.

UNKNOWN FORMS OF ARTERITIS, WITH SPECIAL REFERENCE TO THEIR RELATION TO SYPHILITIC ARTERITIS AND PERI-ARTERITIS NODOSA. F. Harbitz, Am. J. M. Sc. **163**:250 (Feb.) 1922.

Several cases are cited in which certain forms of arteritis are described, the frequency of this pathologic condition being emphasized. While these are apparently different etiologically, they are extremely difficult to diagnose pathologically, especially in syphilitic changes, periarteritis nodosa and tuberculosis.

GASTROHEPATIC SYPHILOMA. Florand and Girault, Presse méd. **29**:841, 1921.

The author reports a case in which there was a gastrohepatic tumor. The gastric tumor was located in the pyloric antrum and was diagnosed by the radiograph. The patient complained of pain after eating, which was followed by vomiting.

A laparotomy was performed and the pyloric tumor was verified. The tumor was the size of a small orange. At the same time a tumor on the left lobe of the liver was discovered; the two tumors were in contact.

The patient gave a history of an old syphilitic infection, and he was immediately put on arsphenamin, mercury and potassium iodid. A roentgenogram was taken after the patient had been under antisyphilitic treatment for a few weeks. at which time it was discovered that the pyloric tumor had disappeared. The author was also unable to find any trace of the hepatic tumor.

CLINICAL ASPECTS OF ARTICULAR SYPHILIS. Broca, Presse méd. **29**:873, 1921.

The author reports nine cases of hydro-arthritis in which the diagnosis lay between tuberculosis and syphilis. The knee and ankle joints were the sites principally attacked. The clinical signs consisted of swelling, pain at all times, fluid in the joints and slight muscular atrophy. A Wassermann test was performed on these patients and all reactions were strongly positive. Treatment with arsphenamin, mercury and potassium iodid was instituted. All of these patients responded quickly to treatment, and were soon able to move around without the aid of a cane.

In all nine cases a history of syphilis was given. At the time that the author saw these patients there were no cutaneous lesions present. The hydro-arthritis was both unilateral and bilateral. At the cessation of antisyphilitic treatment the affected joints were practically normal with the exception of a slight restriction of motion.

THE PHENOMENON OF EXTINCTION AND THE DIAGNOSIS OF SCARLET FEVER. SCHULTZ-CHARLTON, Presse méd. **29**:1001 (Dec.) 1921.

The many differential points of diagnosing scarlet fever are mentioned but not one of them is specific for scarlet fever alone, except the phenomenon of extinction, which the author discusses at great length. The phenomenon of extinction is produced by injecting 1 c.c. of normal human blood serum intradermally at the site where the scarlatinal eruption is most intense. At the end of a few hours this injected area becomes white, and it remains so throughout the disease. Erythemas of other origin are not so affected. The strict specificity of this phenomenon is undeniable. Human blood serum alone, with the exception sometimes of the blood serum from an active scarlet fever patient, is the only serum which will produce this phenomenon. The cause of this phenomenon is still obscure. Reymond considers this extinction as a reaction of local immunity due to the presence of antibodies in the normal serum. It has been suggested that antigen is a germ, living on mucous membranes of all human beings, and that it is perhaps the streptococcus. Therefore, the specific antibody for scarlet fever is present in all subjects. The cause of this phenomenon is by no means proved and, as the author suggests, warrants new researches into the subject.

DIFFERENTIAL DIAGNOSIS OF ALOPECIA AREATA AND TINEA TONSURANS. SABOURAUD, Presse méd. **30**:146, 1922.

The author says that occasionally it is difficult to differentiate these diseases and therefore one must be sure of his diagnosis before roentgen-ray treatment is recommended. Alopecia areata is a disease of all ages, while tinea tonsurans occurs only in children. Tinea may occur on the bearded regions in adults, usually from contact with animals.

In alopecia areata the areas are entirely bald, smooth and shiny; occasionally there are a few hairs remaining when the disease is still progressing, but these hairs are usually from 0.5 to 1 cm. in length. In tinea tonsurans the areas are not entirely bald; one can see and feel many short, broken off hairs. There is also some scaling in these areas.

A microscopic examination should be made in every case. The scales or crusts especially should be examined instead of the hairs. The spores are easily found in the scales, but are not always found in the hair. because not all of the hairs are contaminated.

THE FIRST CLINICAL SIGNS OF SYPHILITIC CHANCRE OF THE MUCOUS MEMBRANE OF THE GENITALS. LACASSAGNE. Presse méd. **30**:245 (March 22) 1922.

The author reports six cases in which the primary lesion had not been present longer than twenty-four hours. according to the history of the patients. all of whom had examined themselves scrupulously daily. None of these lesions had been modified by treatment.

The erosions were round or oval, with a gray or red base, generally well defined, but without a definite border; painless even to instrumental contact. From the surface of the erosions a clear serum exuded in which spirochetes were found in large numbers.

The author desires to emphasize the fact that there is oozing of serum in the early chancres just as in those that have been present several days. Leloir many years ago stated that the principal differential point between a herpetic lesion and a chancre was the oozing of serum which occurred only in herpes, but the writer disproves this fallacy.

He said that the chancres contracted through intercourse differed clinically from those mechanically produced. He also wishes to emphasize the fact that chancres occurring on the mucous membrane were as a rule not indurated. The chief factor in diagnosis is the demonstration of spirochetes.

YAWS. Moss and Bigelow, Bull. Johns Hopkins Hosp. **33**:43 (Feb.) 1922.

The authors give an analysis of 1,046 cases which they studied in the Dominican Republic. They divided the condition clinically into three stages— primary, secondary and tertiary. The primary lesion or mother yaw has an incubation period of from two to four weeks. It appears as a papule which sometimes disappears before the secondary eruption manifests itself but usually overlaps the secondary eruption.

The secondary stage may be divided into the early florid stage and the late secondary stage. The early florid secondary stage begins from one to three months after the primary lesion and is characterized by general eruption of granulomas over the body. The late secondary stage may appear from six months to several years after the early secondary period. In the interval the patient may be entirely free from lesions. The late secondary stage is characterized by a sparsely generalized granulomatous eruption. Some of these late secondary lesions appear on the palms and soles and cause much pain.

The tertiary stage is characterized by gummatous lesions which may be very destructive. There is an absence of visceral involvement. They include under the tertiary stage latent yaws in which gummatous lesions have been present but have undergone spontaneous involution.

Neo-arsphenamin acted as a specific in practically all cases. However, 16 per cent. of the patients treated were unimproved; the others showed marked improvement, and many were cured entirely.

The Wassermann test was made in ninety-one cases and proved positive in eighty-three, while it was negative in eight cases. The negative reactions were obtained in those patients who had had yaws for many years.

McCafferty, New York.

CHEMOTHERAPEUTIC CONSIDERATIONS OF PENTAVALENT AND TRIVALENT ARSENIC. J. F. Schamberg, G. W. Raiziss and J. A. Kolmer, J. A. M. A. **78**:402 (Feb. 11) 1922.

Using white rats infected with *Trypanosoma equiperdum*, the authors determined that neo-arsphenamin had the best therapeutic index, with arsphenamin following. Various other arsenical compounds, both organic and inorganic, were tested, none showing so good a therapeutic index as the foregoing drugs. Trivalent carbon-linked arsenic is a much more powerful trypanocide than is pentavalent.

HEMATOGENOUS STAPHYLOCOCCUS INFECTION SECONDARY TO FOCI IN THE SKIN. D. B. Phemister, J. A. M. A. **78**:480 (Feb. 18) 1922.

Cases of osteomyelitis, renal abscess, perinephritic abscess, myositis, and arthritis have resulted, in the author's experience, from primary foci in the skin. The skin lesions were, for the most part, boils, but acne vulgaris, infected wounds, and various other staphylogenetic dermatoses were the forerunners of these serious visceral infections in some instances.

A DIETARY CONSIDERATION OF ECZEMA IN YOUNGER CHILDREN. E. S. O'Keefe, J. A. M. A. **78**:483 (Feb. 18) 1922.

At the Massachusetts General Hospital, infantile eczema has been treated conjointly by the dermatologic and pediatric departments. This is a rational procedure, since the disease is, in practically all instances, a constitutional disturbance with cutaneous manifestations. An analysis of the cases revealed that 20 per cent. had fat indigestion, and 10 per cent. carbohydrate indigestion.

Of 131 bottle fed and older children, 35 per cent. showed sensitization to one or more of the common food proteins. Of forty-one exclusively breast fed infants with eczema, 60 per cent. showed sensitization. In these patients, eggs, cow's milk, oat, and wheat gave positive reactions in many instances, which would show that sensitization to foreign proteins may occur through mother's milk.

Treatment consisted in improving digestive functions and limiting or excluding the intake of the offending protein. In nurslings, the mother's diet must be properly managed. Combined dietary and local treatment resulted in cure or improvement in 60 per cent. of the cases in less than two months.

ANGIONEUROTIC EDEMA. J. M. Phillips, J. A. M. A. **78**:497 (Feb. 18) 1922.

The author reports two instances of angioneurotic edema in dogs; in one case due to pork and the other to fish. Since these animals acquire the disease spontaneously, they should prove good experimental subjects. The author also reports an experiment in which he attempted passively to sensitize a dog with the serum of a patient who was allergic to pork, but the attempt was a failure.

VACCINIA OF THE LIP. A. Schalek, J. A. M. A. **78**:509 (Feb. 18) 1922.

The patient was vaccinated on the leg. One week later she developed an ulcer on the lip (which was just previously the seat of herpes) resembling a chancre.

ACETONE IN THE TREATMENT OF SYPHILIS. O. Smiley, J. A. M. A. **78**:509 (Feb. 18) 1922.

The author recommends careful cleansing of the skin with acetone before mercurial inunctions.

CONGENITAL SYPHILIS IN INSTITUTIONAL CHILDREN. J. S. Lawrence, J. A. M. A. **78**:566 (Feb. 25) 1922.

In 11,205 children in institutions in New York state, the Wassermann reaction was found positive in 2.3 per cent., and in 28.5 per cent. was doubtful.

Clinical examinations. which were rather superficial, did not allow any definite conclusions. Wassermann tests were performed on the relatives of the children presenting positive or doubtful reactions, with the result that in the adult relatives the positive reactions were, respectively, 82 per cent. and 13 per cent.

This elaborate inquiry reemphasizes the importance of a study of the family in the diagnosis of congenital syphilis.

URTICARIA FROM HABITUAL USE OF PHENOLPHTHALEIN: REPORT OF A CASE. E. F. Corson and D. M. Sidlick, J. A. M. A. **78**:882 (March 25) 1922.

The patient was an habitual user of carbolax, said to contain one grain of phenolphthalein to the tablet. Proof that phenolphthalein was the cause of the urticaria was obtained by withdrawing and readministering the drug.

APLASTIC ANEMIA FOLLOWING NEO-ARSPHENAMIN: REPORT OF CASE. S. M. Feinberg, J. A. M. A. **78**:888 (March 25) 1922.

A woman, aged 46, had been treated with neo-arsphenamin for a supposed syphilis of the liver. Twenty-six injections were given. Shortly thereafter, symptoms of aplastic anemia developed and death resulted. Necropsy revealed no evidence of syphilis in any of the viscera, but confirmed the clinical diagnosis.

The case is reported because of its rarity, and because it points out one of the possible complications of neo-arsphenamin, which has thus far been chiefly overlooked.

KERATODERMA BLENORRHAGICA. Edward C. Gager, J. A. M. A. **78**:941 (April) 1922.

The patient, aged 41, had a gonorrheal urethritis. One week after its appearance he developed a widespread bilateral eruption. Larger lesions presented ostraceous crusts. On the feet confluence led to large, keratotic lesions. In addition, there was fever, polyarthritis, balanitis, and myocarditis.

DERMATITIS HERPETIFORMIS IN CHILDREN: REPORT OF TWO CASES. E. A. Oliver and C. J. Eldridge, J. A. M. A. **78**:945 (April 1) 1922.

The patients were aged 18 months and 10 years, respectively. The infant had two outbreaks of a generalized papulovesicular and bullous eruption, which was pruritic. Liquor potassii arsenitis (Fowler's solution) controlled the outbreaks. The second patient had the disease for two years. The condition presented was typical. These cases are reported because of the rarity of dermatitis herpetiformis in childhood. The youngest reported case is that of Morris in an infant, aged 13 weeks.

TREATMENT AND PREVENTION OF PELLAGRA BY A DAILY SUP-PLEMENTAL MEAL. G. A. Wheeler, J. A. M. A. **78**:955 (April 1) 1922.

At the U. S. Pellagra Hospital, Spartanburg, S. C., an outpatient clinic was established for the purpose of providing a daily supplemental meal to patients with moderately severe pellagra. This clinic has now been in operation five years, and the results show that a supplemental meal of fresh meat, milk, vegetables, fruit, bread and butter was adequate to relieve symptoms and prevent recurrences of the disease.

THE THERAPEUTIC INDEX OF SILVER ARSPHENAMIN: COMPARISON WITH THAT OF ARSPHENAMIN AND NEO-ARSPHENAMIN. A. STRAUSS, D. M. SIDLICK, M. L. MALLAS and B. L. CRAWFORD, J. A. M. A. **78**:632 (March 4) 1922.

Three comparable groups, each composed of twenty-five syphilitic patients, all having strongly positive reactions serologically, were given silver arsphenamin, arsphenamin and neo-arsphenamin. The dosages were 0.2 gm., 0.4 gm., and 0.6 gm., respectively, given twice weekly for four weeks.

The reactions of one patient in the silver arsphenamin group, thirteen in the arsphenamin and nine in the neo-arsphenamin, became serologically negative at the end of the series of injections.

The serologic comparisons prompt the authors to conclude that the spirocheticidal activity of silver arsphenamin is far inferior to that of arsphenamin and neo-arsphenamin in the treatment of syphilis.

MICHAEL, Houston, Texas.

KERATOSIS DIFFUSA FETALIS (ICHTHYOSIS CONGENITA). JULIUS H. HESS and OSCAR T. SCHULTZ, Am. J. Dis. Child. **21**:357 (April) 1921.

In an interesting article the writers report a case of this disease with a very complete résumé of its pathology and a review of the literature. They propose the designation keratosis diffusa fetalis, based on the pathologic condition common to all the cases, for the name ichthyosis congenita and a variety of other terms. The reported cases fall into three groups: In the first, to which this case belongs, the abnormality is so extreme at birth as to be incompatible with a duration of life of more than a few days. In the second group, keratosis diffusa fetalis mitior, the condition is present at birth but is not developed to so extreme a degree as in the first group. The duration of life depends on the rate at which the condition develops after birth and on the degree to which it develops. In the third group keratosis diffusa fetalis tarda evidences of the skin anomaly may not be present at birth. They develop after a variable time, and the degree of development which they reach is also variable. Keratosis diffusa fetalis is a condition having its origin in the fetal period of development, the most striking feature of which is marked increase in the horny layer of the epidermis and abnormal hornification of the epithelial skin structures. Absence of the thyroid or deficiency of thyroid function during intra-uterine life may be a factor in the causation of the epidermal changes which characterize keratosis fetalis.

A CASE OF IDIOPATHIC HEMORRHAGIC SARCOMA OF KAPOSI. STAFFORD McLEAN, Am. J. Dis. Child. **21**:437 (May) 1921.

The author reports a case in which the diagnosis was in doubt, but which it was finally decided more nearly resembled Kaposi's hemorrhagic sarcoma than anything else. The child was 5½ years old, of Jewish parentage and presented on examination a symmetrical deep purplish discoloration of the face not limited to the swollen cheeks but extending above to the lower lids and below to the lower lip and chin. Both cheeks were greatly swollen and hard and tense to the touch. The lips were indurated and pigmented, the lower more so than the upper. The chin was discolored and indurated. There was a slight hemorrhage in the subconjunctiva of the left eye. On the left side of the face there was a marked induration extending from the cheek.

There were a number of subcutaneous masses, not sharply outlined over the frontal region, and a few spots on the scalp about the size of a pea, all of which were purplish. The chest presented some faintly discolored areas of a different character about the same size as those on the scalp. There were also fading spots on the upper part of the chest, arms and forearms, thighs and buttocks. All of the superficial lymph glands were slightly enlarged. Laboratory examination showed a negative Wassermann reaction and urine, a blood picture of 25 per cent. hemoglobin, 1,280,000 red blood cells and 2,400 white blood cells, with marked variation in the size and shape of the red blood cells. The child died twenty-four days after admission to the hospital from anemia with bronchopneumonia.

A STUDY OF THE INCIDENCE OF HEREDITARY SYPHILIS. JEANS and COOKE, Am. J. Dis. Child. **22**:402 (Oct.) 1921.

A study of the placenta and of the Wassermann reaction on the cord blood was made by the authors in a series of 2,030 unselected infants in St. Louis. By examining the blood of 389 of these infants more than 2 months of age, it was determined that the proportion of cases of hereditary syphilis that could be certainly diagnosed by placental examination alone was 27 per cent., while from the Wassermann reaction on the cord 63.6 per cent. could be recognized. By applying these two methods to the entire group, the number of cases could be accurately determined. The incidence of hereditary syphilis thus established is 15 per cent. in the colored race, 1.8 per cent. in the poor of the white race and less than 1 per cent. in the well-to-do classes. By applying these figures to the entire population of St. Louis, it is estimated that the incidence of hereditary syphilis at birth in this city is 3 per cent., of which the colored population, although only 9 per cent. of the total, contributes approximately half the cases.

CALCIFICATION OF THE SKIN IN A CHILD. JOHN LOVETT MORSE, Am. J. Dis. Child. **22**:412 (Oct.) 1921.

The history in this case suggests strongly that the changes in the skin were due to infection. The histology shows no evidence, however, that an infectious process was the cause of the lesions in the subcutaneous fat. The microscopic appearances resemble in many particulars the fat necroses found in the abdominal cavity in acute pancreatitis, in which the lesion is, of course, due to the action of a lipolytic ferment. In spite of the difficulty in accounting for the presence of such a ferment in the subcutaneous tissue, such a possibility must be considered in this instance.

AN UNUSUAL EXANTHEM OCCURRING IN INFANTS. ROY M. GREENTHAL, Am. J. Dis. Child. **23**:63 (Jan.) 1922.

The author reports one of a series of eight such cases he has observed in his practice. Veeder and Hempleman have proposed the name exanthem subitum for this peculiar condition. It is characterized by a preeruptive period of three or four days, with high fever. On the fourth day, there is a sudden drop in temperature coincident with an eruption. The eruption lasts from one to two days and is maculopapular, resembling measles. The etiology is unknown. The blood is characterized by a leukopenia and a high lymphocytosis.

REPORT OF A CASE OF GANGRENE OF THE FEET FOLLOWING DIPHTHERIA. M. B. Gordon and Benjamin Newman, Am. J. Dis. Child. **23**:142 (Feb.) 1922.

This article reports a case of extensive gangrene in the feet of a 6 year old boy, which developed during convalescence from diphtheria. All of the toes of the left foot and the heel of the right foot became gangrenous. Amputation was finally performed on these parts. The case was complicated with a myocarditis, sluggish circulation, low blood. pressure, and insufficient collateral circulation. It is difficult to state positively whether the condition was due to a local thrombus as the result of a local acute arteritis or to a migrating clot originating in the heart.

THE INITIAL EXANTHEM OF SMALLPOX. M. Tsurumi and S. Isono, J. Infect. Dis. **29**:109 (Aug.) 1921.

The authors report their observations on 109 cases of smallpox. Of this number, thirty-nine were seen in adults presenting an initial exanthem. They class this exanthem as three types, the hemorrhagic, the scarlet-fever like. and one resembling measles. The eruption appeared on the outer side of the upper arm in all the cases in this series. There is no direct relation between the initial exanthem and the pock marks. In the vaccinated. the eruption is most marked about the place of vaccination. An initial exanthem does not necessarily guarantee a light attack, they conclude. This is especially true if the exanthem is hemorrhagic.

Oliver, Chicago.

HEREDOSYPHILIS AND NYSTAGMUS. R. Argañaraz, Prensa med. argentina **20**:237 (Dec.) 1921.

The author believes that 95 per cent. of the cases of congenital nystagmus are due to hereditary syphilis. Congenital nystagmus is due to a functional disturbance of the motor centers of the eye, possibly caused by hereditary syphilis. He reports several cases cured with specific therapy.

CHRONIC PERITONITIS DUE TO HEREDITARY SYPHILIS. M. Acuña and A. Casaubón, Prensa méd. Argentina **24**:284 (Jan.) 1922.

Although the spirochetes may attack any tissue or apparatus in the human body, the serous membranes and especially the peritoneum are rarely affected. In the majority of the cases reported peritonitis has been secondary. usually to syphilitic liver disease. The authors report a case of primary syphilitic peritonitis in a Japanese child, 16 years of age. with enormous ascitis and a four plus Wassermann reaction. Specific treatment effected a clinical cure.

RESEARCH ON ANOMALIES AND ALTERATIONS OF CORNIFICATION IN THE HUMAN SKIN. L. Martinotti. Cior. ital. d. mal ven. **56**:681, 1921.

A complete study of the pathology of cornu cutaneum. keratoma plantare. ichthyosis, and acquired ichthyosis. The article is illustrated with four colored plates.

ACANTHOSIS NIGRICANS. Brunetti, Freund and Sturli, Cior. ital. d. mal. ven. **56**:694, 1921.

The authors feel inclined to consider an endocrinous disturbance as a cause of this disease, a case of which is reported, the presence of cancer in many cases being explained by the fact that neoplasms may grow easily in cases of polyglandular deficiency.

XERODERMA PIGMENTOSUM. CHRONIC RADIOLUCITIS ON RADIOSENSITIVE SUBJECTS. H. Gougerot. Prog. Clin. **120**:265 (Dec.) 1921.

A general study is made of this dermatosis, in which the author emphasizes the following points: 1. The cases are not rare; there are many attenuated or late forms that ought to be classified among these cases. 2. It is not exclusively a disease of childhood; there are numerous transitional forms which unite the classical type of the disease with the preepitheliomatous lesions of the aged, peasants, .and sailors. 3. The cause is principally light, and a condition of cutaneous susceptibility. 4. The etiologic rôle of light is evident, and the fact that the lesions are so much like radiodermitis makes the author think that the sunlight acts as does the roentgen ray. 5. The short wave radiations that produce this condition act only on certain skins, which the author classifies as nevic. 6. Hereditary syphilis may be the cause of the susceptibility of the skin.

SYPHILIS AMONG THE NATIVES OF YEBOLA, MOROCCO. J Escobar, Prog. Clin. **121**:1 (Jan., Feb., March) 1922.

The Moroccans call syphilis, hec. The chancre is seldom seen, the patients appearing with secondary or tertiary lesions. Among the secondary lesions, the circinate, pemphigoid and ulcerative forms are common. Among the tertiary manifestations the ulcerative and destructive, especially of the bones, are often observed. Neurosyphilis is extremely rare; the author has not seen a single case of tabes or general paralysis. The number of children with congenital syphilis is enormous.

ARSPHENAMIN AND SYPHILIS. D. Villarejo, Prog. Clin. **121**:59 (Jan., Feb., March) 1922.

Villarejo asserts that syphilis is on the increase in Spain and that this increase is in great part due to the erroneous use of the newest arsenical preparations and the mistaken interpretations of the results obtained. Most of the patients give up all treatment after a few doses of the arsenicals and as soon as their cutaneous lesions clear up. The result is a high percentage of relapses and late neurosyphilis.

MULTIPLE NODULAR TUMORS OF THE SKIN. G. Spremolla, Riforma med. **8**:202 (Feb.) 1922.

This is a histopathologic study of several new growths which the author classifies in four groups: (1) hyperplastic nodules: lipomas, Dercum's disease, fibromas, neuromas and Recklinghausen's disease; (2) blastomic nodules: fibrosarcoma, sarcoma, melanosarcoma and Kaposi's sarcoma; (3) granulomatous nodules: gummas, tuberculosis, leprosy, spirotrichosis and mycosis fungoides; (4) parasitic nodules: cisticercus.

Pardo-Castello, Havana.

MYCOTIC INTERTRIGO: A NEW FORM OF EPIDERMOPHYTON
INFECTION. DUBREUILH and JOULIA, Bull. Soc. franç. de dermat. et
syph. **28**:192, 1921.

The lesions described, in the genitocrural, inframammary and inter-gluteal
regions, are scaly reddish plaques with small outlying satellites. The vegetable organism which was found and cultivated is briefly described.

SEVERE ICTERUS WITH A FATAL STREPTOCOCCIC SEPTICEMIA
FOLLOWING NOMA DUE TO THE EXTRACTION OF SEVERAL
TEETH DURING A COURSE OF ARSPHENAMIN TREATMENT.
M. MILIAN, Bull. Soc. franç. de dermat. et syph. **28**:193, 1921.

The patient was a young man with a syphilitic infection of long standing,
who had undertaken a course of treatment prior to marriage. In preparation,
several carious teeth were extracted. Noma ensued, followed by septicemia.

TWO INSTANCES OF SKIN-GRAFT FOR VICIOUS CICATRICES OF
THE WRIST. ROCHER, Bull. Soc. franç. de dermat. et syph. **28**:249, 1921.

In each case the autoplastic method was used, the flap being taken from
the flank and iliac region. Good motility resulted, and the sensatory recovery
was commendable.

AUTOPLASTIC SKIN-GRAFT IN THE CORRECTION OF INCONTI-
NENCE OF URINE IN A BOY WITH SPINA BIFIDA. ROCHER,
Bull. Soc. franç. de dermat. et syph. **28**:250, 1921.

A patent urachus was obliterated and a new external urethra made, the
result not being reported.

THE INTERSTITIAL RESORPTION OF B O N E IN LEPROSY.
DUBREUILH, Bull. Soc. franç. de dermat. et syph. **28**:253, 1921.

In June, 1919, the author presented before the Society radiographic plates
taken from a leper, which showed metatarsal resorption. Recently, through
pneumonia, the patient came to necropsy, and the remnants of the metatarsal
bones were preserved. Only their proximal ends remained, and the phalanges
were also found to be rarefied.

CONGENITAL LYMPHANGIOMA OF THE RIGHT INGUINOCRURAL
REGION. L. FERRON, Bull. Soc. franç. de dermat. et syph. **28**:253, 1921.

Aside from a fairly extensive lymphangioma of about ten years' duration,
the patient, a young man of 21 years, presented a considerable edematous
enlargement of the corresponding lower extremity. By way of treatment,
Darier favors the destruction of the lymphatic varices by electrolysis and the
reduction of the tumor by filtered roentgen rays.

MULTIPLE BENIGN CYSTIC EPITHELIOMAS. PETGES, Bull. Soc. franç.
de dermat. et syph. **28**:255, 1921.

A woman, aged 25 years, presented many pinhead to bean-sized pink, oval
firm tumors, situated on the face, chest and back. They had increased in size
and number since puberty, and were very disfiguring. In their removal the
roentgen rays were used, and an accidental erythema dose was also disfiguring.

A CASE OF MEDIAN RHOMBOIDAL GLOSSITIS. Dubreuilh. Bull. Soc. franç. de dermat. et syph. **28**:256, 1921.

This condition occurred in a man, aged 51, in whom syphilis could not be diagnosed. Petges comments on its frequency in Asiatics, as observed by him during the war.

CONGENITAL SYPHILIS. Audrain, Bull. Soc. franç. de dermat. et syph. **28**:315, 1921.

Discussing the communication of Milian and Valle, presented at the March meeting, Audrain briefly relates his experiences, supporting and emphasizing the importance of congenital syphilis in the second and even in the third generation.

A CASE OF HEPATIC SYPHILIS, MISTAKEN AT FIRST FOR A HYDATID CYST AND THUS BROUGHT TO OPERATION; LATER TREATED BY ROENTGEN-RAYS. C. Simon and P. Renty, Bull. Soc. franç. de dermat. et syph. **28**:423, 1921.

Although the clinical picture was not that of typical syphilitic hepatitis, the presence of a nasal deformity and a positive Wassermann reaction suggested this diagnosis to the authors, who saw the patient, a man of 39, after surgery and roentgen-ray treatment had failed. Under cautious treatment with neo-arsphenamin there was rapid relief.

THE EXTENSION OF THE ACARUS AND ITS BURROWS TO THE FACE IN A CASE OF INTENSE (NORWEGIAN) SCABIES OF TWO YEARS' DURATION. Gastou and Tissot, Bull. Soc. franç. de dermat. et syph. **28**:425, 1921.

This case, presented because of its unusual severity and because the acarus has been found in lesions on the face, occurred in a child of 7½ years.

TERTIARY SYPHILITIC MYOSITIS OF THE LEFT GENIOHYOID. Hudelo and Boulanger-Pilet. Bull. Soc. franç. de dermat. et syph. **28**:427, 1921.

In a man of 40, whose syphilitic infection was of ten years' duration, an indolent nodule, the size of a small nut, appeared in the substance of the geniohyoid muscle. It disappeared rapidly under antisyphilitic treatment. In a search of the literature, the authors could find no other case of syphilitic affection of this muscle.

ATROPHY AND PIGMENTATION: A CASE FOR DIAGNOSIS. Montlaur and Cailliau, Bull. Soc. franç. de dermat. et syph. **28**:429, 1921.

A boy, aged 9 years, had first shown signs of a cutaneous abnormality at the age of 1 month, when the present condition had rapidly developed, especially affecting the head, extremities, shoulders and genitals, and apparently not progressive. There were many spots of pigmentation, with some telangiectasia and atrophy, recalling the poikiloderma atrophicans vascularis of Jacobi and also xeroderma pigmentosum, but evidently distinct from them. There was a thinning of the epidermis, a degeneration of the connective tissue and a disappearance of the elastic tissue, with changes in the vessel walls and a vascular dilatation, as well as a cellular and pigmentary infiltration in the derma. Two somewhat similar cases had been presented before the Society.

A CASE OF PAPILLOMATOUS TUBERCULOSIS OF THE TONGUE.
LÉVY-FRANCKEL and BLAMOUTIER, Bull. Soc. franç. de dermat. et syph. **28**:434, 1921.

This lesion, situated on the dorsum of the tongue in a patient of 44 years, was of six months' duration, and suggested a diagnosis of epithelioma. However, the patient had pulmonary tuberculosis, and histologic examination of the excised lesion showed it to be tuberculous. There had been no recurrence.

PARKHURST, Toledo, Ohio.

SKIN AFFECTIONS CAUSED BY ACHORION GYPSEUM (BODIN).
C. RASCH, Brit. J. Dermat. & Syph. **34**:1, 1922.

Rasch records four cases of skin affection in which Bodin's *Anchorion gypseum* could be demonstrated. In the first case, a boy of 9 years presented a kerion and developed twenty-five lesions, chiefly about the neck, with some about the hair margin of the forehead; in the second case, a single kerion was observed on the scalp; in the third, the only lesion was an erythematosquamous spot on the cheek; while the fourth patient showed a flat, yellowish, damp, central area surrounded by an erythematosquamous border on the cheek. All responded readily to treatment. The literature reveals only six reported cases of skin disease in man produced by the *Achorion gypseum*. In none of the others had the scalp been affected. No scutula were present either in Rasch's cases, or in four of the previously reported cases. The parasite in its cultural appearance resembles trichophyton of the gypseum group; in its botanical features, a microsporon. It can give rise to scutula like an achorion.

FURTHER REMARKS ON EARLY EPITHELIOMA OF THE SKIN.
LOUIS SAVATARD, Brit. J. Dermat. & Syph. **34**:6, 1922.

Savatard emphasizes the necessity for a prefix to the word epithelioma in order to designate its pathologic character, except in the case of the prickle-cell type, which is always signified when the term epithelioma is used alone. He states that in many cases, when an epithelioma is said to have arisen from a mole, wen, wart or other benign lesion, a histologic examination would disclose that there was evidence of malignancy from the beginning. He feels that in differentiating early epitheliomas from rodent ulcer, the time element should be emphasized.

Benign tumors of the lower lids (tricho-epithelioma, syringo-adenoma of various authors) are more common than is generally supposed, and when well marked are often mistaken for xanthelasma.

The growths resulting from the degeneration of senile keratoses are sometimes rodent ulcers, but are more likely to be prickle-cell epitheliomas.

ON TWO CASES OF EXUDATIVE ERYTHEMA ASSOCIATED WITH MALIGNANT DISEASE OF THE UTERUS. HALDIN DAVIS, Brit. J. Dermat. & Syph. **34**:12, 1922.

In Davis' first case, the patient, suffering with inoperable spindle-cell sarcoma of the uterus of more than a year . . .

circinate patches of erythema, in cases crowned by blisters. In the second case, the patient was admitted to the hospital for a similar eruption, and, on examination, an adenocarcinoma of the uterus was found. In the first case, the eruption persisted till death. In the second, the eruption cleared up when the growth was removed.

Davis then discusses the relation between pathologic conditions of the contents of the female pelvis and their reflection on the skin.

HYPODERMIASIS (OX-WARBLE DISEASE). Noxon Toomey, Brit. J. Dermat. & Syph. **34:** (Feb.) 1922.

Toomey states that the group of diseases known in dermatologic literature as larva migrans includes two eruptions of definite etiology and pathology. The first is due to infestation with the *Gastrophilus,* while the second is caused by nematode worms of the families *Anguillulidae* and *Angiostomidae.* Toomey's paper describes a third type of creeping eruption, differing greatly in pathology and clinical course from the lesions produced by *Gastrophilus* larvae, which is caused by a larval fly of the genus *Hypoderma.*

The disease probably occurs in all cattle raising countries with a temperate or subtemperate climate, and is found only in people who live near herds of cattle. There are three species of the genus *Hypoderma* known to man. The adults are known as heel-flies, and often improperly called bot-flies. The larva enters the body by burrowing directly through the skin, or by being taken into the mouth.

Two types of skin lesions are produced: (*a*) areas of subacute cellulitis along the course of the larvae in the subcutaneous tissues; (*b*) the lesion of the skin at the site of exit of the mature larvae from the body. Both of these types are described in detail.

Treatment consists in the surgical removal of the larvae, although it is often difficult to locate the parasite wandering in the subcutis.

LUPUS TREATED WITH GENERAL CARBON ARC-LIGHT BATHS AS THE ONLY THERAPY: A CLINICAL AND HISTOLOGICAL INVESTIGATION. K. A. Heiberg and Carl With, Brit. J. Dermat. & Syph. **34:**69 (March) 1922.

In view of the fact that patients with lupus treated at the Finsen Light Institute showed a much greater percentage of cures when general light baths were given in conjunction with concentrated light as a local treatment, Heiberg and With determined to investigate how far it is possible to heal skin lupus with general light treatments only. In addition to the clinical observations, numerous histologic examinations were made at various stages in the treatment. They summarize the results of their observations as follows: (1) Carbon arc-light baths without any other treatment can cure lupus. But naturally the cure is hastened by the simultaneous local application of Finsen light. (2) The histologic process of repair eventually involves all the lupus tissue. however deep it is. A condition is thus finally produced which local treatment can also bring about, but only after many repetitions. The way in which the repair takes place seems to be partly dependent on the size of the lesion. (*a*) In the very small lesions the epitheliod cells gradually lose their power of staining, become disintegrated and slowly absorbed. The round cell infiltration is only slightly developed. (*b*) In the larger lesions it will also be found that the epithelioid cells stain poorly and gradually break down, but the most conspicuous feature is usually the considerable increase of round cells in the epithelioid tissue itself, not in the surrounding structures, which is far in excess of what is ordinarily encountered. In some cases also there is a connective-tissue reaction, with many new cells, which is later replaced by young connective tissue rich in cells in which isolated giant cells and some round cells may be found here and there.

Although the connective-tissue changes described can be striking, we consider them of secondary importance in comparison with the dissolution processes in the epithelioid cells.

THE RATIONALE OF THE WASSERMANN REACTION (*Cont.*). J. E. R. McDonagh, Brit. J. Dermat. & Syph. **34**:77 (March) 1922.

In the second part of his paper McDonagh discusses diurnal variation in the serums, the effect of the ingestion of alcohol and anesthesia, the effect of pregnancy, age, heat and other conditions on the Wassermann reaction. Under the heading of changes undergone by the serum in syphilis, he considers the protein particles from the standpoint of increase in number, surface change and mass change. Anticomplementary reactions and various other points are covered, and the special problems presented by the spinal fluid are reviewed.

SENEAR, Chicago.

SKIN ERUPTIONS OCCURRING IN INFLUENZA. V. Janovsky, Ceska Dermat. **3**:33, 1921.

The skin eruptions belong among the rarer complications of influenza. They appear most often in the gastro-intestinal form of the disease—as urticarial and erythematous manifestations, and much less frequently in the respiratory and nervous form. The predominating type of eruption varies in different epidemics. Types of eruption are:

1. Erythematous forms, appearing usually on the second or third day: (*a*) punctate, rapidly· becoming confluent, superficial infiltrates forming spots on the face and trunk, rarely on the extremities; (*b*) exanthem resembling measles but of a brighter red color, and not disappearing on pressure; (*c*) exanthem appearing in stripes on the trunk, parallel with the course of the nerves— similar to scarlatina variegata; (*d*) a diffuse, extensive, scarlatiniform erythema on the trunk, often appearing on the inner side of the thighs. This form presents in many cases great diagnostic difficulties, especially in children.

2. Urticaria, quite common in the gastro-intestinal type; it has no special characteristics, except, perhaps, a longer duration than the ordinary form.

3. Herpes labialis and facialis is most common in the toxic and catarrhal form of the disease and in its pneumonic complications. Zoster is rare. The author reports two cases.

4. Purpura is the rarest and prognostically the most serious skin complication.

The course of the erythematous eruptions is rapid—of two or three days' duration. They have a slight tendency to recurrence. Desquamation never takes place, an important differential point. especially between scarlet fever and the scarlatiniform eruption of influenza. Eruptions on the mucous membranes are rarely seen. They assume the form of red spots on the inner side of the cheeks or of red bands along the border of the soft palate. very different from the congestion of scarlet fever.

The author gives a detailed differential diagnosis between influenzal eruption and drug eruptions. dermatitis scarlatiniformis, measles, and scarlet fever.

CONTRIBUTION TO THE TREATMENT OF PSORIASIS BY MEANS OF THE EXTRACTS OF ENDOCRINE GLANDS. J. Camrda, Ceska Dermat. **3**:38, 1921.

A boy, aged 10 years, presented an extensive psoriasis that resisted all treatment for six years. To give Samberger's theory and treatment another trial, the boy was started on thymus extract. When the supply of thymus preparation gave out, thyroid and testes were substituted. In a little more than two months, the case cleared up completely. It illustrates the beneficial effect of thymus on the increase of cell vitality, and the fact that a similar effect can be produced by administration of extracts of glands which are in correlation with thymus.

ALOPECIA CONFLUENS THYREOGENES. K. Gawalowski, Ceska Dermat. **3**:41, and **3**:69, 1921.

The author cites ten cases of alopecia areata appearing in confluent patches, in persons who showed changes in the eyebrows: seven had a typical Levi-Rothschild's "signe du sourcil," one had no eyebrows at all, and two showed the reversed sign (medial lack of brows). Except two, none had other signs of hypothyroidism. After the administration of thyroid extract, eight of them showed a strikingly .prompt and permanent cure, although all previous treatment was unsuccessful. The medication failed in a boy who undoubtedly did not have hypothyroidism (abnormal bodily development), and there was improvement in a woman with ovarian instability. The best results were obtained with small doses of thyroid (from 0.1 to 1 gm., three times daily). Judging from the response to treatment and from the brow sign, the cases were of the type of mild hypothyroidism. Such authorities as Levi and Rothschild do not consider alopecia areata as a manifestation of hypothyroidism, and Sterling claims that alopecia areata is a syndrome out of which the cases of pluriglandular dysfunction should be excluded. As there is no hypothesis that would completely clear the etiology of alopecia areata, the author concludes that it might be not a clinical entity, but a syndrome resulting from different causes. In the future, it might be necessary to limit our clinical conception of alopecia areata.

Spinka. St. Louis.

Society Transactions

SILVER ARSPHENAMIN AND NITRITOID CRISES. Presented by Dr. Casal.

Dr. Casal stated that after trying various drugs to prevent nitritoid crises, such as epinephrin, sodium hyposulphite and peptone, without obtaining favorable results, a substitution of the arsenical used, silver arsphenamin, for neo-arsphenamin, prevented them completely; i. e., patients having repeated crises when treated with neo-arsphenamin did not have any when the drug was changed to silver arsphenamin.

DISCUSSION

Dr. Barrio de Medina said that Dr. Casal's cases were too few to bear out his point. This insufficiency is further demonstrated by the fact that in one patient treated recently by Dr. Barrio de Medina, this theory failed completely. This patient showed nitritoid crises following neo-arsphenamin injections. As the Wassermann reaction remained positive, the drug was changed to silver arsphenamin, which also caused a crisis. Unless injected hypodermically, epinephrin has no effect. It is effective, however, when it is injected intravenously and the syringe content is also injected after rinsing with 1 c.c. of saline solution. When thus injected, the patient's appearance changes completely and the crisis subsides.

Dr. Sicilia called attention to the fact that he had always had more crises with neo-arsphenamin than with silver arsphenamin. As regards the use of epinephrin, it seemed that Dr. Barrio de Medina had been reading Milian. since this is the method used and advocated by the latter. Dr. Sicilia has also found it successful in the prevention of crises.

Dr. Casal closed the discussion. He said that the crises in Dr. Barrio de Medina's patient might have been due to changes in the tube. His remarks applied only to cases in which crises are caused by the patient's susceptibility. As regarded epinephrin, it had failed only when used as a prophylactic.

CLINICAL AND LABORATORY RESULTS IN PATIENTS TREATED WITH SOLUBLE SALTS OF BISMUTH. Presented by Dr. Sicilia.

Dr. Sicilia said that in cases of syphilis he was still trying soluble salts of bismuth, phosphate, citrate and salicylate of bismuth and cerium. In his more recent cases, their influence seemed rather slow, but progressive The Wassermann test became negative more rapidly with the citrate of bismuth and ammonium. He intended to keep on studying the subject and report in full to the academy.

GLUCOSE HYPERTONIC SOLUTIONS IN DERMATOLOGY. Presented by Drs. Covisa and Bejarano.

Drs. Covisa and Bejarano have continued the studies of Scholtk and Bichter, who employed 20, 30 and 50 per cent. intravenous hypertonic solutions of glucose, and verified the fact that such solutions exerted an endosmotic action on the protoplasm of patients with much skin infiltration, in cases of pemphigus, prurigo, etc. They have observed an apparent antipruritic action and a remarkable decrease in the skin edema.

RARE EARTH SALTS AND SYPHILIS. Presented by Dr. Casal.

Dr. Casal described a case in a patient with a large and hard submaxillary adenitis, without any specific history and with a negative Wassermann reaction. Six injections of rare earth salts were given; following the sixth a general papular syphilid and a strongly positive Wassermann reaction appeared. He reported this case because it was not common and because such salts may have a reactivating power.

SYPHILITIC LYMPHANGITIS. Presented by Dr. Casal.

This was the patient exhibited at a previous clinical session whose condition Dr. Aja diagnosed as phlebitis rather than lymphangitis. Dr. Casal had punctured the vessel and obtained lymph, and presented the patient again in confirmation of his previous diagnosis.

Clinical Session, March 17, 1922

CASE FOR DIAGNOSIS. Presented by Dr. Casal.

Dr. Casal exhibited a patient with lineal keloidal scar lesions on the buttock, trunk, shoulder and arm, probably due to malingering. There was also anesthesia in one zone and delayed sensitiveness in others, attacks occurring for four days previously.

DISCUSSION

Dr. Azua said that, if the history given by the family and patient were correct, the condition was either malingering induced by hysteria or true hysteria without stimulation, i. e., the uncommon lesions seen in hysterical patients. He advised general treatment, as for hysteria; and for the lesions, plain cerate.

Dr. Criado thought it was a perfect case of false dermatitis. The burn had been caused with a piece of cotton soaked in strong lye.

Dr. Sicilia thought it was a case both of malingering and hysteria associated with dysmenorrheic dermatosis.

Dr. Casal, closing the discussion, insisted that the injuries were due to malingering, in view of the lack of lesions on the right side of the face.

LYMPHODERMA. Presented by Dr. Covisa.

Dr. Covisa again presented the patient with lymphoderma shown at a previous session. A blood examination had been made, and the report by Dr. Jimenez Azúa was as follows: "The total increase in the number of leukocytes, together with the predominance of lymphocytes and the presence of considerable pathologic variation of these cells (Rieden cells of a lymphocyte type) and some immature cells (lymphoblasts), justifies the conclusion that it is a case of submaxillary lymphocythemia. The blood has, however, this peculiarity: the other cells (neutrophils) appear in larger numbers than usual in lymphocytosis and the number of eosinophils is not only absolutely high but also relatively so. The signs of anemia are very slight." The treatment had been nine injections of 50 per cent. glucose solution, each injection containing from 8 to 15 gm. of glucose. There had been a definite improvement in the skin infiltration and a decrease of the erythrodermic condition. The furrows on the forehead had regressed. The itching improved with a few injections but it was still present; and, therefore, the improvement has been only partial.

Drs. Azua and Sicilia suggested the addition of arsenic to the glucose serum.

SYPHILITIC SUPERINFECTION. Presented by Dr. Portilla.

Dr. Portilla exhibited a patient who had been infected with syphilis three years previously, having florid secondary manifestations. He was treated with twelve injections of mercuric benzoate, two of neo-arsphenamin and one of mercuric (gray) oil; whereupon all manifestations disappeared. During the last month, a lesion had appeared on the balanopreputial sulcus which seemed to be a new chancre, judging from the surrounding induration and the inguinal gland enlargement on both sides. The fatty film that covered it might suggest either a secondary or a mixed lesion. The case was presented because of doubts as to the clinical diagnosis of the lesion. If it was really a chancre, a superinfection should be kept in mind. The treatment first used justified a belief in the sterilization of the original infection. As there had been recent coitus, the case would fulfil all the necessary conditions for superinfection or, as the French call it, supersyphilization. He thought it wise. therefore, to report the case, as on previous occasions he had been rather conservative in his conception of superinfection, considering it less frequent than it really is, although he had not denied its possibility.

DISCUSSION

Dr. Covisa thought it was a secondary syphilid, indurated because of its localization (sulcus), with a chancrous appearance.

Dr. Sicilia considered it an exulcerated pseudomembranous syphilitic chancre. He thought it was a new infection rather than a superinfection.

Dr. Criado thought it was a diphtheroid secondary infection. He disagreed with the diagnosis of mixed chancre, as no microscopic investigation (for Ducrey's bacillus) had been made. There were no signs of autoinoculation. The syphilitic chancre was excluded because of the lack of gland enlargement. That now present was the remainder of the old infection: therefore. it was a diphtheroid patch.

Dr. Casal agreed with Dr. Criado as to its being a secondary syphilid.

Dr. Portilla closed the discussion. stating that the gland condition was that of a primary lesion. He still thought it was a chancre and not a secondary lesion. since it seemed rather queer to have the patient appear three years after the original lesion with one lesion alone.

MYCOSIS FUNGOIDES. Presented by Dr. Bejarano.

Dr. Bejarano exhibited an interesting case of mycosis fungoides. He pointed out especially the fact that there seemed invariably to be a lesion in the blood-forming organs in this deficiency of splenic function. This was rather remarkable in view of the obscure causation of this disease.

PSORIASIS. Presented by Dr. Covisa.

Dr. Covisa also exhibited a case of psoriasis treated with intravenous injections of sodium salicylate dissolved in hypertonic glucose solution (salicylate, 17 per cent.). However, in spite of the lack of strength, the vein was already indurated (four intravenous injections had already been given).

NEW YORK ACADEMY OF MEDICINE, SECTION ON DERMATOLOGY AND SYPHILIS

Regular Meeting, March 7, 1922

Howard Fox, M.D., *Chairman*

MYCOSIS FUNGOIDES (TWO CASES). Presented by Dr. Lapowski.

B. H., a man aged 51, born in Russia, had been under observation since July, 1916. His first attack occurred fourteen years ago, the whole body being involved. The lesions had appeared at intervals since that time.

In August, 1919, the entire body and extremities were covered with infiltrated erythematous spots, with a few areas of normal skin. In March, 1920, roentgen-ray treatment was begun, and after about fifteen roentgen-ray applications, in June, 1921, practically all the lesions cleared up and itching disappeared. The genital organs which were not exposed to the roentgen ray remained as before and itched a great deal. In December, 1921, lesions began to reappear, but the itching was not so severe.

As presented, there were numbers of dollar-sized, infiltrated patches, scattered over the entire body, intermingled with scars after mycotic lesions.

The patient had been presented previously at the Academy in May, 1916, with a diagnosis of mycosis fungoides.

M. S., a man aged 42, married, was born in the United States. His father died twelve years ago at the age of 58 from a disease which was diagnosed in the New York, Mount Sinai and St. Luke Hospitals as leukemia. His mother was still living.

Fifteen years ago red, pruriginous patches appeared on the body which did not yield to various treatments; they disappeared and reappeared. Five years ago the patient came to the Good Samaritan Dispensary, where a diagnosis was made of seborrheic eczema, which disappeared under resorcin and sulphur ointment and reappeared five months later in aggravated form. Since then the eruption has not disappeared, only occasionally improving and usually reappearing in aggravated forms. As presented, the eruption was reappearing in an aggravated form. It was nearly universal and consisted of pinhead to dime sized slightly infiltrated irregular papules, some discrete, some confluent, forming dime to dollar sized infiltrated hypertrophied plaques. The lesions on the thighs were sharply defined, with raised, infiltrated borders, somewhat resembling psoriasis, but in other places and at other times the lesions were typical of dermatitis seborrheica. At times the itching was negligible; at others marked, especially on the scalp. Some of the spots in time became more infiltrated, harder and enlarged; some of them remained stationary. The Wassermann test was negative. The blood count was negative.

DR. LEVIN said he had seen the first case at varying intervals for four years. When the patient first appeared at the Beth Israel Hospital four years ago. he showed clinically a generalized mycosis fungoides, which was confirmed by biopsy. At that time the skin of parts that were now apparently normal showed typical lesions of mycosis fungoides.

DR. WEIDMAN (Philadelphia) said he had had occasion to study only one similar case. In that instance the histologic appearance was not at all characteristic of granuloma fungoides, and the picture was much like that of psoriasis. Clinically the patch crept over the skin and was followed by scarring. being rather peculiar in that respect.

DR. WISE said that of course the positive biopsy findings in the first case settled any question of diagnosis. Had he not heard the microscopic report. he would have been inclined to say it was not an easy eruption to diagnose. The patient had one infiltrated patch on the back and other lesions that looked like psoriasis.

As to the second case, he had asked the man to wait for reexamination. for it would be interesting to see him again. It was not an easy eruption to diagnose. The color was not characteristic, and the infiltration was applicable to many diseases. The diagnosis was at least debatable. and other conditions should be considered until the diagnosis of mycosis fungoides was proved microscopically.

The second patient (Mr. B.) was again shown, and the psoriatic-like lesions were especially considered.

DR. LAPOWSKI reiterated that the lesions were not psoriatic. but were those of mycosis fungoides; neither the scales. the infiltration. nor the aspect of other lesions and the history of the case even suggested psoriasis. Six years previously the patient came to him from Boston (the Massachusetts General Hospital) with the diagnosis of mycosis fungoides. and since then had been under his observation. The roentgen ray was applied to the upper portion of the body with good results; the lesions disappeared almost completely. and the itching was not as severe. The patient's life was made more bearable. On the places (genitals) where the roentgen ray was not applied. the lesions remained the same, and the itching was intense. But a relapse took place several months after the improvement. as the present condition showed.

• As to the first case. Dr. Lapowski said that it presented an example of that form of mycosis fungoides in which the diagnostic appearance of the lesions suggested seborrheic dermatitis—which was the condition presented in this case. The "seborrheic" patches gradually became more infiltrated and covered with whitish pearly scales, giving occasionally the appearance of psoriasis. During the last eight months only the present infiltrations had appeared.

EPITHELIOMA OF THE ARM?   Presented by Drs. Parounagian and Rulison.

V. L., a man aged 50, an Italian laborer, married, who had eleven living children, twenty years before examination had had gonorrhea. He denied syphilitic infection. His Wassermann test on Feb. 6, 1922, was four plus. On February 23, February 27 and March 2 the patient received 0.2 gm. of silver arsphenamin. The only cutaneous lesion present was on the right forearm. There were no lesions of the mucous membranes. The patient's pupils did not react to light; his knee reflexes were absent; he did not present a Romberg's sign. On the right forearm was a patch the size of a half dollar, oval, with somewhat irregular borders and typical pearly edges. The lesion was reddish-brown, elevated, slightly scaly and dry, and was somewhat indurated. The antisyphilitic treatment given had had no influence on the lesion. The diagnosis was epithelioma. No biopsy had been made.

PEMPHIGUS OF THE MUCOUS MEMBRANES AND OF THE SKIN. Presented by Dr. Lapowski.

B. A., a man aged 44, married, born in Austria, a tailor, was first seen Aug. 8, 1921, with lesions on the lower lip, gums, soft palate and tonsils. The lesions were smooth red patches, some of which looked like burst bullae.

The man disappeared from the clinic, and two months later he was treated in other places for this condition, under various diagnoses. On March 7, 1922, he returned with bullae scattered over the entire body. The pemphigus lesions on the mucous membrane had been present for about two years without involving the skin. Nikolsky's sign was present.

DISCUSSION

Dr. Rosen said he had seen this patient in consultation with an oral surgeon. The patient then presented ulcerating lesions on the gums and on the inside of the cheeks. In such cases it was always safe to make a diagnosis of pemphigus to protect one's self even though occasionally the condition turns out not to be pemphigus. As presented, there were lesions on the body.

Dr. Chargin said he thought that the interesting point in the case was the fact that two years elapsed between the appearance of the eruption in the mouth and that on the body. That was the longest interval he had heard of.

Dr. Wise agreed with the diagnosis.

Dr. Lapowski said that this patient had been treated in many institutions with various tentative diagnoses and various interferences both locally and internally. It was important in bullous cases of the mouth with doubtful diagnosis to avoid all local interference before a diagnosis was arrived at, as by interfering the spreading of the disease was hastened and the life of the patient was shortened. He remembered the instance of a patient who lived ten or fifteen years after he first saw him, in comparative comfort, because he was able to influence the patient not to interfere with the local mouth lesions.

CUTIS VERTICIS GYRATA.   Presented by Dr. Howard Fox.

A. M., aged 43, a salesman, born in Germany, came to the Harlem Hospital for relief of a generalized bullous dermatitis herpetiformis. This eruption had existed for eight months, previous to which time he had not noticed any eruption. The condition for which he was presented was discovered incidentally. It consisted of four parallel depressions and corresponding elevations of the scalp at the junction of the parietal and occipital regions. The depressions varied from 1 to 2½ inches (2.5 to 6.3 cm.) in length, and from one-eighth to one-quarter of an inch (3.1 to 6.3 mm.) in depth. The direction of the lesions was anteroposterior. They were easily palpable in spite of the rather long hair worn by the patient at the time of presentation. Subsequently when the hair was closely cut they were plainly visible and were successfully photographed. The condition had existed as long as the patient could remember, and gave him no inconvenience. Unlike cases previously described, the lesions ran in a straight direction and were not gyrate or curved.

DISCUSSION

DR. WISE expressed the view that it was a typical example of the affection.

DR. LEVIN said that in the cases previously reported either a preceding inflammatory condition or syphilis had been found. In the case reported by Dr. Wise and himself syphilis was present. There was a possibility that the dermatitis herpetiformis, if of long duration, may have predisposed to the condition. He agreed with the diagnosis.

PREFUNGOID STAGE OF MYCOSIS FUNGOIDES. Presented by DR. CLARK.

S. B., aged 26, an Austrian, a porter, who came to the United States eight years before, generally a healthy, strong man. He was married and had one child. He first began to notice flat red spots on his body about six years previously. These would scale off and leave red spots, and he did not believe that any of them had disappeared. During the last six months the lesions had become much more numerous on the body, arms and legs, and some red patches seemed to have become larger. The patient never had had severe itching, but occasionally felt a hot or burning sensation. He now exhibited over the trunk and extremities circumscribed, dull red, scaly patches like a parapsoriasis, some as large as a palm, others the size of a pea. Almost all the hard lesions were without infiltration, but some of the smaller ones in groups on the abdomen and around the waist line were slightly infiltrated. The patient showed no sign of having scratched the lesions and was entirely relieved of itching under treatment with a lanolin ointment. The general physical examination was negative. The pathologic report was that the derma showed groups of small mononuclear cells which in most cases were in the neighborhood of blood vessels or surrounding them. There was a slight amount of acanthosis and hyperkeratosis.

DISCUSSION

DR. TRAUB said the biopsy confirmed the diagnosis of the premycotic stage

LUPUS (?) OF THE NOSE, CHEEKS, UPPER LIP AND NECK. Presented by DR. ROTHWELL. (Previously presented. March, 1919, by Dr. Lane.)

V. B., a man aged 35, an Italian laborer, presented a dark reddish brown infiltration of the nose, adjacent cheeks (more extensive on the left side), upper lip (more especially under the right nostril), with a moderate scale formation on the cheek, adherent and with considerable crusting, rather than scaling, about the left nostril. There was a perforation of the nasal septum. On the left side of the neck at the border of a scrofuloderma-like scar was a similar dark red infiltration covered partially with crusting similar to that on the left nostril. On the right cheek there was an atrophied dime sized area which had succeeded a similar process at that point. In the border of the infiltrated lesion of the left cheek there was a suggestive flattening-down at one point, giving a plateau-like effect suggestive of a beginning lupus erythematosus atrophy.

The history was of three years' duration, progressive involvement, failure of improvement under treatment with drops three times daily during six months and intramuscular injections with mercury for three months. The Wassermann test had been negative repeatedly, and except for a watery discharge from the nose there had been no material subjective symptoms. There was no history of syphilis and the Wassermann test was negative. If permitted, a biopsy would be secured and a report made at a later meeting.

DISCUSSION

Dr. Rothwell said that when the patient was presented in 1919 Dr. MacKee and Dr. Pollitzer considered the condition probably a tuberculous process. He had thought that some one would have suggested lupus erythematosus.

Dr. Highman remarked that the lesions on the cheek looked like those described by Leloir as lupus vulgaris erythematodes.

Dr. Rulison said that when the patient was presented before he had had blocking of the left nostril for sixteen months. Dr. Lane reported that a small section for biopsy had been taken from the nose, but that no tubercle bacilli were found, only staphylococci being demonstrated.

PAGET'S DISEASE OF THE NIPPLE. Presented by Dr. Levin.

Y. K., a woman aged 30, a Galician by birth, was married two years before and had not become pregnant. A scratch on the right nipple four years ago failed to heal, and following the application of salves a moist, red patch developed. This enlarged slowly, but one year ago it began to extend downward. It had never caused pain, but itched.

The region of the nipple of the right breast was covered by a nickel-sized irregularly round, elevated, infiltrated lesion with an everted border. The color was dark red and the surface was scaly. The whole nipple was retracted; the opening was covered by a crust, but there was no discharge. The pectoral glands showed slight enlargement; the cervical and axillary glands were not palpable.

DISCUSSION

Dr. Wise asked how the case was differentiated from epithelioma.

Dr. Levin replied that this was not a typical case of Paget's disease in that it was not so shiny, red and moist. It was also too infiltrated, and it appeared like a case of Paget's disease going on to the formation of carcinoma. The pectoral glands were palpably enlarged. A complete removal of the breast and glands had been advised.

EPITHELIOMA MEATUS PENIS. Presented by Dr. Lapowski.

K. S., a man aged 43, married, born in Russia, a cloak maker, eight years before had had urethral discharge, which lasted four months. During the summer of 1920 (two years before) he noticed redness and itching about the tip of the urethra which gradually increased. There was no painful urination. The meatus urinarius was surrounded by corona-like, hard, indurated tissue,

with an elevated, well-defined smooth border. The lesion was deeply infiltrated, felt almost like cartilage, and extended to a depth of about 5 mm.
The lower part of the growth was more verruco-edematous-like and continuous
with the frenum, which was markedly reddened and was composed of four
pinhead to lentil sized papular edematous elevations. The glans was erythematous with minute glistening papules, due to edema or irritation from applications. The foreskin was markedly edematous. Tne glands were slightly
perceptible.

DISCUSSION

DR. LEVIN said that three things were to be considered—chancre, tuberculosis and epithelioma. The duration of the condition and the absence of acute
signs were against chancre. Against tuberculosis was the fact that the disease
had not spread more rapidly and that there was no ulceration. A distinct
induration on deep palpation was more in favor of epithelioma than anything else.

DR. CHARGIN said he failed to find any induration in the lesion and could
hardly conceive of its being epithelioma. He favored the diagnosis of possible
tuberculosis. Had it been epithelioma, there would have been more infiltration,
more ulceration and more glandular involvement after two years.

DR. ABRAMOWITZ said that it was hard to conceive the lesion at the meatus
as that of an epithelioma. He understood the condition had been present for
two years, yet as presented it seemed to be rather an acute edema with a slight
amount of infiltration such as one would see in a simple irritation. In addition,
the cervical and epitrochlear glands were palpable—the inguinal glands were
not enlarged. There was no cachexia. Certain important facts were omitted in
the presentation of this case. No dark-field examination had been made, and
only one Wassermann test was taken. He had no definite diagnosis to offer.

DR. PAROUNAGIAN said he had observed the case carefully; it was not a
chancre; it was not a gumma, and it was not tuberculosis. Only one thing was
left—epithelioma. He favored the diagnosis of epithelioma.

DR. WISE said that while he admitted that he could offer no diagnosis,
he agreed with Dr. Chargin that there was no sign of epithelioma about the lesion.

DR. ROSTENBERG asked whether the man had had gonorrhea.

DR. LAPOWSKI replied in the affirmative—eight years ago. There was no
history of tuberculosis.

DR. RULISON asked whether the possibility of ioderma had been considered.

DR. LAPOWSKI replied that the man had received 10 per cent. of potassium
iodid once a day for two weeks.

DR. HIGHMAN said the case was as puzzling a one as he had seen. It did
not conform to syphilis, tuberculosis, or epithelioma. It appeared more like a
chronic inflammatory process. He would not call the condition an infiltration
or an induration, such as was seen in any specific condition, but it was slightly
thickened such as any chronic inflammation might be. He agreed with what
Dr. Wise had said.

DR. WISE asked whether the patient had received any antipyrin.

DR. LAPOWSKI replied in the negative. He then said there seemed to be a
great difference of opinion among the members of the Section regarding the
presence or absence of infiltration and hardness in the meatus. When the
patient came for the first time to the clinic, a week previously, Dr. Walzer,
Dr. Schulze and he examined him. The depth of the lesion was measured and
at that time the report said that the hardness extended 5 mm. into the meatus.
At the time of presentation the hardness was less pronounced than it had been.

but it was there, provided the penis was palpated between the two fingers; when the palpation was made with one finger from the upper portion of the meatus down, the hardness was not so pronounced, but even with such a method of palpation, a hard nodule could be felt.

It was unusual to see a tuberculous lesion on the meatus penis without any tubercles, without any subjective symptoms on urination and without even a slight discharge. It was unusual for a tuberculous lesion to remain stationary for two years and if one judged by the clinical symptoms alone, as they were then present, tuberculosis of the meatus could be excluded. Besides epithelioma or sarcoma, the possibility of a gummatous infiltration could be entertained. Dr. Lapowski said he would try to report further development of the case at the next meeting.

ANGIOMA. Presented by Dr. Lapowski.

Y. A., a woman aged 68, married for thirty-seven years, a Russian by birth, twelve years before gave birth to twins. Infection of the bladder followed, lasting, according to the patient's statement, six months. A year and a half before she was in bed for six weeks, suffering with heart and liver trouble (?); eight months before the lesions appeared first on the lower left eyelid, then became scattered over other portions of the body. Some of the lesions had been removed in various hospitals, leaving keloidal scars. The tumors present were scattered all over the body (about twenty), and varied in size from that of a pinhead to that of a cherry-pit. They were raised and angiomatous, and varied in color from red to dark brownish-red. The biopsy made by Dr. Highman showed angioma.

DISCUSSION

Dr. Levin said that he had first seen the patient about six months prior to presentation. At that time the angiomas were more numerous, and some suggested angiosarcoma clinically. The patient was referred to the hospital because of her heart condition, which was poor. The pathologic condition of the tumors was that of angioma. Dr. Levin said that he had observed this form of angioma often in persons who were suffering from hypertension, cardiovascular or renal disease. More recently he had seen the patient at Mount Sinai Hospital. As presented, the lesions were less numerous. A peculiarity of the lesions was the tendency to become dry and form crusts. There was no evidence of infectious endocarditis.

ERYTHEMA AB IGNE. Presented by Dr. Williams.

S. A., a woman aged 21, American born, a student, presented herself in the clinic with an eruption over the anterior aspect of the lower part of both lower legs, of three months' duration. For the past four months she had been doing her studying seated with her legs against a radiator. The Wassermann test was negative. The biopsy showed inflammatory tissue.

ARSPHENAMIN DERMATITIS. Presented by Dr. Rosen.

I. D., a man aged 44, married, born in the United States, presented himself at the Vanderbilt Clinic, Jan. 26, 1922, with a serpiginous syphilid on the left hip. Several Wassermann tests had been four plus; his wife had had about six miscarriages. He was placed on the usual antisyphilitic treatment of mercury salicylate intramuscularly and arsphenamin intravenously. After the fourth injection of arsphenamin the patient became quite ill with nausea, dizziness, etc. In about two hours itching began, and he had a severe burning sensation of the skin. He then presented a diffuse erythematous eruption, which was confined mostly to the trunk and buttocks. In certain places the lesions were moderately elevated and not entirely confluent—closely simulating an urticarial eruption. There was no evidence of jaundice.

DISCUSSION

Dr. Lapowski said that the lesions presented by the patient consisted of scarlatiniform dermatitis with pronounced papular lesions. The papules looked like the classical syphilitic papules seen in cases in which the papules had been present before the arsphenamin dermatitis appeared, and in cases of early syphilis the question would arise whether those papules were not due to syphilis.

LICHEN PLANUS, MOLLUSCUM CONTAGIOSUM AND VERRUCA FILIFORMIS IN THE SAME PATIENT. Presented by Dr. Wise.

P. P., a man aged 27, a Greek, presented typical lesions of lichen planus on the flexor aspects of the wrists and lower part of the forearms. of two months' duration. On the upper and inner side of the left thigh and shaft of the penis, there were about a half dozen shiny, pearl-white, umbilicated lesions of molluscum. The verrucae were located on the lower surface of the glans penis near the frenum.

NODULAR SYPHILID RESEMBLING PSORIASIS IN A NEGRESS. Presented by Dr. Howard Fox.

R. R., aged 18, was presented at the last meeting. The diagnosis of syphilis had been confirmed by the complete disappearace of the eruption under treatment with neo-arsphenamin, no local treatment having been given.

TINEA CAPITIS; TRICHOPHYTID. Presented by Dr. Levin.

E. R., aged 5, born in the United States. was presented at Cornell Medical Clinic, March 6, 1922, with an eruption of the scalp and trunk. The eruption of the scalp had been present for three weeks and consisted of numerous brownish-white scales scattered throughout the scalp. On the occipital region was a half dollar sized, partially bald spot covered with brownish-white scales and a few broken off hairs. Over the posterior part of the neck and shoulders was an erythematous, scaling, infiltrated and ill-defined eruption. which had been present for two weeks. Just beneath the shoulders there was an erythematofollicular eruption, which at a distance looked confluent. but which on close inspection was found to be discrete. A few lesions resembled pityriasis rosea. This patient was shown as presenting a case of trichophytid.

Examination of hairs and scales from the scalp revealed the microsporon. The scales from the body were negative.

MILIARY PAPULAR SYPHILID. Presented by Dr. Parounagian.

ERYTHEMA NODOSUM AND THROMBO-ANGEITIS OBLITERANS. Presented by Dr. Abramowitz.

PITYRIASIS RUBRA PILARIS. (Previously presented.) Presented by Dr. Abramowitz.

GRANULOMA OF CORIUM. Dr. Levin.

Reports on the case of male patient (B.), presented at the January meeting by Dr. Levin. Diagnosis: Syphilis? Epidermoid carcinoma? Tuberculosis?

Both biopsies were made from the same patient. The changes seen in both sections were not identical.

No. 9896: The epidermis was very much thickened, cornification was excessive, and the rete pegs were very long and irregular in shape. Some of the rete pegs had altered staining properties, and giant cells were forming about the deeper epidermal cells. The interpapillary spaces were filled with a granulomatous infiltration and scar made up of lymphocytes, fibroblastic elements and an occasional plasma cell. The papillary vessels were thick walled for the most part, but there were blood channels with wide luminae. No tubercles were to be recognized as such. The hypoderm was very much scarred and in many places hyalinized. The changes seen here resembled very much those seen in early carcinomatous processes and precancerous lesions of the skin described by Ribbert. Analogous inflammatory reactions were seen about early cancer of epidermal origin.

Diagnosis: Granuloma of the hypoderm with precancerous changes.

Section 9901: The changes in the epidermis were not as extensive as in the previous section, but thickening and hyperkeratosis were present. The corium was very much thickened by a poorly vascularized granuloma, consisting of lymphocytes, pale fibroblastic elements resembling epithelioid cells and giant cells of the Langerhans type with peripherally arranged nuclei. The giant cells were not in the most anemic portions of the granuloma, as is usually the case in tuberculosis. No caseation had occurred. The hypoderm was very much scarred, and the vessels of the hypoderm were infiltrated with the cells of the lymphocyte order.

Diagnosis: Granuloma of the corium (probably due to tuberculosis).

(Tissue was removed from the buttock lesion and the material injected into a guinea-pig. After six weeks the pig was killed, and tubercles were found in the spleen.)

Paul E. Bechet, M.D., Secretary.

PHILADELPHIA DERMATOLOGICAL SOCIETY

Regular Monthly Meeting, March 13, 1922

Frank Crozer Knowles, M.D., *Presiding*

Dr. Fred D. Weidman exhibited a number of gross and microscopic specimens. Among the latter were sections from the skin of patients with lupus erythematosus, angiomatous nevi and melanotic carcinoma of the abdominal skin. These were shown to point out certain unusual features.

TINEA CAPITIS AND ECZEMATOID RINGWORM OF THE HANDS. Presented by Dr. Greenbaum.

F. H., a white girl 6 years of age, had pink, scaly, fairly well defined plaques involving the dorsum of both hands. Scales examined microscopically showed spores and mycelia of a trichophyton. This led to an examination of the scalp on which were found furfuraceous areas of partial alopecia. Ringworm was demonstrated. Autoinoculation further demonstrated the nature of the pathogenic cause. Twelve days after inoculation of some scales on a slightly scarified area of the arm, a pink, scaly centrifugally spreading lesion developed in which mycelia were demonstrated.

DISCUSSION

Dr. Schamberg called attention to the sharp margination of the eruption. He had seen the microscopic specimen—many large groups of spores closely packed together. No mycelia were noted. It was unquestionably a case of eczematoid ringworm.

Dr. Strauss asked why these cases were sometimes so difficult to cure. Did the fungus remain in some portion of the eruption or was an eczema sometimes initiated by the irritating fungicides? Was it not possible that many of these cases were eczemas with fungus contamination?

Dr. Schamberg replied that it was possible that the treatment had not eradicated all of the fungus. Where the typical ringworm fungus was found he thought there was more significance than accidental inclusion.

Dr. Weidman said he thought that was particularly true when the fungus definitely invaded the hair-shaft as contrasted to its occurrence in the scales.

Dr. Greenbaum said that in studies of more than 150 patients, apparently not subjects of ringworm diseases, he had found none of the fungi described by Sabouraud. Only molds were found.

Dr. Weidman added that sometimes when the fungus was not present in the scales it could be found in the lanugo. He felt that frequently this fact could be used in connection with the prognosis of a ringworm case.

XANTHOMA TUBEROSUM OF THE FACE ASSOCIATED WITH A PERSISTENT FACIAL ERYTHEMA. Presented by Dr. Schamberg.

A. P., aged 22, presented lesions involving both upper eyelids, consisting of yellowish nodules of the size of peas. They differed from xanthomas in that they were circumscribed and elevated.

Covering the forehead, cheeks, lips and chin was a marked erythema of irregular distribution. The erythema extended over the eyelids and gave to the xanthomatous lesions an orange color.

On the chin in the region of the erythema were small elevations varying in size from that of a pinhead to that of a lentil seed, which were reddish in appearance but which on pressure exhibited a distinct yellowish color. These appeared to be of the same character as the lesions on the eyelids. The patient was apparently in good health. There had been no loss of weight: there was no evidence of liver involvement; the urine was normal, except for a specific gravity of 1.005, the cause of which would be studied further.

DISCUSSION

Dr. Hirschler inquired concerning the blood-sugar content in this case, but was informed that it had not been ascertained.

Dr. Knowles recalled a case of colloid degeneration of the skin shown by Dr. Hartzell. He thought this case resembled that one rather than a fatty change.

DR. SCHAMBERG admitted that this was possible, but when the skin of the patient was put on a stretch, there was a characteristic yellow color as the blood was pressed out of the lesions.

DR. WEIDMAN said that he had a specimen of xanthoma tuberosum of the eyelids—an undoubted case—in the same situation. The eruption further down on the face somewhat suggested colloid.

DR. SCHAMBERG said that colloid milium was not often seen in young persons. A moderate amount was frequently noted in the aged.

DR. WEIDMAN said that xanthoma was a degeneration of the collagen bundles undergoing a fatty change, while colloids indicated a different kind of protein change.

DR. SCHAMBERG said that in xanthoma tuberosum there was a high cholesterol blood finding and that curious connective tissue cells arose as a tissue response.

CASE FOR DIAGNOSIS. Presented by DR. HIRSCHLER.

A white woman, aged 50, presented a condition of twenty years' duration. It started as a "freckle-like" spot on the left temple. Two years before it was desiccated by Dr. Clark and was entirely removed. It had returned, however. The eruption was purely pigmentary, superficial and without depth or infiltration, about 3 by 5 cm. (1.2 by 2 inches) in size. A little white scarring was present on two sides.

DISCUSSION

DR. KNOWLES said it reminded him slightly of the pigmented edge of vitiligo.

DR. SCHAMBERG suggested the employment of carbon dioxid snow which he thought would act deeply enough to remove this condition.

DR. KNOWLES continued that he had two patients with lupus erythematosus who had been treated with carbon dioxid snow by Brocq in Paris. To his surprise only ten seconds had been employed with slight pressure. The results were excellent.

DR. SCHAMBERG said he felt that the results in erythematous lupus were largely dependent on the amount of inflammatory activity in the patch. Such treatments sometimes extended acute outbreaks although resulting in cure in the indolent cases.

CASE FOR DIAGNOSIS. Presented by DR. DENGLER.

J. B., a white man aged 24, a dentist, had had this condition since he was 12 years old. Diffuse, whitish plaques with slightly elevated rough surfaces were present on the roof of the mouth, the buccal mucous membrane and to a lesser extent on the mucosa of the lips, but not extending onto the vermilion surface. There was no cutaneous outbreak, but the presenter considered it a case of lichen planus.

DISCUSSION

DR. SCHAMBERG said it was hard to distinguish leukokeratosis from lichen planus in this situation. He was unable to be more definite. He had recently seen a woman with extensive patches of leukoplakia for which arsenic had been used without avail. If they cleared up under that drug, it was rather confirmatory of lichen planus. Such patches often occurred in nonsmokers as the mucous membrane of the mouth frequently showed a vulnerability to condiments. In other cases it was due to digestive disturbances. We are not yet familiar with all the cases of white patches on the mucous membranes of the mouth. The long duration of the disease was rather against lichen planus. Some white spots were smooth, others showed epithelial proliferation, roughness and elevation. The former, he preferred to call leukoplakia, the latter leukokeratosis.

Dr. Corson inquired concerning the frequency of lichen planus confined solely to the mucous membrane.

Dr. Schamberg replied that it was occasionally seen and most easily recognized when typical papules occurred on the tongue.

MORPHEA. Presented by Dr. Dengler.

H. D., a white woman aged 45, presented an eruption on the inner surface of the right thigh which had lasted six years. A smaller patch was present on the left side of the neck. The patches began as red discolorations of the skin which turned brown and later partly white. Itching was intense. When shown, a violaceous, infiltrated margin was present, but the central pigmented portion was nearly as soft as the normal skin. The larger patch was nearly* double the size of a palm.

DISCUSSION

Dr. Weidman said that some of the patches were only pigmented and had not proceeded as far as the development of fibrous tissue.

Dr. Corson said the central skin was so soft that there could not be much of the fibrous element present.

Dr. Knowles said that in cases of morphea there was no thickening—just the violaceous ring and telangiectases.

MULTIPLE EPITHELIOMAS. Presented by Dr. Dengler.

W. J. E., a white man aged 61, an oyster opener, had had an epithelioma on the left auricle for the past year. At the angle of the jaw was a smaller ulcerating lesion with the same characteristics, which the patient thought had developed from a razor cut.

DISCUSSION

Dr. Schamberg spoke of the metastasis of these conditions as a question recently discussed among surgeons and radiologists. He had never seen a cutaneous growth develop lymphatic metastasis except a single insignificant growth on the eyelid which later recurred in the neck and produced further extensions. It was more likely to occur when other parts were the seat of epitheliomas than when the face was affected. It was remarkable how large and extensive the ulcerations frequently became without metastasizing.

Dr. Knowles felt that this was so on account of the type, almost all of the facial growths being from the basal cell layer of the skin.

Dr. Schamberg said that even when epitheliomas involved the nose or conjunctiva the likelihood of metastasis was not increased, but when the buccal membrane became affected, the chance of metastasis was much greater.

Dr. Weidman raised the question as to the frequency of multiple epitheliomas.

Dr. Knowles said that they were somewhat unusual except in senile keratosis.

Dr. Schamberg said that he believed they were not particularly rare. Sometimes there was a familial tendency; occasionally even in young men multiple growths developed. The skin was usually dry, but that was not essential.

ERYTHEMA INDURATUM AND PAPULONECROTIC TUBERCULIDS.
Presented by DR. GREENBAUM.

F. M., a native born white girl aged 19, with a negative family and personal history, a year before first noticed "sores" on the hands and legs similar to the present lesions. These healed without treatment. Three months before her first visit to Dr. Schamberg's clinic, the "sores" reappeared. The lesions were typically papulonecrotic tuberculids on the hands and erythema induratum (ulcerated type of Hutchinson) on the legs. The patient was presented with healed lesions following the use of tuberculin injections and neo-arsphenamin in small doses with rest in bed.

DISCUSSION

DR. KNOWLES said that he had noted contradictory results from the use of arsphenamin in papulonecrotic tuberculid. One patient especially, had apparently been cured by the injections, while another patient developed them during treatment for syphilis.

DR. SCHAMBERG thought of an interpretation to fit the two cases. Small doses of arsphenamin helped to increase the production of antibodies, while larger doses lowered the formation of the same. In this particular case, the doses were small.

DR. STRAUSS observed that the first patient mentioned by Dr. Knowles had apparently been cured by eight injections, but later had had a relapse, and a second series had not caused improvement. He asked what was considered the proper dose for this condition.

DR. SCHAMBERG said that 0.3 to 0.4 gm. of neo-arsphenamin was about the right dose. If improvement occurred, the arsphenamin must have produced an alteration in the body, allowing it to obtain an ascendency over the disease. As to tuberculin, it was doubtful whether it had helped the condition. In fact, he considered it rather unlikely that it was of benefit in any skin condition.

DR. KNOWLES recalled that he had recently seen records of a postmortem on a case of erythematous lupus. The necropsy report showed that the patient had had generalized tuberculosis. The bovine type of bacillus was nearly always present in cutaneous tuberculosis. He thought that often liquor potasii arsenitis (Fowler's solution) or other arsenic preparations were helpful.

DR. SCHAMBERG said that the whole matter was an open question. It was hard to affirm or deny the various phases of the subject.

DR. GREENBAUM added that there was considerable reaction noted in the skin of this patient following an injection of dry tubercle bacilli of the bovine type.

EDWARD F. CORSON, M.D., Secretary.

CHICAGO DERMATOLOGICAL SOCIETY

Regular Meeting, March 15, 1922

E. A. OLIVER, M.D., *Vice President, Presiding*

ERYTHEMA MULTIFORME. Presented by DRS. ORMSBY and MITCHELL.

A young woman, aged 21 years, when first seen by Dr. Ormsby in 1913 had had erythema multiforme for two years. Three attacks had occurred. The first attack began in May, 1911; the first lesions appeared on the wrists and, according to the patient, resembled mosquito bites. They soon developed into lesions which looked like "bunches of grapes." The feet were soon attacked, then the trunk, and within nine days the entire surface, including the face, became involved. The appearance of lesions was preceded by burning and painful sensations. This attack lasted three months. The second and third attacks each lasted three months. The fourth attack was of three weeks' duration when the patient was first seen. At that time there was a generalized eruption consisting of patches of papules, papulopustules, vesicopapules and crusted nodules. The extremities, trunk and neck, were more markedly affected. During the last nine years the attacks have occurred annually. At the time of presentation the present attack was of three weeks' duration. There were patches of lesions similar to those described. The entire trunk was covered with crusts and weeping. On the extremities were patches of papules, vesicles, pustules and nodules.

Each attack was accompanied by elevation of temperature, nausea and vomiting, which completely incapacitated the patient. No further study had been made as the patient was seen only during the fourth attack a year ago and the present one. The patient was exhibited on account of the interesting history and the severity of the disorder.

DISCUSSION

Dr. Ormsby said that he first saw this patient on May 24, 1913, and again four days later; he had not seen her since. When first seen there were grouped lesions about the body similar to those now present. The disease had then been present for two years, and that was the third attack. Since then she had had attacks twice a year covering a period of nine years, each attack lasting from six to twelve weeks. The present attack was of about three weeks' duration. On Feb. 27, 1922, there were a large number of vesicles and bullae which had now largely disappeared, except on the hands.

Dr. Engman said he thought at first that the condition was lichen planus, but careful examination revealed no lesions of that nature. He did not make the diagnosis from the appearance of the lesions but from the history that the patient had a recurrent bullous eruption. He agreed that it was a case of multiforme erythema.

Dr. Pusey thought it was a case of recurrent multiforme erythema with unusually large lesions.

Dr. Ravitch thought it was a case of lichen planus hypertrophicus and that one could see distinct shiny papules such as are seen in that disorder.

Dr. Ormsby agreed with Dr. Pusey that it was a case of multiforme erythema with bullous lesions. The lesions on the forearms that resembled lichen planus were undergoing involution, producing lesions of that type. He considered the case interesting because of the wide distribution of the lesions, the unusual type and long duration.

HAIRY NEVUS. Presented by Dr. Ravitch.

The patient was an infant, aged 4 months, who was born with heavy, coarse, black hair on the left side of the scalp, while the right side had none. In the beginning the area covered by the hair was elevated, pigmented and slightly fringed by patches of scales. During the last few weeks the pigment and scaliness had cleared up considerably, the hair had become softer, and there was an increase in the growth of hair on the right side of the scalp.

Dr. Mitchell thought the condition was a hairy nevus.

Dr. Stillians thought it was a nevus on account of the pigmentation of the skin under the hair.

Dr. Ravitch said that at birth the child had had much coarser hair, and the area where the coarse hair had been was pigmented. He had used some stimulating oily applications, and the hair had become softer. He believed it to be a case of nevus.

A CASE FOR DIAGNOSIS. Presented by Drs. Senear and Wien.

A man, aged 23 years, four months before presentation had an attack of herpes zoster which involved the left side of the chest, the upper part of the arm and the left scapular region. Following this attack the patient showed grouped comedones at the site of the zoster lesions.

Dr. Pusey said he did not recall having seen comedones following herpes zoster, and he thought it a very unusual occurrence.

Dr. Senear said there was a little itching at times. The patient had used only a calamin lotion for a few days at the beginning of the herpes zoster.

Dr. Ravitch thought the trouble was due to the use of the calamin lotion. The zinc oxid was often impure and likely to cause an eruption.

Dr. Pusey questioned this. He said he had used calamin lotion repeatedly daily for many years, and he did not believe that it ever produced comedones.

PITYRIASIS RUBRA PILARIS. Presented by Drs. Ormsby and Mitchell.

A child, aged 6 years, had an acute disorder which had been present about six weeks, and which was said to have developed shortly after an attack of varicella. The eruption began ón the palms, then it appeared on the joints and within two weeks became generalized.

On presentation the scalp and face presented the appearance of severe seborrheic dermatitis, and the face was encased with seborrheic matter. The extremities presented patches of psoriasiform dermatitis. The entire trunk was covered with discrete, keratotic follicular papules with some psoriasiform scaling patches. The palms and soles were thickened and keratotic. No subjective sensations were present.

Dr. Pusey said he was interested in the rapid development and had never seen a case of this disorder develop in so brief a time.

Dr. Ormsby said that when the patient was first seen three weeks previously the lesions were well defined and limited to the hair follicles. There were a few psoriasiform patches, and the disorder had spread markedly since then. It was the most acute case he had ever seen. There was a history of chickenpox before the development of this disorder.

BROMID ERUPTION. Presented by Dr. Oliver.

The patient was a boy, aged 1 year, who presented an eruption which had been present for four weeks. The child had been in poor health and considerable medicine had been given to him.

The lesions were pea-sized hypertrophic papules on the posterior surface of the legs.

DISCUSSION

Dr. Pusey said he thought the condition was a bromid or iodid eruption.

Dr. Oliver said the baby had been given medicine for about six weeks, but the grandmother, who brought the child to the hospital, did not know what the medicine contained. He had recently seen a child, aged 3 months, whose mother had been taking bromids four or five times a day "for her nerves." The baby's eruption made her nervous, and she took the bromids. Stopping the mother's bromids resulted in clearing up the baby's eruption.

Dr. Ormsby said he had recently had a patient with anthracoid lesions on the face. The mother had been taking bromids which induced the lesions.

Dr. Pusey said he had recently had a baby under his care who had been receiving a mixture containing a small quantity of bromid through the mother, but he did not see many such cases. He asked whether many such cases were seen at the Children's Memorial Hospital.

Dr. Oliver said this was the first case he had seen at the Children's Memorial Hospital.

ARSENICAL KERATOSIS AND DERMATITIS HERPETIFORMIS.
Presented by Dr. Stillians.

An Irishman, aged 35 years, had a dermatitis of several years' duration. The dermatitis had nearly cleared up following extensive and repeated exposures to the Quartz lamp, and no arsenic had been taken for the past year. The patient had taken liquor potassii arsenitis (Fowler's solution) at frequent intervals for eight years and showed marked keratoses on the palms and soles. Several keratotic areas had cleared up under radium therapy. No lesions of dermatitis were present at the time of presentation.

DISCUSSION

Dr. Stillians asked the members of the society to discuss the treatment of such cases with radium or roentgen rays.

Dr. Ormsby said he never employed radiotherapy in such cases.

Dr. Irvine said he had never treated a patient with such a case with radiotherapy, but he had treated roentgen-ray keratosis with good results.

Dr. Lieberthal said that radium as well as the roentgen rays were effective in such cases, but they must be used with caution.

Dr. Stillians said he believed that with a fairly strong dosage the lesions cleared up nicely under radiotherapy.

Dr. Pusey said he did not believe that they would clear up under radiotherapy and said he would be afraid to use it. He did not think there was much danger of carcinoma in the large lesions on the bottom of the feet. He had seen carcinoma occur in a large keratosis, but in those instances they were more like senile keratoses than the heavy plantar variety. He believed there was not much danger of malignant degeneration of the patient's plantar lesions, and thought the treatment would damage the surface. He advised the use of pumice stone or a safety razor. The senile keratoses are a different proposition. The condition in this case was like a callosity and one does not get good results from radiotherapy in such cases.

Dr. Ravitch agreed with Dr. Pusey and said that he had similar lesions. In his own case he had obtained a great deal of relief by immersing the hands in hot water for half an hour. This softened the lesions, and he then applied lanolin.

FAVUS. Presented by Dr. Waugh.

A woman, aged 26 years, had had the disorder for fifteen years. Most of the scalp was involved, and large areas were practically free from hair. One child, 7 years old, had the same disorder. The fungus was demonstrated microscopically.

DISCUSSION

Dr. Engman agreed with the diagnosis of favus, but he thought that there was some intercurrent dermatitis.

Dr. Waugh said he thought the case was interesting not only on account of the extent of the disorder, but because of the acute dermatitis, which was only of three or four weeks' duration. He could not determine what produced the dermatitis on the scalp and neck. There was no history of recent medication.

Dr. Lieberthal recalled a patient with the same disease picture who was shown a few years ago by Dr. Harris. In that instance the neck, forearm and legs were involved with a chronic type of seborrheic dermatitis, and mycelia and spores were found in the scales on the latter regions.

Dr. Engman said that something like this was described in the Norwegian or Swedish literature.

ACRODERMATITIS CHRONICA ATROPHICANS. Presented by Drs. Ormsby and Mitchell.

A man, aged 48 years, had suffered with the disorder for ten years. He was born in Russia and had been in America for eighteen years. The lesions were on the arms, forearms, hands, thighs and legs. The disorder began simultaneously on the hands and feet and gradually extended upward. The skin became dry and scaly, and that in the involved regions was hypersensitive. On examination the patient appeared well nourished. The hands were blue, the dorsa markedly atrophic with a distinctly yellowish crust. A band of reddish atrophy extended from the left hand to the elbow and over the arm to the lower border of the deltoid. The elbows were covered with dry plates of shining scales. Beginning in the lumbar region and extending downward and anteriorly to Poupart's ligament was a sharply démarcated bluish-red scaling atrophy which also covered the lower extremities. The dorsum of the right foot was indented and presented a yellowish waxy crust. On the right thigh in the upper anterior third were several coin sized punched out scars. These were not preceded by nodules or treatment.

DISCUSSION

Dr. Irvine considered this an interesting case of idiopathic atrophy of the skin. He was interested in the little patchy places where the fibrous tissue was interposed, particularly around the ankles.

Dr. Irvine had had an interesting experience recently with a patient presented before the American Medical Association in 1912. The patient, about 70 years of age, had been seen again within the last few weeks. There was not much change in the atrophy, but a great deal in the physical condition. In some places there were ulcers where the fibrous plaques had been, which on one leg extended almost all the way around. This condition had not been studied, but it looked as though it might be malignant. He had tried to get the man into the hospital for observation, but it was impossible to do so.

A CASE FOR DIAGNOSIS. Presented by Drs. Senear and Wien.

A man, aged 62 years, who presented a lesion on the back which had been present for about five months, gave a history of intense itching of the back fifteen years ago and of rubbing his back against the sharp edge of a door to relieve this symptom. The skin pulled off and a sore the size of a dime developed. This itched later, and he again scratched his back against the door. This process repeated itself at frequent intervals, the lesion growing larger. There was a constant stinging and itching sensation. He had been treated with ointments during the last two years.

DISCUSSION

Dr. Mitchell thought it was a case of superficial epitheliomatosus.

Dr. Stillians agreed.

Dr. Pusey said he had taken sections from similar cases and found basal cell epithelioma.

Dr. Senear considered it an example of the Bowen type of precancerous dermatosis. The lesion was moist at times and under the use of ointment, the eczematous aspect had cleared up. There was only one lesion in this instance, while in most cases of this superficial rodent ulcer type the lesions were small and multiple.

A CASE FOR DIAGNOSIS. Presented by Dr. Oliver for Dr. Venn.

A woman, aged 36 years, presented lesions on the flexor surface of the right arm. They were said to have been present for five years, and consisted of large, bluish-red nodules and plaques.

DISCUSSION

Dr. Irvine said he thought it was a tuberculous condition.

Dr. Ormsby said he saw this patient at the Clinic about a year ago. The disorder had been active previous to this time but had cleared up almost entirely under potassium iodid. There was no pus. He had asked Dr. Venn to procure a roentgenogram to ascertain the condition of the bones. No report had been received concerning this matter.

Dr. Engman said he thought the diagnosis lay between syphilis, a fungus infection of some kind and tuberculosis. He would not venture a positive diagnosis.

Dr. Oliver said he first saw the patient in the Clinic a year ago. Dr. Venn had asked him to present her at the meeting, but he knew little of her history. He had been told that careful search for the sporothrix had been made, but Dr. Hektoen had not made a positive diagnosis of that disease.

Dr. Pusey said he thought the condition was an infectious granuloma but believed it was not a sporotrichosis because it was too slow and too old. A tuberculous lesion, he thought, would show some sinuses. The large lesion on the arm had a distinct patch of nodules in semicircular form, and Dr. Pusey believed the most likely diagnosis was syphilis of long standing.

Dr. Lieberthal said he saw the patient two weeks previously, and emphasized the point Dr. Pusey called attention to, namely, the two infiltrated ringed lesions on the arm. The infiltration was raised. Dr. Lieberthal considered it a case of syphilid and suggested that the patient be given arsphenamin.

She had received two injections so far and within this short time the infiltration had flattened down considerably. He did not see any reason why the condition could not have been a syphilid at the beginning.

A CASE FOR DIAGNOSIS. Presented by Drs. Senear and Wien.

A Russian, aged 27 years, presented lesions on the scalp which had been present for one and a half years. The first symptom was loss of hair. There was no scaling or seborrhea and no subjective symptoms were complained of. The patient had been in the United States since 1913, and there was no familial history of favus or similar disorders.

DISCUSSION

Dr. Engman thought it was an old favus.

Dr. Pusey did not agree that it was a new favus and thought the patient was misrepresenting the history.

Dr. Senear asked whether it would be possible for the patient to lose his hair at this late day as a result of an old favus.

PEMPHIGUS WITH LESIONS OF THE MOUTH. Presented by Dr. Stillians.

An Italian woman, aged 38 years, had lesions which appeared five days after a severe fright about June 1, 1921. The primary lesions were bullous. Since then the eruption had fluctuated, never entirely clearing. When first seen by Dr. Stillians, in September, 1921, there were areas of deep pigmentation, although she had taken no arsenic so far as he could ascertain. The patient was presented because of the intense pigmentation and marked itching, the latter coming on in paroxysms and being especially severe at night.

DISCUSSION

Dr. Lieberthal said that he accepted the diagnosis.

Dr. Pusey agreed but thought the itching was rather unusual.

Dr. Stillians said that the itching was so severe that the patient often cried out because of it. The patient had received arsenic at varying intervals since September, 1921.

Dr. Ormsby said he thought it might be a case of bullous dermatitis herpetiformis, as the patients he saw with pemphigus rarely complained of itching. He thought it was difficult to place some of these cases properly.

Dr. Oliver recalled the man shown at the annual meeting in January with lesions on the face and an eruption on the body. This disorder was at first thought to be dermatitis herpetiformis because of the marked itching. The patient's condition went from bad to worse and he died early in March, the entire head and body being covered with a pemphigoid eruption. He had not responded to arsenic or any other medication.

PITYRIASIS LICHENOIDES CHRONICA. Presented by Dr. Mitchell.

A boy, aged 8 years, had an eruption which had been present for five months. It appeared suddenly following a hot bath. No abnormal condition aside from that on the skin was present. The eruption was generalized and of uniform type. The lesions were small, oval, yellowish-red maculopapules and papules. They were most numerous about the axillae and cubital region. Slight scaling was present on some of the lesions. There was no urtication, and the mucous membrane showed no change. There was a slight submaxillary adenopathy. All other glands were normal.

Dr. Irvine said he thought the case suggested an urticaria pigmentosa, but the lesions were not papular, and there was no reaction in the skin. Some of the lesions were flat, and he believed it was a case of parapsoriasis.

Dr. Waugh said he thought it was either an urticaria with pigmentation or an urticaria pigmentosa. The lesions did not respond to irritation as they did in cases of real urticaria pigmentosa. He believed there were more lesions present than are usually found in the latter disorder.

Dr. Senear was inclined to consider the case urticaria pigmentosa rather than parapsoriasis, in spite of the lack of the element of urticaria. There was no response to stimulation.

Dr. Pusey said he did not recall any case of urticaria pigmentosa in which the urticarial element could not be elicited. The lesions in this case did not have enough solidity for urticaria pigmentosa. Those lesions are fleshy. even when thin. He thought it was a case of parapsoriasis of the small, macular type.

Dr. Lieberthal agreed with Dr. Pusey.

Dr. Engman also agreed with Dr. Pusey.

Dr. Mitchell said that he saw the case about a week previously. At that time he tried energetically to produce urtication, but none developed. There are cases of urticaria pigmentosa in which the macules predominate. and he thought it was not a case of urticaria with pigmentation. So far as he was concerned the diagnosis rested between urticaria pigmentosa and parapsoriasis of the lichenoid type, probably the latter because of the lack of urtication. The papules did not respond to irritation or stimulation as do those in urticaria pigmentosa. There was desquamation, which is not present in urticaria pigmentosa.

ICHTHYOSIS—GENERALIZED AND SEVERE. Presented by Drs. Ormsby and Mitchell.

A man, aged 23 years, had a disorder which had been present since birth. One sister was similarly affected while two brothers were normal. The symptoms were modified in summer, but recurred each winter. The patient perspired moderately in very hot weather. Moderate itching was present.

The trunk, upper arms and legs were covered with thick quadrilated. keratotic plates. These were more marked on the knees and elbows. The face. neck, areas in the intrascapular region. forearms and hands were comparatively free from lesions. The hair was not much affected with the exception of a moderate alopecia of the presenile type. The patient was shown on account of the extraordinary development of the disorder.

Dr. Pusey asked whether the man was able to go to work: he said that he had never seen such an extensive case.

Dr. Ormsby said the patient could work during the summer without difficulty. The disease was said to be even more marked in one sister. but two brothers were perfectly well.

A CASE FOR DIAGNOSIS. Presented by Dr. Oliver.

An ex-service man, aged 25 years, had a disorder of three years' duration. The lesion was situated on the dorsal surface of the right leg and was spreading, clearing in the center with some scaling at the periphery. There were no subjective sensations, and the lesion had remained practically stationary since first noticed.

DISCUSSION

Dr. Mitchell said he thought it was the brownish-red, somewhat follicular dermatitis seen on the lower extremities, probably extending peripherally, and clearing in the center.

Dr. Oliver asked for suggestions as to treatment. The condition had not changed since he saw the patient the first time, six months ago; and he had no other lesions.

Dr. Lieberthal suggested that the sensations be tested.

NEW YORK DERMATOLOGICAL SOCIETY

Regular Meeting, March 28, 1922

Fred Wise, M.D., *President*

CASE FOR DIAGNOSIS (ENDOTHELIOMA, XANTHOMA, MYOMA?). Presented by Dr. Wise.

M. F., a girl, aged 14 months, presented on the cheeks and the forehead about a score of soft hemispherical tumors, varying in diameter from an eighth to a quarter of an inch (3.1 to 6.3 mm.). The color of some was yellow, as in xanthoma; others had a brownish tinge, like soft pigmented moles; others resembled molluscum contagiosum, but there was no sign of a central umbilication. The lesions first appeared about five months ago. There were no subjective sensations. A biopsy was refused by the mother. The speaker said that the lesions closely resembled those observed by him in a case of endothelioma cutis, which he had reported in the *American Journal of Medical Sciences* **157**:236, 1919.

LYMPHOCYTOMA. Presented by Dr. Howard Fox.

D. P., a 5-year old girl, born of American parents, had an indefinite history of trauma just preceding the appearance of the tumor which had first been noticed about four weeks before. It had gradually increased in size without causing any subjective symptoms. The lesion was a firm, semisolid hemispherical mass, measuring 1¼ inches (3.1 cm.) in diameter and elevated one-half inch (1.2 cm.). The overlying skin was smooth and of a dull reddish color. The mass was freely movable on the deeper parts. The preauricular glands of the right side were enlarged, firm, and not tender. The child otherwise appeared to be in perfect health. An aspirating needle had been introduced into the tumor, but no fluid was found. A piece of tissue at the center of the tumor was excised under local anesthesia, and the following histologic report was given by Dr. Douglas Symmers:

"Microscopic examination shows the appearance of a richly cellular growth which gives the impression of a neoplasmic rather than an inflammatory process. The growth is made up very largely of small round cells of the lymphocytic type. These cells are arranged diffusely, but on occasions are gathered together into small packets as a result of the interposition of minute connective tissue fibrillae. Mitotic figures are not to be seen. Scattered among the small round cells are minute collections of muscle fibers representing, apparently, the remains of erectors of the hair, hair follicles, sebaceous and sweat glands, etc.

"It seems to me that the most reasonable interpretation is that the growth belongs in the group of lymphocytoma. The skin, like numerous other organs of the body, normally contains minute collections of lymphoid cells which come into view only in certain conditions of disease. It is quite possible that this growth arose from such a focus. The age of the patient also favors the view that the growth belongs in the category of the lymphocytomas. In view of the fact that this variety of tumor only rarely metastasizes, it seems to me that the growth is best interpreted as primary in the situation described.

"Histologically, the growth does not impress one as being particularly malignant. Clinically, growths of this sort vary considerably. As a rule, they grow regionally and infiltrate along tissue planes, in this manner producing, oftentimes, great destruction. Radium and roentgen-ray treatment frequently give favorable results.

"Diagnosis: Lymphocytoma."

DISCUSSION

Dr. TRIMBLE remarked that if he had not heard the histologic report, he would call the tumor a sarcoma. He was not familiar with the term lymphocytoma, and he would prefer to make a clinical diagnosis of such a case, and use the microscopic diagnosis as confirmatory or additional. He was strongly inclined to regard the condition as a malignant growth, regardless of the histologic diagnosis.

Dr. WHITEHOUSE said that Dr. Trimble had brought up an important point. If the tumor was a simple lymphocytic growth without an inflammatory element, why was there such a gland condition accompanying it? He had thought of that when he examined the case.

Dr. HIGHMAN said that the term lymphocytoma did not necessarily exclude a superadded inflammatory process. He had never heard precisely that term applied to a neoplasm, but thought that Dr. Symmers was following the teaching of Borst in more accurately determining the terminology of neoplasms, who recognizes fibroma and fibroblastoma, fibrosarcoma and fibroblastosarcoma, etc. Probably Dr. Symmers meant to imply that this was a neoplasm in the sarcoma group which resembled a lymphocyte growth, and he used the term lymphocytoma instead of the more generic and less descriptive term lymphosarcoma. Certainly there was nothing in this tumor which could be included in the concept of leukemia. Dr. Highman said he though, as Dr. Trimble did, that this was obviously a sarcoma, and with the pathologic evidence furnished by Dr. Symmers, one might consider it a sarcoma made up of cells looking like lymphocytes—a lymphocytic sarcoma. Malignancy, after all, was a relative concept.

Dr. WISE concurred with Dr. Trimble in thinking that the tumor was a sarcoma, and said he would disregard the histologic report with reference t treatment. If he had ever seen a sarcoma, this was one. As for the prognosis, the child would probably die within a year, of metastases.

Dr. Howard Fox said that from his recent observation of this patient he thought sarcoma the most likely diagnosis. The histologic diagnosis of lymphocytoma was arrived at by Dr. Symmers after considerable study. As to treatment, he intended to give an intensive, filtered roentgen-ray application.

Dr. Trimble said he wished to bring out one point without any disparagement of pathology in general: He did not think that dermatologists should defer altogether to a microscopic report. If a man had had many years of clinical experience, and perhaps two or three other clinical observers shared his opinion, they should not all give up and regard the matter as settled because one piece of tissue which had been examined microscopically was reported to show a condition different from that revealed by the clinical diagnosis. That did not always settle it, for after one had had a number of biopsies made it would be found that the chances of a mistake by the pathologist were greater than those by the clinician. Dr. Trimble did not believe that one pathologic examination settled a question.

Dr. Highman said that in the main he agreed with what Dr. Trimble had said, and felt that the trend of dermatology was to rely too much on histopathology; but in the diagnosis of tumors the aid of the microscope was greater than in ordinary dermatoses, and a report like that of Dr. Symmers was of great value in directing attention to the nature of the growth. The fact that he did not mention sarcoma did not necessarily rule it out.

Dr. Howard Fox said that the child was to report to him the next day, and he would have expert surgical advice.

Dr. Wise expressed the opinion that surgery was contraindicated.

Dr. Whitehouse said that he did not favor surgical treatment of this case. Dermatologists generally agreed that even the taking of a biopsy was questionable policy, for there was danger of spreading the disease rather promptly. A sarcoma like this one would yield to radiation, a lymphosarcoma being more amenable to it than some of the hemorrhagic varieties. In his opinion it was wrong to treat them surgically. Neither would save the patient's life, but with radiation one could remove the local lesion, and he had seen some patients live a good while afterward; whereas if excised they were likely to terminate promptly by metastasis.

Dr. Bechet, referring to the surgical treatment of sarcoma, cited the case of a man who came to him seven or eight years previously with a papillomatous-like lesion on the ear. It was not melanotic, and he had clipped it off, and thoroughly curetted and cauterized its base. Six or seven years later the patient was well, and he had had no recurrence. Dr. Highman had kindly made a histologic examination, and had reported that the lesion was a sarcoma.

Dr. Howard Fox asked what the other members thought about the propriety of making a biopsy in this case, as someone had raised this question. He appreciated fully the seriousness of the condition, and would like to know whether they thought he had done right in making a biopsy.

Dr. Trimble said he thought that Dr. Fox had done right in making the biopsy.

Dr. Highman said he thought that Dr. Fox had done right in making the biopsy. Dr. Highman, referring to the case of sarcoma cited by Dr. Bechet, said that there were two reasons why the treatment might have been harmless: First, not all sarcomas were malignant; and second, it was possible that he had made a mistake and that the condition was not a sarcoma.

MONILETHRIX IN MOTHER AND TWO CHILDREN. Presented by Dr. Wise.

These three patients had been presented before the Society previously, and their histories will be found in the article on "Monilethrix" by Drs. MacKee and Rosen in the *Journal of Cutaneous Diseases,* July, 1916, p. 506, and June, 1916, p. 444. One of the children had received a depilating dose of roentgen rays, but when the hair grew there was no improvement in the condition. Other forms of treatment had been of no avail. One other child, a brother of the two children, had normal hair growth.

LICHENOID SCLERODERMA GUTTATA. Presented by Dr. Wise.

E. N., a girl aged 10, presented two distinct groups of lesions. One group was situated just above the manubrium sterni, in the hollow formed by the junction of the clavicles; the other group, about half an inch (1.2 cm.) below the upper, overlying the manubrium. Each group was composed of from thirty to forty millet-seed sized, smooth, rounded, glistening papules, the color of which was slightly lighter than that of the normal surrounding skin. There were no subjective symptoms. The lesions had been present for four years. There was no evidence of lichen planus. The speaker referred to two similar cases observed at the Vanderbilt Clinic, one of them reported by Dr. Rosen and himself (Further Observations on So-Called White Spot Disease, *J. Cutan. Dis.* **35**:66 [Feb.] 1917).

DISCUSSION

Dr. Trimble agreed with the diagnosis, but said the child was 10 years old, and he would be inclined to take into consideration the possibility of the condition being due merely to enlarged sebaceous glands. He had seen a number of such cases in which they were scattered over the chest and one could almost see them through the skin. The fact of the somewhat linear arrangement in this case, however, led him to agree with the diagnosis.

Dr. Whitehouse agreed with the diagnosis, and said he had seen several such cases; the lesions were usually confined to the region of the clavicles or base of the neck.

Dr. Wise said that they had two such cases at the Vanderbilt Clinic, and the microscope showed scleroderma.

FOR DIAGNOSIS: PREMYCOSIS? Presented by Dr. Bechet.

Y. H., a woman, aged 60, born in Hungary, came to the Skin and Cancer Hospital stating that an eruption had appeared on her back and legs seven months previously. There had been a rapid increase of the lesions since that time. She had circinate, infiltrated, pruriginous patches scattered over the body; some of the lesions seemed moist, but on closer inspection were absolutely dry—not the slightest evidence of the presence of vesicles or bullae could be found. There was a slight tendency to grouping. The itching was severe, and some of the lesions were noticeably infiltrated. The histologic examination showed slight hyperkeratosis, parakeratosis, acanthosis, and lengthening of the papillary processes of the derma almost to the stratum corneum, showing congestion of the capillaries with a cellular exudate of mononuclear, small, round cells and of endothelioid cells. This exudate was also present in the superficial derma. There were scattered pigmented cells through these regions at some points. The basal cell layer of the epidermis was encroached on by the exudate, so that the line of demarcation between the derma and epidermis was lost.

DISCUSSION

Dr. WHITEHOUSE said he believed it was mycosis fungoides.

Dr. HIGHMAN said that the gross clinical features suggesting Duhring's disease might indicate leukemia, but he thought the condition was mycosis.

Dr. KINGSBURY thought it was mycosis fungoides.

Dr. HOWARD FOX thought this case was probably one of early mycosis fungoides. He felt that our conception of the disease needed revising. We were accustomed to think of mycosis fungoides as a comparatively rare disease terminating fatally in the fungoid stage. We had of late years seen a large number of cases in which the diagnosis of the prefungoid stage was made, but the number of cases with fungating lesions was extremely small. It would seem that either many erroneous diagnoses had been made or that the number of cases terminating fatally was small.

Dr. TRIMBLE said that though his opinion seemed at great variance with that of the other speakers, he was inclined to view the case as one of pemphigus. This opinion was based on the fact that he had seen two or three such cases that eventually developed into pemphigus. It seemed that deep down in the skin there was some evidence of moisture. The lesions on the chest and back of patients with cases like this on a cursory examination bore a slight resemblance to seborrheic eczema. He thought the case would reveal itself as pemphigus in the near future, probably pemphigus foliaceus.

Dr. WISE agreed with the suggestion of pemphigus, and told of two cases which suggested seborrheic eczema for years, and then suddenly both patients developed pemphigus. Both cases undoubtedly began with clinical lesions indistinguishable from the lesions of seborrheic eczema.

Dr. BECHET said that he had been watching the patient carefully for several weeks and had at first considered the possibility of dermatitis herpetiformis; yet at no time had he been able to observe either moisture or vesiculobullous lesions. Some of the lesions were quite infiltrated and sharply defined. They were very pruritic. The diagnosis of premycosis seemed therefore more tenable. On the other hand, one observed so many cases that were called premycosis, and so few in the advanced stages of the disease, that the conclusion was almost forced that many of the cases of so-called premycosis were not mycosis but some other condition; or that mycosis fungoides was not the severe or fatal disease one had been led to believe in the past.

MULTIPLE TELANGIECTASES FROM EXPOSURE TO EXCESSIVE DEGREES OF HEAT. Presented by Dr. WISE for Dr. STEINKE.

S. K., a man, aged 43, married, born in Poland, a laborer, had been employed in a large oil refinery plant for fourteen years. The duration of the eruption was said to be about ten years.

F. B., a man, aged 39, married, born in Poland, had been working in the same plant fifteen years. The duration of the eruption was said to be four years.

I. Z., a man, aged 44, married, born in Poland, had been working in the same plant for twelve years. The duration of the eruption was said to be ten years.

These three men were employed as "cleaners," their work consisting of scraping away a deposit of carbonaceous matter from the inner surface of oil-refining stills, where they were exposed to great heat. They said that they worked in brief shifts, as it was impossible to remain in the interior of the stills for a prolonged period.

The description of the lesions applies equally to the three men. From the waist line to the face the skin presented numerous more or less scattered telangiectatic macules, varying in size from a sixteenth to a half inch (1 to 12 mm.) in diameter. They were flat, smooth, free of scales, and their color varied from bright pink to purple. Similar lesions were scattered over the upper extremities; only a few were on the face. Some of the vascular spots appeared to be ordinary capillary telangiectases, which disappeared under the diascope with slight pressure; others were distinct venous telangiectases, the branching venules being plainly visible to the naked eye, and these resembled "spider" nevi. The men were exposed to the waist during their work. The parts of the body covered by clothing presented no abnormalities. None of them had epistaxis or other hemorrhages. The mucosae were free from lesions. The speaker suggested the title "telangiectases ab igne" for these eruptions.

DISCUSSION

DR. WHITEHOUSE said that the cases were unique and interesting. The condition was apparently a new form of occupational disease.

DR. HIGHMAN said that they were remarkable cases. It seemed, however, that in addition to the mechanical elements in the occupation of these men that might produce the lesions, one should take into consideration a possible toxic inflammation of the capillaries from whatever chemical elements there might be in their environment. He did not know whether or not the various coal tars, when absorbed, would cause vascular disease, but one could not rule out either mechanical or toxic factors.

DR. HOWARD FOX said that the Society was indebted to Dr. Steinke for enabling them to see three cases of a new occupational disease. It was remarkable to see three cases presenting lesions that were so similar in appearance and distribution.

DR. WISE said that one of the patients presented had said that there were 175 men in the factory with the same kind of lesions. The point made by Dr. Highman was of interest. If these were due to ordinary exposure to heat, why did not stokers have the same condition, for those on warships were exposed to intense heat?

DR. WHITEHOUSE said that these men worked in a relatively small, enclosed space, while stokers did not, which might account for the difference in susceptibility of the two classes of workers.

LUPUS MILIARIS DISSEMINATUS FACIEI. Presented by DR. WISE.

Miss E. G., colored, aged 25, was presented before the Society several years ago, under the same title. Since then the lesions had increased considerably in numbers and in size. A photograph and history of the patient was published in the ARCHIVES OF DERMATOLOGY AND SYPHILOLOGY in an article by Wise and Satenstein entitled "Clinical and Histologic Features of Certain Types of Cutaneous Tuberculosis," July, 1921, p. 586. At one of the other dermatologic societies a controversy had arisen with reference to the identity of lupus miliaris faciei and Barthelemy's acnitis. The speaker contended that these were two entirely different diseases, clinically and histologically. These differences were clearly enunciated in the article referred to. In support his views, the speaker quoted verbatim from Lewandowsky's work on cutaneous tuberculosis, and said that since this authoritative author was a pupil of Jadassohn's, and since his (the speaker's) views on the subject were founded mainly on the work recently done in the laboratory by Dr. Satenstein and himself, his opinion remained unaltered despite the views expressed by others. Briefly stated, acnitis is the deep form of papulonecrotic tuberculid, situated on the face, and almost always associated with folliclis, the superficial form of papulonecrotic tuberculid, occurring on the arms and the hands. The histologic structure is usually that of an ordinary inflammatory reaction; on rare occasions a "tuberculoid" structure is encountered, and still more rarely an occasional tubercle bacillus. Lupus miliaris disseminatus faciei occurs on the face exclusively. It is a lupus vulgaris in spots, and the histologic structure is that of a tuberculoma. Tubercle bacilli have been demonstrated in the lesions.

DISCUSSION

DR. HOWARD FOX agreed with the diagnosis of disseminated miliary lupus. He also agreed with the chairman's conception of the present disease as opposed to acnitis. He did not think, however, that in all cases the differential diagnosis between lupus and acnitis was easy. This point was illustrated by the divergent opinions on a case recently presented before another dermatologic society as one of acnitis.

DR. HIGHMAN did not understand how the two conditions could be confused by students. Telangiectatic acne was a well recognized subvariety of lupus vulgaris disseminatus; whereas acnitis had nothing in common with the other condition. The conditions did not look alike clinically or histologically. One lesion was that of tuberculosis and the other was a tuberculid.

DR. TRIMBLE agreed with the diagnosis and with Dr. Wise's conception of the condition, though he thought there was considerable misunderstanding about the two terms. The term acnitis used by Barthelemy to describe a certain form of tuberculid was fairly well known, though miliary disseminated lupus vulgaris was not so well understood, and in his opinion the latter term was confused quite often. He did not think the various textbooks were as clear as they might be in regard to the last named disease. They were two perfectly distinct clinical entities, but in general they were not well understood.

DR. LANE agreed with Dr. Wise's conception of folliclis, acnitis and miliary lupus.

CASE FOR DIAGNOSIS (ACNE CACHECTICORUM?). Presented by DR. WISE.

M. L., single, a girl aged 20, had been presented previously before the Academy of Medicine. She said that the eruption had been present, with periods of remission and exacerbation, since infancy. She presented a large number of deep-seated scars, situated chiefly on the forehead and the back and arms. On the last named areas there were a few scratched, inflamed papules. The scars on the back were well-defined, and their surfaces were distinctly cribriform. There was distinct pruritus during the stage of active eruption. The condition had improved considerably under roentgen-ray treatment. The speaker thought that the most likely diagnosis was acne cachecticorum.

Dr. Highman said that the point which impressed him was the curious atrophic nature of the lesions with the patulousness of the follicles in the involved areas. The total impression was that of an inflammatory process leading to atrophy, analogous to lupus erythematosus. If the lesions were on the scalp one would not hesitate to make a diagnosis of pseudopelade, and he rather wondered if it was not an atrophy secondary to an unknown type of folliculitis, probably similar to that which occurred in pseudopelade.

Dr. Bechet thought the case was slightly suggestive of dermatitis herpetiformis. There seemed to be much itching, as the tops of some of the papules had been scratched off. There seemed also to be a slight tendency to grouping. The scars, however, were typical of a resolved tuberculoderm.

Dr. Trimble was inclined to consider the condition an atypical tuberculid, and that the patient was 50 per cent., almost 100 per cent., a "picker."

Dr. Highman said that if it were not for the lesions on the back he would agree with Dr. Trimble.

Dr. Lane said that when he first saw the lesions on the arm he had the same thought that Dr. Trimble had just expressed; but some of the scars on the back were almost like vaccination scars—wheel shaped, with distinct radiations from the center. This form of scar did not impress him as resembling that of pseudopelade, which is usually quite irregular. He had also never seen scars of this appearance following self-inflicted trauma.

A CASE FOR DIAGNOSIS: PROBABLE ACRODERMATITIS CHRONICA ATROPHICANS (HERXHEIMER). Presented by Dr. Whitehouse.

E. R., a woman aged 26, presented an eruption which began three and a half years before, and now involved the upper and lower extremities, particularly pronounced about the elbows and knees, palms and backs of the hands, with slight evidences on the chest and face. The lesions consisted of a diffuse dermatitis with slight scaling, but accompanied with telangiectasia and diffuse superficial hemorrhagic lesions with distinct atrophy. There were few or no subjective symptoms; the progression was slow.

IDIOPATHIC ATROPHY OF THE SKIN. Presented by Dr. Whitehouse for Dr. Clark.

W. F., a man aged 21, born in America, a clerk, first noticed the present lesions a year before, when he was asked about them by a physician. These lesions were forgotten until one month ago when a physician again asked him about them, and he decided then to try to find out what they were.

The lesions had never caused him the least discomfort and he did not know whether they had or had not increased in size, or whether any new patches were forming. He was quite sure that none of them were ever infiltrated, like scleroderma, for he would have noticed this while bathing. On examination the patient presented patches of cutaneous atrophy of greater or less size, sharply localized, and with the superficial veins showing clearly throughout the areas. The lesions were on the right side of the body and back of the right shoulder, giving the impression of nerve arrangement such as in herpes zoster distribution. There was, however, one lone patch on the left side of the lower lumbar region. The patient's general health was good, and, as stated, he complained of no local symptoms.

LEUKOPLAKIA IN A NEGRO. Presented by Dr. Howard Fox.

J. B., aged 39, a porter, born in the United States, a full blooded negro, had recently applied at the Harlem Hospital for treatment of nodular syphilis at the corners of the mouth. The Wassermann test was strongly positive, and the eruption had promptly disappeared under treatment with neo-arsphenamin. He was presented on account of a moderate amount of typical leukoplakia affecting chiefly the buccal mucosa near the angle of the mouth. The disease was also present in a mild form on the sides of the tongue. He was not aware of having been infected with syphilis. He had always been a heavy smoker, chiefly of cigarets. He had been a moderate drinker.

LEPRA (TWO CASES). Presented by Dr. Bechet.

J. R., a man aged 38, born in Russia, came to the Skin and Cancer Hospital stating that he had first noticed the eruption six years before. He had been living in New York for sixteen years. The case was of the mixed type, presenting various sized macules over the trunk, and tubercles and nodules on the arms, particularly about the elbows. The face already presented leonine changes. The ulnar nerves were markedly enlarged.

J. C., a man aged 42, a Sicilian, stated that he first noticed the eruption fifteen years before. He had lived twenty-one years in the United States, with the exception of a six months' trip to his home in Sicily ten years previously. The eruption was of the macular type and consisted of various sized noninfiltrated patches of a brownish color and rounded contour, distributed generally over the trunk. They were numerous, and a few on the back were markedly anesthetic. The face presented no changes. The ulnar nerves were enlarged. There were no subjective sensations. The Wassermann test was positive.

TUBERCULOSIS OF SKIN. Presented by Dr. Schwartz.

M. C., a man aged 48, born in Holland, a butcher, complained of an eruption of ten months' duration on the right buttock. This had spread slowly, and itched slightly. He had had diabetes for three years. He had had a chancre twenty years before, but gave no history of secondary syphilis. On the left buttock was a large lesion 5 inches (12.7 cm.) from above downward and 3 inches (7.6 cm.) wide, made up of a slightly scaly middle zone surrounded by a border which was elevated, dark red and scaly. Just above this main lesion there were two small tubercles. General examination showed the presence of diabetes. The Wassermann test was negative. The urine showed a strong reaction for sugar, and the blood sugar was 250 mg. per hundred c.c. Histologically the lesion was a chronic granuloma, made up of many lymphocytes and a few small giant cells. The lesion did not respond to roentgen-ray therapy.

DISCUSSION

Dr. Whitehouse said that according to the man's description the condition began around the anus. It was tuberculosis developing from the mucous surface.

Dr. Trimble said he would not hesitate to call it syphilitic had it not been questioned by the men present, for whose views he had a high opinion. A lesion of such characteristic appearances should be regarded as syphilitic regardless of the Wassermann test, or even its histology. The test that would prove the diagnosis in this case was the therapeutic, not the Wassermann test nor the microscopic examination. Further study would bring forth the proper diagnosis, of course; but viewing the case for the first time as presented, so far as he could see there was not one sign of any form of tuberculosis that he was familiar with.

DR. HOWARD FOX said he could not refrain from repeating what he had recently said, namely, that cutaneous syphilis and tuberculosis were at times almost indistinguishable clinically. He was certain that the serpiginous character of the eruption did not rule out tuberculosis, as he had seen a number of such cases. In his opinion the present case was one of tuberculosis, and it seemed quite possible that its origin might have been in an ischiorectal abscess.

DR. WISE agreed with what Dr. Fox said.

DR. SCHWARTZ said that he had seen the case for the first time that day, and could only report that the histologic examination revealed chronic granuloma of the skin, probably tuberculosis, and that the Wassermann test was negative. The patient had not received syphilitic treatment. He recognized, of course, that a negative Wassermann test did not exclude syphilis, but he agreed with Dr. Fox that the two conditions were easily confused, and he cited another case which he at first thought to be syphilis and in which the histologic report was quite confusing. That patient was put on antisyphilitic treatment without any result whatever; later guinea-pig inoculation showed that he had tuberculosis. This patient would be given arsphenamin and mercury.

MINNESOTA DERMATOLOGICAL SOCIETY

April Meeting

JOHN BUTLER, M.D., *Chairman*

SCHAMBERG'S PIGMENTARY DERMATOSIS. Presented by DR. OLSON.

A man, aged 32, had received mercury and arsphenamin injections for syphilis during the last year. Seven months ago a follicular eruption was noted occurring in circumscribed areas over the shins and inner aspect of the ankles. The lesions at the onset were definite follicular papular lesions resembling in color spots of cayenne pepper. There was considerable inflammatory reaction. Within a few weeks the lesions became confluent in some areas and showed some scaling. They healed slowly and were followed by pigmented spots. The patient remained under treatment for syphilis, with no untoward results from arsphenamin and mercury, although he believed that the lesions were somewhat worse while the mercury salicylate injections were being continued.

PSORIASIS (EXFOLIATIVE DERMATITIS). Presented by DR. IRVINE.

R. M., a man, aged 40, first seen in April, 1917, had had psoriasis for seventeen years and had just recovered from an exfoliative dermatitis which confined him to the hospital for nearly six months. He was free from the condition for short periods after this, but the eruption was again becoming general. At this time he responded well to diet, baths and mild ointments. Until the spring of 1921 he remained comparatively free from the condition by following a low protein diet. During the winter of 1921 his skin cleared up under sun exposures in Colorado, and then indiscretion in diet was followed by recurrence. He was seen in March, 1921, and during the next two or three months the condition improved but was not cured, and in the latter part of April the patient lost weight and became very weak and short of breath. Examination by an internist revealed no organc trouble, but the patient was put on full diet. The lesions became worse and the roentgen-ray was resorted to in an effort to clear them up. The patient went to Arizona and tried sun baths without much improvement; he then went to Los Angeles, and was under Dr. Frost's care again. He was confined to the hospital with exfoliative dermatitis for nearly two months. The thymus was treated with roentgen rays. He returned to Minneapolis the latter part of February; lesions were again appearing. He made some progress on diet, baths and mild salves, but after two weeks he began to lose weight and felt weak; then suddenly the exfoliative dermatitis started again, and only a few small patches on the legs and hands remained free. The rest of the body was affected, including the scalp, face, palms and soles. On March 18 treatment was begun with the violet ray. Improvement began at once, and during eighteen days he improved remarkably and lost no time from his work. During the course of his disease the patient had received almost every kind of treatment, including removal of sources of focal infections. He was presented on account of his resistance to treatment, because he had had three attacks of exfoliative dermatitis and finally on account of the marked benefit to the entire body from the violet ray.

CASE FOR DIAGNOSIS. Presented by Dr. Odland.

A girl, aged 9, who was born in the United States, two and one-half months ago developed a small scaly spot on the scalp. A home antiseptic had been applied, and about a month later the family physician had prescribed salve. Since then, six weeks ago, the hair had been falling out rapidly, beginning as a small spot progressively enlarging at the periphery. At the time of presentation there were several areas, round to oval, the larger being 5 cm. in diameter. They were covered with gray scales, the deeper scales being quite adherent to the underlying epidermis. There was no apparent hyperemia nor any signs of inflammation, and a few lusterless hairs remained in the areas. Several examinations for fungi had proved negative.

DISCUSSION

There was general agreement that the condition was ringworm, in spite of negative microscopic findings.

PITYRIASIS LICHENOIDES CHRONICA. Presented by Dr. Michelson.

A trained nurse presented a diffuse, scaling reddish-brown macular and papular eruption, situated on the arms,, chest, abdomen and legs. She stated that the eruption appeared three years ago following injections of typhoid vaccine. She had been treated by the presenter a year ago with heliotherapy, which brought about a complete disappearance of the lesions, but they gradually returned. On presentation the predominating lesions were of the papular, psoriasiform type. The Wassermann reaction had been negative twice.

MYCOSIS FUNGOIDES (PREMYCOTIC STAGE). Presented by Dr. Butler.

A farmer, aged 47, who had always lived in Minnesota, first noticed an eruption on the leg in March, 1921. It was at that time 1 inch (2.5 cm.) in diameter, red and flat. Within a few weeks similar spots had appeared on the arms, then on the back, over the shoulders, then on the chest and later on the back of the neck. At first there had been only moderate itching, but during the latter part of the summer the spots had become thicker and padded in appearance, spreading peripherally; they were accompanied by itching, preventing sleep at night. The patches became thicker and scaly. The older patches had begun to clear up at the sixth month, leaving a white clear skin, while new patches were forming continuously. When presented he had lesions on the trunk, neck, arms, legs, abdomen and penis; the hands and face were free with the exception of a new lesion on the forehead. The lesions were multiform, large, irregular, raised, padded plaques, showing erythema and scaling. Microscopic section showed marked acanthosis and a diffuse exudate of small round cells of the lymphoid type in the subpapillary layer of the corium. Intermingled with these were imperfectly developed connective tissue cells and occasional irregularly shaped giant cells with centrally placed nuclei.

CASE FOR DIAGNOSIS (ADULT URTICARIA PIGMENTOSA). Presented by Dr. Gager.

A single man, aged 28, had had an eruption on the trunk for several years. The individual lesions began as an erythematous spot which progressed to a papule and after several weeks became a pigmented macule. 0.25 cm. in diameter. The pigmented macules were scattered over the body and had existed for over four years, new ones appearing constantly. A diagnosis of syphilis had been made from chancre four years ago. The patient was treated for over a year, and there was no apparent relation between the present skin condition and the syphilitic infection. No subjective symptoms accompanied this skin condition.

DISCUSSION

Dr. Olson said that he thought the condition was clinically urticaria pigmentosa, because these pigmentary macules became edematous and were palpable after rubbing. A section would show mast cells if this were the condition.

Dr. Irvine said he did not feel that he could definitely make a diagnosis of urticaria pigmentosa because the lesions were too small and there was no itching.

Dr. Michelson said that itching did not necessarily accompany urticaria pigmentosa, and he asked to have a pathologist's report at the next meeting. (At a later meeting it was reported that mast cells were present, and it was agreed that the diagnosis was urticaria pigmentosa.)

BROMODERMA TUBEROSUM. Presented by Dr. Odland.

E. E., a woman, aged 36, when presented had several large tuberous lesions on both legs. The lesions were purplish, vegetating and covered with thick crusts, and were of one year's duration. She had suffered from epilepsy for many years, and had taken large doses of bromids.

LINEAR NEVUS. Presented by Dr. Turnacliff.

EPITHELIOMA, MULTIPLE IN SCAR TISSUE. Presented by Dr. Turnacliff.

A man, aged 45, born in Holland, at the age of 4 had had some destructive process on the right side of the face and down below the chin, leaving a scar of irregular margin with some scaling. An accurate history was not obtainable, but apparently since early childhood he had had some scaling on this area, and three years ago new lesions began to appear at the margin and within the scar itself. At the time of presentation there were five lesions 0.75 cm. in diameter and one 1.5 cm. in diameter, which were raised, ulcerating and with a regular margin covered with a heavy crust. The Wassermann reaction was negative. From the appearance of the scar and the lesion a clinical diagnosis of epithelioma in an old lupus vulgaris scar was made. Sections had been made but were not ready.

DISCUSSION

Dr. Butler remarked that the scar did not have the usual corded appearance of an old lupus vulgaris scar, and from the warty appearance of the lesion he felt that tuberculosis verrucosis cutis should be considered.

Dr. Wright did not feel that a definite opinion as to the cause of the scar could be given, but clinically it was an epithelioma on an old scar tissue. (Section showed squamous cell carcinoma.)

PEMPHIGUS CHRONICUS. Presented by Dr. Freeman.

A man, aged 65, who had always been in good health, noticed some spots under his arms six months ago. Two months ago bullae had developed on the forearms and later lesions had appeared on the face and body and in the mouth. There had been intense itching when the lesions appeared. When first seen by the presenter he had had several bullae on the forearm and one cheek and one on the back, as well as several crusted lesions.

GRANULOMA ANNULARE. Presented by Dr. Sweitzer.

A girl, aged 4, when presented had an annular lesion on the right wrist and one over the knuckle of the left hand. They had begun some months ago, appearing first on the leg. The older lesions had disappeared at the time of presentation.

CHRONIC URTICARIA. Presented by Dr. Sweitzer.

COPAIBA ERUPTION. Presented by Dr. Sweitzer.

SEBORRHEIC DERMATITIS. Presented by Dr. Sweitzer.

Miss S., aged 26, when presented had a scaly eruption on the face, arms, axilla, parts of the trunk, and practically all of the lower extremities. The hands and feet showed that the skin was very much thickened. Her legs were edematous. The patient said that the eruption had started in November, 1921, with a swelling on the eyelids, and had spread over the face and later began to involve the body and extremities. Itching was quite severe at times. Blood examination showed a mild anemia and an increase in the eosinophils. The urine and heart were normal.

D. D. Turnacliff, M.D., Secretary.

Index to Current Literature

DERMATOLOGY

Leg. Twenty Cases of Ulcer of the Leg Treated by Electrical Methods. C. A. Robinson, Arch. Radiol. & Electroth. **26**:253 (Jan.) 1922.

Leprosy, Rat, Studies on. M. Uchida, Japan Med. World **2**:4 (Jan.) 1922.

Leukoderma, Case of. N. Ghosh, Indian M. Gaz. **57**:100 (March) 1922.

Lipoma of Finger. Martin and Grenier, Paris méd. **12**:303 (April 8) 1922.

Lupus Erythematosus. J. M. H. MacLeod. Practitioner, London **108**:236 (April) 1922.

Lupus. Tuberculin Treatment in Extensive Lupus. W. Bohme, Wien. klin. Wchnschr. **35**:180 (Feb. 23) 1922.

Lupus. "Tuberculin Treatment in Extensive Lupus," Reply. M. Strassberg, Wien. klin. Wchnschr. **35**:181 (Feb. 23) 1922.

Lymphogranuloma, Malignant. I. Allende, Semana méd. **1**:321 (March 2) 1922.

Lymphogranulomatosis. H. von Hecker and W. Fischer, Deutsch. med. Wchnschr. **48**:482 (April 14) 1922.

Melanotic Growths; Researches of Alterations in Melanoblastic Layer of Vertebrates Explain Structure and Origin of These Growths. H. W. Acton, Indian J. M. Res. **9**:464 (Jan.) 1922.

Oidiomycosis: Coccidioidal Granuloma: Cutaneous Blastomycosis. C. R. Burkhead, Kansas M. Soc. J. **22**:101 (April) 1922.

Oriental Sore, Cutaneous Herpetomonas. Note on Behavior of Herpetomonas Tropica Wright, the Parasite of Cutaneous Herpetomonas (Oriental Sore) in the Bed Bug Cimex Hemiptera Fabr. W. S. Patton and S. Rao, Indian J. M. Res. **9**:240 (Oct.) 1921.

Oriental Sore, Non-Ulcerated, Histopathology of. J. W. Cornwall, Indian J. M. Res. **9**:545 (Jan.) 1922.

Oriental Sore Problems and Kala-Azar. W. S. Patton, Indian J. M. Res. **9**:496 (Jan.) 1922.

Penis. Epithelioma of Glans Penis: Report of Case. R. C. Lonsberry, Missouri State M. A. J. **19**:176 (April) 1922.

Radiodermatitis, Professional. P. Degrais, Paris méd. **12**:293 (April 8) 1922.

Roentgen Rays in Dermatology. H. C. Semon, Practitioner, London **108**:259 (April) 1922.

Roentgen-Ray Skin Reactions, Relation of Temperature Changes to. C. L. Martin and G. T. Caldwall, Am. J. Roentgenol. **9**:152 (March) 1922.

Scarlet Fever in Adults. C. Saloz and P. Schiff, Bull. de l'Acad. de méd. **87**:386 (April 4) 1922.

Scarlet Fever in Rome. P. Sorgente, Policlinico, Rome **29**:353 (March 13) 1922.

Scarlet Fever Problems. K. Kisskalt, Klin. Wchnschr. **1**:181 (Jan. 21) 1922.

Sclerema Neonatorum. A. Brinchmann, Norsk Mag. f. Lægevidensk. **83**:269 (April) 1922.

Skin, Arsenical Pigmentation of. D. W. Montgomery and G. D. Culver, Med. Rec. **101**:655 (April 22) 1922.

Skin in Relation to Tuberculosis Immunity. W. Böhme, München. med. Wchnschr. **69**:306 (March 3) 1922.

Skin Manifestations in Hemoblastosis. Martinotti, Tumori **8**:448 (March 15) 1922.

Skin, Multiple Nodular Tumors in. G. Spremola, Riforma med. **38**:202 (Feb.) 1922.

Skin Reactions, Roentgen-Ray. Relation of Temperature Changes to. C. L. Martin and G. T. Caldwell, Am. J. Roentgenol. **9**:152 (March) 1922.

Skin, Relations of, to the Whole Organism. B. Bloch, Klin. Wchnschr. **1**:153 (Jan. 21) 1922.

Skin. Reticulation in Normal Human Skin. H. Homma, Wien. klin. Wchnschr. **35**:149 (Feb. 16) 1922.

Skin. Tabes Dorsalis Plus Tertiary Cutaneous Syphilis. B. Barker Beeson, J. A. M. A. **78**:1537 (May 20) 1922.

Smallpox and Vaccination. G. Dock, Missouri State M. A. J. **19**:163 (April) 1922.

Smallpox, Treatment of, in Its Last Stage. R. L. Fraser, Arkansas M. Soc. J. **18**:220 (April) 1922.

Tongue, Actinomycosis of. G. B. New and F. A. Figi, Am. J. M. Sc. **163**:507 (April) 1922.

Tuberculosis Immunity, Skin in Relation to. W. Böhme, München. med. Wchnschr. **69**:306 (March 3) 1922.

Ulcer of Leg, Twenty Cases of, Treated by Electrical Methods. C. A. Robinson, Arch. Radiol. & Electroth. **26**:253 (Jan.) 1922.

Xanthoma Diabeticorum: Report of Case. D. M. Lyon, Edinburgh M. J. **28**: 168 (April) 1922.

SYPHILOLOGY

Anesthesia, Wassermann Reaction After. L. Domenici, Policlinico, Rome **29**: 92 (March 20) 1922.

Arsenical Pigmentation of the Skin. D. W. Montgomery and G. D. Culver, Med. Rec. **101**:655 (April 22) 1922.

Arsphenamin and Its Limits. Lehnhoff-Wyld, Ann. d. mal. vén., Paris **17**:261 (April) 1922.

Arsphenamin Death with Cerebral Symptoms. Henneberg, Klin. Wchnschr. **1**:207 (Jan. 28) 1922.

Arsphenamin, Endolumbar Injections of. L. Fuchs, München. med. Wchnschr. **69**:271 (Feb. 24) 1922.

Arsphenamin, Jaundice After. G. Stümpke, Med. Klin. **18**:295 (March 5) 1922.

Arsphenamin Plus Calcium Therapy in Syphilis. Pulay, Deutsch. med. Wchnschr. **48**:223 (Feb. 16) 1922.

Arsphenamin Questions. Arndt, Med. Klin. **18**:226 (Feb. 26) 1922.

Bismuth in Treatment of Syphilis. P. de F. Parreiras Horta and P. Ganns. Brazil-med. **1**:81 (Feb. 18) 1922.

Bismuth to Promote Tolerance of Mercury. A. Stagnetto López, Semana méd. **29**:315 (Feb. 23) 1922.

Bismuth Treatment of Syphilis. Jeanselme and Blamoutier, Bull. méd. **36**:317 (April 22) 1922.

Bladder, Syphilis of. P. Ghiso and J. J. Puente. Semana méd. **1**:426 (March 16) 1922.

Bones, Long, Inherited Syphilis of. L. A. Tamini, Rev. Asoc. méd. argent. **34**: 1702 (Dec.) 1921.

Calcium Plus Arsphenamin in Syphilis. Pulay, Deutsch. med. Wchnschr. **48**: 223 (Feb. 16) 1922.

Chancres, Extragenital, Prevention of, in the Army, Based on Study of Syphilitic Registers on File at Army Medical Schools. J. S. Lambie. Mil. Surgeon **50**:261 (March) 1922.

Chancres, Soft, Protein Therapy for. L. M. Bonnet and P. Juvin, Lyon méd. **131**:91 (Feb. 10) 1922.

Chondrocalculosis. Inherited Syphilis with Separation of Epiphyses and Chondrocalculosis. M. Divella, Policlinico, Rome **29**:143 (March 1) 1922.

Diabetes Insipidus, Syphilitic. J. Lhermitte, Ann. de méd. **11**:89 (Feb.) 1922.

Epiphyses. Inherited Syphilis with Separation of Epiphyses and Chondrocalculosis. M. Divella, Policlinico, Rome **29**:143 (March 1) 1922.

Eye. Ocular Manifestation of Syphilis. E. F. Garraghan, Illinois M. J. **41**:272 (April) 1922.

Gate and Papacostas' Formol-Gel Test for Syphilis, Reliability of. as Compared with Wassermann Reaction. S. Ramakrishnan. Indian J. M. Res. **9**:620 (Jan.) 1922.

Gumma, Syphilitic, of the Ovary. Von Kubinyi and Johan. Zentralbl. f. Gynäk. **46**:57 (Jan. 14) 1922.

Hydrarthrosis, Syphilitic. J. Montpellier and A. Lacroix. Ann. d. mal. vén. Paris **17**:294 (April) 1922.

Jaundice After Arsphenamin. G. Stümpke, Med. Klin. **18**:295 (March 5) 1922.

Keratitis, Antisyphilitic Treatment of. Langendorff. Deutsch. med. Wchnschr. **48**:290 (March 2) 1922.

Meinicke and Sachs-Georgi Tests. L. Philippson, Policlinico, Rome **29**:155 (March 1) 1922.
Meinicke and Nonspecific Wassermann Reactions. K. Bauer, Wien. klin. Wchnschr. **35**:173 (Feb. 23) 1922.
Meningitis, Febrile Syphilitic, Case of. Bock, Med. Klin. **18**:340 (March 18) 1922.
Mercury. Bismuth to Promote Tolerance of Mercury. A. Stagnetto Lopez, Semana méd. **29**:315 (Feb. 23) 1922.
Mercurial Treatment, Valvular Insufficiency Develops Under. G. Causade and A. Foucart, Bull. Soc. méd. d. hôp. de Paris **46**:437 (March 10) 1922.
Neo-Arsphenamin, Late Accident Due to. Van Winsen, Arch. méd. belges. **75**: 121 (Feb.) 1922.
Neo-Silver-Arsphenamin in Neurosyphilis. G. L. Dreyfus, München. med. Wchnschr. **69**:268 (Feb. 24) 1922.
Neo-Silver-Arsphenamin, My Experiences with. E. Galewsky, München. med. Wchnschr. **69**:352 (March 10) 1922.
Neurosyphilis, Latent, Case of. C. I. Urechia, Ann. de méd. **11**:158 (Feb.) 1922.
Neurosyphilis, Neo-Silver-Arsphenamin in. G. L. Dreyfus, München. med. Wchnschr. **69**:268 (Feb. 24) 1922.
Neurosyphilis, Some Present-Day Opinions Concerning. J. D. Gable, Florida M. A. J. **8**:164 (March) 1922.
Neurosyphilis, Treatment of. H. J. Farback, Kentucky M. J. **20**:235 (April) 1922.
Ovary, Syphilitic Gumma of. Von Kubinyi and Johan, Zentralbl. f. Gynäk. **46**:57 (Jan. 14) 1922.
Pigmentation, Arsenical, of the Skin. D. W. Montgomery and G. D. Culver, Med. Rec. **101**:655 (April 22) 1922.
Precipitation Reactions in Syphilis. A. Sordelli and C. E. Pico, Rev. Asoc. med. argent. **34**:1651 (Dec.) 1921.
Protein Therapy for Soft Chancres. L. M. Bonnet and P. Juvin, Lyon méd. **131**:91 (Feb. 10) 1922.
Sachs-Georgi and Meinicke Tests. L. Philippson, Policlinico, Rome **29**:155 (March 1) 1922.
Sachs-Georgi Test. J. Parthasarathy, M. M. Barratt and J. C. G. Ledingham, Brit. M. J. **1**:594 (April 15) 1922.
Spermatozoa of Syphilitics. V. Widacowich, Rev. Asoc. méd. argent. **34**:1564 (Dec.) 1921.
Spirochaeta Pallida, Microbiology of. P. I. Elizalde, Rev. Asoc. méd. argent. **34**:1455 (Dec.) 1921.
Spleen, Syphilis of. A. Furno, Policlinico, Rome **29**:123 (March 1) 1922.
Striate Body Syndrome of Syphilitic Origin in the Elderly. J. Lhermitte and L. Cornil, Presse méd. **30**:289 (April 5) 1922.
Syphilis, Bismuth in Treatment of. P. de F. Parreiras Horta and P. Ganns, Brazil-med, **1**:81 (Feb. 18) 1922.
Syphilis, Bismuth Treatment of. Jeanselme and Blamoutier, Bull. méd. **36**: 317 (April 22) 1922.
Syphilis, Campaign for Prevention of. A. W. Stillians, Illinois M. J. **41**:268 (April) 1922.
Syphilis, Comparative Serodiagnostic Tests for. A. Versari, Riforma méd. **38**: 175 (Feb. 20) 1922.
Syphilis: Course in Venerologic Technic. M. Joseph, Deutsch. med. Wchnschr. **48**:491 (April 14) 1922.
Syphilis, Early, Treatment of. G. A. Rost, Med. Klin. **1**:175 (Jan. 21) 1922.
Syphilis, Early, Treatment of. G. A. Rost, Klin. Wchnschr. **1**:223 (Jan. 28) 1922.
Syphilis, Etiology and Social Prophylaxis of, in Argentina. G. Sirlin, Semana méd. **29**:101 (Jan. 19) 1922.
Syphilis, Flocculation and Turbidity Reactions in. E. Meinicke, Deutsch. med. Wchnschr. **48**:219 (Feb. 16) 1922.

Archives of Dermatology and Syphilology

VOLUME 6	AUGUST, 1922	NUMBER 2

DERMATOLOGIC TRAINING AND PRACTICE *

OLIVER S. ORMSBY, M.D.

CHICAGO

The annual meetings of the American Dermatological Association are the milestones on which are inscribed the results of the year's activities in scientific research. The high standard set by the founders of this Association has been maintained by the diligent work of their successors. The responsibility of presiding at this, the forty-fifth annual session, is keenly realized and words cannot convey to you my deep appreciation of the honor you have conferred on me. The brilliant record of achievement of the Association has been recorded by my predecessors, so I shall today briefly discuss two topics that have occupied much of my thought for some time.

In the past there has been no organized effort to train men in the practice of dermatology and syphilology. The major portion of the men now engaged in this practice selected the method of acquiring their knowledge themselves. Some began as assistants to established dermatologists and added to their knowledge later by doing work abroad in the various European clinics, and continued their education by attaching themselves to the teaching institutions at home. In fact, a great factor in the education of many of the men now engaged in this practice has been the teaching of undergraduate students. Another important factor in the continued development of many men has been the local dermatologic society. The educational value of the clinical meetings of these societies is high, and the advancement of American dermatology is shown by the number of new societies organized comparatively recently. The dermatologic group probably gains more through its society meetings than any other group in medicine. There are at present ten such societies in this country, having a total active membership of 250.

During the past seventeen years many facts have been added to our knowledge which have materially changed the practice in our particular field of medicine. Before the discovery of *Spirochaeta pallida* and the

---

* President's address, read at the Forty-Fifth Annual Meeting of the American Dermatological Association, Washington, D. C., May 2-4, 1922.

complement-fixation test for syphilis, the diagnosis of this disease was made solely by examination of the patient and the lesions present. Often the evidence was meager and much skill was required to arrive at proper conclusions. There is no doubt, however, that the responsibility of having to rely on this examination produced careful and accurate observers. On the other hand, little mechanical equipment and no assistance, human or otherwise, was required. With the discovery of arsphenamin added difficulties arose. The use of vaccines, roentgen therapy, radium therapy, phototherapy and other electrotherapeutic measures, including electrolysis and fulguration, still further complicated matters.

If all these diagnostic and therapeutic measures are carried out in a single office, assistants become necessary. This requirement is valuable in two ways. First, it keeps all the work under single supervision and therefore the component parts can be better correlated; and second, it serves the useful purpose of giving special training to young men wishing to enter this field.

At present there are approximately 300 men practicing dermatology and syphilology in this country. This number will probably be increased in the future somewhat more rapidly than it has been in the last twenty years, for several reasons. First, the recent war demonstrated to a number of the younger men in the service the broad scope of this special field and created a desire for more to enter it than had hitherto done so. Second, the establishment of group practice, which, in spite of much opposition, is growing, will call for more men especially trained to enter these groups. Finally, as we as a nation grow older, specialization in all departments of activity increases, and this will add to our field as it will to all others.

There are approximately 148,800 physicians now practicing in this country. With 300 in our field, our present proportion is 1 to 500. This year 2,700 will be added to the general field through graduation from the various colleges. This is much below the normal average, as this class entered college as we were entering the war. If we maintain our proportion, nine would need to be added, six to maintain the general average and three on account of retirement and mortality. A total of nine added this year would keep up the present average. It would, therefore, appear that the addition of eighteen dermatologists annually would be ample to supply the demand, even with the possible new requirements. From a survey of the present facilities in this country it appears that this number can be adequately trained with a moderate amount of reorganization in some institutions. A few are now so organized, and the adequacy of the training is well shown by the character of the work now being done by the young men trained in dermatology and syphilology.

The importance of graduate instruction is now generally recognized, and recently at the seventeenth annual conference of the Council on Medical Education and Hospitals, committees representing the various specialties made recommendations for training men in their respective departments. The following was the report submitted by Dr. Pusey, chairman of the committee on dermatology and syphilology:

GENERAL TRAINING

As a preliminary to taking up the practice of dermatology and syphilology, the student should have, after graduation, at least one year in a general hospital with either a service in internal medicine, or a rotating service in which internal medicine and the medical specialties are the chief part. General medicine and neurology play such an important part in this specialty that one year in a general hospital must be regarded as an absolute minimum. An internship of two years is not an excessive preliminary general training and an internship followed up by a general practice for a few years—not more than five—makes the best preliminary training for this specialty.

It is desirable that the student should graduate from a Class A medical school; that he should have a reading knowledge of French and German; and that as an intern he should have had some work in general pathology, particularly in mortuary pathology.

SPECIAL TRAINING

Clinical Training.—Familiarity with skin diseases and the ability to differentiate them requires visual memorizing of a large number of clinical pictures. It is, therefore, the first essential for the dermatologist to have an opportunity to see an extensive dermatologic material. This can be obtained in two ways: First, as an assistant in a hospital or dispensary which has an abundance of dermatologic cases; or, second, exceptionally, with a specialist of established ability in dermatology who has a large amount of skin disease and syphilis in his practice. This assistantship should not be in a place where there are less than a thousand new cases of skin disease and syphilis a year.

Laboratory Training.—This opportunity for the clinical study of skin diseases and syphilis is the first essential of training in this specialty. The next and not less important, in order to make a thorough dermatologist, is a proper laboratory training in this specialty, and a training in the technic of treatment. This training should be obtained at the same time as, and in connection with, his clinical training. A minimum requirement for laboratory clinical training should include a working knowledge of cutaneous pathology and bacteriology, ability to recognize and demonstrate the bacteria and the animal and vegetable parasites that are commonly found in the skin. With these should be included a working knowledge of the dark field and at least a theoretical knowledge of the Wassermann reaction.

TRAINING IN PRACTICE OF DERMATOLOGY

He should become familiar with the technic of diagnosis and treatment of skin diseases, including the therapeutic use of roentgen rays and radium, and the various dermatologic procedures. He should be trained in the intravenous administration of drugs and the performance of spinal punctures.

For the training which it will give him in exactness, in the thorough study of clinical and laboratory material, in the use of literature and in other ways, he should be encouraged, during the last half year of his training, to do a piece of research work in some subject in dermatology or syphilology. The simplest form, and perhaps the best for the beginner, is the thorough working up of one, or a group of, unusual cases.

It is assumed that the training outlined is to be obtained either as an intern or as an assistant in a hospital or dispensary, or with a specialist in dermatology or syphilology, where the student is an actual participant in the work and is not simply an observer.

TIME REQUIREMENTS

The length of time necessary for such training depends on the opportunities of the student, his industry, and his ability. It must be long enough for him to become well grounded in the essentials of dermatologic training as outlined, if he is to be made competent to proceed independently on his special career after this training. For an adequate training of this kind two years is a reasonable time; for a thorough seasoned training three years should be given.

CERTIFICATES

If an authoritative responsible body can be devised to give the student, after examination, a certificate of efficiency in this specialty, it may be desirable that he be given such a certificate. But certificates are a cheap form of distinction, easily imitated and open to many abuses, and there are many safeguards that should be thrown around the giving of certificates in the specialties. If such a course as outlined in the foregoing is given by a university it might well be recognized by a degree or a diploma which should be a Master's degree or a degree of Doctor of Philosophy—not something new. A thorough course leading to such a degree in dermatology and syphilology should be not less than three years in duration, and the university giving it should have not only adequate laboratory facilities for giving the course, but also adequate clinical facilities; and there are few universities which can at the present time meet these requirements. For adequate training in this specialty at the present time opportunities are afforded chiefly by a few university clinics, a few special hospitals, a few hospitals with special departments and in the practice of established specialists.

The foregoing suggestions were concurred in by the committee and accepted by the conference, and they will serve as a guide for those on whom will rest the responsibility of providing this instruction in the future.

FACILITIES FOR DERMATOLOGIC TRAINING

The question now confronting us is, Are these facilities sufficiently available to meet the requirements and furnish enough men for the work in this country? It would have to be answered in the affirmative, with the reservation that some reorganization would be necessary. All that will be required is for members of this Association to take advantage in their various localities of the unorganized material to make it available for this particular instruction.

In the institution with which I have been connected for some years, postgraduate instruction on a rather large scale is to be undertaken in all departments of medicine and surgery soon, and a part of this instruction will include the training of specialists. Naturally, the number of men trained as specialists will be few, as they cannot be instructed through lectures, recitations and clinics in the way the ordinary medical student is taught the science of medicine. The instruction here will be in the form of practical work in the departments as assistants under the supervision of capable instructors. With clinical facilities such as exist at Rush Medical College and the Central Free Dispensary, four students could be properly trained in our department in a two years' course. On the completion of this course some kind of degree, not special, could be given. For students wishing to remain an extra year, special work, including teaching, will be arranged. and on its completion a more advanced degree will probably be offered. The first two years may be divided into four periods of six months each:

1. Laboratory work.
2. Clinical dermatology and radiotherapy.
3. Clinical syphilology and treatment of syphilis.
4. Investigative work and paper.

During the portion of the course devoted to laboratory work sufficient time will be allowed for the student to become fairly familiar with the histopathology of the skin. A large number of examinations for *Spirochaeta pallida* will be a part of the work, as well as a sufficient number of examinations for ringworm fungi, *Acarus scabiei*, and other vegetable and animal parasites, to make the student familiar with the work. The selection of proper material for examination from infected patients is important, and this work also will be done by the student.

In the clinical department the study of individual diseases will be made by the writing of a clear history and description of the lesions found. This work will include the examination of several patients daily over a period of six months. From our standpoint it is essential that radiotherapy be understood from practical experience in this department, and considerable time is necessary to acquire proper knowledge. In the early part of the work the treatment will always be given under the direct supervision of the instructor. Later, independent work will be done.

In the section on syphilis individual cases will be studied as noted in the foregoing for the department of dermatology. and in addition a large number of intravenous and intramuscular injections will be administered by the student, in addition to practical experience in intraspinal therapy.

During the last six months a piece of investigative work will be undertaken in addition to some of the routine work outlined.

It is obvious that when such a plan is in operation the work in a large outpatient clinical department can be successfully carried on with a comparatively small teaching force.

No mention has been made of post-graduate instruction for practitioners of medicine, the so-called "brush up courses," as the present discussion concerns only the training of men as specialists.

The question of having an examining board for dermatology and syphilology to issue certificates to competent men should be studied further. The Board of Ophthalmic Examiners has been functioning for several years and has accomplished much. Such certificates have no legal value, but they represent professional attainment and can be made a valuable asset.

DERMATOLOGIC PRACTICE

During the last several years the question of the position of syphilology, both in the curriculums of colleges and in practice, has been largely settled by its being attached to the department of dermatology. There are, however, some contingencies arising in practice that are worthy of our consideration. Within the last two years a group of highly respected business men has organized an institution for the treatment of venereal diseases, which has been a successful enterprise. They did this on the assumption that the venereal disease problem was not being adequately handled, and some of them having had war experience, where they saw this problem handled in wholesale fashion, decided to put similar methods into operation in civil life to help eradicate, or at least control, these diseases. On their continued success will probably depend the organization of similar institutions in various localities throughout the country. How far this will go and to what extent it will affect this particular practice can only be conjectured.

The great disadvantage placed on the medical profession is readily shown by the phenomenal growth of the institution mentioned, which obtains a large portion of its patients through advertisements in the daily press.

Through the activities of many organizations, both lay and professional, the problem of venereal disease has assumed a public character which is upsetting the relation of the medical profession to this class of patients. A public opinion is being formed that demands a different method of dealing with this problem, and it may be well for the medical profession to recognize this and act accordingly. If an organized attack is to be made on venereal disease through more comprehensive and efficient treatment, this should be done by physicians and not by groups of business men. The possibilities of what can be done by laymen are well illustrated by the example quoted. The method of procedure whereby the medical profession may accomplish the desired result is not clear at present, but the problem merits our careful study and consideration.

There has been much agitation recently concerning the practice of medicine in all departments, and apparently this has only begun. Group practice, pay clinics, and the time honored general practitioner have been chiefly discussed. That this unrest will affect us all to some extent, there seems to be no doubt, but no matter what the outcome may be, specialties will continue, and it is perfectly right and proper that they should, as progress in scientific medicine would be greatly curtailed if intensive work were not done by specially trained groups. The outlook for our own specialty is bright. The opportunities for the development of a school of American dermatology in the future are good. American contributions have received little recognition abroad, while foreign contributions have been welcomed and studied intensively here. This gives us advantages that are important and favorable for our development. The large amount of original research being done here is illustrated in the ARCHIVES OF DERMATOLOGY AND SYPHILOLOGY, which is now being so admirably managed by Dr. Pusey and his collaborators. Institutions and individuals are collecting facilities and are arranging methods whereby much more will be done in the near future. The time is not far distant when men will be trained just as well here as elsewhere, and the scientific contributions will have such merit as to command the respect of the whole scientific world. The comparatively large number of young men now earnestly working for the advancement of our knowledge, the large amount of work already accomplished by the older members whose ideals for American dermatology have always been of the highest character, together with the several institutions and societies devoted to this work, place American dermatology on an unassailable and firm foundation.

SEROLOGIC STUDIES ON THE EXUDATE OF SYPHILITIC CHANCRES *

CESAR FUENTES. M.D

HAVANA, CUBA

When an animal is inoculated with a pathogenic bacillus a struggle occurs at the site of inoculation between the toxin secreted by the foreign bacteria or their endotoxin and a cellular element—phagocytes and white cells—and its secretions, that is, between antigens and antibodies. In other words, besides histologic changes and the appearance of substances not existing before, biochemical changes occur due to the presence of new cells.

In a general way this is what happens in infections with the usual bacterial organisms. Now let us consider what happens when *Spirochaeta pallida* is inoculated into man or experimental animals. The organism spreads through the capillaries in large numbers. We find the bacilli in the blood capillaries as well as in the surrounding spaces, and undoubtedly new substances—lipoids—appear from the cells in the tissue which has borne the noxious action of *Spirochaeta pallida*. The invading bacillus and the cell products then pass into the lymph and blood circulation.

In the case of man, *Spirochaeta pallida* invades the body chiefly through the lymphatic vessels, although it is possible that the organisms may also do so through the blood stream. It is believed that they struggle against the different barriers offered by the lymphatic system until they overcome them, when they enter the general circulation, which carries them to every part of the organism. They establish foci in the different tissues toward which they display some degree of tropism. In the tissue in which they develop, the same cell reaction occurs and identical chemical substances are produced.

It is therefore easy to understand why, in the period of primary inoculation, it is not possible to demonstrate the presence of the lipoids in the blood. This is due to the fact that only one focus, the chancre, is available, and here they do not develop in an amount sufficient for detection in the blood stream. When the general invasion is at its height, however, the number of local foci becomes enormous, the blood stream is flooded with these bodies, and it is easy to demonstrate them. The Wassermann test enables us to prove their presence.

We know that the blood of patients with secondary syphilis has the power of deviating the complement because of the presence of

* From the Calixto Garcia National Hospital Laboratories and the Covadonga Sanatorium.

bodies which, when in their colloidal stage, carry an electric charge equal (but with different tension) to that of the other lipoid used as antigen in the test. While this is an established fact, the source of these substances has only been surmised.

The statement that their source lies in the foci in which spirochetes develop is a theoretical conception. This led us to undertake our experimental work to find out whether it was possible to demonstrate these complement-binding substances in the exudate of chancres, that is, in the foci of *Spirochaeta pallida.* The Wassermann test enabled us to demonstrate this fact.

When we began our efforts to find a practical and simple way to stain the spirochetes, it was observed that many chancres, after serum had been expressed, still exuded fluid to such an extent that it was possible to obtain over fifteen samples, while in some favorable cases the fluid came out spontaneously. The fluid was therefore present. Our problem was to measure it, as otherwise it would have been impossible to make a complement-fixation test without the possibility of gross errors.

The amount of fluid necessarily is very small, so that the usual quantities of 0.1 and 0.2 c.c. used in the routine Wassermann test were not applicable in this case. Therefore, it was necessary to adjust the proportions to the amount of exudate available, in such a way that there would always be the same proportion of antigen, fluid in which the amboceptor was sought, complement and hemolytic system.

As it was not intended to determine the quantity of amboceptor and antigen contained in the fluid from the chancres, but only to demonstrate their existence or nonexistence, we employed the usual proportions used in our Wassermann tests. Had they been too large or too small, they would have been submitted to further investigation.

In any liquid in which it is intended to demonstrate the presence of amboceptors, it is necessary to determine three things: first, whether it is hemolytic in itself; second, whether it has any anticomplementary power in the quantities used in the test; and third, its specific power.

Before recording the final notes for this study, we carried out a series of preliminary tests in order to determine the hemolytic power. We assumed that a chancre fluid would contain complement since all body fluids contain it. After determining its existence, we ascertained whether the quantity would be sufficient to influence the test.

It is evident that heating the fluid to 56 C. (132 F.) would have been sufficient for our purpose, namely, the demonstration of the presence of amboceptors; but as we were working on an unknown subject, and as it was possible that the quantity of amboceptors might be very small, the destruction of complement through exposure to the temperature mentioned might bring about a decrease in the quantity of amboceptors.

DETERMINATION OF HEMOLYTIC POWER

In order to ascertain whether there was complement or not, we took two parts of complementary fluid from a chancre. In one tube we placed two parts of chancre fluid mixed with ten parts of sensitized sheep cells. We placed this in the incubator at 37 C. (98.6 F.) and made readings every fifteen minutes.

In the other tube we placed one part of antigen, two parts of the fluid to be examined, one half part of complement and after half an hour's incubation we added ten parts of sensitized cells.

In the first tube, both after intervals of two hours and twenty-four hours, we noted only slight hemolysis.

In the second tube we discovered no hemolysis in thirty minutes or in two hours. This showed that the complement or the substance, whatever it might be, which had stained slightly the supernatant fluid, did not interfere with the test.

In both these tubes the quantity was brought up to 0.1 c.c. with saline solution.

DETERMINATION OF ANTICOMPLEMENTARY POWER

As regards the demonstration of the anticomplementary power, it may be stated that if each of the tubes of the routine Wassermann test is compared with those used in our investigation of the chancrous fluid, it will be evident that the components of the various tubes are not identical; in fact, in the routine Wassermann test, the first tube contains saline solution, antigen, patient's serum and complement, and in the second, saline solution, patient's serum and complement but no antigen. The inhibition of hemolysis in the first tube shows that the serum contains a complement-binding substance, completing the chain of antigen, complement and amboceptor, while there will be no hemolysis at all in the second tube. This inhibition of hemolysis in the second tube shows that the patient's serum must contain a complement-binding substance, and therefore there is anticomplementary power.

In the case of a Wassermann test with the chancre exudate, it is not possible to give the same interpretation to this second tube, since, besides the amboceptor, there is a substance that acts as an antigen, and through the fixation of the complement, we will have a second tube without hemolysis. The presence of this antigen has been demonstrated in the ten cases in which it was investigated.

It is evident, then, that we cannot state that there is anticomplementary power when there is no hemolysis in the second tube, and therefore we cannot make a determination of the anticomplementary power under such conditions.

Both in the syphilitic chancre and in the serum from it, there are the three elements that form the specific system of the Wassermann test, namely, antigen represented by the spirochetes themselves or substances derived from them, amboceptor from the chancre cells, and the complement found in all body fluids.

As stated, our study is concerned with the first two elements, antigen and amboceptor, especially the latter. The method followed for this study of the amboceptor was to make the Wassermann test, adjusting the reagents to the amount of serum available. As regards the antigen, we used the serum of a proved syphilitic patient selected from among those found positive in our weekly tests, complement and the fluid to be examined.

In cases in which we did not have a sufficient quantity for both tests we studied the amboceptor alone. If among the cases reported there is not a larger number of antigen tests, it is because we did not have on hand a serum probably syphilitic and a normal serum.

METHOD OF STUDY

In this investigation the following procedure was followed: (1) a clinical diagnosis of the chancre was made; (2) a bacteriologic diagnosis; (3) an investigation of the amboceptor; and (4) an investigation of the antigen.

In the clinical diagnosis of the chancre we considered: age, number, pain, induration, readiness with which the exudate came out, amount of swelling and use of local treatment. In doubtful cases the patient was questioned as to the history of previous syphilitic infections.

Bacteriologic Diagnosis.—This is made by dark-field examination and through impregnation with silver nitrate, using a modification of Fontana-Tribondeau's method. The dark-field examinations were made by Dr. Alberto Recio. The silver nitrate impregnations were made by the author, and they always agreed with the results reported independently by Dr. Recio.

Two or three specimens were examined under the microscope. As to the reliability of this silver salt staining method of the spirochete, it is enough to recall the papers published so far on Fontana-Tribondeau's technic, important modifications such as Hollande's, and our own personal experience with its use, including a comparative statistical table with dark-field examinations in which both results harmonized. This work was done last year.

In our study we depended on clinical diagnosis of the chancre and bacteriologic demonstration of *Spirochaeta pallida*, besides the determination of antigen and amboceptor. In these experiments we employed as control: first, normal serum; second, syphilitic serum; and third, hemolytic system.

As the immense majority of the cases referred to the laboratory were clinically specific, we were swamped by the enormous quantity of positive results in spite of controls. We tried, therefore, to study some chancres that seemed clinically negative. These showed the same agreement between clinical and serologic results as clinically specific chancres.

TECHNIC

Collection of Material.—All patients who came to the laboratory had stopped their daily local treatment the day before the exudate was collected, and had washed the lesion with sterile water or saline solution only. If the chancre presented an adherent crust, this was removed and the lesion squeezed. After discarding the serum obtained in the first two or three expressions, some time elapsed before collection in order that the chancre might be covered with fluid.

In those types of chancre that did not present a depression but a smooth or protruding surface, we pressed the sides with the finger, creating in this way a fold, at the bottom of which was the chancre, from which we aspirated the fluid.

Chancres in the frenulum caused most difficulty because of their painfulness.

Material.—The following material was employed: (1) Tubes 0.5 cm. wide and 6 cm. long, of domestic manufacture, made of glass and closed by the flame at one end. As these tubes have a triangular bottom the column of fluid used in the test seems higher than it actually is. (2) A device to collect and measure the fluid; we used Potain's mixer because it has a calibrated capillary tube. (3) The usual 1 c.c. pipets divided into tenths. (4) Cover glasses and slides for the examination of the spirochetes.

This procedure was followed: Five tubes were used in each test, one for the antigen, the second one for the amboceptor and the three others as controls, holding, respectively, known syphilitic serum, known normal serum and the hemolytic system. Therefore we used practically two tubes for each patient, in one of which was placed one tenth of saline solution. In the antigen tube there was placed one or two units of serum measured in the capillary portion of Potain's mixer, one or two units of syphilitic serum and one half or one fourth unit of complement.

In the amboceptor tube, we placed one part of antigen and one or two parts of serum and complement, and, after keeping in the incubator for thirty minutes at 37 C. (98.6 F.), added five or ten parts of red cells, the quantity depending on whether one fourth or one half unit of complement was used.

In the control tube of syphilitic serum were placed one part of antigen, two of serum and one half or one fourth unit of complement. In the normal serum the same quantities were used and in the hemolytic system tube, one fourth unit of complement. In the normal serum the same quantities were used. Finally, in the hemolytic system tube, one fourth unit of complement was used to five units of red cells, one half unit of complement or the required amount according to the use of either five or ten parts of red cells.

The total number of experiments was twenty, only nineteen of which are taken into consideration since in one a technical error was suspected. As we were unable to check this experiment, we have discarded the results.

In the nineteen experiments were found ten clinically positive chancres, six clinically negative chancres, one clinically mixed chancre, two clinically doubtful chancres, six with *Spirochaeta pallida*, eleven with amboceptor and nine with antigen.

REPORT OF CASES

CASE 1.—E. M. had one chancre, located in the balanopreputial sulcus. It was hard and painless and secretion oozed readily. There was specific bilateral gland enlargement. The patient had received fifteen injections of red mercuric iodid.

TABLE 1.—OBSERVATIONS IN CASE 1

Spirochetes						
Dark-Field Negative	Staining Negative	Antigen Positive	Amboceptor Positive	Syphilitic Serum Positive	Normal Serum Negative	Hemolytic System 1v
5 in 0.1 C.c.						5 in 0.1 C.c.
Exudate........................... 5				Exudate........................... 5		
Antigen........................... 5				Syphilitic Serum................... 5		
Complement....................... 1¼				Complement....................... 1¼		
Red cells.......................... 25				Red cells.......................... 25		
Result: Hemolysis 0–30–60				Result: Hemolysis 0–30–60		

CASE 2.—S. G. had a slight induration of the glans: it secreted pure lymph with relative difficulty. Bilateral enlarged glands were present. Previous gonorrhea had been insufficiently treated.

TABLE 2.—OBSERVATIONS IN CASE 2

Spirochetes					
Stain Negative	Antigen Positive 30v and 60v	Amboceptor Positive 30v and 60v	Syphilitic Serum Positive 30v and 60v	Normal Serum Negative 12v	Hemolytic System 1v
Exudate........................... 3/4				Exudate........................... 3/4	
Antigen........................... 1				Syphilitic serum.................. 1	
Complement....................... 1/2				Complement.......................	
Red cells.......................... 10				Red cells..........................	

CASE 3.—S. G. had a chancre in the meatus which was hard and painless, discrete and oozed readily.

TABLE 3.—OBSERVATIONS IN CASE 3

Spirochetes					
Stain	Antigen	Amboceptor	Syphilitic Serum	Normal Serum	Hemolytic System
Positive	....	Positive	Positive	Negative	10ʹ

Exudate............................	3	Comment: After 24 hours in the incubator the same result was obtained as after 20 minutes
Antigen............................	1½	
Complement........................	½	
Red cells...........................	10	

CASE 4.—The patient had a phagedenic chancre of the urethra which was hard and painless and oozed readily.

TABLE 4.—OBSERVATIONS IN CASE 4

Spirochetes					
Stain	Antigen	Amboceptor	Syphilitic Serum	Normal Serum	Hemolytic System
Positive	....	Positive ++ 60ʹ	Positive 60ʹ	Negative	10ʹ

Exudate............................	9	
Antigen............................	4½	Comment: After 24 hours the same result was obtained as after 30 minutes.
Complement........................	½	
Red cells...........................	10	

CASE 5.—R. S. The patient had: a slightly indurated lesion in the left groove, bilateral enlarged glands, periadenitis on the left side, with hard mobile glands, painless, of fifteen days' duration. There was a discrete rash on the chest. The blood Wassermann test was positive. The patient was hemophilic. Some years ago the Wassermann test had been negative.

TABLE 5.—OBSERVATIONS IN CASE 5

Spirochetes					
Stain	Antigen	Amboceptor	Syphilitic Serum	Normal Serum	Hemolytic System
Positive	Positive ++++ 30ʹ and 60ʹ	Positive ++++ 30ʹ and 60ʹ	Positive ++++ 30ʹ and 60ʹ	Negative	10ʹ

Exudate............................	1	Exudate............................	1	
Antigen............................	1	Syphilitic serum....................	1	
Complement........................	½	Complement........................	½	
Red cells...........................	10	Red cells...........................	10	

CASE 6.—E. G. had a slightly indurated chancre in the meatus. which was 4 days old. There was hardly any secretion.

TABLE 6.—OBSERVATIONS IN CASE 6

Stain Negative	Spirochetes			Syphilitic Serum Positive ++++ 30′ and 60′	Normal Serum Negative	Hemolytic System 1·′
	Antigen Positive ++++ 30′ and 60′	Amboceptor Positive ++++ 30′ and 60′				

Exudate.........	¼	Exudate...........................	¹₁
Antigen............................	1	Syphilitic serum....................	2
Complement.......................	½	Complement........................	¹½
Red cells...........................	10	Red cells...........................	10

CASE 7.—J. M. had a chancre on the frenulum and one on the balanopreputial sulcus; the chancres had indurated bases. The one chosen was 15 days old and painless. The patient had bilateral adenitis. There was no history of gonorrhea or treatment for syphilis.

TABLE 7.—OBSERVATIONS IN CASE 7

Stain Negative	Spirochetes			Syphilitic Serum Positive ++++ 30′ and 60′	Normal Serum Negative	Hemolytic System 10′
	Dark-Field Negative	Antigen Positive ++ 30′ and 60′	Amboceptor Positive +++ 30′ and 60′			

Exudate.........	1	Exudate.........	1	Comment: The investigation was repeated
Antigen..........	1	Syphilitic serum.	1	in 48 hours, on amboceptors, using the
Complement......	½	Complement.....	½	same quantities. The result was —+—.
Red cells.........	10	Red cells.........	10	In 2 hours hemolysis was almost complete; the same result was obtained in 4 hours. Hemolysis complete in 8 hours.

CASE 8.—C. G. had only one chancre on the frenulum. It was 8 days old. somewhat painful and indurated. It oozed readily. Bilateral adenitis was present.

TABLE 8.—OBSERVATIONS IN CASE 8

Stain Negative	Spirochetes			Syphilitic Serum Positive — — — 30′ and 60′	Normal Serum Negative	Hemolytic System 1·′
	Dark-Field Negative	Antigen	Amboceptor Positive ++++ 30′ and 60′			

Exudate...	3
Antigen...	1½
Complement..	1½
Red cells..	1·

CASE 9.—A. I. had a chancre on the foreskin with a virulent serum coating and slight induration, discrete, not very painful, 20 days old, which oozed readily. The patient had a few not very enlarged inguinal glands. There was no history of gonorrhea. Local treatment had been given.

TABLE 9.—OBSERVATIONS IN CASE 9

Spirochetes						
Stain Negative	Dark-Field Negative	Antigen	Amboceptor Negative 10′	Syphilitic Serum Positive 30′ and 60′ ++++	Normal Serum Negative	Hemolytic System 10′

Exudate...	2
Antigen..	1
Complement...	½
Red cells..	10

CASE 10.—A. G. had a chancre on the balanopreputial sulcus. It was slightly indurated, not very painful, oozed readily, and was 5 days old. Two or three glands in both groins were enlarged.

TABLE 10.—OBSERVATIONS IN CASE 10

Spirochetes						
Stain Negative	Dark-Field Negative	Antigen Negative 10′	Amboceptor Negative 10′	Syphilitic Serum Positive 30′ and 60′	Normal Serum Negative 10′	Hemolytic System 10′

Exudate............................	1	Exudate............................	1
Antigen............................	1	Syphilitic serum....................	1
Complement........	½	Complement........................	½
Red cells...........................	10	Red cells...........................	10

CASE 11.—J. G. had four chancres on the margin of the foreskin. He had congenital phimosis, gonorrhea and suppurating right adenitis. The chancres were painless, indurated and discrete. The chancre selected was 20 days old, oozed readily, and had an indurated and somewhat painful base.

TABLE 11.—OBSERVATIONS IN CASE 11

Spirochetes						
Stain Negative	Dark-Field Negative	Antigen 30′ and 60′ Positive ++++	Amboceptor 30′ and 60′ Positive ++++	Syphilitic Serum 30′ and 60′ Positive ++++	Normal Serum Negative	Hemolytic System 10′

Exudate............................	2	Exudate............................	2
Antigen............................	1	Syphilitic serum....................	1
Complement........................	½	Complement........................	½
Red cells...........................	10	Red cells...........................	10

CASE 12.—I. M. had one chancre, with a slightly indurated base, somewhat painful, 8 days old, which had been treated with peroxid and phenol during five or six days. He had had a chancre four years ago and another ten years ago. Three years ago he injected into himself two doses of neo-arsphenamin, 0.6 and 0.75 gm., respectively. Later, he took red mercuric iodid. There was no enlargement.

TABLE 12.—OBSERVATIONS IN CASE 12

		Spirochetes				
Stain Negative	Dark-Field Negative	Antigen Positive ++++ 30′ and 60′	Amboceptor Negative	Syphilitic Serum Positive ++++ 30′ and 60′	Normal Serum Negative	Hemolytic System 10′
Exudate......... 1		Exudate......... 1		Comment: This test was made on a very busy day. The test was made together with Test 14. We were unable to check it. It is believed an error was made.		
Antigen......... 1		Syphilitic serum. 1				
Complement..... ½		Complement..... ½				
Red cells......... 10		Red cells:........ 10				

CASE 13.—E. G. had one chancre, an indurated, painless, balanopreputial sulcus, 8 or 10 days old. He had received treatment for four days. There was specific bilateral gland enlargement.

TABLE 13.—OBSERVATIONS IN CASE 13

		Spirochetes				
Stain Positive	Dark-Field	Antigen Positive +++ 30′ + 60′	Amboceptor Positive ++++ 30′ +++ 60′	Syphilitic Serum Positive ++++	Normal Serum Negative	Hemolytic System 10′
Exudate......... 2		Exudate......... 2		Comment: Eight days later the chancre was still suppurating profusely. However, pure lymph was obtained. The test was repeated, yielding identical results. No spirochetes were found the second time. He had already received 0.3 gm. of neo-arsphenamin, and local treatment during twelve days.		
Antigen......... 1		Syphilitic serum. 2				
Complement..... ½		Complement..... ½				
Red cells......... 10		Red cells......... 10				

CASE 14.—M. F. had a chancre on the balanopreputial sulcus. It was indurated, and painless and oozed readily. There was bilateral gland enlargement. The chancre was indurated, painless, nonadherent and 12 days old. The patient had received local treatment for nine days.

TABLE 14.—OBSERVATIONS IN CASE 14

		Spirochetes				
Stain Negative	Dark-Field	Antigen Positive ++++ 30′ and 60′	Amboceptor Positive ++ 30′ + 60′	Syphilitic Serum Positive + + + +	Normal Serum Negative	Hemolytic System 10′
Exudate......... 1		Exudate......... 1		Comment: Repeated in 72 hours with amboceptor −+++; antigen −−−−		
Antigen......... 1		Syphilitic serum. 1				
Complement..... ½		Complement..... ½				
Red cells......... 10		Red cells......... 10				

CONCLUSIONS

1. In the exudate from chancres which are clinically syphilitic there is a substance that acts as amboceptor in the Wassermann test.

2. There has been found also in the exudate of the same chancres another substance that acts as antigen in the Wassermann test.

3. In the exudate from chancres which are clinically negative with no spirochetes, no antigen or amboceptor has been found.

4. While only one mixed chancre was studied, both antigen and amboceptor were found besides spirochetes.

5. The substance that acts as amboceptor and the substance that acts as antigen were found together when their presence was demonstrated.

6. While both substances appeared together, it has been possible to demonstrate their presence independently using the Wassermann test for this purpose.

7. In all the exudates from the chancres examined which contained spirochetes both antigen and amboceptor have always been found.

8. No case was positive for spirochetes and negative for antigen and amboceptor.

9. Exudates from chancres that were clinically positive but in which no spirochetes were found contained both antigen and amboceptor.

10. The amount of complement in these exudates is not sufficient to change the positive or negative reaction.

THE CLINICAL EVALUATION OF THE WASSER-
MANN REACTION

ROBERT A. KILDUFFE, A.M., M.D.

Director, Laboratories, Pittsburgh and McKeesport Hospital;
Serologist, Providence Hospital

PITTSBURGH

In the sixteen years which have elapsed since the introduction of the Wassermann reaction as a diagnostic aid in syphilis the procedure has undergone the common fate of all innovations in medical science. The first disposition to accept the test more or less blindly with unquestioning faith as a pathognomonic indication of syphilitic infection has been followed by a critical and even hypercritical survey of its possibilities and limitations, until now, as has been pointed out by Strickler,[1] the medical profession may be divided, according to its attitude, into three groups: (1) those who place absolute dependence on the Wassermann reaction as a means of diagnosis; (2) those who consider it as a gross test the findings of which must be considered and correlated with the clinical findings, and (3) those who consider the test so liable to error as to be entirely unreliable.

In view of this lack of agreement, the existence of which must be admitted, it seems timely, perhaps, to review the salient features of available data with a view to ascertaining, if possible, the consensus of thought as to the clinical evaluation of the Wassermann test in general practice.

In thus establishing the purpose of this paper, certain general premises must be frankly admitted and clearly understood. No attempt will be made to present an exhaustive or complete survey of the literature, nor to carry the discussion into the specialized realms of the syphilographer or serologist. To these the subject will be familiar ground and the data herein grouped that which they have already submitted to keen and analytic scrutiny—a necessity if they are to remain in the forefront of their respective fields.

It is for that larger group for whom the Wassermann test must stand or fall as a means of diagnosis that this paper is largely written: for the man who, in his hastily-snatched moments of reading and study, is apt to be confronted with diametrically opposed statements and who, without exhaustive study, is apt to be confused as to the exact merits of each.

---

1. Strickler, A.: A Review of the Clinical Significance of the Wassermann Reaction. J. A. M. A. **78**:962 (April) 1922.

The Wassermann test was originally introduced as a means of diagnosis; its more recent application as a means of following the efficacy of treatment is a later development, the application of which is not always clearly manifest. It is as a means of diagnosis that it finds, perhaps, its widest use in general practice, and it is in this connection that the significance of the reaction will mainly be discussed.

It is impossible, however, to avoid discussion to some extent of certain features of technic, both because certain variations in technic are directly associated with variations in the reaction, and because the intelligent interpretation of the reaction requires at least an elementary understanding of the principles on which the test is based.

While the introduction of this reaction constituted an epochal advance in the study of syphilis, it cannot be regarded as without some disadvantageous effects. Recollecting the infinite variety of the manifestations of this disease, an understanding of which requires an understanding of so many related and nonrelated phenomena; recollecting the difficulty with which a satisfactory history and, at times, even a satisfactory examination is obtained, it is not to be marveled at that this test which can be made even without the knowledge of the patient has, to a preceptible degree, under certain circumstances supplanted the exhaustive history and clinical examination.

As Broeman [2] has emphasized, there is a prevalent tendency in the study of syphilis to rely largely on laboratory methods rather than to endeavor to coax or drag forth a history from the patient; and, as succinctly said by Smith,[3] "A product of our modern methods of diagnosis and treatment is the pseudosyphilographer. To him the clinical study of syphilis is unnecessary. The public Wassermann laboratory makes the diagnosis without charge and a few injections of arsphenamine clear up the lesions."

So much emphasis has been laid on the Wassermann test that perhaps the estimation of its value has been distorted or unduly magnified. It is essential to realize that its significance is quite definitely affected by the care and technic with which the reaction is performed, and it is equally essential that the clinician should be so far familiar with the generalities of the technic as to enable him to estimate closely the reliability of the serologist to whom he refers his specimens.

The reaction is not infallible, and, as pointed out by Rhodenburg and his associates,[4] it is of the greatest value when its limitations are clearly

2. Broeman, C. J.: A Thorough History an Important Factor in Syphilis. Am. Jour. Syph. **4**:565 (Oct.) 1921.

3. Smith, C. M.: The Treatment of Early Syphilis, Arch. Dermat. & Syph. **4**:724 (Dec.) 1921.

4. Rhodenburg, Garbat, Spiegel and Manheims: The Wassermann Reaction and Its Limitations in Diagnosis and Treatment. J. A. M. A. **76**:14 (Jan. 1) 1921.

understood, some of which are dependent on technical variations, with which the clinician must familiarize himself, and others on the biologic processes involved.

From the foregoing generalizations it should be evident that no intelligent consideration of the significance of the Wassermann reaction is possible without an understanding of the fundamental principles on which the test is based, and these will, therefore, be considered briefly.

THE MECHANISM OF THE WASSERMANN REACTION

As originally devised, the test was thought to be a variation of the Bordet-Gengou phenomenon, biologically specific in nature, and requiring a syphilitic antigen before complement could be fixed by the syphilitic antibody. Very soon, however, it was found that complement fixation could be obtained in syphilis with an "antigen" consisting of an extract of normal organs, and, moreover, after the discovery and culture of *Spirochaeta pallida*, that antigens made of such cultures—and, therefore, biologically specific—were far less delicate than the nonspecific normal extracts.

It is now almost universally recognized that the Wassermann reaction is not a true biologically specific test indicating an interaction between a specific antibody and its specific antigen, but a reaction the exact nature of which is not known other than that, in its production, lipoid bodies are intimately concerned.

In spite of all the work which has been done, all that is known of the mechanism of the test can be thus expressed: "While lipoidal extracts, as well as normal and syphilitic serums, may separately absorb or fix a small amount of complement, a mixture of a suitable extract and a syphilitic serum is capable of fixing large amounts of complement.[5]

In this connection, however, it must be noted that there are occasional observers who still cling to the biologic specificity of the reaction, among whom is Laird,[6] who holds that extracts of spirochete-containing tissue are "the only proper antigens with the highest degree of accuracy," and Durupt,[7] who believes the Wassermann test to be of a two-fold nature: (a) a nonspecific, physical chemical reaction, and (b) a strictly biologic reaction.

This worker uses two antigens, an extract of syphilitic liver containing spirochetes, and an extract of normal heart. He believes the former gives about 15 per cent. more positive reactions than the latter with the serum of patients with active syphilis. When reactions with both extracts are equal, he considers the reaction nonspecific in character though indicative of syphilis.

---

5. Kolmer, J. A.: Infection, Immunity, and Specific Therapy. Ed. 2 Philadelphia, W. B. Saunders Company, 1920, p. 429.

6. Laird, J. P.: Bull. Penn. Dept. of Health, No. 104, p. 171.

7.   922

It is fair to state, however, that these views are not in accord with those of the majority, who now regard the Wassermann reaction as a biologically nonspecific phenomenon and who use the term "antigen" with a full realization that the extracts so denominated are not true antigens in an immunologic sense; the substance in syphilitic serums interacting with such extracts, until its true nature is known, being perhaps best spoken of as a "reagin."

It is of interest to note that Wassermann,[8] reporting the results of investigations into the mechanism of the test, claims to have demonstrated in the blood of syphilitic patients a substance which, in the presence of complement, enters into a reversible combination with the antigen. This substance, which he claims to have isolated, is produced by or related to the lipoid substances which must be present in large quantities in the blood of the patients, and he holds that the "syphilitic suffers from an inversion (Umstellüng) of lipoid metabolism which explains why the reaction is positive not only with extracts from the organs of syphilitic children, but also with all organs containing lipoid-like substances."

ANTIGENS AND THEIR INFLUENCE

Following the discovery that extracts of normal organs could be used as antigens, a great variety of such extracts came into use. While this, of course, enters the realm of technic, because of the varying delicacy of various extracts; because different antigens and combinations of extracts are used by different workers, which sometimes accounts for the varying reports from different laboratories on the same serum, and because reports of Wassermann tests should always—as they often do—contain a statement as to what antigens were used, it behooves the clinician to know something of prevailing opinions as to the delicacy and reliability of the antigens in common use.

These may be divided into these main groups:

1. Alcoholic extracts of organs containing spirochetes.

2. Alcoholic extracts of normal organs.

3. Alcoholic extracts of normal organs reinforced by the addition of cholesterin.

4. Acetone-insoluble lipoids of normal organs.

Extracts of Syphilitic Organs.—The most commonly used is an extract of syphilitic fetal liver. The use of such extracts originated with the idea of retaining a biologic specificity despite the fact that the coincident presence of liver tissue extractives introduced a nonspecific factor. While such antigens are useful and reliable, it must be recog-

---

8. Recent Experimental Investigations on Syphilis, Berlin Letter, J. A. M. A. **76**:463 (Feb. 2) 1921.

nized that there is a limit to their delicacy and, moreover, that the mere presence of spirochetes in a tissue does not necessarily indicate that its extract will be a good antigen; in fact, the antigenic property may be nil.

These are, probably, the weakest antigens of the series though reference has been made to contrary opinions.[9]

Alcoholic Extracts of Normal Organs.—These are extensively used and are, in most cases, extracts of beef, human or guinea-pig hearts, the former usually producing a very good antigen. The use of a fresh beef heart is preferable to a human heart which has undergone any perceptible degree of decomposition, though extracts of fresh human hearts are especially efficient.

These antigens are quite reliable and delicate and not infrequently give positive reactions when syphilitic liver extracts have failed to detect the syphilitic reagin.

"Cholesterinized" Extracts of Normal Organs.—These consist of an alcoholic extract of a normal organ to which has been added chemically pure cholesterin to saturation or half-saturation. These antigens are highly sensitive and widely used. There has been much discussion as to the exact degree to which they will react with normal, non-syphilitic serums, thus giving false positives, and this question will be taken up later.

Acetone-Insoluble Lipoids.—These are the lipoids precipitated from an alcoholic extract of a normal organ by acetone and redissolved in ether and methyl alcohol, and form quite sensitive, reliable and satisfactory antigens.

In discussing the subject of antigens it must be borne in mind that none of those in common use are biologically specific and that all are of varying degrees of delicacy. It is essential to remember that the reliability of an extract depends, not on its nature as much as on the care with which it has been prepared and with which it has been titrated, checked and controlled before being put into use.

Until a standard technic is generally adopted the clinician should refuse to accept reports which read merely "positive" or "negative" and should insist that the report embody a statement as to the antigens used and the degree of reaction to each. Only in this way can the reports of different laboratories be compared and correlated.

THE SPECIFICITY OF THE WASSERMANN REACTION

It is now recognized that a positive reaction may be obtained in conditions other than syphilis.

Conditions generally admitted to give complement fixations with the antigens in common use are:

1. Leprosy, for reasons at present unknown.

2. Frambesia (yaws), the reason being also unknown though it is of interest to note that the cause of this disease, *Spirochaeta pertenuis*, is morphologically indistinguishable from *Spirochaeta pallida*.

3. Pneumonia, if the blood is taken during the febrile period.

4. Anesthesia or alcoholism may cause false positive or negative results.

Obviously any reaction in which positive results may be obtained in conditions other than that for which it was devised cannot be looked on as absolutely specific; but, because the conditions in which such positive results are obtained are readily differentiated from syphilis, no confusion need arise; and, when properly checked, controlled and carefully correlated and interpreted in conjunction with the other findings in the patient, the Wassermann reaction may be looked on as a highly specific and reliable means of diagnosis.

Pollitzer [10] says: "A *strongly* positive reaction is found only in syphilis (barring yaws and leprosy), and a strongly positive reaction means syphilis."

This is, perhaps, an extreme view, unless we tacitly assume that the specimen has been appropriately and carefully collected and that the technic of the test is accurate to a high degree.

It is unfortunate that the shadow of the first conception of the Wassermann reaction as absolutely biologically specific still hangs over the test and that there are still clinicians for whom the result of a single positive or negative reaction constitutes the ultima thule on which dogmatic assertions as to the presence or absence of syphilis can be safely predicated. It is equally unfortunate that so many clinicians consider it unnecessary to bother with any study of serologic technic.

It certainly seems justifiable to maintain that if, as is often the case, the clinician is to constitute the sole arbiter in the interpretation of the test, he should be familiar with the technic—beginning with the collection of the specimen—in a sufficient degree to correlate intelligently and carefully the results of the examination with the results of other examinations which are—or should be—made.

If, on the other hand, the responsibility of the proper interpretation of the reaction is to be borne solely by the serologist, then he should be looked on as a consultant in relation to the patient and furnished with all the data available to other consultants.[11]

---

10. Pollitzer. S.: General Prognosis of Syphilis in the Light of Recent Progress. J. A. M. A. **74**:12 (March 20) 1921.

11. Kilduffe. R. A.: The Function of the Pathologist as a Consultant, J. A. M. A. **76**:54 (Jan. 1) 1921.

As has been noted elsewhere,[12] "It is a common practice to have Wassermanns performed as a matter of routine by laboratory assistants trained in the work. While these, often of the laity, may have been carefully trained and their manipulations possess a high degree of mechanical accuracy, the weight of direct evidence would force the conclusion that the preparations for the test, their performance, and the reports based upon them should not be left to laboratory assistants however skilled they may be in manipulation. The responsibility attaching to any imperfection or slovenliness of technic is so great, and the results of a false diagnosis may bear so heavily upon the patient and his family, that the whole weight of responsibility for the reports should be borne by a fully qualified pathologist, and, under no circumstances, should the reputation of the pathologist be used as a cloak for the work of an assistant, no matter how great his manipulative skill."

THE WASSERMANN TEST IN CONDITIONS OTHER THAN SYPHILIS

The early literature abounds in reports of positive Wassermann reactions in a great variety of conditions, which our present knowledge shows to have been due largely to technical errors.

Nevertheless, there are certain nonsyphilitic conditions in which positive reactions may be obtained and others in which, with syphilis a possibility, perhaps, the correct interpretation of the results presents a matter of some difficulty necessitating careful study.

While there are extensive statistical data concerning the Wassermann test in syphilis, similar data are not available to the same degree as concerns the test in nonsyphilitic conditions. The data following, therefore, cannot be looked on as exhaustive nor is it to be dogmatically interpreted; it is simply an attempt to note the consensus of experience as far as recorded.

1. Frambesia and leprosy consistently give a positive Wassermann reaction as usually performed, and the reaction is of no value for the diagnosis of syphilis in the coincident presence of these conditions.

2. Pneumonia, if the blood is taken during the febrile stage, will frequently give a positive Wassermann reaction, becoming negative during the afebrile stage; in this condition the test should always be repeated during convalescence if there is any possibility of syphilis.

3. In relapsing fever, due to the *Spirochaeta obermeirii*, a transient positive reaction may be found in the acute stage. The transient character of the reaction serves to distinguish it from the reaction due to

12. Kilduffe, R. A.: The Practical Value and Utilization of the Wassermann Test in General Practice. Arch. Diagnosis. January, 1920.

syphilis. If the positive result is observed on every occasion in a particular patient it may be suspected that he has syphilis also.[13]

4. In scarlet fever the reaction is uniformly negative, and a positive reaction is strongly presumptive of coincident congenital syphilis.[5]

5. Occasional transient positive reactions may be obtained after ether or chloroform anesthesia; alcoholism may give rise to a false negative reaction.

6. Malaria: It has been stated that malaria will produce a positive reaction per se, but this contention is not borne out by recent investigations. Johnson,[14] after the examination of a large series of various types of malarial infection, each serum having been tested with the Wassermann test by four different methods, concludes that the blood in active benign tertian, malignant tertian, and mixed malarial infection does not give a positive Wassermann reaction. Positive reactions, when they do occur, are due to latent syphilis or errors of technic. If, on retesting, after an interval, the serum is persistently positive, the reaction indicates syphilis.

INFLUENCE OF CHOLESTEREMIA ON THE WASSERMANN REACTION

Henes [15] has advanced the opinion that an increase in the cholesterin content of the blood may, at times, be the direct cause of positive reactions. This opinion, however, is controverted by the work of Craig and Williams,[16] who increased the blood cholesterin in rabbits by as much as 680 per cent. without producing a positive Wassermann reaction.

The subject is, perhaps, worthy of extensive investigation but, on the basis of evidence at hand, cholesteremia cannot per se be looked on as producing a positive Wassermann reaction. These findings are in accord with those of de Villa and Ronch [17] after an extensive investigation into the results of the Wassermann reaction in children.

Of interest is the recent work of McFarland [17a] who concludes, as a result of his studies, that blood cholesterol is not uniformly increased

13. Road, H. E.: The Wassermann Reaction in Relapsing Fever, J. Exper. Path., London **3**:59 (Feb.) 1922.

14. Johnson, J. P.: The Diagnosis of Syphilis in Malarial Patients by the Wassermann Reaction, J. Path. and Bacteriol. **24**:145, 1913.

15. Henes, quoted by Craig, C. F., and Williams, W. C.: Experimental Observations on the Effect of Cholesteremia on the Results of the Wassermann Test, Am. J. Syphilis **4**:685, 1920.

16. Craig, C. F., and Williams, W. C.: Experimental Observations on the Effect of Cholesteremia on the Results of the Wassermann Test, Am. J. Syphilis **5**:392 (July) 1921.

17. De Villa, S., and Ronch, A.: The Wassermann Reaction in Children, Policlinico, Rome **29**:185 (Feb. 6) 1922.

17a. McFarland, A. R.: Studies on Blood Cholesterol in Syphilis, Arch. Dermat. & Syph. **6**:39 (July) 1922.

in syphilis and that the positive Wassermann reaction apparently does not depend on a high cholesterol value and that there is apparently no relation between cholesterol values and the clinical and serologic response of the patient.

THE WASSERMANN REACTION IN DIABETES

Williams [18] in a study of 337 diabetic patients, encountered a positive Wassermann reaction in sixteen, or 4.8 per cent., seven of whom without any treatment for syphilis later gave a negative reaction. Similar results have been reported elsewhere,[19] the tests being repeated with identical results.

Unless diabetes can be looked on as syphilitic in origin, which yet remains to be proved, the explanation of these findings is a matter of some difficulty. Coincident hypercholesteremia, which was noted in some of the cases reacting positively, is apparently not a factor of importance. Williams comments that the reaction may indicate a relation either between syphilis and diabetes in some cases, a possibility deserving serious consideration, or between the nutritional state and the Wassermann reaction because large amounts of fats and lipoids are mobilized on a low diet, substances which probably enter into the mechanism of the Wassermann test.

It is of interest to note the work of Warthin [20] who says that "diabetes may be associated with the more marked degrees of syphilitic pancreatitis, and in all our autopsy series all of our diabetic cases were so associated; but a number of cases of syphilitic pancreatitis of similar severity have not presented the clinical symptoms of diabetes. It seems probable, therefore, that latent syphilis is the chief factor in the forms of pancreatitis frequently associated with diabetes, but that diabetes is not always associated with severe degrees of this type of pancreatitis."

The work of Leman [21] must be noted in this connection. This investigator, starting with the premise that syphilis was a prevalent disease in the negro and that, therefore, if syphilis was a frequent cause of diabetes the latter disease should also be frequent in the negro.

18. Williams, J. R.: A Study of the Wassermann Reaction in a Large Group of Supposedly Non-Syphilitic Individuals, Including Large Groups of Diabetics and Nephritics, Am. J. Syphilis **2**:284 (April) 1921.

19. Kilduffe, R. A.: Incidence of Positive Wassermann Reactions in Four Hundred and Eighty-Four Supposedly Nonsyphilitic Patients Admitted to a General Hospital, Arch. Dermat. & Syph. **5**:207 (Feb.) 1922.

20. Warthin, A. S., and Wilson, U. F.: The Coincidence of Latent Syphilis and Diabetes, Am. J. M. Sc. **58**:157, 1916.

21. Leman, I. I.: Diabetes Mellitus, Syphilis, and the Negro, Am. J. M. Sc. **162**:226 (Aug.) 1921.

analyzed 160,044 hospital admissions for the incidence of both diseases in the negro race. He found that diabetes occurred in 0.47 per cent. per thousand cases, while syphilis was found in the proportion of 50 per cent. of all syphilitic admissions. He concludes, therefore, that either there is no connection between the two diseases or else that the negro has an unexplained relative immunity to syphilitic pancreatitis just as he has to locomotor ataxia.

THE WASSERMANN TEST IN NEPHRITIS

Williams,[18] Kilduffe [19] and other observers find the reaction only rarely positive so the condition is not one in which nonspecific fixations are likely to be encountered.

THE EFFECT OF INTRAVENOUS MEDICATION

In a recent paper, Strickler, Munson and Sidlick [22] have raised the question of the influence per se of intravenous injections of arsphenamin on the Wassermann test in normal persons and contend that, in the absence of syphilis, a positive reaction may be obtained as the direct result of intravenous arsphenamin therapy. These results, however, have not been confirmed by Stokes [23] and are disputed by Kolmer,[24] who calls attention to the fact that if the intravenous administration of arsphenamin can cause a positive Wassermann reaction in a non-syphilitic person, a similar result should be obtained in a syphilitic person, whereas clinical experience shows that, in the latter, following arsphenamin therapy, the reaction becomes negative. Moreover, the "Wassermann-fast" cases, which Strickler contends may be so as a result of intravenous administration of arsphenamin, frequently show involvement of the central nervous system and require thorough investigation. Further reference will be made to this type of case later.

In connection with the increase of the strength of the Wassermann reaction following treatment, as in the "provocative" Wassermann reaction, Kolmer looks on this as a serologic Herxheimer reaction due to the influence of the drug on the spirochete, and, finally, the Wassermann reaction in syphilis may become negative, to be later positive after a cessation of treatment, whereas if Strickler's contention were correct the reverse would occur.

---

22. Strickler, A.; Munson, H. G., and Sidlick, D. M.: A Positive Wassermann Test in Nonsyphilitic Patients After Intravenous Therapy, J. A. M. A. **75**:1486 (Nov. 27) 1920.

23. Stokes, J. H.: The Treatment of Late Syphilis and of Syphilis in the Mother and Child, a Résumé of Principles. Arch. Dermat. & Syph. **4**:778 (Dec.) 1921.

24. Kolmer, J. A.: The Question of Positive Wassermann Reactions Caused by Intravenous Administration of Arsphenamin, J. A. M. A. **75**:1796 (Dec. 25) 1920.

The failure of experimental intravenous administration of arsphenamin, neo-arsphenamin and mercury to produce a positive Wassermann reaction in rabbits has been reported by Kolmer and Kilduffe.[25]

THE WASSERMANN REACTION IN PREGNANCY AND CONGENITAL SYPHILIS

The present intensive interest in syphilis has focused attention on the problem of congenital syphilis and its early recognition. It is a problem presenting peculiar difficulties. As noted elsewhere,[26] the ideal method of investigation involves a serologic examination of both parents before delivery and of the infant after delivery and some months later. This, unfortunately, is rarely possible and the usual method rests on a serologic test of the mother before delivery and of the cord blood at the time of delivery.

The results are conflicting. Fordyce and Rosen [27] believe that the blood of the normal pregnant woman may be faintly positive to cholesterinized extracts, a finding corroborated by the work of Stühmer and Dreyer [28] who, as a result of examination of a series of 1,000 pregnancies with 2,500 controls, conclude that the findings in pregnancy are unreliable in fully 10 per cent. of all cases and that the retroplacental and cord bloods are especially unreliable. This view is also held by Williams,[29] after a careful analysis of 4,564 cases.

The work of Jeans and Cooke [30] and other observers,[26] however, would indicate that simply because of a certain percentage of unreliable tests the cord Wassermann reaction should not be neglected if no other means of examination is feasible, but that the results should be interpreted with care and corroborated by further and more extensive examinations of parents and child.

It is obvious that the use of the Wassermann reaction in pregnancy and congenital syphilis must be safeguarded with extreme care and

25. Kilduffe, R. A.: Effect of Intravenous Administration of Arsphenamin. Neo-Arsphenamin and Mercury on the Wassermann Test in Normal Serums. J. A. M. A. **76**:1489 (May 28) 1921.

26. Kilduffe, R. A.: Concerning the Wassermann Test in Its Relation to Prenatal and Congenital Syphilis. Am. J. Med. Sc., to be published.

27. Fordyce, J. A., and Rosen, I.: The Treatment of Congenital and Antenatal Syphilis. Arch. Dermat & Syph.. **5**:1 (Jan.) 1922

28. Stühmer, A., and Dreyer, K.: Serologic Tests in Pregnancy. Ztschr. f. Geburtsh. u. Gynäk. **84**:289 (Nov. 12) 1921.

29 Williams, J. W.: The Value of the Wassermann Reaction in Obstetrics. Based upon a Study of 4.547 Consecutive Cases. Bull. Johns Hopkins Hosp. **21**:356 (Oct.) 1920.

30. Jeans, P. C., and Cooke, J. V.: Incidence of Hereditary Syphilis. Am. J. Dis. Child. **22**:402 (Oct.) 1921.

that the results of the test must be closely correlated with the history and clinical findings. Both positive and negative reactions must be closely scrutinized.

Cornell and Stillians [31] were unable to show any relation between a positive Wassermann reaction and repeated abortions in their series, and they hold syphilis responsible for not more than 10 per cent. of abortions.

Mills [32] notes that in hereditary syphilis both parents may give positive reactions, or the father may give a positive and the mother a negative reaction. He has not yet seen a father with a negative reaction and a mother with a positive. He calls attention to the fact that many cases of inherited syphilis have none of the cardinal signs usually described, and that there may be no history of rash, snuffles or condylomas. The condition may be manifested in a variety of ways and only recognized by the "therapeutic test." In the young child syphilis may produce a condition indistinguishable from tuberculous peritonitis, or an anemia not improved by iron may be the sole manifestation.

Rolleston [33] emphasizes the fact that it is impossible to accept as absolute the proposition that in the presence of syphilitic stigmas a negative blood Wassermann reaction eliminates the possibility of syphilitic infection; and Ross and Wright [34] note that congenitally syphilitic babies tend to give a negative Wassermann reaction until a month or so after birth. Fordyce and Rosen believe such babies should be kept under observation for at least two years.

In congenital syphilis, therefore, repeated serologic examinations are advisable for at least one or two years in a suspected case, combined with, if possible, examinations of both parents.

THE "CHOLESTERIN-PLUS" WASSERMANN REACTION

Following the introduction of cholesterinized antigens, reports soon accumulated of cases reacting positively to such antigens but negatively to the extracts of syphilitic liver and acetone-insoluble lipoids, with resultant discussion concerning the reliability of such reactions as indicative of syphilitic infection.

At first, in the absence of clinical or historical evidence of syphilis, it was customary to look on these as nonspecific and to feel that the

31. Cornell and Stillians: Syphilis in Pregnancy and Labor, Am. J. Syphilis Nov. 20, p. 342.

32. Mills, A.: Wassermann Test in General Practice, Edinburgh M. J. **29**:19 (June) 1922.

33. Rolleston, H.: Sequels of Congenital Syphilis. Lancet **1**:5088 (March) 1921.

34. Ross, S. M., and Wright, A. F.: The Incidence of Congenital Syphilis Among the Newly Born. Lancet **1**:321 (Feb. 12) 1921.

cholesterinized antigens would react positively with a definite proportion of normal serums. Later study and evidence, however, seem to indicate that these reactions cannot be thus summarily dismissed.

The subject has been discussed at length in a previous communication [35] and can be briefly summed up here.

Experience has shown that in the primary stages of syphilis a positive reaction may be obtained with cholesterinized antigens before any of the other extracts react, and in latent and neurosyphilis such reactions may occur in the blood, other antigens being negative, corroborated by strongly positive spinal fluid findings. In the treated cases, also, the cholesterin plus reaction can be obtained long after a clean-cut negative occurs with liver and acetone extracts.

The absence of history or clinical evidence must be considered with care for venereal histories are notoriously unreliable and syphilis may be asymptomatic.

Experience also seems to indicate that, during pregnancy, cholesterin plus reactions may be obtained which are undoubtedly nonspecific and which do not indicate syphilis; but the nonspecific reactions obtained in normal serums with a carefully prepared and titrated extract are beyond doubt far more infrequent than has hitherto been supposed.

If cholesterin plus reactions, uncorroborated by clinical or historical evidence, are to be held of dubious value, it is obvious that Wassermann reactions should not be conducted with these as the sole antigens. Nevertheless, the Wassermann test, as performed in the American Expeditionary Forces; the "standardized" technic adopted for the British Expeditionary Forces; and the technic of such institutions as the Boston City Hospital, Boston Board of Health, Massachusetts General Hospital, Peter Bent Brigham Hospital, and others, rely on cholesterinized antigens as the sole criterion of the presence or absence of syphilis, even though some of their results must be "weakly positive" reactions, or those most prone to be considered nonspecific and unreliable.

The present status of the question may be thus summed up:

1. Cholesterinized antigens are highly delicate and sensitive and superior to the plain extracts or artificially prepared lipoids.

2. Under certain circumstances, their exact nature being as yet unknown, faint positive reactions may occur with nonsyphilitic serums. Such reactions, however, with a carefully controlled, checked and titrated antigen are relatively rare, and their occurrence necessitates a careful clinical and historical study before concluding that they are nonspecific.

35. Kilduffe, R. A.: Concerning the Specificity of Cholesterinized Antigens in The Serologic Diagnosis of Syphilis. Arch. Dermat. & Syph. **3**:598 (May) 1921.

3. In pregnancy cholesterin plus reactions occur frequently, and these antigens should not be relied on for diagnosis under these conditions.

4. In the known case of syphilis, treatment should be continued until a negative reaction is obtained with a cholesterinized antigen.

5. In the unknown case tested for diagnosis, a cholesterinized plus reaction should form the basis of an exhaustive clinical, historical, and laboratory study fortified by repeated serologic blood and possibly spinal fluid Wassermann reactions. Under such circumstances corroboratory evidence will be obtained in a large percentage of cases.

6. On the basis of past experience,[36] the writer would look on a $+ +$, $+ + +$ or $+ + + +$ reaction with a cholesterinized antigen, barring pregnancy or pneumonia, as strongly presumptive evidence of the presence of syphilitic reagin in the blood, and on any reaction below $+ +$ as at least suspicious and necessitating further and exhaustive examinations, clinical, historical and laboratory.

7. To pass over a cholesterinized plus reaction, in the absence of fixation with other antigens, as generally nonspecific is an attitude certainly not justified by the data available.

ANTICOMPLEMENTARY REACTIONS

The reading of the Wassermann reaction depends on the presence or absence of hemolysis. Under certain conditions, such as bacterial contamination, the presence of fat, bile, chyle, and other substances the exact nature of which is unknown, the serum tested may be able of itself to prevent completely the hemolytic action of the complement. Therefore, since all the tubes in the test contain a dose of serum, it will be impossible to tell whether the absence of hemolysis is due to its utilization in the union of antigen and reagin, or to the preventive (anticomplementary) action of the serum. Such a test cannot be read and must be repeated with a fresh specimen of serum.

"WASSERMANN-FAST" REACTIONS

In the literature of the Wassermann reaction a class of cases in which no amount of treatment suffices to produce a negative reaction is not infrequently mentioned. For a time it was thought that such cases were "Wassermann-fast" because of some property other than syphilitic reagin in the blood. It is now realized, however, that such cases require extensive study and lifelong observation. Stokes and Bushman [37] find no evidence to prove that the fact that a person is

---

36. Kilduffe, R. A.: Footnotes 19, 25 and 35.

37. Stokes, J. H., and Busman, J. A.: A Clinical Study of Wassermann-Fast Syphilis with Special Reference to Prognosis and Treatment, Am. J. M. Sc. **160**:658, 1920.

Wassermann-fast indicates an infection with any special strain of spirochete, and they believe that such a reaction indicates a grave infection. Such a patient, they think, should not be discharged from careful periodic reexamination throughout life with special reference to the cardiovascular and central nervous system, in which opinion numerous observers concur.

THE WASSERMANN REACTION IN SYPHILIS

In spite of the enormous literature which had accumulated, there are still clinicians willing to hazard a dogmatic statement on the results of a single Wassermann test on the blood alone.

While it is true that the Wassermann reaction is the most constant and delicate single symptom of syphilis, it has been abundantly proved, however, that in syphilis a single negative reaction is not sufficient nor definite evidence that a cure has been effected, for the disease may recur after treatment, at least to the extent that the Wassermann reaction reappears followed by clinical manifestations.

It is necessary, therefore, that successive examinations be made during a period of at least two years and at intervals during the remainder of life.[5]

The disappearance of Wassermann bodies from the blood of a syphilitic person with a consequent negative reaction indicates merely the cessation of interaction between the organisms and the tissues. A negative reaction only means that there are no foci of spirochetes sufficiently active to bring about the formation of a detectable amount of reagin in the blood; hence, "as an indication of complete removal of treponemata at a given moment a single negative Wassermann is useless. On the contrary, however, as an indication of failure to eradicate the treponemata, a positive Wassermann reaction has the greatest value."[1]

In certain stages of syphilis the Wassermann reaction may be negative, at least for a time; on the other hand, the possibility of asymptomatic syphilis must be considered.

In the primary stages of syphilis only a small proportion of cases will react before the third or fourth week, and in those reacting early, the reaction is prone to be weak or to occur only with cholesterinized antigens, such reactions having been obtained as early as the tenth day.

In the initial stages the weaker reactions are of greater diagnostic value than in the later stages of the disease. After the third week following the appearance of the chancre, about 50 per cent. of cases react positively with all antigens and about 75 per cent. with cholesterinized antigens only.

In the secondary stage about 95 per cent. of all cases are positive, and dependence should not be absolute on a single negative in this stage.

In neurosyphilis the blood Wassermann reaction may be negative while the spinal fluid is positive, a condition possibly dependent on the fact that the interchange of antibodies between the blood and spinal fluid is slow and, apparently, difficult.

Of late much attention has been paid to the incidence of neurosyphilis, and the opinion is growing that syphilitic persons should not be released from observation until the results of examination of the spinal fluid are known.

This position is advocated by numerous investigators, among whom may be noted Gay,[38] and Fordyce and Rosen,[39] who call attention to the fact that the absence of clinical signs and symptoms does not exclude syphilis of the central nervous system.

In this connection the work of Jackson and Pike [40] is of interest as pointing out that, in the presence of mental disease, a positive Wassermann reaction does not necessarily indicate its syphilitic origin and that syphilis may be merely coincidental. Their work also indicates that the diagnosis of neurosyphilis should be based on definite neurologic signs and spinal fluid reactions, irrespective of blood serum readings. These observers note that neurosyphilis is rarely, if ever, superimposed on a well-developed psychosis.

Attention must also be called to the work of Thaysen,[41] who has shown that in syphilis the Wassermann reaction may show wide variations from time to time, both as to degrees of positiveness and even as to its occurrence or absence without definite cause.

In the ultimate analysis, the clinical value of the Wassermann reaction is in direct proportion to the realization that it constitutes only a single method of phase of examination and that it should always be carefully correlated with and interpreted in the light of all the other findings—however obtained—in the individual patient.

---

38. Gay, H.: Latent Neurosyphilis in Eight Per Cent. of Medical Cases Ignored Owing to Neglect of Lumbar Puncture, Am. J. M. Sc. **163**:600 (March) 1922.

39. Fordyce, J. A., and Rosen, I.: Laboratory Findings in Early and Late Syphilis. Review of 1064 Cases, J. A. M. A. **77**:1696 (Nov. 26) 1921.

40. Jackson, J. A., and Pike, H. V.: Interpretation of Wassermann Reaction of Blood Serum in Mental Disease, J. A. M. A. **76**:360 (Feb. 5) 1921.

41. Thaysen, T. E. H.: Spontaneous Variations in the Strength of the Wassermann Reaction, Acta Med. Scand. **55**:281 (June 17) 1921.

POTASSIUM PERMANGANATE AS A CURATIVE AGENT IN DERMATOLOGIC DISEASES

SAMUEL FELDMAN, M.D.

Adjunct Attending Dermatologist, Bronx Hospital; Chief of Clinic, Lebanon and Bronx Hospital Dispensaries, Departments of Dermatology and Syphilis

AND

BENJAMIN F. OCHS, M.D.

Associate Dermatologist, Lebanon Hospital; Chief of Clinic, Harlem Hospital

NEW YORK

It was early in 1918, while the late Dr. W. S. Gottheil instructed a class of students at the Lebanon Hospital Dispensary, that a patient who had extremely foul smelling eczematoid lesions on and between the toes of both his feet, was presented to him for demonstration. He refused to show the patient to the students and advised a potassium permanganate dressing in order to do away with the foul odor. When the patient returned to the clinic three days after the dressing was applied, the results appeared startling. Not only had the foul odor disappeared, but the lesions had cleared up also to a great extent. The case was subsequently diagnosed as eczematoid ringworm, *Epidermophyton inguinale* being found in the scrapings of the lesions. Desirous of ascertaining whether the drug had any special action on the lesions or whether improvement was coincidental, the treatment was continued until the case was brought to a successful termination within a period of about four weeks.

During the last four years we have treated a comparatively large number of patients with epidermophytosis in four dispensaries in this city according to the method described in the foregoing, and we have obtained uniformly good results. At first, every patient so treated was alternated with one treated with Whitfield's ointment as a control. We soon found that the results obtained from the employment of the former method were so much superior to those obtained with the latter, that further checking was considered unnecessary.

The strength of the solution to be employed depends on the character of the lesion. In general, it may be said that the more acute the lesion is the milder and the more dilute the solution should be. The strength commonly employed is 1:1,000, and the solution is applied in the form of wet dressings. In patients with a considerable amount of irritation it may become necessary to reduce the concentration to 1:2,000 or even as low as 1:5,000. Exudation and maceration always call for a mild application, except in the intertrigenous form of epidermophytosis found on the webs of the fingers and toes. In spite of the maceration and moisture which usually are present, the patient can bear strong solutions very well. Our method of treating these patients was to soak a pledget of cotton in a solution of the drug varying from 1 per cent. to full saturation and to insert it between the toes or fingers once every twenty-four hours. One week is usually sufficient to clear up the lesions. Out of a large number of cases of this class treated, we cannot recall a case in which we failed to obtain favorable results. One thing, however, must be borne in mind—namely, that the lesions may apparently be cured, yet the fungus may persist and cause a recurrence at some future date. For that reason, it is advisable to keep up the treatment for a long time after the lesions have disappeared.

In cases with infiltration and lichenification, as is often the case in eczematoid ringworm and in eczema marginatum of long standing, we had occasion to use a saturated solution of the drug in the form of daily paintings, without causing any irritation.

The cases of epidermophyton infection most resistant to treatment are found among the dyshidrotic group. In the early stages of the disease, when the deep-seated vesicle is unbroken and is covered with a thick layer of horny epidermis, there seems to be no way of attacking the fungus. In these cases a wet dressing of a 1 per cent. aqueous solution of salicylic acid, which can readily be made up by the addition of about four times its weight of borax, is at first applied to the parts until maceration occurs. The lesions are then attacked by the potassium permanganate solution.

REPORT OF CASES

CASE 2.—*Eczematoid Ringworm.*—Dr. B., an intern at the hospital, was treated with Whitfield's ointment and various other applications for a period of about four months, without any improvement. Later he received about a dozen roentgen-ray treatments and, although he felt relieved owing to its use, he was forced to abandon it on account of the appearance of a slight erythema. When he came for advice in June, 1921, he had marked eczematoid lesions in the interspace between the second and third fingers of the right hand. They were moist and, in places, there were bleeding fissures which were quite annoying, especially on the hands of a physician.

One of us (Feldman) tried iodin cataphoresis on the lesions. This method of treatment is quite effective in ordinary body ringworm, but, in this case, it failed to give appreciable results after six applications. As the lesions, at this stage, were dry and not exuding, the patient was ordered to paint the parts once daily with a saturated solution of potassium permanganate. There was almost immediate improvement. The fissures healed promptly, the infiltration gradually disappeared, and the entire condition was apparently cured within a period of about one month. He remained asymptomatic for four months; then there was a slight recurrence of the disease. The fresh lesions cleared up a few days after the resumption of treatment, and the patient was advised not to discontinue the applications for several months.

Case 3.—*Intertrigo.*—Mrs. G., the wife of a local physician, suddenly developed an erythema in the folds under both breasts and on the upper part of each thigh. Portions of the lesions soon became finely vesicular, followed by exudation and maceration. The burning sensation was so severe that she was deprived of sleep. Most of the usual remedies, including a 5 per cent. anesthesin ointment, were tried and failed to give her any relief until a wet dressing of 1 : 5,000 potassium permanganate was applied. The relief was almost immediate, and the patient slept that night for the first time in six days. The lesions cleared up completely after four days' treatment by this method.

Case 4.—*Eczema Marginatum.*—Dr. R., one of the physicians on the dispensary staff, came to our clinic with eczematoid lesions on the upper part of both thighs and extending upward to the groins. The edges were sharply outlined, the surface was moist and, in places, presented a granulating appearance. He complained of itching and burning, which could not be relieved by ordinary treatment. A wet dressing of 1 : 2,000 potassium permanganate caused a prompt drying of the lesions. The subjective symptoms quickly disappeared, and the whole condition cleared up in less than two weeks' treatment by this method.

Case 5.—*Dyshidrotic Form of Epidermophytosis.*—Mr. H. was referred to us by Dr. Hochman. He presented on the soles large, translucent, pearl-like vesicles which were deep-seated and covered with a thick horny layer of epidermis. There was intense itching, and the patient found relief only in rupturing the vesicles. In the left axillary pit, there was a brownish moist patch with sharply defined margins. Epidermophyton mycelium was obtained from this lesion, but, after repeated examinations of scales from the lesions on the feet, no fungus was found. The lesion in the axillary region was successfully attacked by 1 : 1,000 solution of potassium permanganate, and it was practically healed within ten days. The lesions on the soles, however, were first prepared by the application of a wet dressing of salicylic acid in order to produce maceration of the vesicles. This occurred within two weeks. After exfoliation of the macerated epithelium, the lesions were treated with 1 : 1,000 potassium permanganate, and the disease was brought to a successful termination before the month was over by painting the surface with a 1 per cent. solution of this drug.

COMMENT

From the results of treating the cases herein cited and numerous others with potassium permanganate solutions, there seems to be no doubt that, in this drug, we have a remedial agent more potent than any of the drugs that we have hitherto employed. No mention is made in the literature of this form of treatment, except in a recent paper by White and Greenwood,[1] which is quoted here verbatim. "In most cases fomentations fifteen minutes twice a day of 1 : 5,000 potassium permanganate constitutes one of our best methods of attack." We rarely saw good results from the use of Whitfield's ointment, in spite of the fact that it is so extensively used. Iodin, so effective in trichophytosis, seems to yield no beneficial results in this disease.

1. White, C. J., and Greenwood, A. M.: Epidermophytosis, J. A. M. A. 77: 1297 (Oct. 22) 1921.

Chrysarobin, which is readily borne by patients with ordinary ring-worm, is too irritating in most cases' of epidermophytosis to give it sufficient trial.

The manner in which the drug acts has, so far, not been ascertained. From clinical observation, however, there seems to be an indication that the beneficial action takes place by means of changes produced in the cells of the epidermis rather than by the direct action of the drug on the fungus. This may partially be deduced from the fact that it exerts a beneficial action on some distinctly nonfungoid diseases, such as chronic eczema and seborrheal dermatitis, especially when associated with lichenification. Experimental work along these lines has recently been instituted, and we hope shortly to be able to report further results.

CONCLUSIONS

Potassium permanganate in our hands has, so far, yielded better results in the treatment of epidermophytosis than any drug or combination of drugs hitherto employed.

It can be used in strengths ranging from 1:5,000 to the full saturated solution, the former in early, moist and irritated lesions, the latter in those associated with deep infiltration and lichenification.

Cases of intertrigo of the mammary folds and on the upper thighs yield readily to very dilute solutions (1:5,000), while in the intertrigenous type of epidermophytosis occurring between the fingers and toes stronger solutions may be employed with equally good results.

Unmistakable results are obtained in eczema marginatum by wet dressings and, in old lesions, by paintings with strong solutions of the drug. Patches situated on the flat surface of the body are occasionally resistant to treatment.

In eczematoid ringworm, far better results are obtained by this method of treatment than is seen with the use of Whitfield's ointment. These cases require a longer period of treatment in order to obtain a cure than those enumerated in the foregoing and the treatment must be kept up a long time after the disappearance of the lesions in order to make the results permanent.

The dyshidrotic form is the most resistant to treatment, especially in the presence of deep-seated vesicles and a thickened epidermis. Even here good results are obtained after the lesions are prepared by some keratolytic agent.

1955 Grand Concourse—310 Concord Avenue.

DERMATOSCOPY

JEFFREY C. MICHAEL, M.D.

HOUSTON, TEXAS

Dermatoscopy may be defined as the examination of the skin by means of the slit-lamp microscope, or dermatoscope. Credit for the introduction of the method is due to Saphier,[1] who in January, 1921, presented the first formal report on it. That paper, covering the subject in an inclusive manner, has been followed by articles dealing with detailed observations of particular diseases, as well as pathologic and normal phenomena of special interest and particular applicability for examination.

The slit-lamp microscope has been in use by ophthalmologists for several years and in that department of medicine a fairly large literature about it is being accumulated. The eye is particularly well suited for examination by an instrument which allows observation of the intact organ, and yet magnifies as high as 172 times.[2]

Dermatoscopy is comparable to ophthalmology in that direct observation forms the most important feature of diagnosis, and so dermatologists aid natural vision with magnifying apparatus with the desire to see the minutiae of lesions. On the one hand, lenses of low magnification are in daily use for examination of the surfaces of efflorescences; on the other hand, biopsy gives opportunity for detailed observation of the microscopic architecture of diseased tissue. With the slit-lamp microscope it is possible to obtain magnifications comparable to that of low power microscopy and yet examine lesions in their intact condition. This method of examination is still in its infancy. and the subject, at present, has hardly reached the point of practical utility, yet it requires no further statement to arouse the interest of dermatologists in a method of examination which. falling midway between ordinary visual and microscopic examination. contains something of each and adds something of its own.

My own acquaintance with the instrument and its use in dermatoscopy is only of several months' duration. during which time I have not worked with a more definite object in mind than routine examination of as many cases as possible. so as to orient myself in the possibilities of the method. Therefore, the object of this communication is to discuss the method in general and to record certain preliminary observations made with it.

1. Saphier, J.: Die Dermatoskopie, Arch. f. Dermat. u. Syph. **128**:1. 1921.

2. Vogt, A.: Atlas of the Slitlamp Microscopy of the Living Eye. (Trans. by von der Heyt.) Julius Springer. Berlin. 1921. (The chapters on technic and methods of examination are valuable.)

INSTRUMENT

The slit-lamp microscope (Fig. 1) consists of an illuminating device and a binocular microscope. These are mounted on a suitable base, depending on the purpose to which the instrument is to be put; that is, either for examination of the skin or the eye. The observations detailed herein were made with the apparatus mounted for eye examination (corneal microscope of Zeiss), which, because of the arrangement of the stand, practically permits only examination of lesions of the face, hands and upper extremities. It is possible to examine other parts of the

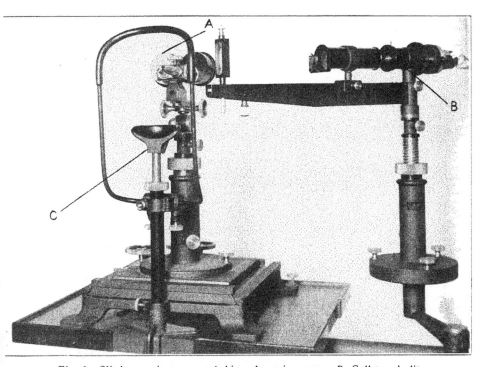

Fig. 1.—Slit-lamp microscope: *A*, binocular microscope; *B*, Gullstrand slit-lamp; *C*, head rest.

body with the apparatus, but the arrangements for doing so are too difficult for practical use and I have not attempted it. The dermatoscope proper, according to Saphier's description, is mounted so as to lend itself more readily, though with some difficulty, to the examination of all parts of the body surface.

The microscope is binocular. It is supported on a pillar which is set in a heavy movable base. The pillar contains several joints and micrometer screws which allow movements of the microscope in various directions.

There are three objectives and four oculars. These give magnifications from 8 to 172 times. Magnifications over 100-fold are unsatisfactory because of insufficient illumination and poor definition. The most useful magnifications are 40 and 67 times; the latter permits distinct inspection of the blood flow and gives good general pictures.

The tubes carrying the oculars can be adjusted to any interpupillary distances.

The illuminating device is the Gullstrand slit-lamp. This utilizes the principle of focal illumination to the utmost. It consists of a small nitrogen lamp enclosed in a hard rubber cylinder mounted on a movable bar. The light escapes through a rectangular aperture in a rubber diaphragm, and then passes through an adjustable lens by means of which it may be focused on the part under observation as an intense linear bundle of light.

The lamp can be raised or lowered, and moved about on its support. It cannot be tilted. To overcome this drawback, I have had a joint inserted into the supporting pillar so that the lamp can be tilted to any desired angle. The lamp is attached to a rheostat which permits the use of any ordinary lighting current.

For dermatologic use it would be better if the microscope and slit-lamp were made as a unit, and the combined apparatus mounted on a lighter base. An arrangement of this kind would greatly facilitate examination of all bodily surfaces.

TECHNIC

It may be said here that the technic is at present elementary. This, of course, is to be expected in such a new method, but there is no doubt that human ingenuity will eventually solve many of the problems that present themselves.

Clearing.—The skin is a semi-opaque medium; even with the strongest illumination thrown on it, it is not possible to see far into its depths. Strong illumination will, however, penetrate a certain distance; and this relative opacity depends on various factors which are not clearly understood. Whether the horny layer (Kromayer) or the keratohyaline layer (Unna) hinders illumination most, need not be discussed. Saphier [1] mentions this important problem, and recalls the investigations of Spalteholz on the clearing of dead hardened tissues. A few observations with the slit-lamp microscope will show any observer that the irregularities of the horny layer hinder the penetration of light. These irregularities may be due to a number of factors: dryness, entrance of air, hyperkeratosis, and other factors. Whatever the cause of the surface irregularities, it is the numberless facets so formed which, reflecting the light in various directions, hinder its passage and prevent a view of the deeper tissue. One need only call to mind the surface of a polished glass plate and that of a frosted glass to grasp the problem raised by the horny layer.

This problem has been surmounted easily and in an obvious manner. It is merely necessary to obliterate the surface irregularities and thus prevent light refraction. For this purpose an oil is most useful. I have found cedar immersion oil best, after trying water, glycerin and anilin oil.

The oil is applied in a thin layer, and this process, designated clearing by Saphier, is completed. Clearing is effected almost immediately, proving that it is not the penetration of the oil which effects it, but the obliteration of the surface irregularities. My personal observations are that the visibility of the deeper tissues is the same several minutes or as late as two hours after the surface has been cleared by cedar oil.

Illumination.—So far as the light is concerned, the tissue may be examined in various ways. Thus, the bundle of rays may be thrown directly on the field to be examined; or it may be made to enter the skin obliquely at various distances. In the former instance, the intense glare evoked prevents an examination of the area on which the light falls, but the strongly illuminated surrounding parts can be advantageously seen. The second method gives an effect of transillumination, in which there is a gradual gradation from an intensely illuminated area to a duller one. Most information can be gained by arranging the field in this way.

It is desirable, indeed almost necessary, to make examinations in a dark room, since sources of light other than the lamp obscure the picture.

Routine of Examination.—The dermatoscope allows direct observation of only three things in the skin: (1) the horny layer, (2) the blood vessels, and (3) the pigment. Excepting red blood cells, individual cells cannot be seen; and therefore infiltration, which constitutes such a conspicuous feature of histologic examination, is lacking. At times, however, by the observation of other elements, notably the blood vessels, its presence may be inferred. The limitations noted in the foregoing are at first glaring to one accustomed to examining prepared material under the microscope, and, without doubt, detract considerably from the value of dermatoscopic examination. It is to be hoped that in this field, as in histopathology, an Unna will arise whose genius will solve these problems.

In the examination proper, the skin, without preparation, is observed under low power, and then under higher magnifications. In this way, scales, crusts, surface hemorrhages, skin markings, follicular openings and follicular plugs may be examined in their natural state. To me, so far, it has been the least important part of the examination, though observations of the sweating skin, of Auspitz's sign in psoriasis, of comedones and other phenomena are best observed, or at least, should be examined first in this way. And, it may be added, they are very interesting.

Following this the skin is cleared with cedar oil. The oil may be applied by means of an ordinary wooden applicator, and allowed to flow over the surface. Prior to this, scales, crusts, and other impedimenta may be removed if desired.

With the clearing of the horny layer, the blood vessels and pigment come into prominence. The blood vessels themselves cannot be seen; they can be observed only because red blood cells are visible. Through this fact, the number, form, arrangement and position of the vessels may be noted; and in addition, hemorrhage, if present, is discernable.

The vessels that come into observation are the capillaries of the papillae and in certain favorable instances, the vessels of the papillary body (superficial plexus).

So far as the pigment is concerned, its color, arrangement and position may be observed.

Besides these tissue constituents, which are always observable, it is possible at times to note the sweat pores when sweat secretion is occurring. The illustration (Fig. 2) is a happy chance which presented itself during the artist's observations.

OBSERVATIONS ON NORMAL AND DISEASED SKIN

Normal Skin.—The description of the various conditions observed will be given in a rather fragmentary manner, because it is not my purpose, at present, to enter into detailed discussion of the changes noted.

The hair follicles appear as irregular, funnel-shaped depressions containing a hair, or as slightly raised epidermal mounds closely embracing the hair shaft. Coil gland openings are much harder to discern; they appear as cup-shaped depressions fairly regularly spaced. According to Saphier, a capillary is closely adjacent as one usually accompanies the duct.

In a sweating skin, the epidermal portion of the duct can be plainly observed. It appears as a gradually mounting, obliquely placed series of highly refracting circles (Fig. 2). By shifting the focus, the spiral course of the duct can be made out. The sweat collects in a head on the surface and then runs along the skin grooves.

Under comparatively low magnification ($\times$ 40) the capillaries appear as fine red points, loops, lines or in bizarre forms. They are fairly spaced, of fairly uniform dimensions with an occasional vessel of larger lumen, and do not anastomose. The capillaries that are seen no doubt are papillary vessels, and indicate the approximate center of a papilla. The deeper vessels (superficial plexus) are just discernable as nebulous reddish streaks. With higher magnifications ($\times$ 67 and over), the circulatory flow is distinctly seen. In normal skin, the blood vessels are observed best just above the epionychium of the little finger.

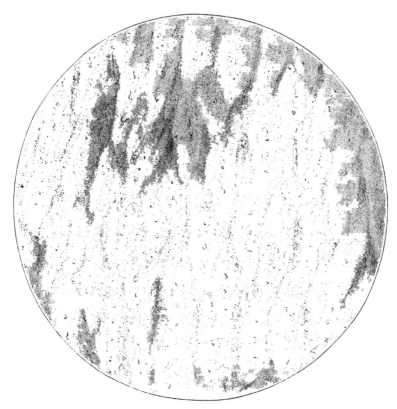

Fig. 2.—Normal skin showing the capillaries, skin markings and epidermal portions of the sweat ducts. The skin markings are erroneously portrayed. being considerably more prominent in the illustration than in nature. ($\times$ 40; Obj. A₂, Oc. 4.)

The normal white skin does not show pigment in granular form. So far as my personal observations go, it is only when pigment accumulation is pathologic (lentigines, chloasma, pigmentary nevi, etc.) that it occurs in discernible granules, or in homogeneous but distinct masses.

Dermatoses.—My observations unfortunately do not include the two disease states in which dermatoscopic examination is said to be of distinct diagnostic value. These diseases are lupus vulgaris and the

lenticular syphilid. Lupus vulgaris and, indeed, tuberculosis of the
skin in all its forms, appears to be an extremely rare disease in this
part of the country; so rare that only the merest chance will afford
an opportunity to examine a case by this new means.

According to Saphier, the diagnostic differentiation of these diseases
lies in the appearance of the blood vessels. The lupus nodule contains "numerous branching vessels forming branch-like (dendritic)

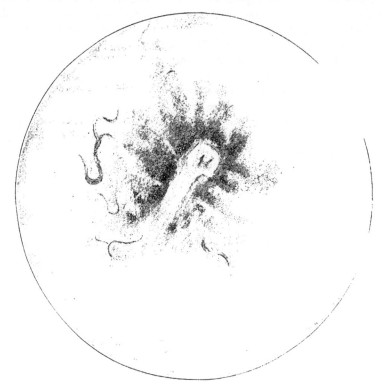

Fig. 3.—A small pigmented nevus to show pigment, a hair follicle and blood
vessels at this magnification. The circulatory flow was distinctly observed in
these vessels. The entire vascular supply is not portrayed. (×67: Obj. A:.
Oc. 15 mm.)

ramifications. . . . Numerous fine anastomoses connect these vessels to
each other and with deeper invisible vessels." On the other hand, the
lenticular syphilid shows "numerous expanded capillary loops. The
dilatation, as a rule, is quite considerable; so that the lesion is sharply
defined from the surrounding tissue. Moreover, we do not find the
dendritic ramifications, as in lupus vulgaris." He mentions several
cases in which dermatoscopic examination led to the correct diagnosis.

A phenomenon, personally observed, has been noted that may be important. It concerns the differential diagnosis between urticaria (including angioneurotic edema) and the group closely allied to it: the erythemas of the multiform type and their allies. Clinically, there are certain faits de passage between these two that are not easily differentiated.

With the dermatoscope, urticaria is characterized by the lack of definite outline of the capillaries. The vessels are blurred even to the margin of the wheal, and in the center appear only as nebulous red strands, or may be entirely invisible. It seems reasonable to conclude that the lessened visibility of the vessels is due to the edema; the increased lymph content of the tissue, which hinders or diffuses the refraction of light. On the other hand, in the erythemas, the vessels are sharply defined, dilated and more distinct than in normal tissue.

The difference of appearance between these two groups of diseases has been of some importance in differential diagnosis. In this particular, one very interesting case may be briefly described.

A man of 41 complained of an eruption of three years' duration. It disappeared while he slept, but with almost chronological exactness appeared in the morning an hour after he bestirred himself. It developed by successive appearance of lesions and was at its height in midafternoon. It was attended at times with mild itching. The eruption was composed of three types: (1) wheal-like efflorescences; (2) irregular oval nodules with intensely red margins and lighter colored centers, and (3) small, firm, dark red, split-pea sized papules, which occasionally formed small arciform lesions. These were intermingled on the cutaneous surface in irregular order with the exception that on the face and neck macules alone appeared, while on the extremities the papular lesions predominated.

The patient has been under observation for five months and, despite treatment, there has been no effect on the eruption.

The appearance of the eruption is that of erythema multiforme, but the behavior of the condition precluded that disease and the alternative diagnosis of urticaria was made. Dermatoscopic examination, which has been made on a number of occasions and at various times of the day, lends its testimony to this conclusion. The lesions show an absence or blurring of the vessels. In the margin of the lesion they become distinct and dilated. This picture seems characteristic for urticaria with the reservation that too few observations have been made to permit a definite conclusion.

In psoriasis, early patches (after removal of scales and clearing) show strikingly distinct capillaries. They appear close to the surface, as was to be expected from histopathologic findings. The circulation appears brisker than normal. The edge of the spot may be determined ith precision by the sudden increase in number and size of the vessels

Involuting lesions present a different picture. Hyperkeratosis is noted, and both the number and size of the capillaries are less than in early patches.

It is interesting to watch the appearance of Auspitz's sign under the dermatoscope after scraping the surface of the patch. From the tops of the capillary loop closest to the surface, there is a slow trickle of red cells, which take a tortuous course through the epidermis and collect on the surface as a small pool of blood. It is to be understood that this is a description of the smallest hemorrhages; those that are hardly discernable by the naked eye.

Three cases of leukoderma have been examined. Two were of the type with intensely hyperpigmented borders; while one did not have this feature. It was rather surprising to note that the transition from the depigmented area to the normal or hyperpigmented skin was not sharply defined. The pigmented areas showed scattered pigment dust, and the color was light gray. From these observations it would appear that pigment is only strikingly noticeable under the dermatoscope when it is present in abundance, or when the granules are of comparatively large size, as in pigmented nevi or lentigines. The blood vessels of the depigmented areas did not appear with appreciably more distinctness than in normal skin.

A case of ichthyosis of mild degree in a 4 year old child showed marked follicular plugging with horny masses. This was similar to the picture in keratosis pilaris. Another feature in this case was the abnormally long and straight capillaries which after clearing showed up prominently, and could be traced for some distance. This is consonant with the histologic findings in this disease, of flattening of the papillae, and the formation of a straight or undulating line between the epidermis and corium.

A number of pigmented moles have been examined. So far a typical melanotic mole has not been observed, but a dark brown pigmented mole on the forehead of a young girl was carefully studied. This lesion was about 4 mm. in diameter and to unaided observation appeared flat. Because of its appearance and a suspicion of impending malignancy aroused by a history of a recent noticeable but slight enlargement, it presented an opportunity to determine what value dermatoscopy might have in such circumstances.

The picture presented was remarkable. Without clearing, the epidermis showed many small follicular elevations from which projected fine lanugo hairs, with several larger hairs interspersed among them. It was also noted that the pigmented area was really slightly raised and supported on a base of normally colored skin with sloping walls. About the hairs the epidermis was slightly roughened, while the depressions presented a smooth appearance.

After clearing, it could be seen that projecting out of the depths were numerous translucent, pale brownish cones with larger bases than summits. They were hair follicles, because from the tops projected lanugo hairs. Around the base of the follicles, dark brown, dustlike pigment was scattered, forming as it were, encircling walls. The pigment was not uniformly distributed nor was it entirely confined to the peripilar regions. There were streaks of it scattered at random in the interfollicular regions. The situation of the pigment appeared to be both epidermal and dermal. The dermal situation could be definitely made out by observations of the blood vessels. These were larger than normal, but not so numerous. They came up from the deeper tissue and curved about the base of the follicular cones, forming occasional anastomoses. By focusing it could be determined that the blood vessels were surrounded, and in places somewhat obscured by the pigment. The perivascular pigment, of course, must have been as deep, at least, as the papillary body. On examination of the sloping nonpigmented walls of the lesion, granules were found beneath the epidermis. There the pigment lay in bundles and extended more deeply than it could be followed. The latter feature and the dermatoscopically observed elevation of the lesion were considered portents of impending, if not already present, malignancy. The patient passed from my hands and I, unfortunately, have not been able to confirm these observations by histologic examination.

Early basal cell epithelioma of the superficial nodular type with central atrophy presents, before clearing, thin scales attached by one border, while in places greater cavities extend into the deeper parts. The floor of these depressions appeared to be formed of very thin epidermis and comparatively large tortuous vascular trunks lay immediately beneath, even seeming to form part of it occasionally. After clearing, the vessels showed clearly through the thin epidermis. Large vascular trunks ramified through the upper cutis, giving off branches, which ascended to the surface or coursed toward the deeper parts.

The capillaries did not form loops as in normal tissue, but coursed in straight or zig-zag lines. At the raised periphery the vessels were obscure; they could be discerned, but lacked sharp outline. The epidermis was evidently thicker here. In this region, diffuse grayish or brownish collections were noted. These, in places blotted out the underlying parts. They were, most probably, both pigment deposits and infiltration.

A typical case of lupus erythematosus was examined. Before clearing, the features were the follicular plugs, which stood out prominently, and the pitlike depressions, which remained after the plugs were removed. When the lesions were cleared, strikingly distinct dilated blood vessels were observed. From these trunks numerous ramifying branches were given off. There was no regular capillary arrangement. Moderate pigment deposits were observed in the periphery of the lesions. From the distinctness of the blood vessels and the unusual transparency of the tissue it was possible to deduce that atrophy was present; a fact which ordinary examination had left in some doubt.

Verruca vulgaris shows, after clearing, a translucent keratotic plate overlying a base in which large papillae each containing an enlarged capillary are distinctly seen. The tops of some papillae are close to the surface. This is the only condition in which it has been possible to observe the papillary outlines with unmistakable distinctness.

Besides the observations detailed in the foregoing, observations have been made on a number of other dermatoses. Among these acne. tatoo marks, nevus flammeus and dermatitis seborrheica presented nothing of unusual interest in the few cases examined.

Several different onychoses, among them mycotic infections. pigmentations and leukonychia traumatica proved interesting. Under the dermatoscope leukonychia traumatica appears as a milk-white. highly refracting cloud on the nail substance, made up of an aggregation of minute white irregular fractures resembling a certain type of frosted glass which has been treated so as to produce innumerable chippings. The leukonychial spots appear to be situated nearer the nail bed than the upper surface. The central spot is always surrounded by small collections or single minute satellite spots. In studying the latter. it appears that they are minute nail plane faults. in the geologic sense. the nail plane having been displaced in various directions. but mainly in either a transverse or a vertical way. The ultimate conclusion in this is reserved, especially as Heidingsfeld has apparently so thoroughly proved the origin of leukonychia traumatica as due to incomplete keratinization of the areas presenting the phenomena.

Observations of onychomycoses have not reached a point worthy of further remark.

DISCUSSION

The slit-lamp microscope has created an histology of the living skin. Elementary as this histology is at present, it can hardly fail to develop. That the slit-lamp microscope renders it possible to observe pigment. discern papillae, and see the blood circulating in the skin is sufficient to convince any one of the potentialities inherent in this means of examination.

The apparatus needs improvement. It should be made more adaptable for the examination of all parts of the body surface and the illumination and lenses should be improved so that the higher magnifications can be used advantageously.

The skin itself presents difficulties that will be harder to solve. In the first place, individual cells cannot be observed. It is unlikely that they ever will be, because the preparation of a transparent, differentially stained and yet viable area of skin is hardly within the bounds of the practicable. For this reason dermatoscopy will never replace biopsy. However, another defect may be remedied eventually. This concerns the inability to see the deeper parts of the cutis.

The present value of the dermatoscope in diagnosis is small. Saphier appears to have established an important differentiation between lupus vulgaris and the lenticular syphiloderm. Again, the difference in the vascular appearance in urticaria and in erythema multiforme may be of value.[3]

Carter Building.

3. In addition the following references will be found of interest (these are only available to me in abstract):

Saphier, J.: Die Dermatoskopie, II, Arch. f. Dermat u. Syph. **132**:69, 1921. Die Dermatoskopie, III, Arch. f. Dermat. u. Syph. **134**:314, 1921. Die Dermatoskopie, IV, Arch. f. Dermat. u. Syph. **136**:149, 1921.

Kumer, L.: Dermatoscopic Observations in Some Skin Diseases, Dermat. Ztschr. **34**:127 (Sept.) 1921.

Müller, O.: Mein Capillar Mikroskop, Med. Klin. **17**:1448 (Nov. 27) 1921.

ULCER OF THE LEG

ITS LOCALIZATION AS A POINT CF DIFFERENTIAL DIAGNOSIS

HERMAN GOODMAN, B.S., M.D.

NEW YORK

After service at several of New York City's larger dispensaries, and having a special interest in syphilitic manifestations, I gained the impression that the localization of ulcer of the leg as a point in differential diagnosis between syphilitic ulcer and varicose ulcer had been overestimated as to location on the limb, and entirely neglected as to whether it was on the right leg or the left leg. At first glance, the importance of the latter would seem negligible, and it became my aim to collect a series of fifty cases of ulcer of the leg for analysis. However, with ulcers of both legs appearing, the number was extended, and I have records of sixty-four patients with ulcers of the lower part of the legs. The cases are divided as follows: ulcers of the lower part of the right leg, twenty-five; of the left, twenty-six; of both legs, thirteen. This series was a continuous one from the surgical outpatient departments of Bellevue Hospital, and represents unselected patients as they came in.

ANALYSIS OF ULCERS OF THE RIGHT LEG

The clinical diagnosis of ulcer of the leg does not always follow the textbook descriptions. Still, the diagnosis of syphilitic gumma was made in a patient with a single punched out ulcer of the middle of the tibia. a horseshoe ulcer of the lower third of the back of the limb, multiple gummas of both the upper and lower thirds of the right leg of one patient, and scars from former ulcerations in about the same location in another patient. There were two patients not included in the ulcer group with serpiginous gummas of the right leg, one of the dorsum of the foot, and the other of the lower part of the leg. A positive clinical diagnosis of syphilis could not be made from other ulcers. The Wassermann reaction was performed on this series of twenty-five ulcers of the right leg. Thirteen were reported positive, two as anticomplementary. and ten serums were negative.

ANALYSIS OF ULCERS OF THE LEFT LEG

There were twenty-six patients with ulcers of the left leg. It was not possible to make a definite clinical diagnosis of syphilitic ulcer in any patient of this group. The Wassermann reaction was reported negative nineteen times; and it was anticomplementary once. There were two patients with reports of slightly positive Wassermann reactions. One of these two patients had a perforating ulcer of the foot. He did not improve with intensive antisyphilitic treatment. Four were reported as having strongly positive Wassermann reactions. One of these patients had a traumatic ulcer of twenty years' duration about the left knee and contiguous portions of the lower part of the leg. Intensive antisyphilitic treatment did not heal this ulcer. The other patients of this group with strongly positive Wassermann reactions did not present lesions which were clinically syphilitic. In a number of patients with negative Wassermann reactions mixed treatment, mercury and iodid,

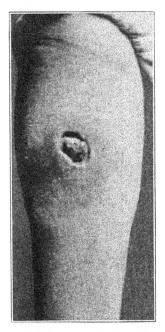

Fig. 1.—Ulcerated gumma in the middle of the lower part of the right leg.

was given by mouth. Some improvement could be noted in certain cases, but the result could not be considered a positive therapeutic test. The so-called "alterative" properties of the mixture had probably asserted their effects. Provocative Wassermann reactions in this group were also negative.

There were two patients with a negative Wassermann reaction and ulcer of the left leg deserving of further mention. Both were clinically examples of Marjolin's ulcer, or cancerous degeneration of chronic ulcers. Other ulcers in this group were undoubted nonsyphilitic ulcers, such as circular ulcer, variose ulcer, diabetic ulcer, tuberculous ulcer, senile ulcer, ulcer of thrombosis obliterans and filth ulcer. An effort was made to differentiate further these ulcers by means of roentgen-ray examinations of the underlying bones, but the changes were about the same in all cases. Seemingly, as pointed out by Dudley Morris,[1] any chronic ulceration of the leg means an associated periostitis and changes in the deep arteries of the leg.

ANALYSIS OF ULCERS OF THE LOWER PART OF BOTH LEGS

Thirteen patients had ulcers on the lower part of both legs. The clinical diagnosis of syphilitic ulcer could not be made in this group.

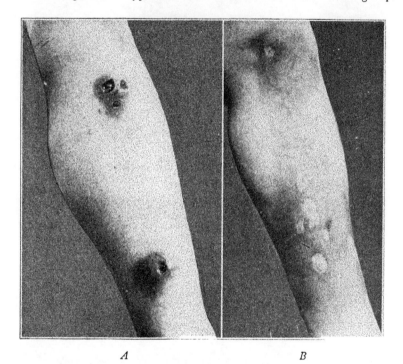

A   *B*

Fig. 2.—Multiple gummas of the upper and lower thirds of the right leg: *A*, before treatment; *B*, scars in another patient.

The Wassermann reaction was positive in two patients of this group. The most exaggerated ulcers occurred in patients with a negative Wassermann reaction. One patient, a woman, who weighed considerably over 200 pounds (90 kg.), was a cook and stood all day. She came from a suburb as no hospital nearer than ours would treat her. There was one pair of ulcers with an associated periostitis, and the right leg seemed more affected than the left.

1. Morris, D. H.: The Deeper Structural Changes Arising from Varicose
    C   922

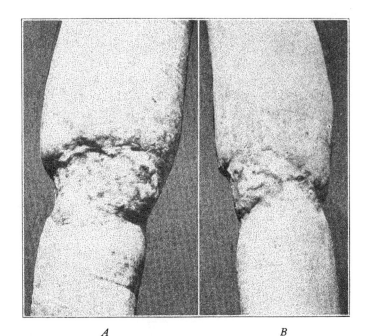

A   B

Fig. 3.— Circular ulcer of the left leg; *A,* front view; *B,* view from the back.

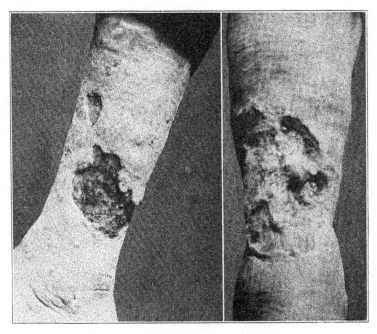

Fig. 4.—Nonsyphilitic ulcers of the left leg.

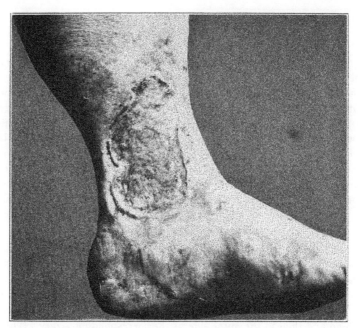

Fig. 5.—Nonsyphilitic ulcer of the left leg with overgrowth of epithelium at edges.

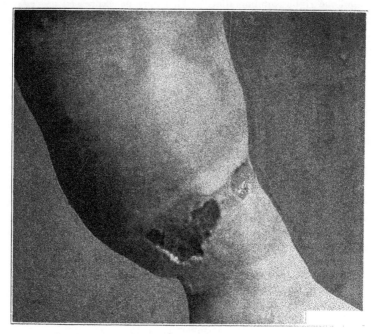

Fig. 6.—Ulcer on leg of cook (case mentioned in text).

COMMENT

The most cursory examination of the figures shows that ulcers of the right leg are more apt to be syphilitic than those of the left leg, when the ulcers are limited to one leg, and that, on the contrary, patients with ulcers of the left leg gave 73 per cent. negative Wassermann reactions as compared to 40 per cent. negative Wassermann reactions obtained in patients with ulcers of the right leg. As far as I have been able to learn, there is nothing in the nature of the syphilitic process to cause this predominance of right side syphilitic ulcers. It was necessary to seek an answer by looking for the cause of predominance of nonsyphilitic ulcers on the left leg, and such causes were not difficult to find.

COMPARISON OF SALIENT ANATOMIC FACTORS

The static relation of the two lower limbs is very different, owing to the dissimilarity of the veins and arteries. Although the superficial and deep crural veins are almost alike, the common iliac veins are very different. According to Gray's "Anatomy": "The right common iliac is shorter than the left, nearly vertical in its direction, and ascends behind and then to the outer side of the corresponding artery. The left common iliac, longer than the right, and more oblique in its course, is at first situated on the inner side of the corresponding artery, and then behind the right common iliac." This may be expressed as regarded from the arterial relation, in that the right common iliac artery compresses the left common iliac vein against the body of the fifth lumbar vertebra and intervertebral disk. The left internal iliac artery crosses the left external iliac vein at a right angle which is in marked contrast to the relations of the vessels on the right side. Further, according to Gray: "Each common iliac receives the ilio-lumbar, and sometimes the lateral sacral veins. The left receives in addition, the middle sacral vein. No valves are found in these veins. In the list of peculiarities, the left common iliac instead of joining with the right in its usual position, occasionally ascends on the left side of the aorta as high as the kidney, where after receiving the left renal vein, it crosses over the aorta, and then joins with the right vein to form a short inferior vena cava. In these cases the two common iliacs are connected by a small communicating branch at the spot where they are usually united."

According to Riedl,[2] "The right iliac vein crosses the right iliac artery at a very acute angle. The artery gradually pushes itself past the vein to emerge above Poupart's ligament to the lateral side of it and then rests in the median line. The same artery higher up crosses the left iliac vein almost at a right angle exerting greater pressure

---

2. Reidl, quoted by Royster in discussion of Kestler, H. D.: Thrombophlebitis of the Left Leg. J. A. M. A. **59**:437 (Aug. 10) 1912.

on the left than on the right vein. At this point, anteriorly, the quite large median sacral artery passes downward to the spinal column so that the left iliac vein is to a certain extent enclosed within the acute angle formed by the crossing of the right iliac artery and the median sacral. Still lower down, the hypogastric artery passes obliquely in front of the left iliac vein. The left iliac vein is therefore subjected to a three-fold arterial pressure while the right iliac vein is subjected to but a single pressure."

McMurrich[3] has described also an interesting peculiarity found in ten of thirty-seven cadavers examined, of which nine were in the left iliac vein. The peculiarity observed was an adhesion of the anterior and posterior walls of the common iliac just below its termination in the inferior vena cava. The adhesion was of small extent, not measuring more than 2 mm. as a rule in either the lateral or vertical position and also in its height. In some cases it appeared as if the two walls of the vein came in direct contact; in others the adhesion took the form of a column, 2 mm. high, extending from one wall to the other. As to its horizontal position, it was found sometimes almost in the center, but more usually somewhat toward the outer side of the vein, and indeed sometimes quite at the outer side of the vein, when it took the form of what appeared to be a linear thickening of the wall of the vein of slight extent longitudinally. In the majority of cases, however, it was far enough away from the outer border to divide the lumen of the vein, the outer of the two lumens, so formed, usually being the smaller.

CONCLUSION

It would seem, then, that there is much anatomic ground for changes in the left leg due to static conditions, and that the right leg is comparatively free from such possibilities. It should not be surprising, therefore, that the left leg is subject to diseases dependent on retarded venous circulation more often than the right. It is only necessary to recall that 90 per cent. of all cases of thrombophlebitis occur on the left leg; that milk-leg is much more common on the left than on the right; and that a patient with failing circulation is likely to have edema of the left leg rather than of the right leg. The greater frequency of nonsyphilitic ulcerations on the left leg may, then, be expected. That they should be twice as frequent, as my short series would indicate, justifies the reverse proposition, that the syphilitic ulcer is encountered twice as infrequently on the left leg. To carry the proposition farther leads to the conclusion that the syphilitic ulcer is encountered twice as often on the right leg as on the left. At

---

3. McMurrich: Brit. M. J. 2:1699, 1916.

first thought such a conception seems foolhardy, but on deliberation based on the facts as set forth in the body of this paper, the reasoning becomes more clear.

Although I recognize that the number of cases used in the analysis is small, it should be remembered that it bears out an impression gained from the study of a large number of patients with ulcer of the leg seen at one time or another at various hospitals and clinics about New York City. More recently, as the reported series took form and substance, this matter has been broached in the discussion of diagnosis of ulcers of the leg before clinic classes. The publication of this paper at this time should serve as an impetus for additional information from others, and it is hoped that evidence concerning the significance of this differential diagnostic point, not previously stressed, will be forthcoming.

News and Comment

THE CANCER QUACK

The Fool Killer was evidently just as active one hundred and fifty years ago as he is now, and the problems of the medical profession in dealing with him were just as real. In illustration of this we publish below the "Epitaph on a Patient Killed by a Cancer Quack," written by Dr. Lemuel Hopkins. It is interesting to see that more than a hundred and fifty years ago, at a time when we are prone to regard medicine as being in the dark ages, an intelligent physician's view of the quacks' treatment of cancer differed in nowise from the view of the physicians of the present day.

Dr. John E. Lane, who numbers among his other scholarly attainments that of medical antiquarian, gives the following account of the author:

Dr. Lemuel Hopkins was born in Naugatuck, Conn., June 19, 1750. He began to practice. in Litchfield in 1776. He served in the army for a short time in 1776 as a volunteer. He moved to Hartford in 1784, and made a name for himself there. Among his pupils, Elisha North was the most prominent. He belonged to a small coterie of literary men known as the "Hartford Wits." The others were Joel Barlow, Timothy Dwight, John Trumbull, Richard Alsop and Theodore Dwight. He wrote "The Cancer Quack," "Ethan Allen," "The Hypocrite's Hope."

These poems were published in a volume entitled "American Poems." selected and original, volume 1 (pp. 137-142), Litchfield: Collier and Buel.

Elihu H. Smith was the editor of this volume, though his name does not appear on the title page. It did not receive the support expected and Smith never got out the second volume.

EPITAPH

On a Patient Killed by a Cancer Quack

DR. LEMUEL HOPKINS

Here lies a fool flat on his back.
The victim of a Cancer Quack:
Who lost his money and his life.
By plaister, caustic, and by knife.
The case was this—a pimple rose.
South-east a little of his nose:
Which daily redden'd and grew bigger.
As too much drinking gave it vigour:
A score of gossips soon ensure
Full three score diff'rent modes of cure:
But yet the full-fed pimple still
Defied all petticoated skill:
When fortune led him to peruse
A hand-bill in the weekly news:
Sign'd by six fools of diff'rent sorts.
All cur'd of cancers made of warts:
Who recommend, with due submission.
This cancer-monger as magician:
Fear wing'd his flight to find the quack.
And prove his cancer-curing knack:

But on his way he found another,—
A second advertising brother:
But as much like him as an owl
Is unlike every handsome fowl;
Whose fame had rais'd as broad a fog,
And of the two the greater hog:
Who us'd a still more magic plaister,
That sweat forsooth, and cur'd the faster.
This doctor view'd, with moony eyes
And scowl'd up face, the pimple's size;
Then christened it in solemn answer,
And cried, "This pimple's name is CANCER."
"But courage, friend, I see you're pale,
"My sweating plaisters never fail;
"I've sweated hundreds out with ease,
"With roots as long as maple trees;
"And never fail'd in all my trials—
"Behold these samples here in vials!
"Preserv'd to shew my wond'rous merits,
"Just as my liver is—in spirits.
"For twenty joes the cure is done—"
The bargain struck, the plaister on.
Which gnaw'd the cancer at its leisure,
And pain'd his face above all measure.
But still the pimple spread the faster,
And swell'd, like toad that meets disaster.
Thus foil'd the doctor gravely swore,
It was a' right rose-cancer sore;
Then stuck his probe beneath the beard,
And Shew'd them where the leaves appear'd;
And rais'd the patient's drooping spirits,
By praising up the plaister's merits—
Quoth he, "The roots now scarcely stick—
"I'll fetch her out like crab or tick;
"And make it rendezvous, next trial,
"With six more plagues, in my old vial."
Then purg'd him pale with jalap drastic,
And next applies th' infernal caustic.
But yet, this semblance bright of hell
Serv'd but to make the patient yell;
And, gnawing on with fiery pace,
Devour'd one broadside of his face—
"Courage, 'tis done," the doctor cried.
And quick th' incision knife applied:
That with three cuts made such a hole,
Out flew the patient's tortur'd soul!

Go, readers, gentle, eke and simple,
If you have wart, or corn, or pimple;
To quack infallible apply;
Here's room enough for you to lie.
His skill triumphant still prevails,
For DEATH'S a cure that never fails.

Abstracts from Current Literature

LATENT NEUROSYPHILIS IN EIGHT PER CENT OF MEDICAL PATIENTS IGNORED OWING TO NEGLECT OF LUMBAR PUNCTURE. H. Gray, Am. J. Med. Sc. **163**:384 (March) 1922.

Among sixty-two patients, eight had unrecognized syphilis, and of these five had definite involvement of the central nervous system which had not been observed previously. It is recommended that lumbar puncture be performed on all syphilitic patients and, if the fluid is positive, repeated at least annually until found negative for a year. To guard against recurrence it should be repeated every two years thereafter.

AN ENDOCRINAL FACTOR IN GENERAL PARESIS. T. K. Davis, Am. J. Med. Sc. **163**:425 (March) 1922.

Eighty-two unselected cases of general paresis were examined for status lymphaticus, two outspoken cases being found. The remaining eighty were classified according to their degree of trichosis. It was found that the average duration of the paresis was appreciably shortened in those showing the most marked hypertrichosis, this condition of excessively hairy growth being interpreted by the author as indicating a heightened suprarenal function. Status lymphaticus is associated with a suprarenal cortex hypoplasia. It is rare among male paretic patients and necropsy examinations have shown that it is less frequent among paretic than among other patients. He thinks, therefore, that there is some relation between hyposuprarenal and hypersuprarenal function and the occurrence and duration of general paresis.

ACTINOMYCOSIS OF THE TONGUE. G. B. New and F. A. Figi, Am. J. Med. Sc. **163**:507 (April) 1922.

The authors found only three cases of primary actinomycosis of the tongue among 437 tumors of the tongue of all types. The greater frequency among animals is due to the greater amount of contact with infected material, most cases showing foreign particles in the tongue, especially in recent cases. Trauma of the tongue caused by carious teeth harboring the fungus may also be the cause.

The condition is more common among farmers and usually is manifested by a single isolated nodule, often near the tip of the tongue, and may follow injury to that organ. The process may be acute or may develop slowly for a few months or years and may be accompanied by adenitis, which is due to staphylococci, not actinomycoses.

The lesion is a small nodule enclosed in a fibrous capsule which may become infected and form an encapsulated abscess or rupture spontaneously. The overlying mucous membrane may be normal, yellowish or elevated and tense, but rarely ulcerates.

The treatment of choice is complete excision, potassium iodid internally and iodin locally with radium. Early cases and tumors situated near the tip of the tongue have a more favorable prognosis.

A report of the authors' cases and a review of the previously reported cases accompany the article.

Jamieson. Detroit.

DOSAGE IN RADIUM THERAPY. G. Failla, Am. J. Roentgenol. **8**:674, 1921.

It is suggested that doses of radiation be reckoned according to the amount of energy absorbed by the radiated tissue. The latter includes not only the pathologic tissue which one is trying to obliterate but also the surrounding normal tissue which must not be unduly injured. The success of the treatment depends on the relative amounts of radiation absorbed by the healthy and diseased tissue as well as the absolute amount of radiate energy absorbed by the pathologic tissue. The intensity of a treatment which may be measured by the duration of the exposure or the strength of the radioactive source is not without influence on the final result and must be taken into account.

The physical constants which enter into a complete specification of a dose are: (1) the strength of the radioactive source, (2) its distribution, (3) the total filtration used, (4) the duration of the irradiation, and (5) the relative positions and distances of the source of radiation, pathologic tissue and normal tissue.

Having the above data, the dose may be expressed in any unit. Since the biologic effect must be due to the radiant energy absorbed by the tissue, it is suggested that this be taken as a measure of the dose administered and that it be expressed in calories. At the present time it is not possible to express doses in calories for all forms of radium treatment because some of the data necessary for such calculations are not available.

Some examples are given in the paper and show the advantage of the method of dosage suggested.

INTENSIVE X-RAY THERAPY AS PRACTICED IN THE CLINICS IN EUROPE. S. Stern, Am. J. Roentgenol. **8**:741, 1921.

There seems to be a unanimity of opinion on only two of the essentials of carrying out intensive roentgen-ray therapy: (1) the necessity of having apparatus that is able to deliver at least 200,000 volts, (2) the essential employment of heavy filters. On all other important and even vital questions of technic there seems to be the greatest divergence of opinion. The details of treatment at a number of European clinics are given.

In the roentgen-ray treatment of skin diseases Stern thinks Americans do at least as well, and mentions seeing "them epilate the beard of a patient with sycosis which took fifty minutes. This epilation here is usually done in eight or nine minutes."

AMERICAN LITERATURE ON RADIUM AND RADIUM THERAPY PRIOR TO 1906. C. Chase, Am. J. Roentgenol. **8**:766, 1921.

Chase reviews the early literature on radium up to Jan. 1, 1906. He says that the study of the early literature has some other value than its purely historical interest as it gives the student a certain perspective that it is difficult otherwise to obtain.

RADIODERMATITIS. G. T. Pfahler, Am. J. Roentgenol. **8**:781, 1921.

Every possible precaution should be taken for the prevention of radiodermatitis. The production of any type of dermatitis should be guarded against, except where it is definitely indicated. Detailed and complete records should be kept of what is done. Careful attention should be given to prevent the patient from applying any irritant to the skin following roentgenization.

It is important to eliminate the term "x-ray burn" from the vocabulary. It is in no sense a burn. The expert roentgenologist should be most cautious about drawing conclusions as to neglect or incompetence. The very evidence that the expert uses may be turned against him when some patient of his has an unfortunate end-result even though it may not be the fault of the roentgenologist himself.

GOODMAN, New York.

A REPORT OF THE WORK OF THE RADIUM DEPARTMENT OF THE UNIVERSITY OF CALIFORNIA HOSPITAL BETWEEN APRIL, 1920, AND APRIL, 1921. L. R. TAUSSIG, Calif. State J. M. **20**: 50 (Feb.) 1922.

This report embraces the records of treatment in 420 cases. The end-result in metastasizing malignancies cannot be given as the plant has been in operation for too short a time. In general, the results have been satisfactory and conform to those usually obtained in comparable cases.

MICHAEL, Houston, Texas.

A CASE OF SPOROTRICHOSIS IN CONNECTICUT. C. T. NELLANS, J. A. M. A. **78**:802 (March 18) 1922.

This is the first case reported from Connecticut. There were no particularly unusual features.

SYPHILIS AND TRAUMA: THE WORKMEN'S COMPENSATION ACT, THE INDUSTRIAL PHYSICIAN AND THE SYPHILITIC EMPLOYEE. J. V KLAUDER, J. A. M. A. **78**:1029 (April 8) 1922.

The author reviews the literature pertaining to the influence of trauma on the development of syphilitic lesions, and adds several illustrative cases of cutaneous manifestations as well as of post-traumatic paresis. Particular attention is called to the delayed union of fractures and the increased liability to fractures in syphilitic persons.

The question of the bearing of syphilis on the Workmen's Compensation Act is discussed in some detail. Klauder advises the industrial physician to have a Wassermann test performed as a routine in all accident cases.

The author reports two interesting cases in which a previously negative serologic test became positive following trauma. Klauder tried, without success, to produce syphilitic lesions by traumatizing syphilitic rabbits in various ways.

THE TREATMENT OF LUPUS VULGARIS WITH SOLUTION OF MERCURIC NITRATE. E. P. ZEISLER, J. A. M. A. **78**:1045 (April 8) 1922.

The results in six cases of lupus vulgaris in which the patients were treated with acid nitrate of mercury have been excellent. The action of the acid is enhanced by a preliminary course of roentgen-ray therapy.

CAROTINOID PIGMENTATION OF THE SKIN RESULTING FROM VEGETARIAN DIET. H. HASHIMOTO, J. A. M. A. **78**:1111 (April 15) 1922.

In certain parts of Japan, squash forms a large part of the diet. The result is that adult cases of carotinemia are not uncommon. The author has seen about thirty-five patients with this condition.

PURPURA FULMINANS: REPORT OF CASE. H. L. Dwyer, J. A. M. A. **78**:1187 (April 22) 1922.

A boy, aged 3 years, suddenly became ill with pain in the abdomen and vomiting. A few hours later various sized ecchymotic areas appeared in the skin. The patient was very toxic. Death occurred within twenty-four hours of the appearance of the initial symptoms. Necropsy revealed the fact that the hemorrhages were limited to the skin.

THE DETERIORATION OF NEO-ARSPHENAMIN. G. B. Roth, J. A. M. A. **78**:1191 (April 22) 1922.

Lots of neo-arsphenamin kept in ampules for about two years show a change in color, solubility, mobility in the ampule, odor and toxicity. These changes may render the drug useless or dangerous to life. Warmth hastens the deterioration of the drug.

Roth advises that neo-arsphenamin be kept at icebox temperature.

A HISTOPATHOLOGIC STUDY OF POSITIVE CUTANEOUS TESTS: PRELIMINARY STUDY. Albert Strickler, J. A. M. A. **78**:1287 (April 29) 1922.

Positive tuberculin and endermic food tests show similar pathologic pictures characterized by a mononuclear cellular infiltration in the superficial cutis. Positive luetin tests show an intense inflammatory reaction in the deeper cutis with polymorphonuclear cellular infiltration.

As a positive tuberculin reaction is generally considered a specific response, the finding of a similar tissue reaction in positive food tests implies that such reactions are specific. The explanation of the histopathologic picture in positive luetin tests must await further investigation.

DEMONSTRATION OF LEPRA BACILLI BY ASPIRATION OF NODULES. S. S. Greenbaum and Jay F. Schamberg, J. A. M. A. **78**: 1295 (April 29) 1922.

The procedure is similar to the well known acupuncture of lymph glands for the detection of *Spirochaeta pallida.*

It may be useful in the deeper forms of nodular leprosy when biopsy is unobtainable, for immediate confirmation of the provisional diagnosis, when examination of the discharge or scraping of the nasal mucosa fails, and possibly in macular leprosy.

MADURA FOOT, MORE PROPERLY CALLED MYCETOMA. G. A. Pagenstecher, J. A. M. A. **78**:1363 (May 6) 1922.

Two typical cases are reported. The patients were laborers, and the disease followed an injury to the foot. Light yellow granules were present in the discharge.

The author advises amputation only when the patient has become crippled by the disease.

ERYTHEMA BULLOSUM. J. S. Eisenstaedt, J. A. M. A. **78**:1365 (May 6) 1922.

The five cases reported herein were of the rare type with serious visceral manifestations. Treatment consisted in alkalinizing the patient to the utmost and in giving large doses of salicylates. All recovered. Study of the cases indicated that the disease is due to toxic substances probably derived from foci of infection.

PRIMARY ACTINOMYCOSIS OF THE SKIN. M. J. BASKIN, J. A. M. A. **78**:1367 (May 6) 1922.

The patient was a trapper who developed a granulomatous lesion of the dorsum of the left hand, in which the organism was found. Treatment with surgical solution of chlorinated soda led to cure in two weeks.

TABES DORSALIS PLUS TERTIARY CUTANEOUS SYPHILIS. B. B. BEESON, J. A. M. A. **78**:1537 (May 20) 1922.

The patient, aged 57, had serpiginous syphilid and moderately advanced tabes. He had contracted syphilis in 1898, and the only medication was pills and potassium iodid for six months.

MICHAEL. Houston, Texas.

STUDIES ON X-RAY EFFECTS. X. THE BIOLOGICAL ACTION OF SMALL DOSES OF LOW FREQUENCY X-RAYS. W. NAKAHARA and J. B. MURPHY, J. Exper. Med. **35**:475 (April) 1922.

Using a special tube, a point spark gap of ½ inch (1.27 cm.), 11 milliamperes and a 6 inch (15.2 cm.) distance for one minute, mice showed an increase in lymphocytes beginning twenty-four hours later, gradually increasing for fourteen days and then subsiding. These mice also showed a greatly increased resistance to cancer transplants, the time of greatest resistance being about ten days following the treatment.

STUDIES ON X-RAY EFFECTS. XI. THE FATE OF CANCER GRAFTS IMPLANTED IN SUBCUTANEOUS TISSUE PREVIOUSLY EXPOSED TO X-RAYS. J. H. LIU, E. STURM and J. B. MURPHY. J. Exper. Med. **35**:487 (April) 1922.

Erythema doses of roentgen rays administered directly to subcutaneous tissue will produce protective changes similar to those produced in the skin. This resistance of subcutaneous tissue to the growth of implanted cancer cells is only local and does not follow erythema doses administered to the intact skin. A few days after the exposure there is a marked lymphoid infiltration which may even include the muscle layers.

A CUTANEOUS NEMATODE INFECTION IN MONKEYS. H. F. SWIFT. R. H. BOOTS and C. P. MILLER, JR., J. Exper. M. **35**:599 (May) 1922.

A parasite to which is given the name of *Trichosoma cutaneum*, 1922, was found to have caused subcutaneous nodules with edema about the joints, and blisters of the palms and soles of experimental monkeys. Larval forms were found in the subcutaneous nodules. while in the blisters the eggs were laid and subsequently discharged.

PATHOLOGY OF THE DERMATITIS CAUSED BY MEGALOPYGE OPERCULARIS. A TEXAN CATERPILLAR. N. C. FOOT. J. Exper. M. **35**:707 (May) 1922.

All stages of the larvae of the caterpillar are capable of producing stings with a dermatitis consisting of a localized painful burning area with erythema followed by small vesicles. The investigations of the writer disclosed the fact that the dermatitis is not due to the hair or tissue juices of the caterpillar, but that the poison is introduced by hollow specialized setae of its cuticular tubercles. The venom producing the dermatitis can be rendered inert by boiling and when injected into man produced localized necrosis with vesicle formation.

JAMIESON, Detroit.

PROGRESS REPORT ON THE TREATMENT OF LEPROSY BY THE INTRAVENOUS INJECTION OF CHAULMOOGRA OIL. PHILIP HARPER, J. Trop. M. **25**:2 (Jan. 2) 1922.

In thirty-eight patients who had been under treatment for varying periods up to eleven months, twenty-eight had improved, one died of intercurrent influenza, three were worse and six showed no change.

The author believes that in many of the cases showing improvement the same result could have been obtained by other modern methods of treatment, but he thinks his procedure is safer, more effective and less painful.

NOTES ON A PECULIAR TYPE OF EPIDEMIC DERMATITIS. OSBORNE BROWN, J. Trop. M. **25**:4 (Jan. 2) 1922.

This dermatitis has appeared in British Honduras since the return of troops from Mesopotamia and Egypt. It is highly contagious and has an incubation period of from one to two months.

The onset is abrupt with itching and the appearance of urticarial lesions on the buttocks or abdomen. These lesions become crusted and appear in successive crops during the course of the disease and are accompanied by intense pruritus. No area is exempt; there is more or less exfoliation of the skin in general, and alopecia may also accompany the disease.

The intensity of the disease gradually lessens in a few months. Treatment of all kinds may be used, but is, of no particular value except symptomatically. It is believed to be a systemic infection of unknown origin.

ANTIMONY IN THE TREATMENT OF LEPERS AND HYDATID DISEASES. F. G. CAWSTON, J. Trop. M. **25**:27 (Feb. 1) 1922.

Several cases of ulcerative leprosy are cited in which prompt healing resulted after the intramuscular injection of a colloidal preparation of antimony.

JAMIESON, Detroit.

CHRONIC CIRCUMSCRIBED NODULAR LICHENIFICATION. PAUTRIER, Ann. de dermat. et syph. **6**:49 (Feb.) 1922.

The author describes a case of lichen obtusus corneus, the involvement being generalized, and he gives a detailed analysis of the clinical and histologic features of this condition and of lichen planus, showing that the two conditions are far from identical and should not be classified together. The publications of Schamberg and Hirschler and of Charles J. White are cited (*Jour. Cutan. Dis.*, 1906-1907).

DISSOCIATIONS OF THE PATHOLOGIC SPINAL FLUID REACTIONS IN SYPHILIS OF THE NERVOUS SYSTEM. CESTAN and RISER, Ann. de dermat. et syph. **6**:63 (Feb.) 1922.

In a series of 200 cases examined at Toulouse, the authors found a positive Wassermann reaction, an increased amount of albumin (more than 0.3 gm. per liter) and an increased. lymphocyte count (more than 5 cells per cubic milli-meter). in 157 cases. In thirty-seven cases there was a dissociation of these reactions, as follows: In thirty-one patients, some of whom had been treated, there was a normal or a very low lymphocyte count; in one case of cerebral gumma the albumin content of the fluid was normal in the presence of a lymphocytosis; in four cases the positive Wassermann reaction was the only sign present, the other two features being normal. The extent of the involve-ment seems to bear no relation to these reactions.

CUTANEOUS ATROPHY IN DISSEMINATED PLAQUES OF TUBER-CULOUS ORIGIN. CHATELLIER, Ann. de dermat. et syph. 6:76 (Feb.) 1922.

A man, aged 20 years, presented numerous scars, lentil-sized on the average, some depressed and others keloidal, scattered over the thorax, abdomen, thighs and buttocks. There was a history of the occurrence of ulcers, probably tuber-culous, in. these locations, but the biopsy examination revealed only the pres-ence of scar tissue and did not reveal tuberculosis. The author considers the condition to be a healed tuberculosis cutis.

A TEMPORARILY POSITIVE AND OSCILLATING BORDET-WASSER-MANN REACTION IN THE COURSE OF AN AFFECTION CALLED SUBACUTE INGUINAL LYMPHOGRANULOMATOSIS. P. RAVAUT and RABEAU, Ann. de dermat. et syph. 6:80 (Feb.) 1922.

In a study of twenty-three cases of this condition, the authors found a positive Wassermann reaction at times in three. This reaction was fleeting, disappearing spontaneously and reappearing as the accompaniment of a brief febrile reaction. The positivity of the reaction seemed to vary with the severity of the other symptoms. Considering the clinical manifestations of this affection. it is imperative that this possibility be kept in mind. especially when the more delicate laboratory technic is used, in order that false diagnoses of syphilis may be avoided.

MYCOTIC INTERTRIGO: A NEW FORM OF EPIDERMOPHYTON INFECTION DUE TO A YEAST. DUBREUILH and JOULIA. Ann. de dermat. et syph. 6:145 (April) 1922.

The authors describe .the microscopic appearance and cultural character-istics of a vegetable parasite which they have found in erythematosquamous plaques involving the inguinal, genitocrural, perianal, intergluteal and sub-mammary regions, describing nine cases as examples. The organisms were recovered from the lesions of a supposed diabetic intertrigo, and in another case the condition was apparently transmitted by conjugal relationship. Whit-field's ointment. one-half strength, is especially recommended. also dilute tinc-ture of iodin for exuding lesions and 2 per cent. chrysarobin ointment in suit-able locations.

NEW TRIALS WITH AUTOHEMOTHERAPY IN THE DERMATOSES. NICOLAS, GATÉ and DUPASQUIER. Ann. de dermat. et syph. 6:163 (April) 1922.

This treatment. described by the authors in a previous communication (*Ann. de dermat. et syph.* 6: No. 3. 1921). has been used by them in prurigo. in which they had originally found it useful, and also in various dermatoses. such as eczema, urticaria, Duhring's disease and neurodermite, as well as in a case of furunculosis, with encouraging results. In lichen planus it was of no avail. The theories of its action are discussed.

FOLLICULAR ELASTIC DYSTROPHY OF THE THORACIC REGION POSSIBLY HEREDITARY. CARL WITH and A. KISSMEYER, Ann. de dermat. et syph. **6**:169 (April) 1922.

This condition, the first example of which was presented by With before the Scandinavian Dermatologic Congress at Copenhagen, in 1919, has since been called "nevus elasticus" by Lewandowsky, who saw three cases and described their histology. The authors again describe their original case, including a histologic study with elastic tissue stains. The elastic tissue of the papillae and upper corium is rarefied, showing elastorrhexis (Darier).

SYPHILIS BEGINNING IN THE LYMPH NODES. SEARCH FOR SPIROCHETES IN THE LYMPH NODES. CHATELLIER, Ann. de dermat. et syph. **6**:174 (April) 1922.

With Audry, the author has recently reported five cases of this type (*Ann. de dermat. et syph.* **6**:380 [July] 1921), and he now records another instance in which the bubo seemed to be the earliest sign of the disease, there having apparently been no chancre. Figures are given to show the advantage gained by looking for the organisms in the juice from the lymph nodes.

MERCURIAL HEPATITIS AND ANEMIA DUE TO THE CYANID. A. NANTA, Ann. de dermat. et syph. **6**:177 (April) 1922.

A man, aged 40 years, who had received arsenical and mercurial treatment since 1918, including a considerable amount of mercuric cyanid, finally developed a hepatitis and an aplastic anemia, from which he recovered. In 1915 he had had icterus following the use of chloroform.

PARKHURST, Toledo, Ohio.

THE WASSERMANN REACTION IN TUBERCULIDS. SACHS, Arch. f. Dermat. u. Syph. **123**: No. 5, 1917.

In two cases with numerous eruptions, the Wassermann reaction was positive. In one of the cases cod liver oil medication turned the reaction negative in four weeks.

MERCURY AND ARSPHENAMIN IN VARIOUS DOSES IN SECONDARY SYPHILIS. SCHOLTZ and KELCH, Arch. f. Dermat. u. Syph. **123**: No. 5, 1917.

The authors secured their best results in the secondary stages of syphilis, by using mercury for eight days, and arsphenamin on the two succeeding days. The arsphenamin was given as follows: from 0.2 to 0.25 gm. at 9 o'clock in the morning; at 1 o'clock, from 0.25 to 0.3 gm., and at 9 o'clock on the following morning, 0.3 gm.

BLOOD PICTURE IN EPIDERMOLYSIS BULLOSA HEREDITARIA. SPIETHOFF, Arch. f. Dermat. u. Syph. **123**: No. 5, 1917.

The cases examined concerned members of one family all of whom showed a pathologic blood-picture, i. e., increased number of mononuclear cells and lymphocytes, also pathologic forms of the latter and alteration of the neutrophils. On the whole, the picture somewhat resembled that seen in endocrine disturbances. There arises the question whether epidermolysis bullosa hereditaria is not in some way connected with endocrine disturbances.

CUTIS REACTION IN LEPRA AND ITS RELATION TO THE LEPRA-ERYSIPELOID. STEIN, Arch. f. Dermat. u. Syph. **123:** No. 5, 1917.

During an intense attack of erysipeloid several lepra patients gave a positive cutis reaction with an extract gained from lepra lymph glands.

A WIDESPREAD BROMID ERUPTION IN A PSORIATIC. STRANDBERG, Arch. f. Dermat. u. Syph. **123:** No. 5, 1917.

Small doses of potassium bromid given to a neurasthenic psoriatic caused the development of extensive polymorphonuclear eruptions.

THE LEUKOCYTE FORMULA OF VARIOUS SKIN ERUPTIONS. HECHT, Arch. f. Dermat. u. Syph. **125:** No. 3, 1918.

The author found typical leukocytosis in the lesions of lupus vulgaris. Hoke and Deal had already found an increase of lymphocytes, compared with body blood, in tuberculous lesions.

CIRCULATION OF MERCURY IN THE SYSTEM. LOMHOLT, Arch. f. Dermat. u. Syph. **126:** No. 1, 1918.

Absorption of mercury is quicker than elimination; mercury accumulates in the system. The kidneys and intestinal tract do most of the eliminating, while the coli and salivary glands do but little. Mercury is found in small quantities in the spinal fluid. The largest quantities are found in the kidneys, liver and bile. Large quantities pass from the mother to the fetus.

CONTRIBUTION TO THE KNOWLEDGE OF THE CALCIFICATIONS OF THE SKIN. KERL, Arch. f. Dermat. u. Syph. **126:** No. 1, 1918.

Myositis ossificans and calcinosis interstitialis represent a primary disorder of the collagenous tissue which subsequently leads to calcification.

SOME EXPERIMENTS AND REMARKS ON BLACK SKIN-PIGMENT. WINTERNITZ, Arch. f. Dermat. u. Syph. **126:** No. 1, 1918.

Extracts of horse skin and uvea stain black with solutions of tyrosin. Tyrosin therefore possibly accounts for the black skin pigmentation.

DERMATOLOGY. SAPHIER, Arch. f. Dermat. u. Syph. **136:** No. 2, 1921.

This article contains illustrations of sweat pores magnified 112 times; also a description of molluscum contagiosum nodules and sclerodermas.

ARTIFICIAL PURPURA IN A TUBERCULOUS PATIENT. FISCHL, Arch. f. Dermat. u. Syph. **136:** No. 2, 1921.

The author describes the provocation of purpura by the injection of physiologic sodium chlorid solution. In one case a papulonecrotic tuberculid developed on the purpura. The author believes that tuberculosis causes a hemorrhagic diathesis which, however, remains latent and only occasionally becomes activate

A CONTRIBUTION TO THE CLINICAL KNOWLEDGE AND ETIOL-
OGY OF SKIN ATROPHIES. Singer. Arch. f. Dermat. u. Syph. **136:**
No. 2, 1921.

The cause of skin atrophies is a disturbance of the endocrine equilibrium.

XANTHOMA. Siemens, Arch. f. Dermat. u. Syph. **136:** No. 2, 1921.

The author distinguishes two forms of cholesterin disease—simple hematogenous cholesteremia (Xantoma) and inflammatory-degenerative cholesteremia (pseudoxanthoma; Aschoff, Kammer). A hypercholesteremia is not
absolutely necessary for the development and progress of a xanthoma.

PROPRIETY OF FIXING CHARACTERISTIC GOLD FLOCCULATION
CURVES OF THE SPINAL FLUID IN SYPHILITIC CONDITIONS
OF THE CENTRAL NERVOUS SYSTEM. Arzt and Fuhs, Arch. f.
Dermat. u. Syph. **136:**207, 1921.

The authors state that it is not possible to diagnose a syphilitic condition
of the central nervous system from the type of gold reaction curve. Progressive paralysis curves were seen in tabes and cerebral syphilis.

IMPORTANCE OF SPINAL FLUID ALTERATIONS IN CERTAIN
SYPHILITIC MANIFESTATIONS. Arzt and Fuhs, Arch. f. Dermat.
u. Syph. **136:**212, 1921.

Basing their investigations on a large amount of material, the authors
answer three questions: 1. Does the spinal fluid in syphilis become pathologic,
and of what importance is this? 2. Does the location on the skin in late syphilis protect the central nervous system? 3. What relation have alopecia and
leukoderma to disease of the central nervous system? 1. The authors state
that patients with primary syphilis thoroughly treated never develop syphilis
of the central nervous system, nor do primary sores on the face, owing to their
location, in any way dispose to syphilis of the nervous system. 2. Contrary to
Finger, Hoffmann, Matzenauer and others, the authors state that projection
of syphilis onto the skin does not protect the central nervous system in any
way from being attacked. 3. There exists a close relation between alopecia,
leukoderma and the central nervous system.

CRITICISM OF THE DOPA REACTION. Bloch, Arch. f. Dermat. u. Syph.
136:231, 1921.

The author states that the silver reaction and Dopa reaction are not
identical. The silver reaction is positive, the Dopa reaction negative in cells
with strong pigmentation. Bloch proved that previous treatment with silver
dioxid, hydrocyanic acid, hydrogen sulphid vapors and acids hinders the Dopa
reaction, while the silver reaction is not influenced.

CIRCUMSCRIBED AMYLOID DEGENERATION IN A CASE OF
DERMATITIS ATROPHICANS DIFFUSA. Kenedy, Arch. f. Dermat.
u. Syph. **136:**245, 1921.

A case is described in which for the first time the amyloid degeneration
was already clinically visible. Histologic examination (van Gieson stain)

revealed a yellowish gray appearance of the collagenous parts within the lesions. The author believes that in this case the acrodermatitis was the cause of the amyloid degeneration.

A CASE OF PSEUDOLEUKEMIA WITH CHANGES IN THE SKIN. LEHNER, Arch. f. Dermat. u. Syph. **136**:251, 1921.

The vesicular infiltrations showed a degeneration (histologically) of the epithelium terminating in a coagulation necrosis, similar to the changes in herpes zoster and variola. The symmetry of the location of the lesions, as well as the simultaneous constitutional involvement (rise of temperature, etc.) in the author's opinion point to a hematogenous origin of the dermatosis in question.

THE CUTANEOUS TUBERCULIN REACTION (PIRQUET) WITH REGARD TO VARIOUS DERMATOSES AND TO THE COURSE OF SYPHILIS. SIMULTANEOUS PHARMACODYNAMIC CUTANEOUS REACTION (GROVER-HECHT) IN SOME OF THE CASES GUTMANN, Arch. f. Dermat. u. Syph. **136**:255, 1921.

Certain dermatoses, as well as secondary syphilis, considerably influence (hamper) the Pirquet reaction. The vasoconstrictory reaction following epinephrin, as well as the vasodilatation reaction following morphin administration, has little influence on the Pirquet reaction. In syphilis the epinephrin reaction is very strong. The author believes that experiments along these lines will reveal the etiology of certain diseases.

SMALL CYSTS CAUSED BY PATHOLOGIC SINKING OF THE EXTERNAL SKIN. TAKASUGI, Arch. f. Dermat. u. Syph. **136**:265, 1921.

In the regio scapularis of a girl the skin showed cribriform perforations due to numerous cysts, containing cholesterin, lanugo hairs and corneous material. The author believes that the disorder is due to a folding (Einstülpung) of the skin in late intra-uterine life.

A NOTE ON SARCOMATOSIS AND SOLITARY SARCOMA OF THE SKIN. VOLLMER, Arch. f. Dermat. u. Syph. **136**:273, 1921.

In young persons there is a tendency toward the formation of sarcoma in a skin exposed to constant irritation. These tumors heal spontaneously. There is no metastasizing, though relapses occur, and different parts of the skin may be affected simultaneously.

THE BASIS OF A NEW FLOCCULATION REACTION IN SYPHILIS. HECHT, Arch. f. Dermat u. Syph. **136**:296, 1921.

Hecht claims to be the first to prove that the Wassermann reaction is based on a precipitation. He succeeded in rendering this precipitation visible in the form of one large floccula. The technic of the new Hecht flocculation reaction must be read in the original paper. A colloid-chemical process accounts for the formation of the floccula which is completely soluble in alcohol. The nucleus of the floccula most likely consists of the antigen-lipoids which are covered by serum substances. The new reaction is as sensitive as the Wassermann reaction but cannot yet be utilized as a substitute.

SEROLOGIC AND CLINICAL OBSERVATIONS ON PRIMARY SORES WITH SPECIAL REFERENCE TO THE KAUP METHOD OF WASSERMANN REACTION AND THE FLOCCULATION REACTION AFTER SACHS-GEORGI. Gross, Arch. f. Dermat. u. Syph. **136**:304, 1921.

Kaup's modification of the Wassermann reaction proved to be the most sensitive method for demonstrating positive fluctuations during abortive treatment. In primary sores the alcoholic liver extract is the most sensitive antigen, in contradistinction to latent syphilis and the tertiary stages, in which cholesterinized ox heart is preferable.

EFFECT OF THE SERUMS ON SARCOID-BOECK AND LUPUS-PERNIO PATIENTS ON TUBERCULIN. Martenstein, Arch. f. Dermat. u. Syph. **136**:317, 1921.

Experiments showed that the serum of two patients suffering from lupus pernio weakened the Pirquet reaction in tuberculous patients while the serum of three patients suffering from Boeck's sarcoid increased the reaction. The study of more cases is necessary to warrant the forming of conclusions.

Ahlswede, Hamburg, Germany.

THE HUMAN TUBERCLE. Heiberg, Zentralbl. f. allg. Path. u. path. Anat. **32**:6, 1921.

This article contains illustrations of "preepithelioid" cells (preliminary stages of ordinary epithelioid cells). The nuclei are still oval in this stage and only later when they "grow older" assume an irregular shape with sharp edges.

Ahlswede, Hamburg, Germany.

THE CONTRACTILITY OF THE HUMAN SKIN CAPILLARIES. Parrisius, Pflueger's Arch. f. d. ges. Physiol. **191**:217, 1921.

This article contains a description of five cases in which there were alterations in the capillaries in patients with vasomotor disturbances. Mueller's skin capillary microscope was used. Peristaltic contraction and spasm were observed. Epinephrin (subcutaneous injection) caused interruption of the blood current.

Ahlswede, Hamburg, Germany.

NATURE'S CURE AND DRUG CURE OF SYPHILIS. Blaschko, Berl. klin. Wchnschr. **58**:1206, 1921.

In a syphilitic person there is a struggle between the "surviving spirochetes" and the tissue. The result and the sign of this struggle is the Wassermann reaction which expresses the defensive action of the body and therefore in itself is not an unfavorable omen. Blaschko states with Lesser that mercury treatment might disturb the defensive action of the body as the defensive inflammations of the system are too quickly broken up under this treatment. Long practical experiences and statistics, however, have proved beyond doubt the superiority of mercurial treatment to the expectant treatment (Naturheilmethode).

ROENTGEN-RAY TREATMENT OF LEUKEMIA. Oppenheimer, Berl. klin. Wchnschr. **58**:1351, 1921.

An attempt was made to cure leukemia with the roentgen rays and arsenic medication combined. Permanent cure was not possible.

Ahlswede, Hamburg, Germany.

NUMMULAR ERYTHEMATOSCLEROTIC LESIONS. Milian, Bull. Soc. franç. de dermat. et syph. **28**:488, 1921.

In a girl, aged 13 years, with asymptomatic congenital syphilis and a negative Wassermann reaction, there were nummular lesions on the legs, of six months' duration, atrophic and extending peripherally with central crusting which later became sclerotic. The biopsy examination suggested the diagnosis of tuberculid. A second similar case is shown and a third reported.

DESENSITIZING AUTOSERUM THERAPY FOR RECURRENT HERPES. Tzanck, Bull. Soc. franç. de dermat. et syph. **28**:489, 1921·

Successful results following this treatment are reported in three cases of regularly recurring herpes of the type which always returns in the same location, the hand, face and buttock having been involved here in these cases. Two cubic centimeters of the serum were injected at intervals of three days, ten injections being given.

RECURRENT HERPES PROGENITALIS; A POSITIVE INOCULATION OF THE CORNEA OF THE RABBIT. Flandin and Tzanck, Bull. Soc. franç. de dermat. et syph. **28**:491, 1921.

Fresh fluid inoculated intracorneally in the rabbit produced positive results in four days. There was photophobia, soon followed by hemiparesis, convulsions and coma.

GONORRHEAL KERATOSIS LIMITED TO THE GLANS PENIS. Jeanselme and Blamoutier, Bull. Soc. franç. de dermat. et syph. **28**:493, 1921.

The patient's infection was of five years' duration, arthritis and endocarditis having appeared. The diplococci were found in the lesions, which were permanently removed by the curet. The authors believe that these lesions arose from local inoculation, due to a urethral discharge, and were not bloodborne. In the *Journal of Cutaneous Diseases* (**36**:225, 1918), Brown and Davidson reported a case with lesions in the same location.

CUTANEOUS DYSTROPHY WITH ATROPHY DUE TO AGENESIS OF THE ELASTIC TISSUE. Hudelo, Boulanger-Pilet and Gailliau, Bull. Soc. franç. de dermat. et syph. **28**:496, 1921.

A girl, aged 10½ years, presented areas somewhat suggesting the final stage of epidermolysis bullosa, but there were no bullae nor epidermal cysts. and Nikolsky's sign was not present. Trauma determined the location of the lesions. There was a considerable lack of elastic tissue in the walls of the blood vessels and throughout the derma.

LINGUAL LEUKOPLAKIA IN A WOMAN. Marcel Pinard and Declaire, Bull. Soc. franç. de dermat. et syph. **28**:499, 1921.

In this case the condition was apparently of syphilitic origin.

AUTOPLASTY IN TWO CASES OF SYPHILITIC PERFORATION OF THE PALATE. Lemaitre and Aubin, Bull. Soc. franç. de dermat. et syph. **28**:500, 1921.

The author briefly describes his technic, reporting two successful instances. The syphilologist prepares the patient for operation by giving thorough treatment.

A CASE OF LEPRA IMPROVED UNDER THE INFLUENCE OF TREATMENT WITH THE MANGANATE OF CALCIUM AND POTASSIUM. Loiselet, Bull. Soc. franç. de dermat. et syph. **28**:502, 1921.

This drug was used with apparent success in the treatment of an advanced case of lepra of the mixed type, with ulcerations. Ampules of 5 c.c. were employed and ten intravenous injections constituted a series, each injection being given as soon as the febrile reaction from the preceding one had subsided.

FREQUENCY OF APPARENTLY BANAL GASTRO-INTESTINAL DISTURBANCES POSSIBLY CAUSED BY SYPHILIS. Pathault, Bull. Soc. franç. de dermat. et syph. **28**:505, 1921.

The author briefly describes fourteen cases, the symptoms being those of secretory alterations, atony at times, and often pain. He urges that the diagnosis of syphilis be considered at first, on an equal footing with other possibilities, instead of being a matter of last resort. Persistent headaches and a history of syphilis in the parents are held to be most suggestive, and failure to respond to local gastro-intestinal treatment also points toward a syphilitic etiology. The advantages of a correct diagnosis, if syphilis is present, are felt by the patient and by the community at large.

AN EXTENSIVE PRURIGINOUS ERUPTION CAUSED BY FELINE ITCH. G. Thibierge, Bull. Soc. franç. de dermat. et syph. **28**:511, 1921.

In the author's case nearly two thirds of the skin surface was occupied by an intensely pruritic eruption, not unlike the prurigo of Hebra. The organisms were easily found on the pet cat, and the lesions readily vanished under treatment with a simple mentholated paste.

A CASE OF FELINE ITCH. W. Dubreuilh and Joulia, Bull. Soc. franç. de dermat. et syph. **28**:513, 1921.

In this case the lesions, as usual, were limited to the areas formerly in contact with the cat, the anterior trunk and arms being affected. The parasites were found on the cat.

A CASE OF COLLOID MILIUM. W. Dubreuilh, Bull. Soc. franç. de dermat. et syph. **28**:515, 1921.

The eruption, in a man of 43 years, was of six years' duration, consisting of many small pseudovesicles situated on the cheeks, behind the ears and on the left hand. A biopsy could not be obtained, but microscopic examination of the contents of the lesions confirmed the diagnosis.

UNGUAL GRANULOMA PYOGENICUM. W. DUBREUILH, Bull. Soc. franç. de dermat. et syph. **28**:516, 1921.

A recurrent tumor as large as a small pea appeared through a fissure in the finger nail. One intensive roentgen-ray treatment was followed by its disappearance.

CUTANEOUS, OSSEOUS AND ARTICULAR TUBERCULOSIS. SCHEFFER, RIETMAN and LIX, Bull. Soc. franç. de dermat. et syph. **28**: R. S. 57, 1921.

A woman, aged 46 years, who had had phlyctenular keratitis in early childhood, said that she had first noticed the presence of a pruritic papule on her nose sixteen years previously. At present there were numerous scattered lesions, erythematous, ulcerated and infiltrated, as well as sinuses leading from bone involvement and three ankylosed joints. Biopsy examination confirmed the diagnosis.

SECONDARY SYPHILIS IN A PERSON WITH CONGENITAL SYPHILIS. J. ROEDERER and R. CAMUS. Bull. Soc. franç. de dermat. et syph. **28**: R. S. 62, 1921.

A patient, in whose bones roentgenograms showed definite signs of congenital syphilitic changes, presented a fresh maculopapular eruption, with inguinal adenopathy and the possibility of an anorectal chancre. The organisms were not found.

DISSEMINATED MILIARY LUPOID OF THE TRUNK AND EXTREMITIES. PAUTRIER and ELIASCHEFF, Bull. Soc. franç. de dermat. et syph. **28**: R. S. 64, 1921.

The eruption, of two years' duration, in a woman aged 22 years, consisted of many small nodules and cicatrices. microscopically shown to be miliary lupoid. Several intravenous injections of neo-arsphenamin (novarsenobenzol) were given, and rapid recovery ensued. Bloch reports the case of another patient similarly cured.

PARAPSORIASIS LICHENOIDES APPROACHING THE CUTANEOUS ATROPHIES. PAUTRIER, Bull. Soc. franç. de dermat. et syph. **28**: R. S. 68, 1921.

In a woman, aged 57 years, there was a dermatosis of six years' duration, fairly generalized and somewhat suggesting the poikiloderma atrophicans vascularis described by Jacobi. The case is described and discussed in detail.

NEW INVESTIGATIONS CONCERNING THE PROBLEM OF CUTANEOUS PIGMENTATION. B. BLOCH, Bull. Soc. franç. de dermat. et syph. **28**: R. S. 77, 1921.

By impregnating the tissues with dioxyphenylalanin, which he briefly designates as "Dopa," the author has shown to his satisfaction that the pigmentation of the skin of the higher mammals is of epidermal origin. produced by the action of an oxidase on some substance similar to "Dopa" or identical with it. probably brought to the cell through the blood stream. Under various conditions, notably after exposure to the sunlight, to roentgen rays and to other physical agents, this process of pigment manufacture is speeded. The residual pigment extruded after the break-down of cells is engulfed by dermal phagocytes, which may retain it for long periods of time.

An extensive bibliography is appended.

PARKHURST, Toledo, Ohio.

THE HAIR IN ALOPECIA AREATA. SABOURAUD, Bull. Soc. franç. de dermat. et syph. **29**:2 (Jan.) 1922.

Sabouraud discusses in some detail the various stages of the hair in alopecia areata. At the periphery of the alopecic area the hair resembles an exclamation point. One can usually observe the beginning of an area because of its extreme rapidity of development. At the periphery of the area one finds numerous short hairs not much longer than 4 to 6 mm. (one-eighth to one-quarter inch).

Sabouraud explains the formation of the hairs in alopecia areata as follows: The hair becomes thinner and thinner, principally at the level of the bulb; the pigment gradually disappears from the hair, and there is also a disappearance of the medullary substance; lateral erosions are found along the hair similar to trichorrhexis nodosa. The loss of pigment will explain the appearance of white hair on the areas. However, some pigment is found within the pilaric orifice. Sabouraud concludes by stating that we do not know the etiologic factor of alopecia areata, but we do know the mechanism of its formation.

McCAFFERTY, New York.

SUBCUTANEOUS NODOSITIES COEXISTING WITH TUBERCULIDS OF THE FEET TREATED AND CURED BY TUBERCULIN INJECTIONS. CHEVALLIER and BLAMOUTIER, Bull. Soc. franç. de dermat. et syph. **29**:3, 1922.

Gummatous nodules, with and without ulceration, papulonecrotic tuberculids and lupus pernio, all located about the feet and ankles of a 17 year old girl, showed surprising improvement after twelve days of tuberculin treatment, and were soon apparently cured.

BISMUTH STOMATITIS. MILIAN and PERIN, Bull. Soc. franç. de dermat. et syph. **29**:7, 1922.

The treatment of syphilis by bismuth salts is fraught with difficulties. Pigmentation of the oral mucosa, especially in the form of a line along the gingival margin, appears in an overwhelming percentage of cases, and ulcerations are of frequent occurrence. The frequency of these symptoms varies directly with the dosage and inversely with the interval between treatments. Ptyalism does not occur, and the stomatitis disappears within fifteen days after the treatment is discontinued. The pathology is described.

BISMUTH STOMATITIS. HUDELO, BORDET and BOULANGER-PILET, Bull. Soc. franç. de dermat. et syph. **29**:10, 1922.

Among fourteen patients treated, the authors found stomatitis in 30 per cent. It seemed to appear even when the dental condition was excellent, being dependent on the intensity of the treatment and disappearing soon after the bismuth had been discontinued.

Others have also observed this stomatitis.

THE USE OF THE SOLUBLE TARTROBISMUTHATE IN TREATING
SYPHILIS. E. Jeanselme, Pomaret, Blamoutier and Joannon, Bull.
Soc. franç. de dermat. et syph. **29**:13, 1922.

Other preparations produced local tenderness, so the soluble salts of potassium and sodium in aqueous glucose solution were employed, the intramuscular
route being used; injections were given every other day; a series of seventeen
had already been given. All stages of the disease were treated and the results,
satisfactory but somewhat slower than those from the use of the arsenicals,
are recorded. Some degree of stomatitis occurred in 40 per cent. of the cases,
depending apparently on the oral hygienic habits of the person.

It should be emphasized, as was especially brought out in the discussion,
that great care must be used, for the accidental intravenous injection of small
amounts of the drug has resulted fatally.

WHAT IS THE NORMAL LYMPHOCYTE COUNT OF THE CEREBRO-
SPINAL FLUID? Leredde, Rubinstein and Druet, Bull. Soc. franç. de
dermat. et syph. **29**:22, 1922.

The authors believe it to be not over one lymphocyte per cubic millimeter,
and in only thirty of 100 suspected cases did the count even slightly exceed
this figure.

THE TRANSMISSION TO MAN OF THE SARCOPTIC ITCH OF THE
DOG. D. Thibierge, Bull. Soc. franç. de dermat. et syph. **29**:26, 1922.

In a physician's family the man, wife and son were affected, the source of
infection being a small dog. The eruption was pruriginous, involving chiefly
the forearms, mammary regions, back and the inner surfaces of the thighs.
as well as the abdomen and axillae.

CHANCRE AND CANCER OF THE LIP. Goubeau, Bull. Soc. franç. de
dermat. et syph. **29**:29, 1922.

The alleged epithelioma on the lower lip of a man, aged 40 years, appeared
coincidently with the healing of a chancre at the same site, in which the
organisms were found. Four arsenical injections and a short course of mercury
benzoate had been given. Histologically, syphilis was still present in the lesion,
but on careful examination of an imperfect specimen, the diagnosis of epithelioma could not definitely be confirmed.

A CASE OF ANGIOLUPOID. Burnier and Bloch, Bull. Soc. franç. de
dermat. et syph. **29**:33, 1922.

A woman, aged 50 years, presented several small telangiectatic nodules
about the eyes and nose, which had begun to appear in 1915. The diagnosis
of angiolupoid was confirmed histologically.

THE REACTIVATION OF COMPLEMENT. L. Chatellier, Bull. Soc.
franç. de dermat. et syph. **29**:34, 1922.

Guinea-pig serum whose complement has been enfeebled or destroyed by
heat or lapse of time may apparently be perfectly reactivated by the addition
of a small amount of fresh serum.

DERMATOLOGIC USE OF THE TAR AND ESSENCE OF MOROCCAN CEDAR (CEDRUS ATLANTICA). E. Lepinay and R. Massy, Bull. Soc. franç. de dermat. et syph. **29**:35, 1922.

The tar is said to be superior to oil of cade, but the essence of cedar is inferior to the essence of cade employed in France. Their properties are given.

Parkhurst, Toledo, Ohio.

CANCER AND CHANCRE OF THE LOWER LIP. M. Goubeau, Bull. Soc. franç. de dermat. et syph. **29**:40, 1922.

The author reports the case of a primary lesion of the lower lip with a one plus Wassermann reaction. Antisyphilitic treatment was begun; the primary lesion involuted slightly and the general state improved, but owing to the delayed process of regeneration of the primary lesion a biopsy was performed and revealed a squamous cell epithelioma.

Repeated operations were performed, but the progress of the condition was not stopped. It is the author's belief that syphilis played a prominent rôle in the evolution, invasion and rapidity of the epithelioma.

POROKERATOSIS OF MIBELLI. Milian and Lefèvre, Bull. Soc. franç. de dermat. et syph. **29**:41, 1922.

A woman, aged 25 years, presented three interesting conditions: first, there was a narrow, elevated, hyperkeratotic band, extending from the nail of the index finger to the nail of the thumb forming an uninterrupted line. There was a short band on the last phalanx of the middle and third fingers similar to the one above. This condition was present only on the dorsal surfaces and was symmetrical. The second interesting feature was the palmar curving of the nails of the affected fingers, so that the nails resembled a parrot's beak. The nails were thickened and striated both transversely and longitudinally. The third interesting feature was a hard, fibrous, annular band around the middle and index fingers of the right hand and middle finger of the left hand.

The hyperkeratotic bands went through a peculiar cycle. The keratotic period usually lasted three weeks; then a period of desquamation which lasted ten days; a period of relative cure for fifteen days; then the corneous layer reforms and soon the process is at its height.

The condition is probably porokeratosis of Mibelli associated with ainhum. It is interesting to note that several authors attribute ainhum to a form of leprosy and that Mibelli described his original porokeratosis in a leper country. Darier thought the fibrous band was annular scleroderma instead of ainhum, which was found usually in negroes.

McCafferty, New York.

CONGENITAL VERRUCOUS ERYTHROKERATODERMA IN PLAQUES, SYMMETRICAL AND PROGRESSIVE. Hudelo, Boulanger-Pilet and Caillau, Bull. Soc. franç. de dermat. et syph. **29**:45, 1922.

This condition, in a boy, aged 15 years, occupied the entire head and neck as well as the extremities, being accompanied by several pigmented nevi. There was no palmar hyperhidrosis. There was no familial element.

Parkhurst, Toledo, Ohio

CUTANEOUS ATROPHIC SYPHILID. CHEVALLIER and JOANNON, Bull. Soc. franç. de dermat. et syph. **29**:50, 1922.

Two patients were presented with colorless, atrophic, macular or linear lesions which were undoubtedly of syphilitic origin. The patients had never observed these lesions until they were examined. However, they had noticed the crusted and ulcerated serpiginous lesions. The atrophic lesions were numerous, closely grouped with normal skin intervening; the lesions were ivory white, smooth, without any lines of normal skin; they were not depressed; the periphery was less discolored. The lesions ranged in size from that of a dime to that of a quarter. On palpation no infiltration was felt, but a certain degree of laxity. The lesions had a mosaic appearance. The linear lesions were very similar. These lesions developed independently without any premonitory signs. The Wassermann reaction was positive in both cases.

RECURRENCE OF ALOPECIA AREATA CONSECUTIVE TO SOME ATTACKS OF ANOSCROTAL PRURITUS. REGROWTH OF HAIR ON CURE OF PRURITUS. THIBIERGE and COTTENTOT, Bull. Soc. franç. de dermat. et syph. **29**:54, 1922.

The patient had had five attacks of alopecia areata. Each attack was preceded by pruritus of the anoscrotal region. Local treatment was instituted for the pruritus which disappeared, and with its disappearance there was a regrowth of the hair in the peladic regions.

Sabouraud believes the association of alopecia areata with pruritus is a mere coincidence. He states that the recurrence of alopecia areata often coexists with dermatologic conditions of nervous origin. The pruritus is quite rare, but he has observed it a few times. The cure of the alopecia areata by curing the pruritus is also a coincidence as the alopecia areata cures itself.

McCAFFERTY, New York.

ATYPICAL PRECOCIOUS MALIGNANT SYPHILIS; ARREST BY BISMUTH; A LINGUAL LESION OF UNDETERMINED NATURE. LERI, TZANCK and WEISMANN-NETTER, Bull. Soc. franç. de dermat. et syph. **29**:56, 1922.

A course of six injections of a compound of quinin and bismuth was given, intervals of three days elapsing between treatments. A yellowish plaque on the tongue, which appeared during treatment, may have been due to the drug.

PARKHURST, Toledo, Ohio.

A CASE OF MALIGNANT SYPHILIS TREATED BY IODO-BISMUTH OF QUININ. AZOULAY, Bull. Soc. franç. de dermat. et syph. **29**:57, 1922.

Azoulay reports on the beneficial action of iodo-bismuth of quinin which he believes is the best combination. It is insoluble in water, but soluble in alcohol. He employs the drug in a 10 per cent. oil-suspension. The dose is 0.3 gm. given two or three times a week intramuscularly and is not followed by pain, abscess or stomatitis. The author cites a case of precocious malignant syphilis which resisted mercurial injections but responded quickly to this preparation. Two weeks after the initial injection the deep ulcerations were nearly cured. Other cases are cited with results comparable to our best results with arsphenamin compounds.

McCafferty, New York.

ULCERATING AND HYPERTROPHIC SYPHILOID INFLAMMATION OF THE PERINEUM AND VULVA. Pinard, Bull. Soc. franç. de dermat. et syph. **29**:60, 1922.

These lesions, first appearing as pustules and then as moist hypertrophic papules, fairly symmetrical in location, appeared five days after the last venereal exposure. The staphylococcus and an organism resembling the pneumococcus were found in the discharge, and a biopsy examination showed a superficial inflammatory process. As Darier suggests, it may have been genital herpes.

SPONTANEOUS ULCERATIONS APPEARING IN ANIMALS AFTER SUBCUTANEOUS HYPERTONIC INJECTIONS. Levy-Franckel, Bossan and Guieysse, Bull. Soc. franç. de dermat. et syph. **29**:63, 1922.

Subcutaneous injections of a 10 per cent. sodium chlorid solution, given every three days for a ten-day period, were followed by the appearance of necrotic lesions at some distance from the point of injection. A biopsy examination confirmed the impression of necrosis. The urinary output was simultaneously diminished, suggesting a possible renal involvement.

Parkhurst, Toledo, Ohio.

TREATMENT OF LUPUS BY ETHER BENZYL-CINNAMIC. Jacobson. Bull. Soc. franç. de dermat. et syph. **29**:64, 1922.

The ether benzyl-cinnamic radical when injected intramuscularly has a marked effect on the involution of all forms of cutaneous tuberculosis. It is suggested that 1 c.c. of the radical be given daily for five days; then increased to 1.5 c.c. for five days; the last two days 2 c.c. may be given, or in other words, twelve days' treatment comprises one series. An interval of fifteen days should elapse before another series is given; three series of treatments are usually given and then a month's rest, whereupon the same routine is repeated.

Jacobson reports a case in which the patient was treated according to this method. The infiltration disappeared even in places where the roentgen-rays had failed. The suppuration disappeared entirely. The ulceration healed, and the lupus tubercles involuted. The glands were also favorably influenced.

Drs. Jeanselme and Darier spoke enthusiastically of the treatment and bore witness to the admirable results in this case.

IMPROVEMENT IN THREE CASES OF TABETIC PAPILLARY ATROPHY AS A RESULT OF ARSENO-MERCURIAL TREATMENT. Balina, Bull. soc. franç. de dermat. et syph. **29**:69, 1922.

Balina reports three classical cases of tabes dorsalis associated with double papillary atrophy of the optic nerves. There was little vision in each case; the visual fields were much restricted.

He emphasizes the importance of mercuric cyanid intravenously, the dose averaging from 1 to 2 cg., daily if possible, until from ten to fifteen injections have been given. This should be followed by intensive neo-arsphenamin treatment; he recommends beginning with 0.075 cg., carrying the dosage up to 0.75

decigrams. In one case the author gave thirty intravenous injections of neo-arsphenamin spaced two days apart, beginning with a very small dose and working up to the maximum dosage. The mercuric cyanid was given between the doses of neo-arsphenamin.

The treatment in all three cases has been similar to that in the foregoing case. All patients have improved. Vision has improved and the visual fields have been enlarged. The author believes the improvement is the result of the arsenomercurial treatment restoring the partially affected nerve fibers. Those that have been definitely destroyed, nothing can improve; but those that are partially damaged can be restored and perhaps give some vision.

Darier spoke enthusiastically of these most important results.

McCAFFERTY, New York.

SYPHILITIC SEQUELAE EXTENDING THROUGH FOUR GENERATIONS. AUDRAIN, Bull. Soc. franç. de dermat. et syph. **29**:77, 1922.

The author has made a thorough investigation to confirm an observation which he presented before the society one year ago, and it is here given in detail. In the first generation the lesions were especially cardiovascular, and later the involvement affected mainly the endocrine glands.

A PAPULAR ERUPTION OF THE BEARDED REGION CAUSED BY INGROWING HAIRS. DUBREUILH, Bull. Soc. franç. de dermat. et syph. **29**:80, 1922.

Two cases are reported, in young men, the eruption being composed of miliary papules and pustules occurring at points at which the free ends of cut hairs turned back and pierced the skin.

LEUKODERMA APPEARING AROUND NEVI. MONTPELLIER, Bull. Soc. franç. de dermat. et syph. **29**:81, 1922.

In a boy, aged 14 years, there were three pigmented nevi on the trunk which, according to the mother's statement, had recently been surrounded by lenkodermic rings, still present. In a review of the French and British literature on this subject, eight similar cases are cited and briefly reviewed.

EMOTIONAL LEUKODERMA. L. QUEYRAT, Bull. Soc. franç. de dermat. et syph. **29**:84, 1922.

A girl, aged 17 years, presented plaques of leukoderma of four years' duration, with some symmetry of distribution; the scalp and hair were extensively involved. In the center of some patches were pigmented nevi. At the time of presentation the patches were growing smaller and the hairs were regaining their normal color, the free end strangely becoming pigmented first. The original outbreak occurred fifteen days after a war-time shock. Two similar cases, Darier's and Leloir's, are briefly described for comparison.

The question of the alleged sudden occurrence of canities following severe emotions is brought up, and Sabouraud considers these cases of leukoderma, when they actually occur.

A DERMATITIS FROM WEARING A WAIST DYED WITH "KABILINE." HUDELO and DUMET, Bull. Soc. franç. de dermat. et syph. **29**:92, 1922.

A woman who had recently dyed her waist showed an erythematous eruption in the areas which had been in contact with it. A chemical analysis of the dye is given.

CONCERNING DYSHIDROSIS. Sabouraud, Bull. Soc. franç. de dermat. et syph. **29**:102, 1922.

According to the author, there are occasional cases of this disease which are not of parasitic etiology and may therefore be called dyshidrosis. He cites cases in which cultures have been constantly negative.

THE "HEMODIAGNOSIS" OF CONGENITAL SYPHILIS. Leredde, Bull. Soc. franç. de dermat. et syph. **29**:104, 1922.

A number of cases are cited to show the blood picture which may be found in congenital syphilis. with a diminution in the number of red corpuscles, some alteration in the color index, and a relative lymphocytosis. Treatment of the syphilis is said to be followed by an improvement in this picture. which may be the only tangible symptom of the disease, in the absence of a positive Wassermann reaction.

TREATMENT OF SYPHILIS WITH BISMUTH SALTS. Cable, Bull. Soc. franç. de dermat. et syph. **29**:113, 1922.

Using the oily preparation. the author has found the injections too painful, and the frequent stomatitis is troublesome. The therapeutic results do not seem sufficiently good to override these serious objections.

RESEARCHES CONCERNING ACIDOSIS IN THE COURSE OF POST-ARSENICAL ERYTHRODERMAS. Pomaret and Blamoutier, Bull. Soc. franç. de dermat. et syph. **29**:115, 1922.

The hepatic condition has considerable importance here, according to the authors. They found acidosis accompanying severe postarsenical eruptions.

SYPHILITIC REINFECTION; THE POSITIVE SERUM REACTION: IS IT DEPENDENT ON THE SOIL OR THE GERM? Lacapere, Bull. Soc. franç. de dermat. et syph. **29**:120, 1922.

The patient had had a typical Hunterian lesion of the penis in 1918, which resisted local treatment but responded at once to antisyphilitic treatment;. the Wassermann reaction had never become positive. After a fair amount of treatment with neo-arsphenamin and mercury the patient was discharged, and in December, 1921, he returned with a new penile lesion in which spirochetes were easily demonstrated. This time, in spite of treatment, his Wassermann reaction became temporarily positive. In the discussion it is agreed that the manifestations of the disease usually depend on the soil rather than on the seed.

SYPHILITIC REINFECTION. Lepinay, Bull. Soc. franç. de dermat. et syph. **29**:124, 1922.

In 1917, the patient had had a chancre which was immediately excised; a thorough course of treatment was given, and at length the Wassermann reaction became negative. In November, 1921, two erosions appeared on the penis, and the dark-field examination revealed the presence of numerous spirochetes. The patient's consort was found to have a secondary roseola and vulvar mucous patches.

GENERALIZED PEDICULOSIS PUBIS. Dubreuilh, Bull. Soc. franç. de dermat. et syph. **29**:126, 1922.

A man, aged 70 years, and supposedly very cleanly, complained of itching. Examination revealed the presence of nits on all the hairs of the body excepting the eyelashes.

THE HAIR IN ALOPECIA AREATA. Sabouraud, Bull. Soc. franç. de dermat. et syph. **29**: R.S. 2, 1922.

The author describes the "exclamation-point" hairs found in variable numbers about the margins of actively spreading patches of alopecia areata. These hairs are rarely longer than 1 cm., and the distal end is hyperpigmented. A study of a large number of hairs about the borders of these patches has shown the presence of lateral abrasions and lesions apparently identical with those of trichorrhexis nodosa; at these points the hairs break off, and thus the presence of the short hairs is explained. The basic fault seems to be a temporary follicular dystrophy, best explained as being due to a disorder of the sympathetic nervous system.

LEUKOPLASIC GINGIVAL LESIONS POSSIBLY CAUSED BY A FUNGUS. Pautrier and Scheffer, Bull. Soc. franç. de dermat. et syph. **29**: R.S. 12, 1922.

A woman, aged 44 years, whose gums were partially edentulous, had complained of some gingival tenderness for several months. The gums were stippled with white punctae on erythematous bases, chiefly grouped, from which an ordinarily nonpathogenic fungus was recovered.

A CASE OF PARTIAL SCLERODERMA. Hugel, Bull. Soc. franç. de dermat. et syph. **29**: R.S. 15, 1922.

A man, aged 28 years, whose right foot and ankle had been injured three times prior to 1914, first noticed, in 1920, an edema of this leg. True scleroderma, proved histologically, soon developed, involving the right leg alone. The intramuscular administration of thiosinamin-sodium salicylate was followed by great improvement. The author has used this treatment before, and thinks well of it.

A CASE OF VON RECKLINGHAUSEN'S DISEASE WITH PIGMENTARY LESIONS IN THE SKIN OF THE PATIENT'S DAUGHTER. J. Roederer, Bull. Soc. franç. de dermat. et syph. **29**: R.S. 17, 1922.

A woman, aged 49 years, had first noticed the appearance of the tumors in 1909, and she soon developed the classical signs of von Recklinghausen's disease, excepting the usual mental impairment. Her daughter, aged 19 years, presented a number of hyperpigmented areas, and both mother and daughter had a low blood pressure, suggesting the presence of suprarenal deficiency, which has been demonstrated in previous cases of this disorder.

Parkurst, Toledo, O.

Society Transactions

PURPURA ANNULARIS TELANGIECTODES MAJOCCHI. Presented by DR. NOBL.

This disorder, as first described by Majocchi in 1905, appeared in a woman. Her arms, chest and back were covered with pink and brownish-red, round and oblong spots and yellowish-red eruptions. There was slight scaling but no pronounced atrophy. Etiologically, syphilis and tuberculosis were excluded. Atrophic damage to the vessels was assumed, that is, a neurogenous origin of the disorder.

AFTER-EPILATION METHOD FOR FUNGUS DISEASES OF THE SCALP. DR. FUHS.

After roentgen-ray epilation of the scalp, the hair still remaining is removed by a warm mixture of colophony and wax. A thick layer of this mixture is spread on a piece of cloth and then placed on the scalp and left to cool. It is then removed, with the hair adhering to the sticky mixture.

RARE FORMS OF AN ARSENICAL ERUPTION FOLLOWING THE ADMINISTRATION OF SILVER ARSPHENAMIN AND SODIUM. DR. ULLMANN.

In the discussion of this case it was stated that intravenous administration of arsenic does not encourage eruptions, particularly hyperkeratoses, as much as medication by mouth does, as the elimination is quicker and there is no storing in the liver. The frequent arsenical eruptions observed recently in connection with arsphenamin medication are due to the large and frequent doses given.

Session, Dec. 1, 1921

PIGMENTARY SYPHILIS. Presented by DR. KRUEGER.

Specific treatment removed secondary symptoms in a case of syphilis, but left strong pigmentation on the site of the healed papules. There also developed a concentric depigmented zone around the pigmented site; also lenkoderma colli. In the discussion Kyrle pointed to a possible central origin of these pigmentations (leukoderma, alopecia) due to an irritation of the meninges. The positive spinal fluid also pointed to this.

ACNE CONGLOBATA ET INDURATA WITH SUBSEQUENT DEVELOPMENT OF TUBERCULOID SKIN ERUPTIONS AND PAPULO-NECROTIC TUBERCULIDS. DR. OPPENHEIM.

This patient was treated with tuberculin injections of increasing strength, which caused brownish-red papular eruptions with central scaling and crust formation. Two days after each injection the acne lesions were surrounded by bright pink rings, 2 to 3 mm. in diameter, which disappeared in three days.

TRANSMISSION OF HERPES GENITALIS. Dr. Lipschütz.

Vaccination of the cornea of rabbits with material taken from herpes febrilis and herpes genitalis eruptions proved that these two disorders are of different origin. The etiologic factor of herpes febrilis and of herpes genitalis is not identical, as has been assumed in recent publications.

FOREIGN-BODY TUMORS AFTER INJECTIONS OF MERCURY. Dr. Planner.

A woman, aged 57, developed palm-sized, tough, painless tumors near the anguli scapulae. These had persisted for years. Fifteen years ago she had received injections of mercury, which were assumed to be the cause of the tumor development. In the discussion Oppenheim said that one of his patients developed similar tumors seven years after the injection of mercuric salicylate.

SKIN HEMORRHAGES AFTER SLIGHT TRAUMA IN A SYPHILITIC PATIENT. Dr. Arzt.

A syphilitic patient responded to three injections of neo-arsphenamin with a strong Herxheimer reaction, toxic exanthems, chills and vomiting. The slightest pinching of the skin immediately provoked pinpoint hemorrhages. In the discussion no definite explanation was agreed on. Oppenheimer said that the arsphenamin damage to vessels required particular attention.

Session, Jan. 26, 1922

Dr. Oppenheim, in the Chair

APLASIA CUTIS CONGENITA WITH PERIPHERAL ANGIOMA CAVERNOSUM. Dr. Oppenheim.

This case supports the opinion of the presenter that atrophodermas should be classified as nevi. The concomitant cavernoma in this case was caused by a disturbance of the circulation in the surrounding area.

PITYRIASIS LICHENOIDES CHRONICA, BEGINNING AS A GENERALIZED SPOTTED ERYTHEMA. Dr. Oppenheim.

Oppenheim presents his third case, in a woman, aged 22, in whom, without cause, there was a sudden development over the whole body of a spotted erythema with slight itching. In fourteen days a part of these spots developed into yellowish red papules and the rest into slightly scaling brownish spots

PIGMENTED SYPHILIS. Dr. Bruenauer.

This patient presented distinct hyperpigmentation of unhealed syphilitic eruptions.

ARSENICAL HYPERKERATOSIS. Presented by Dr. Porias.

A patient had pronounced hyperkeratosis on the palms and soles caused by oral medication of solution of potassium arsenite (Fowler's solution). It had been administered in 5 drop doses three times during a period of several weeks; later, over a period of two or three months, three different times in 10 drop doses. The disorder had developed during the last two weeks of medication.

PAPULONECROTIC TUBERCULID. Dr. Kumer.

A woman, aged 27, had papulonecrotic tuberculids with atypically located lesions in the palms.

PEMPHIGUS PRURIGINOSUS. Dr. Kumer.

In a man, aged 63, pea to coin sized vesicles developed on an erythematous basis. Nikolsky's sign was present and 10 per cent. eosinophilia.

LYMPHOGRANULOMATOSIS WITH SECONDARY INVOLVEMENT OF THE SKIN. Dr. Arzt.

Histologic examination of a nodule taken from the skin of the left thorax showed a progressing granulation tissue which infiltrated the cutis and was composed of various forms of cells; there were numerous Paltauf-Sternberg giant cells.

SCLERODERMA AND SCLERODACTYLIA WITH SUSPICIOUS ALTER-ATIONS OF THE BUCCAL MUCOSA. Dr. Arzt.

The patient had pale yellowish buccal mucosa and numerous thin vessel branches. The disorder resembled the conditions of the mucosa of the mouth observed by Kren in combination with scleroderma.

Session, Feb. 9, 1922

URTICARIA PIGMENTOSA OR EXANTHEM-LIKE SKIN ERUPTION OF NEVUS CHARACTER. Presented by Dr. Oppenheim.

A man of 64 developed on the chest and back, pea-sized, round, dark brown eruptions with a normal surface which did not change under glass pressure. Histologically there was acanthosis and edema of the papillae. The basal cells contained pigment. There were mast cells in the papillae. These also abounded in the collagenous tissue of the cutis. There were no subjective symptoms. The Wassermann reaction was negative. The blood was normal. A definite diagnosis was not agreed on.

ULCUS PHAGEDENICUM CRURIS. Dr. Brünauer.

A round ulcer appeared on the leg of a woman. The Wassermann and luetin tests were negative. Gram-negative bacilli were found.

SKIN LESION CAUSED BY ELECTRIC CURRENT. Dr. Fuhs.

The vola of right hand and bend of the arm in a laborer showed brownish-red coloring caused by impregnation with metal dust from an electric arc.

In a second case there was superficial necrosis of the vola and sharply defined loss of substance on the dorsum of the hand, caused by a strong electric current.

ERYTHEMA EXUDATIVUM MULTIFORME ATYPICUM. Dr. Arzt.

A woman, aged 47, suffering from fever and arthritis, developed a polymorphous exanthem on the arm, cheek and dorsum of the hand. There were also numerous disseminated hemorrhagic eruptions on the trunk.

ISOLATED PSORIASIS ERUPTION. Presented by Dr. Sowade.

A patient, aged 30, developed a small isolated patch of psoriasis on the penis. Repeated negative Wassermann reactions excluded syphilis. There was no question of any other diagnosis. An uncle of the patient suffered from psoriasis.

NEUROTIC ECZEMA. Dr. Sowade.

Eczema appeared in the region of the third cervical to fourth dorsal segment in a woman aged 46. As a child she had suffered from endocarditis and St. Vitus' dance. In 1915 she developed zoster-like vesicles on the right arm. Since 1921 there had been a skin eruption in this region, which was sharply defined, frequently oozed and had a distinct eczematous character. The neurotic etiology of eczemas was hypothetic. In the discussion histologic examination was advised.

RABBITS WITH SECONDARY SYPHILIS. Dr. Frühwald.

Dr. Frühwald showed two rabbits which had been vaccinated (intra testes) with *Spirochaeta pallida*. One developed keratitis parenchymatosa in nineteen weeks and finally iritis, the other secondary papules on the prepuce.

NEW STAININGS OF SPIROCHAETA PALLIDA. Dr. Lennhoff.

The new stain consisted of tannin oxalic acid after treatment with ferric chlorid. This stain reveals a larger number of granules in the body of the spirochetes than other staining methods. No conclusions were drawn as to the vital structure of the spirochete.

CHANCRE OF THE TONSILS. Dr. Hayn.

Dr. Hayn gave a report on thirty cases. He said that the tonsillar chancre is the most frequent extragenital chancre. The prognosis is unfavorable as chancre is generally diagnosed too late, that is, when the head and meninges are flooded with spirochetes. Neurorelapses are frequent. Three cases of meningitis, one case of oculomotorius paresis and one case of recurrent iritis were seen in spite of combined syphilitic treatment.

KERATODERMA OF THE PALMS AND SOLES. Dr. Callomon.

A case occurred in a man aged 49 who developed chronic disseminated cornifications chiefly on parts exposed to mechanical irritation. There were no symptoms of inflammation. The Wassermann reaction was negative. A genodermatosis was not probable, though some relation was assumed to the keratoderma maculosa disseminata symmetrica of Buschke and Fischer. Treatment, including roentgenotherapy, had no effect.

URTICARIA. Dr. Baum.

The case was in the climacterium. The only treatment which proved successful was bleeding. (In two sessions during forty-eight hours 50 c.c. of blood were removed.)

Session, Feb. 23, 1922

MICROSPORON AUDOUINI OF THE SCALP IN THREE BROTHERS. Dr. Fuhs.

In one of the patients there was herpes tonsurans vesicopustulosus resembling kerion. The clinical pictures of trichophytina and of microsporon are so similar in some cases that clinical diagnosis becomes impossible.

STOMATITIS ULCEROSA AFTER TEN PER CENT. WHITE PRECIPITATE OINTMENT. Presented by Dr. Riehl.

A psoriatic patient had been treated with 10 per cent. white mercuric ointment followed by 10 per cent. lenigallol. This provoked a severe stomatitis. In the test tube a weak alkalin solution of lenigallol and white mercuric ointment forms a gray-green deposit of colloidal mercury. In this case mercury had evidently been liberated by the effect of lenigallol on the mercuric ointment in the skin. This method could perhaps be used wherever the action of free mercury is desired in a tissue.

PEMPHIGUS VULGARIS. Dr. Kumer.

The bullae were strictly limited to the scrotum.

LEUKEMIA CUTIS. Dr. Rusch.

Dr. Rusch presented a patient with an interesting palm sized lesion on the flexor side of the arm resembling idiopathic atrophy. The disorder was considered as a postleukemic skin atrophy, a special type of atrophy which has probably not been described.

MOSCOW VENEREOLOGICAL-DERMATOLOGICAL SOCIETY

Session, Dec. 4, 1921

LIVEDO SYPHILITICUM. Presented by Dr. G. Mestschersky.

A case of this disease was reported in a woman of 67 who had never been treated specifically. The symptoms disappeared after treatment.

THE ADMINISTRATION OF NORMAL HORSE SERUM FOR CURING SKIN DISEASES. Dr. S. Selitzky.

In several cases of pruritus gravidarum, furunculosis, pemphigus vulgaris, urticaria chronica, urticaria papulosa and lichen ruber planus he saw satisfactory results. Dr. Selitzky said that a rise in temperature should not occur in nonspecific protein treatment.

LEPRA TUBEROMACULOSA. Dr. Iwanow.

Two leprous brothers were presented, one suffering from the tuberomaculo-anesthetic form. In the discussion W. Iwanow called attention to the acute course of some lepra cases. In two cases at the Mjasnitzky Hospital the lepra eruptions resembled those of lichen planus and lichen scrofulosorum.

Session, Jan. 15, 1922

CANCROID AND CUTANEOUS TUBERCULOUS SYPHILIS Dr. F. Grintschar.

The patient had a three plus Wassermann reaction. Microscopically the tumor, located on the temple, was a basocellular carcinoma. Syphilitic symptoms improved under specific treatment but it stimulated the development of the cancroid.

CASE FOR DIAGNOSIS. Dr. A. Wewiorowsky.

The patient had a plus Wassermann reaction. Two injections of neo-arsphenamin improved the symptoms. The condition was either lupus erythematosus faciei et mucosae oris or cutaneous tuberose syphilis.

A. Brytschow discusses the new French antisyphilitic drug 'Trepol.'

BERLIN DERMATOLOGICAL SOCIETY

Session, Jan. 10, 1922

The president, Dr. Rosenthal. called attention to the recent death of Drs. Lewandowski and Schaeffer.

VERRUCOUS DERMATITIS CAUSED BY PETROLATUM. Dr. Heller.

Sharply defined. black, warty and hyperkeratotic lesions developed on a seborrheic eczema after a short period of treatment with petrolatum and lanolin substitutes.

MULTIPLE FIBROMAS IN THE URETHRAL CANAL. Presented by Dr. Langer.

A patient with typical Recklinghausen's disease had a sudden attack of retention of urine caused by multiple fibromas in the urethra. Four injections of fibrolysin distinctly diminished the size of tumors.

SOCIETY OF MIDDLE GERMAN DERMATOLOGISTS

Third Session
Jan. 22, 1922

SARCOID OF BOECK. Presented by Dr. Grouven.

Old tuberculin and roentgenotherapy improved the condition considerably. The former effected distinct local reaction.

PEMPHIGUS CONJUNCTIVAE. Dr. Grouven.

Two cases with shriveling of the conjunctiva were presented. In one there was also repeated vesicular eruption on the buccal mucosa. Therapeutic measures, including arsphenamin, had no success, though the latter had proved very effective in several other cases of pemphigus foliaceus. In one of the cases symptoms disappeared after ten years.

ANGIOKERATOMA. Dr. Grouven.

A case of this disease was concomitant with erythema induratum and congelation in a young girl. The erythema responded well to large doses of old tuberculin (2.5 mg.), though no local reaction became visible.

PITYRIASIS RUBRA PILARIS. Dr. Peters.

Treatment in this disease included the use of arsenic, cignolin (synthetic chrysarobin) and the roentgen rays and resulted in improvement.

SCLERODERMIE EN PLAQUES. Dr. Peters.

There were two round flat tough lesions on the extensor side of the leg in a girl, aged 13. Treatment consisted in softening of the patches with pepsin and caseosae compresses. The disorder was believed to be independent of a concomitant struma.

Ahlswede, Hamburg. Germany.

DERMATOLOGIC CONGRESS IN STRASBOURG

Session, July 10, 1921

ADENOMA SEBACEUM. Presented by Dr. L. Gèry.

The patient had a typical lesion on the scalp (épithélioma sébacé typique). There was also a small spindle cell epithelioma on the nose.

LICHEN OBTUSUS CORNEUS. Dr. L. M. Pantrier.

The case was an abnormal form of lichenification. The disorder had persisted for thirty-two years, covering the whole body with the exception of the scalp. This condition is entirely different from the lichen planus of Wilson. There were no lichen planus eruptions; however, the patient had pre-eruptive pruritus, with attacks of intense itching three or four times daily. The histologic picture also differed.

CASE OF ADENOMA SEBACEUM, PRINGLE TYPE. Dr. M. Huegel.

There were numerous tumors the size of a pea on the cheeks, nose and chin.

URTICARIA PIGMENTOSA. Dr. Mandel.

Dr. Mandel spoke of the danger of mistaking this disorder for secondary syphilis.

SUBCUTANEOUS SARCOID IN A SYPHILITIC PATIENT WITH MUL-
TIPLE GUMMAS CURED BY SPECIFIC TREATMENT. Drs.
Pautrier and Zimmerlin.

A complete cure was effected by combined antisyphilitic treatment. This
case supports the assumption that etiologically sarcoids must be in some way
connected with tuberculosis and syphilis.

SILESIAN DERMATOLOGICAL SOCIETY

Session, Jan. 28, 1922

SKIN LEISHMANIOSIS. Presented by Dr. Jessner.

A case of oriental sore was demonstrated. Microscopic smears and sections
abounded in *Leishmania tropica*. A dog was vaccinated (nose and eyebrows)
with material from the lesion. During two months it developed specific lesions.
During the discussion Dr. Kuznitzky said that in his experience arsphenamin
treatment had proved ineffective. He had seen complete and definite disappearance of all symptoms, however, after treatment with arsenophenylglycin.

A NEW FORM OF NAIL MYCOSIS (LEUKONYCHIA TRICHO-
PHYTICA). Dr. Jessner.

This disorder, of which three cases have been reported, is located on the
nails of the toes, on which white sharply defined, smooth spots are formed.
In all cases fungi were found; in Jadassohn's case, *Trichophyton gypseum
asteroides*. In a second case the fungus resembled *Trichophyton equinum*.

PSORIASIS PUSTULOSA COMBINED WITH ARTHRITIS ("PSORIASIS
ARTHRITICA"). Presented by Dr. Hoffman.

A patient, aged 37, suffering from arthritis, had an eruption which was
diagnosed as "curious psoriasiform universal dermatosis" or "atypical
psoriasis." This was followed by the development of vesicular and pustular
eruptions on the trunk and extremities. The contents of the pustules were
sterile. A case of this kind has not been reported in the literature. This
case is remarkable on account of the acute sterile pustular eruption developed
on "psoriasis arthritica."

ROSACEA OR TUBERCULID? Dr. Heymann.

Dr. Heymann reported a case which clinically resembled rosacea and whose
history suggested tuberculosis. Tuberculin reactions were positive. Dr.
Heymann believes this case belongs to those described by Lewandowsky as
"rosacea-like tuberculids."

FOUR CASES OF GRANULOSIS RUBRA NASI. Dr. Trost.

The question whether granulosis rubra nasi belongs to the tuberculids has
not yet been settled. While Ritter says that granulosis rubra nasi cannot
heal spontaneously, Dr. Trost says that this is not correct and that the lesions

generally disappear in later life. He has seen eleven cases, in seven of which the tuberculin test was positive. Of the four patients presented, two suffered from hereditary tuberculosis.

RHINOSCLEROMATOID LUPUS. Dr. Martenstein.

In a woman, aged 34, the left half of the nose was hard, with lupus granulations in the vestibulum and introitus nasi.

PEMPHIGUS OR DERMATITIS HERPETIFORMIS IN A WOMAN AGED FORTY-ONE. Presented by Dr. Leschinski.

The case is interesting with regard to the therapy. Quinin medication, intravenous injections of silver compounds, as well as serum injections (according to Linser), all failed. Painting with 2 per cent. acriflavine solution distinctly improved the condition. Vesicle formation was reduced and inhibited, deodoration was effected and the general constitution improved.

TUBERCULOSIS MUCOSAE RESEMBLING SYPHILIS. Dr. Glaser.

Dr. Glaser presented a case in which there was complete disappearance of the uvula and cicatrization of the adjoining tissues resembling a lesion of tertiary syphilis. Yet the process was distinctly of a tuberculous nature. (The Wassermann reaction was negative; all tuberculin tests positive). In the discussion Jadassohn said that in these regions (pharynx and uvula) the lupus has evidently a tendency to spontaneous (syphilis-like) cicatrization.

MONILETHRIX OR APLASIA PILORUM INTERMITTENS. Dr. Braendle.

The condition was congenital. The hairs were dry, short and brittle, the disorder resembling lichen pilaris. Microscopically, the individual hair showed a sequence of thin and thick parts: an "aplasia intermittens."

NEW YORK ACADEMY OF MEDICINE, SECTION ON DERMATOLOGY AND SYPHILIS

Regular Meeting, April 4, 1922

Howard Fox, M.D., Chairman

LUPUS VULGARIS DISSEMINATUS. Presented by Dr. Parounagian.

J. V., aged 17, was presented because of the extensive eruption and the history, which was considered of special interest. The patient gave a negative history of diseases of childhood. The first record of anything unusual occurred at 8 years of age, at which time the patient was run over by an automobile. No serious injuries were said to have been received. A year later there was an operation for "water" over the right scapula. After the operation a sinus persisted for a year and then healed. About two years later a boil was noticed on the right flank which contained "matter." This opened by itself and drained for a year and a half. When this sinus began to heal some lesions of the skin in the neighborhood of the sinus were noticed, also lesions on the face. All of these spread, and new ones appeared at intervals of four months or so. The latest one appeared about five months ago. Examination revealed a sinus over the right femur; ulceration of the right foot, dorsal aspect; serpiginous healing scarring lesions of both cheeks about the eyes, around the legs and shoulders, the trunk, both anterior and posterior, the buttocks, elbows and forearms. The boy gave the general impression of not being more than 9 years of age. He weighed only 85 pounds (38.5 kg.), and was about the height of boys of 8. He said that he had not grown since he was 9. There were no pubic, axillary or beard hairs. There were no stigmas of congenital syphilis either in the eyes, ears or teeth. The mother had married when 16; she had three children by the first husband, the patient being the third. There were eight children by the second husband. All were healthy, and there had been no miscarriages. The Wassermann test (cholesterin antigen) was reported one plus on the patient's blood. Other tests on the patient and mother had not been reported. A biopsy had been made, but had not yet been reported on. Medical and roentgen-ray examinations would be made later.

ACQUIRED SYPHILIS IN A BOY OF FIVE YEARS. Presented by Drs. Parounagian and Rulison.

R. S., aged 5, came to the hospital the afternoon of presentation. He was said to have had a sore on the left side of the sulcus about two and a half months previously. On March 23, a rash was noticed, and the patient had a severe cough. The Wassermann test on this date was four plus. The patient presented a macular eruption, mucous patches of the tongue, and marked enlargement of the cervical and suboccipital glands. The inguinal glands were only slightly enlarged, and the epitrochlears were not palpable. The scar of the initial lesions was still noticeable.

A CASE FOR DIAGNOSIS (CIRCINATE MACULOPAPULAR LESIONS). Presented by Dr. Williams.

E. H., aged 27, a housewife, presented herself in the clinic of the Skin and Cancer Hospital with an eruption which had been present for about one and a half years. Though never free from the rash at any time, during this period it had spread from one point to another, remaining only a short time in a given spot. The eruption was characterized by an irregularly spreading, slightly raised inflammatory rash, clearing up in the center and scaling peripherally. Most of the lesions formed complete circles, but a fair number were horseshoe or semicircular in shape. No vesicles could be demonstrated about the periphery or in any part of any of the lesions, which were practically confined to the chest and back, with a few new lesions just appearing on the shoulders and upper arms. Local applications of calamin lotion. dieting, and thorough purging had no effect. Applications of tar or Whitfield's ointment cleared the lesions, leaving a tan pigmentation New lesions appeared elsewhere as the old ones disappeared, and some even returned to the same areas. The Wassermann test was negative. A section taken from the indurated border of a lesion on the back suggested the diagnosis of the premycotic stage of mycosis fungoides.

Dr. Highman said he did not know of anything particularly characteristic in the epidermis of mycosis, and barring hyperkeratosis and an indeterminate perivascular round cell infiltration he saw nothing striking in the section, certainly nothing on which a plausible diagnosis of mycosis might be made. He did not like to suggest mycosis; the condition which seemed most likely was that particular subvariety of seborrhea which Unna considered the petaloid type. Etiologically, he did not see how, without further investigation, a fungus infection could be ruled out, but the condition was probably either a seborrhea or an atypical tinea.

Dr. Levin said the first clinical impression was that of tinea. However, the border was elevated, infiltrated, and on palpation was found to be present in the skin as well as on the surface. It resembled the lesions of a case (tuberculosis cutis) previously presented by him before the Section. The diagnosis in his opinion was a superficial form of tuberculosis cutis.

Drs. Scheer, Rulison, and Parounagian said they thought the condition was tinea.

PHENOBARBITAL (LUMINAL) ERUPTION ON TONGUE, CHEEKS AND LIPS. Presented by Dr. Chargin.

C. S., a woman, aged 22, single, a houseworker, had been the subject of essential epilepsy since early childhood. Up to two years ago, for a period of eight years, she had been taking bromids. She gave no history of a bromid eruption. Two years ago she began to use luminal, at which time bromids were discontinued. At first she took 1½ grains (0.09 gm.) three times daily; later four doses of 1½ grains a day. In the last few months she had been taking 2½ grains (0.14 gm.) a day. The patient denied having any general eruption while taking the luminal. The mouth condition began six months ago, and during this period the mouth was never normal. She came under observation, Jan. 3, 1922, when she was admitted to Mount Sinai Hospital, the service of Dr. Goldenberg. Except for pediculosis capitis with a consequent dermatitis on the neck and upper part of the back, the skin was normal. The mouth was unclean, and emitted a fetid odor, with dribbling of saliva. The hard palate was normal; along the teeth on the gums was a red line. The tongue was from two to three times its normal size, and showed marked indentation along the border; the border was thin. The surface of the tongue was uneven and showed areas denuded of epithelium. It was raw and beefy looking, and presented alternate patches of red and gray, resembling healthy and unhealthy granulations. There were several thin walled blisters filled with a bloody fluid; these blisters ruptured readily, either spontaneously or on the slightest trauma. The condition extended to the under surface of the tongue, which it affected for about three-quarters of an inch (12.7 mm.) along its margin. The line of demarcation between the normal and abnormal mucous membranes was sharply defined but of irregular outline. The floor of the mouth was entirely normal. The upper lip showed a few lesions resembling mucous patches; the lower lip was covered with a blood crust. The soft palate showed numerous erythematous patches which varied in size and configuration. The throat, nose, pharynx and esophagus were entirely normal. Luminal was promptly withdrawn; this was followed by a gradual improvement. At the end of three weeks the mouth was almost well. Resumption of the luminal resulted in the reappearance of the eruption after 36 grains (2.3 gm.) had been administered. The skin tests for luminal were negative. Luminal was demonstrated in the urine on two occasions. On account of the epileptic attacks, luminal was continued off and on, and at the time of presentation the patient still showed a triangular patch on the upper surface of the tongue which bore the characteristics noted in the foregoing.

DISCUSSION

DR. ROSEN said he had seen four different types of phenobarbital eruptions: the pemphigoid type, with lesions on the mucous membrane; a morbilliform type; a scarlatiniform type, and an erythema multiforme type.

DR. CHARGIN, in response to an inquiry from Dr. Wise, said that pheno-barbital was chemically ethyl-phenyl-barbituric acid. The eruption was said to be due to the amido or phenyl radical, which presumably broke up certain of the proteins in the system that acted much like foreign proteins. Erup-tions on the mucous membranes from phenobarbital had been reported, but mostly in the fauces (tonsils) and not on the tongue. Many of the cases show-ing mucous membrane lesions had a rise of temperature, but this patient had none. This was apparently the first reported case of phenobarbital eruption on the tongue; he had not been able to find reports of other cases in the literature.

TUBERCULOSIS CUTIS. (Presented in March at the Manhattan Dermatological Society as acnitis.) Presented by DR. LEVIN.

L. M. B., aged 37, unmarried, a salesman, applied for treatment at the Cornell Clinic ten weeks ago. The skin condition had been present for four months. The lesions first appeared on the chin and upper lip, and gradually extended involving the cheeks, nose and eyelids, forehead and scalp. When first seen there were three types of lesions. Scattered over the face, particu-larly on the upper lip, cheeks, chin and eyelids, there were about two dozen brownish red, soft, elevated, rounded papules; some of these were arranged in circinate groups. A second type of lesion resembled the first type, but seemed to be more follicular in character and was surrounded by pustules. A third type consisted of subcutaneous, firm, pea-sized tubercles which were more evident on palpation than on inspection, and tended to become confluent. The skin over the last type appeared normal in color but after two to three weeks became purplish. On the scalp there were several lentil to pea-sized follicular papules which tended to become pustular and form adherent crusts. Complete medical, ophthalmologic and neurologic examinations were negative. The first Wassermann test was one plus, but several later tests were negative. Eight arsphenamin and eight mercury injections were without effect on the lesions. A study of a section taken from a lesion on the cheek showed tuber-culosis. Further studies on the pathology, bacteriology, and guinea-pig inocu-lations were being made, and would be reported on. Electro-desiccation had been performed locally.

DISCUSSION

DR. WISE said that according to modern conceptions, acnitis was the deep form of papulonecrotic tuberculid, occurring on the face; while lupus miliaris disseminatus facei was a non-necrotic scattered tuberculoma of the face.

DR. LAPOWSKI asked whether it corresponded to lupus.

DR. POLLITZER said that the present case corresponded fairly well with a case which he had published under the name of hidradenitis suppurativa about the same time that Barthelemy published his paper on acnitis and folliclis. In this case, as he had pointed out in the case he had published, some of the lesions were deep seated and could be palpated but not seen. These lesions gradually made their way to the surface and appeared as a papule which broke down in the center, discharged a little pus, and healed with a small depressed scar. These cases were subsequently grouped with the tuberculids, this particular form constituting the papular or papulonecrotic tuberculid.

Dr. HIGHMAN said that lesions justifiably called tuberculids should not be considered anything but cutaneous tuberculosis, if actually of a tuberculous nature. There were lesions that clinically resembled tuberculosis in which tuberculous structure was never found; or if found, it might be because of the attenuated bacilli or toxins rather than viable bacilli. Such an asumption might be dangerous. In syphilis the lesions which are known to be due to spirochetes are called syphilids, while tuberculids are lesions not containing tubercle bacilli. This is inconsistent. If one were satisfied from the microscopic structure that these lesions were due to the tubercle bacilli, and further evidence from inoculation proved it, then Dr. Highman agreed with Dr. Wise that this case was not what was called acnitis in the past. Whether or not we choose to call it acnitis in the future is a different matter. Clinically, any one who wanted to call it acnitis was justified in his belief. This very discussion showed how confused the profession was on the subject. Personally he expressed the wish that all had the courage to call all forms of cutaneous tuberculosis "tuberculosis." In the old sense, tuberculids should be eliminated from consideration as related to tuberculosis unless proved to be related. It was perhaps permissible to regard lesions that histologically were not tuberculosis as tuberculosis, but this was at present theoretical, although in the development and differentiation of lesions there might be a period when they became histologically typical, before and after which they were atypical. A great deal of loose talk and unscientific discussion had been indulged in which could not bear the test of scientific and astute scrutiny, which revealed an elementary attitude toward the conception of the appearance, disappearance and nature of lesions. Without knowing more about the subject from the newer angle, he did not understand how such a case as this could be discussed with the intelligence that the sons' and grandsons of the present generation would bring to their aid in their conception of the matter; but if this was histologically tuberculous and clinically acnitis, then some lesions resembling acnitis were tuberculous. This should be the attitude in general until more was known about it.

Dr. POLLITZER said that the group of skin lesions which were called tuberculids had a distinct tuberculous structure, as the pathologist understands that term, yet did not show under careful examination any tubercle bacilli and did not produce tuberculosis when inoculated. Such lesions might properly be called tuberculids; as soon as the tubercle bacilli were discovered or successful inoculations made into a guinea-pig, producing tuberculosis, they were no longer tuberculids but were properly grouped with the tuberculoses. The conception of a tuberculid group was therefore only a temporary arrangement and subject to extinction with increase in our knowledge.

Dr. HIGHMAN responded that that was the very point he had been making; a "syphilid" was a lesion in which the spirochetes were present; the term "tuberculids" ought to be applied to those caused by the tubercle bacilli. There might be some reason for calling nontuberculous lesions tuberculids, but there was no sense in the word tuberculid as employed at present. He was aware of the distinction that Dr. Pollitzer mentioned, but it seemed illogical.

Dr. Levin said that clinically there were two main groups of lesions: First, the lesions which were dark red and firm which after persisting for some time tended to become necrotic and form pustules on the summits. The lesions of the other main group were soft, apple-jelly in color, did not form pustules and resembled lupus vulgaris. The first suggested acnitis. Another type of lesion present was found mainly on the forehead and appeared first as hard tubercles in the hypoderm without any change in the overlying skin. These gradually developed toward the surface, became more prominent and the skin over them became purplish-red. The pathology of this type was that of tuberculosis. Further studies were to be made and reported later.

CASE FOR DIAGNOSIS (LUPUS VULGARIS?). Presented by Dr. Halperin.

H. W., aged 4, with a negative family history, presented several brownish lesions on both cheeks and ears, which had existed for more than one year. The mother said that similar lesions had previously appeared on the arms and legs, all of which had completely disappeared except one near the right elbow which had left a brown stain.

DISCUSSION

Dr. Abramowitz said he thought that the eruption was the sarcoid of Boeck.

Dr. Levin said the lesions were soft and apple jelly in color, and thought the diagnosis was either lupus vulgaris or sarcoid.

Dr. Pollitzer was inclined to consider it a case of sarcoid.

Dr. Halperin said he did not know the mother had said that the child had taken bromid. He had asked her again about it, and she said she was not sure it was bromid that the child had taken, but that some doctor had suggested it. The mother also said that at certain times the patient had taken cathartics which contained phenolphthalein.

PARAKERATOSIS VARIEGATA. Presented by Dr. Bechet.

E. J., a boy, aged 10, born in the United States, came to Dr. Whitehouse's clinic on the day of presentation. The mother asserted that the eruption had been present for about a month. It consisted of well-defined purplish red patches, semi-confluent, oval and round, enclosing areas of apparently healthy skin, giving a reticulated, network-like appearance; this was most marked on the arms and legs. There were some lesions on the trunk. Slight scaling was also present. The lesions were not pruritic. The family history was negative.

DISCUSSION

Dr. Pollitzer said he had seen the case and noted the diagnosis with which it was presented. He did not like the term "lichenoid" applied to the case for he could see nothing resembling that disease. If it were a parapsoriasis or belonged to that group it belonged rather to the guttate than the lichenoid form. He had examined the patient carefully with that in mind, and he did not find that the condition conformed to parakeratosis variegata.

Dr. Highman thought the case looked like parapsoriasis, but he did not know whether the diagnosis was tenable or not.

Dr. Rosen agreed with Dr. Bechet in classifying the case as parakeratosis variegata, and cited a similar case seen at the Mount Sinai Hospital with the same netlike reticulation and violaceous color of the lesions.

Dr. Wise suggested that it would be a good case in which to eliminate all external and internal treatment and present the patient again at the May meeting in order to decide on the actual diagnosis. The duration of only one month threw a wet blanket on the diagnosis. If it were a parapsoriasis one would not expect well marked manifestations in a month.

Dr. Bechet agreed with Dr. Wise that it was most unusual to have a case of parapsoriasis develop to such an extent in one month, but the mother might have been mistaken in stating the duration of the disease. Dr. Rosen had brought out the point he had in mind; he had believed the term parakeratosis variegata to be the correct one because of the reticulated, lacelike distribution of the eruption. Stelwagon had described such lacelike, reticulated eruptions under the heading of parakeratosis variegata, but he agreed fully with Dr. Pollitzer that there were no lichenoid lesions.

Dr. Pollitzer said that the first case described by Unna and himself had been sent to the Hamburg Clinic by Besnier as an aberrant type of lichen planus. The lesions were distinctly lichenous, and the condition was named variegata because the lesions on the upper part of the body were a vivid red and those on the lower part of the body were dusky. These variations in color, with the reticulated arrangement of the shining lichenoid lesions, gave a variegated appearance to the entire surface. Some time later Juliusberg published a case which he called pityriasis lichenoides chronica, and which was identified as similar to the first case published. What Dr. Pollitzer wished to emphasize was that these cases had distinctly lichenoid lesions, whereas the case presented by Dr. Bechet was in no respect lichenoid; he objected to calling it parapsoriasis variegata because the main characteristic of that disease was the lichenoid lesion.

SARCOID (BOECK). Presented by Dr. Rothwell. (Previously presented by Dr. Fraser, January, 1921.)

Mrs. R. F., a white woman, aged 44, presented on the bridge and sides of the nose contiguous thereto a plaque of infiltration, dark reddish, only slightly elevated, and showing only slight effect of various treatments applied. The condition had existed sixteen months. The Wassermann test was negative.

FOR DIAGNOSIS (ECZEMA SEBORRHEICUM OF EYELIDS). Presented by Dr. Rothwell.

S. C., a girl, aged 7, presented on the upper and lower lids of both eyes a symmetrical, noninfiltrated (?), greasy appearing brownish eruption, sharply defined at the borders, with slight scale formation (when salves were abstained from) which had existed for six or seven weeks. Efforts to obtain scales for examination were unsuccessful. A 5 per cent. salicylic acid salve seemed to cause disappearance, and the condition returned on discontinuance of its use.

DISCUSSION

Dr. Abramowitz said he thought it was a rash due to phenolphthalein. The lesions were sharply limited with a pink border and a slight play of color. He had questioned the mother, but it was difficult to obtain anything definite from her; but he thought that if Dr. Rothwell would let the lesions subside under a nonirritating dressing and then give the patient phenolphthalein, the eruption would break out again.

Dr. Scheer agreed with the diagnosis of phenolphthalein eruption and added that the mother gave a history of having given the child Ex-Lax on several occasions.

Dr. Wise said that it required a good deal of courage to make a definite diagnosis of phenolphthalein eruption, although he believed it to be that type of eruption. However, it was unusual to see it limited to both eyelids. He had seen it on the eyelids, but with other lesions on the body; of course then the diagnosis could be made very easily. In all probability, however, this was a phenolphthalein eruption.

Dr. Pollitzer said that he also had questioned the mother; she was rather vague about the history, but said she had been giving the child Ex-Lax from time to time. The lesions corresponded in appearance to those produced by phenolphthalein, and that diagnosis was probably correct.

Dr. Bechet said that he had seen the case in the clinic the day before, and that the child had at that time practically no eruption on the eyelids. The mother was told to discontinue the antiseborrheic ointment she had been using, because it had been noticed that the eruption almost disappeared on its use, to recur when it was discontinued. The lesions were limited to the upper eyelids; there were no lesions on the body. The mother had told him that she had not administered Ex-Lax to the child for two months previously. Discounting the history, the fact that the eruption was located on the eyelids only and responded to antiseborrheic treatment, was rather against the diagnosis of phenolphthalein rash and in favor of an atypical form of seborrheic eczema.

GENERALIZED NEURODERMATITIS AND ICHTHYOSIS. Presented by Dr. Wise.

C. A., aged 21, born in the United States, had had a mild ichthyosis since birth. Six years ago an itching developed on the forearms and face, followed by an eruption. There was a generalized erythroderma on the face, neck and upper extremities. The back presented an ichthyosis and the legs a mild keratosis pilaris. The patient was sensitive to horse dander, which manifested itself by asthma; simultaneously the eruption became aggravated.

DISCUSSION

Dr. Wise said that probably the French term, pruritus with lichenification. was the better name, but the name neurodermatitis seemed to be all right. It was probably some form of anaphylactic phenomenon manifested in the skin of patients suffering from asthma and hay fever, as did this one.

Dr. Pollitzer said that Dr. Wise might have stressed a little more the ichthyosis from which this patient suffered and the rather unusual association of lichenification with ichthyosis.

Dr. Highman agreed that it was a generalized ichthyosis with a secondary dermatitis and lichenification.

Dr. Wise said that he was unable to satisfy Dr. Highman in regard to the justifiableness of the name. Even the Frenchmen who proposed it were very vague; they said, however, that it occurred in neurotic persons. With regard to the ichthyosis, he could not agree with Dr. Pollitzer's interpretation. The patient had had the ichthyosis since childhood and neurodermatitis for only five or six years, and had asthma caused by horse dander—a very suggestive complication of the skin disease.

Dr. Levin suggested the administration of thyroid.

PAPULAR SYPHILID OF GLANS PENIS AFTER INTENSIVE SPE-CIPIC TREATMENT. Presented by Dr. Bechet.

P. J., a man, aged 34, born in Denmark, from Dr. Stetson's service at the New York Skin and Cancer Hospital, said that fifteen years previously he had had a primary lesion followed by secondary eruptions. He first came to the hospital on April 6, 1920, complaining of vague general pains. His family history was negative. The spinal fluid findings were negative, but the blood Wassermann was four plus. There were no mouth or skin lesions. From April 6, 1920 to Aug. 18, 1921, he received thirty arsphenamin injections, varying in dose from 0.2 to 0.4 gm., and thirty-four intramuscular injections of mercuric salicylate of 1 grain each. The Wassermann reaction on July 17, 1920, was two plus; Dec. 2, 1920, negative; April 6, 1921, negative; Jan. 1, 1922, negative; March 3, 1922, negative. The last Wassermann test was made five months after the last injection of arsphenamin, and two months after the last mercury injection. The lesions first appeared on the glans four weeks previously, and consisted of several raised, copper colored indurated papules. There were no subjective symptoms.

DISCUSSION

Dr. Parounagian agreed with the diagnosis of nodular syphiloderm.

Dr. Highman inquired whether since the appearance of the lesions the treatment had had no effect. Clinically the lesions did not look like syphilis but like lichen planus.

Dr. Bechet, in reply to Dr. Highman's inquiry as to whether treatment had had any effect on the lesions, said that the man had had no specific treatment for six weeks previous to the occurrence of the eruption, four weeks previously. The last specific treatment was given on Aug. 18, 1921.

Dr. Pollitzer said that clinically the lesions were not syphilis but lichen planus. They were distinctly umbilicated; one especially had an almost quadrilateral appearance, while the syphilitic papule was conical or spherical in shape. Moreover, it seemed almost impossible that a syphilitic papule should appear fifteen years after infection, and especially after several months of such treatment as this man had had.

Dr. Abramowitz thought the lesions on the penis were those of lichen planus. He had seen five or six similar cases within the last few years, all the patients having had syphilis for a long time and having recently been receiving arsphenamin. There seemed to be a predisposition for such patients to develop lichen planus, or lichen-planus-like lesions on the genitals.

Dr. Wise agreed with what Dr. Abramowitz had just said. There were five or six articles in the literature relating to lichen planus appearing as the result of arsphenamin injections. That might have some bearing on this case.

Dr. McCafferty said he had a patient who developed lesions resembling lichen planus following arsphenamin treatment, but said there were many points for and against lichen planus. The papules strongly suggested lichen planus. The arsenical keratoses suggested chronic arsenical poisoning. Such men as Buschke and Freymann were of the opinion that perhaps all of their cases were arsenical dermatoses. It had been known for many years that arsenic could produce lesions resembling lichen planus; occasionally such lesions appeared on the buccal mucosa and tongue. The histopathologic picture was characteristic of lichen planus.

Dr. Bechet said he could not see any connection between the administration of arsphenamin and the lesions, as the eruption had appeared six months after the last injection. In his estimation the lesions resembled syphilis rather than lichen planus. He would give the man active specific treatment, and show him at the next meeting.

DUHRING'S DISEASE FOLLOWING VACCINATION (SMALLPOX AND TYPHOID). Presented by Dr. Abramowitz.

J. B., a private patient, aged 25, single and American born; had not been working for the past four years. The skin disease had existed for the past five years, and was said to have followed vaccination against smallpox, and injections of typhoid vaccine. The eruption had been present all over the body, including the mouth. The present distribution of the lesions was on the face, arms, penis, thighs, legs and feet. In these locations a circinate and serpiginous eruption was present, made up of vesicles, papules and erythematous plaques. No pigmentations were noted from previous eruptions. During the past few days a pinhead sized vesicle had appeared on the conjunctiva of the left lower eyelid. Several Wassermann tests had been taken, and were all negative. The patient had received all kinds of treatment from various dermatologists throughout the country, the administration of arsenic being about the only measure that afforded any relief. This had to be discontinued because of palmar keratoses. He was recently under the care of Dr. Thornley of the Public Health Service.

MYCOSIS FUNGOIDES. Presented by Dr. Rothwell for Dr. Trimble. (Previously presented at the December meeting.)

K. Y., a woman, aged 67, a widow, presented the reticulated skin and nodular condition shown at the time of presentation last December, but modified by roentgen-ray therapy still being applied.

DISCUSSION

Dr. Scheer asked for some discussion on the case of mycosis which had previously been presented.

Dr. Wise expressed the opinion that the reticulated area on the woman's breast had nothing to do with the disease. She had mycosis fungoides, but the reticulation and telangiectasis on the chest was probably an angioma serpiginosum.

PEMPHIGUS. Presented by Dr. Levin.

Mrs. M. G., aged 48, was a Russian Jewess. The disease began eleven months ago, with a bulla on the right conjunctiva and marked inflammatory reaction. One month later she developed bullous lesions in the throat, causing hoarseness and painful swallowing. Then numerous lesions appeared on the tongue, cheeks and lips. Six months ago the patient noticed a bleb under the left arm, which was followed by an outburst of numerous blebs over the trunk. These shriveled up after several days and formed crusts. The patient felt no itching, burning or pain. For the last two months she had been practically covered with crusts and blebs. The mouth was constantly raw and painful from the lesions therein. She had developed bullae in the vagina. The crusts on the body were somewhat adherent, and when removed left a red.

infected surface. The patient had lost 20 pounds (9 kg.) and was greatly exhausted. She had become bent and old looking. She had always been healthy and able to do her work efficiently. Her family history was negative to pemphigus or any chronic disease so far as she knew. The Wassermann test was negative.

ACRODERMATITIS CHRONICA ATROPHICANS. Presented by Dr. Levin.

R. S., aged 28, married, an Austrian, had had the condition of the skin for ten years. First appearing about the ankles, it had gradually extended to include the feet, legs, lower thighs and buttocks. The eruption was symmetrical, and showed atrophy with a purplish discoloration and prominence of the veins on both legs. The skin of the ankles was purplish, swollen and hard, suggesting scleroderma. Both buttocks showed a bluish-red discoloration. The skin of the fingers and hands was bluish-red and cold.

ERYTHEMA PERSTANS (PHENOLPHTHALEIN). Presented by Dr. Levin.

M. W., a woman, aged 23, married said that she had been having recurrent itching eruptions for six years. When first seen two weeks previously she presented an eruption of three days' duration. Two days prior to the development of the rash she had taken Partola. On the right arm, and on the back near the right posterior axillary fold, there were two quarter-dollar sized, irregularly round, slightly elevated, brownish-red patches. Three days prior to presentation she took two Ex-Lax tablets. This was followed by enlargement of the old lesions, increased pruritus, generalized, evanescent wheals, and a new quarter-dollar sized round, erythematous patch on the inner aspect of the upper part of the left thigh.

PAGET'S DISEASE OF THE NIPPLE. Presented by Dr. Rothwell for Dr. Trimble.

Mrs. M. McC., aged 50, a widow, presented about the nipple a reddish plaque of infiltration, circular in outline, about 1½ inches (3.8 cm.) in diameter, covered with fine scales, the border sharply outlined and slightly raised, a suggestive waxy appearance being present at places in the border. There had been no subjective symptoms, no response to local treatment, and the condition had been present for four years.

LUPUS ERYTHEMATOSUS. Presented by Dr. Levin.

The patient was presented to show the good effect of roentgen-ray therapy in a condition usually not responsive to this form of treatment.

F. G., aged 37, a native of the United States, was first seen on March 22, 1921. He complained of an obstinate eruption of the face of eight years' duration. It had resisted all forms of therapy. When first seen, he showed a large patch of lupus erythematosus covering the outer two-thirds of the left cheek, and a smaller patch on the right cheek; small scattered lesions were present on and in the neighborhood of the nose. An unusual feature was the marked elevation of the border. As presented following the use of the roentgen rays, the cheeks showed areas of atrophy with slight brownish pigmentation and atrophy. Small active lesions were present near the nose.

LEPRA. Presented by Dr. Rothwell.

B. G., aged 24, a Spaniard, presented profuse citron-colored nodules on the face, though less profuse in number and smaller in size than at the time of last presentation. The case was again shown to demonstrate that apparently injections of the ethyl esters of the fatty acids of chaulmoogra oil had a better effect than injections of the usual chaulmoogra-camphorated oil-resorcin mixture.

SUPERINFECTION; SYPHILIS. Presented by Dr. Levin.

The patient was presented at the March meeting of the Manhattan Dermatological Society. G. P., aged 27, a Greek busman, had a chancre of the penis followed by secondary symptoms of syphilis in 1916. The Wassermann test of the blood was four plus. During the following sixteen months he was given fourteen intravenous injections of arsphenamin and thirty-eight intramuscular injections of mercury. In March, 1918, the Wassermann test of the blood was four plus and the spinal fluid showed a four plus Wassermann test, 130 cells per cubic millimeter, and a two plus globulin reaction. In 1919, while in the army, he received eight arsphenamin and six mercury injections. The blood Wassermann reaction was subsequently negative. Since that time the blood was negative on three different occasions. Eight weeks ago he was exposed to infection. Six weeks ago a lesion appeared on the penis. Spirochetes were found in the secretion from this lesion, but not in the material obtained from the inguinal glands. He presented at that time a typical chancre of the shaft of the penis about the size of a five-cent piece, adjacent adenitis, and a one plus Wassermann test of the blood. Since. the lesion had grown to the size of a quarter and looked as though it were secondarily affected by pyogenic micro-organisms. There was a generalized adenopathy, and the Wassermann had become four plus.

LEUKEMIDS; CHRONIC MYELOGENOUS LEUKEMIA. Presented by Dr. Levin.

I. H., a man, aged 60, married, a Russian, complained of an intense generalized pruritus, with an eruption which had been present for ten years and which had resisted all forms of treatment. For years he had suffered from severe headaches, which had been somewhat relieved by glasses. There was a slight blurring of vision. He had had a deformed chest since childhood. Three years prior to presentation he had a profusely discharging abscess of the left axilla for five weeks. The skin condition appeared ten years ago. with itching lesions under the arms which spread within a year to the rest of the upper extremities, then to the lower extremities, and finally to the trunk and the rest of the body. The pruritus was constant, but worse at night.

Examination revealed a well nourished man, coughing occasionally. slightly cyanosed and of a sallow complexion. The tonsils were small. cryptic and congested. Herpes labialis was present. There was a large lymph node under the right subclavian muscle. The chest showed a marked enlargement of the right side with greater expansion on breathing. A scar was present in the left axilla. The right lung was hyper-resonant, with puerile breath sounds and sibilant and sonorous ronchi. The left lung showed diminished resonance above, dulness to flatness posteriorly and in the axilla. generalized fremitus. diminished breath sounds. exaggerated spoken and whispered voice. coarse and whistling râles. The spleen was firm, smooth, and was felt 8 cm. below the costal margin. The liver was firm, smooth and palpable four fingerbreadths below the costal margin. The eyegrounds showed tortuosity of the vessels and pallor of the disk outlines. The skin showed a generalized eruption made up of crops of wheals, firm papules and excoriations. Patches of pigmentation were evident, and there were areas of lichenification and infiltration. Exaggerated dermatographia was manifested. At points of pressure and irritation there appeared groups of wheals. The temperature was normal, the pulse varied between 72 and 100, the respirations were normal. The urine showed a trace of albumin and no Bence-Jones bodies. The protein skin sensitization tests were all negative. The roentgenogram of the left side of the chest was obscured by a dense shadow extending from the sixth rib in the axilla to the base in the lateral half of the lung. Fluoroscopy showed a fixed mass and no fluid wave. Radiographic diagnosis was pleural tumor or encapsulated empyema. Two blood examinations were made. The first revealed 44,000 leukocytes, polymorphonuclear neutrophil cells, 36 per cent.; eosinophils, 2 per cent.; basophils, 3 per cent.; myelocyte neutrophils, 18 per cent.; myelocyte eosinophils, 12 per cent.; stimulation forms, 2 per cent.; large mononuclears, 4 per cent.; transitionals, 4 per cent., and lymphocytes, 19 per cent. The second examination revealed: White blood cells, 60,000; polymorphonuclears, 55 per cent.; eosinophils, 1 per cent.; basophils, 5 per cent.; myelocyte neutrophils, 19 per cent.; myelocyte eosinophils, 2 per cent.; myelocyte basophils, 3 per cent.; lymphocytes, 10 per cent.; transitionals, 4 per cent. The urea nitrogen of the blood was 21 mg. per 100 c.c., and the blood sugar was 150 mg. per 100 c.c.

Under benzene in drop doses internally and radium applied to the chest the pruritus was relieved; the eruption faded until when presented again about 10 per cent. of the lesions were present. A biopsy of the skin lesions revealed the pathology of an exudative nonvesicular eruption.

PIGMENTATION AND KERATOSES FROM ARSENIC. Presented by Dr. Levin.

V. C., aged 34, married, a decorator, complained in January, 1922, of recurrent ulcers of the legs, of fourteen years' duration. He had been taking arsenic at varying intervals for years. He presented then several clean, punched out ulcers, varying in size from that of a pea to that of a five-cent piece, as well as old purplish scars on the front of the right leg. Examination revealed brownish pigmentation covering the trunk and neck, and thickened, scaly, hyperkeratosis of the palms and soles. The Wassermann test was twice negative, and the urine did not show arsenic.

ERYTHEMA BULLOSUM. Presented by Drs. Howard Fox and B. F. Ochs.

H. S., aged 14, a school boy, a full-blooded negro born in the United States, first noticed the eruption two weeks previously. It was confined to the mouth and lips, and to the backs of the hands and the forearms. There was an extensive bullous eruption of the buccal mucosa and of both lips, causing considerable pain on eating. The lips were swollen and covered with dirty, yellowish crusts, and there was an ill smelling purulent discharge. On the backs of the hands and forearms there was a sparse eruption of pea to dime sized maculopapular erythematous lesions, some of them presenting a characteristic "iris" arrangement. On the palms there were a few pea sized macular lesions, similar to the macules seen in early palmar syphilis. There were no other symptoms suggesting syphilis. There was no apparent cause for the eruption, the patient being well nourished and in apparent good health.

LICHEN PLANUS ANNULARIS. Presented by Dr. Maloney.

J. M., a man aged 28, born in Italy, a tailor, had syphilis in 1918. He was treated with arsphenamin and mercury (intramuscularly). He had had four negative Wassermann tests during the last year. He presented a group of small, discrete lichen planus lesions on both forearms, neck, and over the sacral and lumbar regions; large patches of confluent, somewhat infiltrated lesions on the inner surface of both legs and many annular lesions on the penis.

ULCERS OF THE TONGUE; TERTIARY SYPHILIS. Presented by Dr. Levin.

This patient was presented to show evidence of active clinical and serologic syphilis, notwithstanding almost constant treatment for more than five years.

G. V., aged 28, married, a pedler, had an initial lesion and secondary lesions of syphilis in July, 1916. He had been under almost constant observation and treatment since then. The Wassermann test had varied; at times the reaction would be negative, and at other times from two to four plus. On Sept. 6, 1921, it was four plus. Since then he had received six arsphenamin and eight mercury injections. Altogether he had received forty-three intravenous injections of arsphenamin and ninety-six intramuscular injections of mercury. The lesion of the tongue appeared about two weeks ago. On the dorsum of the tongue near the right border he showed two pea sized, punched out infiltrated ulcers. These were situated on a quarter-dollar sized, slightly elevated, dark red patch. There were no teeth or dental work which could have irritated the tongue.

LICHEN PLANUS ATROPHICANS. Presented by Dr. Abramowitz.

EPITHELIOMA OF THE CHIN. Presented by Dr. Levin.

MULTIPLE CIRCUMSCRIBED LIPOMAS; MARKED IMPROVEMENT UNDER THYROID THERAPY. Presented by Dr. Levin.

LUPUS VULGARIS OF CHEEK (CHILD). Presented by Dr. Levin.

LUPUS VULGARIS: LOBULE OF EAR. Presented by Dr. Maloney.

PIGMENTED ATROPHY. Presented by Dr. Levin. (Previously presented).

STRIAE ATROPHICAE IN A MALE. Presented by Dr. Bechet.

Paul E. Bechet, M.D., Secretary.

PHILADELPHIA DERMATOLOGICAL SOCIETY

Regular Monthly Meeting, April 10, 1922

Frank Crozer Knowles, M.D., *Presiding*

SYPHILIS. Presented by Dr. Hirschler.

A male colored baby, 3 months old, had been observed for two days only. No history was available. Skin lesions were present on the buttocks, legs and knees, especially. They consisted of definite rings, distinctly raised and firm to the touch. Some of them had coalesced with others and presented a serpiginous outline. There were similar lesions on the buttocks, some eroded but none fissured. The Wassermann reaction was negative. The rings had flattened out markedly during the last forty-eight hours.

DISCUSSION

Dr. Schamberg said the absence of a positive Wassermann reaction did not negative the diagnosis. The glazed and peeling condition of the soles, together with the other lesions, strengthened the supposition that the condition was syphilis. Occasionally, when positive at birth the reaction changed later, possibly owing to a carrying over of antibodies from the syphilitic mother. Usually the eruption persisted, but it sometimes disappeared without treatment.

Dr. Knowles considered the lesions on the knees quite typical of syphilis.

PAPULONECROTIC TUBERCULID. Presented by Dr. Strauss.

This patient, alluded to at the last meeting, was a white girl of 24. The eruption first broke out in the summer of 1920, lasting until it was apparently cured by administration of arsphenamin, which was begun in January, 1921. Ten treatments were necessary to cause its disappearance. In January, 1922, the outbreak reappeared, mainly on the hands and forearms, and again improved under arsphenamin. At first the remedy appeared to make it worse, but later it always improved.

DISCUSSION

Dr. Schamberg mentioned the fact that warm weather usually caused an abatement of the condition. This eruption, however, started in summer. Arsphenamin had a nonspecific action of forming antibodies in various infections and was frequently useful in cases of septicemia and puerperal sepsis.

Dr. Strauss said he wondered whether the season or the arsphenamin had cured this patient.

DERMATITIS HERPETIFORMIS. Presented by Dr. Schamberg.

A young man, white, had a widespread, slightly elevated, gyrate and festooned eruption, accompanied by severe itching. The space enclosed by these irregular borders was deeply pigmented. Many areas of skin were normal. The eruption for the most part occurred on the trunk.

DISCUSSION

Dr. Knowles said he had had the patient under observation at the Philadelphia Hospital for three months and had considered the case one of lichen planus. The appearance then had been quite different; where pigment was now present, there had been violaceous plaques, formed by aggregations of papules. The pigmentation was possibly due to arsenic. As Dr. Schamberg remarked, the case now markedly resembled dermatitis herpetiformis, but from the previous history and appearance he held to the earlier diagnosis.

Dr. Weidman said the case strongly reminded him of a case of granuloma fungoides in a female subject whom Dr. Schamberg also had seen.

Dr. Corson said he thought some of the small annular lesions on the breast resembled lichen planus.

DR. SCHAMBERG said that festoons were not uncommon in dermatitis herpetiformis, which he felt strongly was the correct diagnosis. The eruption affected only certain parts. Lichen planus annularis had, as a rule, a broader border.

DR. WEIDMAN added that it almost suggested erythema perstans in its more active portions or erythema multiforme of atypical form.

CASE FOR DIAGNOSIS. Presented by DR. WEIDMAN.

P. J. R., a white laborer, aged 60 years, had complained of burning and an erysipelas-like swelling around the eyes intermittently for eight weeks. Both hands were somewhat livid and the backs were studded with minute keratoses. He had multiple telangiectases on the scrotum but no overlying keratoses. The sections showed an unusually heavy mantle of lymphocytes around the blood vessels, particularly in the deepest part of the corium, where the sweat glands were similarly and most heavily affected. The tubules were broadened and the lining cells degenerated. There was no necrosis. The presenter believed the condition on the hand was a tuberculid (lupus pernio) at a very early stage—too early to show any equivocal tuberculous architecture. He felt that the facial condition suggested erysipelas faciei perstans of Kaposi.

DISCUSSION

DR. SCHAMBERG agreed that there was marked infiltration around the sweat glands in the section.

DR. WEIDMAN called attention to the peculiar granules in the epithelium of the sweat glands. There was no history of a dermatitis antedating the present condition.

DR. KNOWLES said he felt that there were two conditions here—a chronic one with an acute outbreak associated.

DR. SCHAMBERG added that the eruption on the face was hard to distinguish from an eczema.

CHLOASMA. Presented by DR. CORSON.

A colored woman, aged 28, who did housework, first noted, a year ago, pin-point to pin-head sized pigmented spots on the backs of her wrists. These slowly spread up her arm, in places becoming confluent, and involved the upper part of her chest, anteriorly, her face and neck. Where the macules were still discrete the follicles alone were pigmented. There was no associated ill health of any kind or pregnancies. Gynecologic and general medical examinations had thrown no light on the cause, but the Wassermann reaction was four plus. At present the areas affected were jet black, appearing as though stove polish had been used on them, giving a rather lurid hue. The presenter had seen three of these cases and was puzzled as to both cause and treatment. The others had negative Wassermann reactions.

DISCUSSION

DR. SCHAMBERG remarked that he was at a loss to answer these questions. If the patient had been asthenic, one might consider Addison's disease. The condition was certainly due to an involvement or compromise of the sympathetic system of the abdominal cavities.

DR. WEIDMAN said he thought, in explanation of the follicular phase of the pigmentation, that it spread from the surface by a continuation of the coloring matter down into the follicles.

Dr. Corson said he had seen a much more pronounced case in which, in a year, the entire body of a comparatively light colored negress had become jet black. It spread from follicular macules just as in this case. In none of these cases had subjective symptoms played a prominent part.

CICATRICES. Presented by Dr. Greenbaum for Dr. Klauder.

A young white man showed about twenty lima bean sized depressed, soft scars which, according to his history, had each been preceded by papules. The scars resembled vaccination marks, with numerous small follicular pits. The presenter spoke of them as "vergetures." The epidermis was wrinkled and gave a false impression of elevation to the spots.

DISCUSSION

Dr. Schamberg commented on these scars as being areas of circumscribed atrophy. Whether the previous lesions were syphilitic or not, was a question. It would seem that this was probably the case. Local causes could produce elastic tissue loss and disturbance of the collagen.

Dr. Weidman suggested the substitution of the term "fovealated" as a word descriptive of the lesions.

DHOBIE ITCH. Presented by Dr. Greenbaum.

F. G., a colored man, developed an extremely itchy eruption in the groins two years ago while stationed with troops at Key West. When first seen three days before there were two large eczematoid patches extending from the groin half way down the inner surface of the thighs. At fairly numerous points moderately infiltrated lesions were palpable. On the left wrist and dorsum of the hand was an irregular patch, infiltrated and eczematized, like the groin lesions. Microscopic examination of the scrapings revealed mycelia and spores.

PITYRIASIS RUBRA PILARIS (?). Presented by Dr. Weidman.

H. McC., aged 4 years, had had a disease for six months which consisted of fairly well circumscribed patches of minute horny follicular papules with graterlike feel, and of uniform size, distributed not only over the extensor surfaces of the buttocks, arms and shoulders, but also over the flexor surfaces, sternum and both sides of the chest and abdomen. There were none on the backs of the fingers. They were not itchy. There was no redness or scaliness. The lesions had markedly regressed under boric acid treatment and had become flat-topped. Dr. Weidman had seen several such cases during the last year or two, and he wondered whether we were experiencing pityriasis rubra pilaris in America in a form modified by not being so red, brawny or extensive. Except for its patchy arrangement and presence apart from the extensor surfaces, the eruption resembled keratosis pilaris.

DISCUSSION

Dr. Knowles looked on the case as one of lichen urticatus.

Dr. Weidman opposed this diagnosis as the lesions did not itch and were not large enough.

Dr. Schamberg regarded the papules as scarcely acuminate and keratotic enough for the tentative diagnosis of Dr. Weidman. They were undoubtedly lichenoid but not classifiable as lichen planus or lichen acuminatus. He rather hesitated to place the condition definitely.

CANITIES. Presented by Dr. Dengler.

A child, aged 3, and his father were presented as patients. The former had a white tuft of hair growing from an area the size of a silver dollar over the frontal portion of the scalp. The history showed that the father, grandfather, the latter's sister and her two children and several other relations on the paternal side of this child all had exactly the same lesion.

MICROSCOPIC SLIDES AND SPECIMENS. Dr. Weidman.

Dr. Weidman had several exhibits of microscopic slides and specimens.

A binocular, monobjective microscope was shown for its application to ringworm culture work. Dr. Weidman demonstrated reversed hanging drop cultures of microsporons to bring out the stereoscopic effect which could be secured by this microscope.

XANTHOMA TUBEROSUM. Presented by Dr. Weidman.

The presenter had performed a necropsy examination on an unclaimed pneumonia subject and had preserved the head, hands and several slabs of skin in formaldehyd. These were exhibited. There were no visceral lesions and only three or four of the "tumors" in the tendo patellae. The disease was extensive, distributed over the usual locations, and the nodules ranged up to the size of a soup bean. Particular attention was called to the eyelids. The right bore a typical xanthoma planum lesion, while the left bore several strictly nodular ones along the usual zone. Sections were demonstrated from the tendon, eyelid and skin. Frozen ones brought out in addition to the usual features, neutral fat *within* the connective tissue corpuscles, as stained by Sudan III and copper hematoxylin. Some of the collagen bundles in the tumor were crowded with cholesterol plates which Dr. Weidman believed to be a new observation.

Dr. Knowles expressed sorrow over the death of Dr. Maurice L. Mallas. one of the younger members of the society, who had shown great promise as a dermatologist and radiotherapist.

Edward F. Corson, M.D., Secretary.

Regular Monthly Meeting, May 8, 1922

Frank Crozer Knowles. M.D., *Presiding*

KERATOSIS PALMARIS ET PLANTARIS. Presented by Dr. Ludy.

An Italian girl, aged 3½ years, exhibited on her soles and palms an eruption which had been present since the child was 3 months old. No other case was known to have occurred in the immediate family. the parents and grandparents, and the brother and sister, aged respectively. 6 years and 14 months. being free of the disease. The regions affected were covered with thick, yellowish, rough. keratotic integument, bordered by a bright pinkish zone which continued entirely around the thickened area. It was probably preceded by a hyperhidrosis. The Germans laid stress on the color of the border. especially when there was cyanosis about the keratotic patch. They also considered it a sign of atavism. In some of these cases, abnormalities in the sella turcica, the epiphyses or the thymus, were to be considered. Undoubtedly, certain glands in the skin were deficient.

GRANULOMA PYOGENICUM. Presented by Dr. Weidman.

F. C., aged 13 years, presented a classical case of this disease. The present lesion was located over the deltoid muscle, the size of a pea, projecting, soft, red, and of three weeks' duration. A similar lesion was excised and cauterized three weeks ago, and the present one was a recurrence. Sections from the first, excised, lesion showed the usual richly vascular plexus with no important leukocytic infiltrate and no bacteria except in the overlying crust.

DISCUSSION

Dr. Knowles remarked that these cases were noteworthy because they were extremely difficult to eradicate. They usually tended to appear at muco-cutaneous margins or where the skin was smooth.

Dr. Klauder said he had treated a case successfully with roentgen-ray, giving two erythema doses at one time. During the three months that had elapsed since that time there had been no recurrence.

CRETINISM WITH SYPHILIS. Presented by Dr. Klauder.

A native white girl, aged 18 years, a dwarf in stature and obviously a cretin, had a four plus Wassermann reaction. She had been a puny, weak child but without marked cerebral deficiency. She had completed the work of the seventh grade in school. There were no stigmas of congenital syphilis. The bones and joints were negative. There was apparently a gumma in the septum nasi with perforation. This child was the eldest of ten living children, the other nine being apparently normal. An eleventh child was born dead and the twelfth and thirteenth members of the family had died in early childhood of diphtheria.

DISCUSSION

Dr. Knowles asked what percentage of cretins gave positive Wassermann reactions. As far as he could tell, this patient had no Hutchinson's teeth, old scars, defective hearing, bone involvement or interstitial keratitis. In his opinion, it was certainly not a case of congenital syphilis.

Dr. Klauder answered that he was uncertain about the percentage but that it was low. He believed this to be an accidental infection.

Dr. Weidman called attention to the myxedematous condition of the patient's skin.

BLASTOMYCOSIS (?). Presented by Dr. Sidlick.

A colored woman, aged 60, presented an eruption on the back of her left hand and the contiguous portions of the forearm. It consisted of two separate granulomatous areas elevated about 5 mm., surrounded by old and, in some cases, recent scarring. While part of the outline of these cicatrices was crescentic, there was no striking similarity to syphilitic scarring. The active areas were itchy, slightly larger than a silver dollar, somewhat cyanotic and with a tendency to fungation. The condition had been present for four years and had once healed under medication by mouth. The Wassermann reaction was negative. No fungi or blastomycetes were found.

DR. HIRSCHLER suggested a resemblance to a bromid eruption, but there was no history to bear out the supposition that the patient had been taking that drug. Others felt it was a case of blastomycosis.

LICHEN SIMPLEX. Presented by DR. SIDLICK for DR. KNOWLES.

A Jewish girl, aged 19, presented an eruption of four years' duration, limited to the back of the neck, including an inch (2.54 cm.) of hairy scalp, and a separate area over the top and front of the left shoulder. The lesions were discrete, flat, shiny papules, quite itchy and light pinkish. There was no coalescence at any point. A papular eczema (lichen simplex) was to be considered.

DISCUSSION

DR. CORSON suggested the diagnosis of neurodermatitis with markedly lichenoid lesions.

DR. GREENBAUM considered it lichen simplex chronicus.

Microscopic sections were exhibited by Dr. Fred. D. Weidman, including the following conditions: camphor oil tumors in lymph nodes, xanthoma planum of the eyelids and leukoplakia of the tongue.

EDWARD F. CORSON, M.D., Secretary.

CHICAGO DERMATOLOGICAL SOCIETY

Regular Meeting, April 12, 1922

E. A. OLIVER, M.D., *Presiding*

A CASE FOR DIAGNOSIS. Presented by DR. F. NICHOLS for DR. RAVITCH.

A man, aged 44, an American, had first consulted Dr. Ravitch one week previously because of lesions of the scalp, upper lip and outer canthus of the right eye. He gave a history of having had an eruption on the scalp for over seven years, which had resisted all treatment. The scalp presented many yellowish patches, cup-shaped crusts, which on disappearing left red, well-marked depressions. Pruritus was not intense but always present to a greater or less degree. The patient attributed the trouble to a Polish friend who had the same disorder.

DISCUSSION

DR. PUSEY thought the condition was unquestionably erythematous lupus.

DR. RAVITCH said that the history of the man's companion having the same complaint suggested favus, but the clinical picture, excluding the lesions on the upper lip, suggested lupus erythematosus.

SPOROTRICHOSIS. Presented by DRS. SENEAR, FINN and WIEN.

A woman, aged 50, said that during November, 1921, she cut her thumb on the bone of a rabbit, which she was dressing. On December 26, she developed a sore at the site of this injury. About a month later a tumor appeared on the forearm, and subsequently she developed several more on the forearm and upper arm, the last one being in the region of the anterior axillary fold. She had been treated with potassium iodid for several weeks which resulted in healing of the abscess.

Cultures were negative. The blood agglutinated a number of different strains of sporothrix.

DISCUSSION

Dr. ORMSBY said he thought it was interesting to see a patient presented with a definite history of trauma. Whether the infection came from the rabbit injury it was difficult to say, but the history of the case and response to treatment seemed to place it in the category of sporotrichosis.

Dr. PUSEY thought the positive agglutination test left no doubt of the diagnosis. He believed roentgenotherapy would cure the lesions on the hand.

Dr. RAVITCH asked whether iodid had been continued and how much she had received.

Dr. SENEAR said that the lesion of the hand, when he first saw the patient, was of the eczematous type described as an occasional primary lesion in sporotrichosis. It had involuted somewhat but had remained stationary for the last month. She had been taking about 25 drops of potassium iodid three times daily for about three months.

GENERALIZED ERUPTION. Presented by DRS. STILLIANS and OLIVER.

A man, aged 47, had a generalized eruption which began in April, 1921, following the use of pills containing iodin. It had persisted in spite of the discontinuance of the pills. At the time of presentation there was a generalized maculopapular and pustular eruption. The Wassermann reaction was positive.

DISCUSSION

Dr. SENEAR said it seemed to him that the man showed an acne cachecticorum.

Dr. ORMSBY said he was interested in the fact that the man had taken iodin, but as the eruption was not in the place where an iodin eruption was usually located he thought it unlikely that the drug had anything to do with it.

Dr. PUSEY said that the lesions were abundant in the locations of acne cachecticorum. The nodules were dark red and there was scarring. He believed the condition was acne cachecticorum.

Dr. STILLIANS said that the man had had an eruption in the spring of 1921 which cleared up promptly under medication. In the fall the present eruption appeared and had persisted. The Wassermann reaction was positive. It has been suggested that the patient had syphilis in the spring and developed this eruption in the fall. In his opinion the lesions were papulonecrotic tuberculids. The lesions came in successive crops and were present in all stages—from papule to scar.

Dr. OLIVER said the man told two different stories on different occasions. He first said that he had taken pills called "iodex" and that the eruption came out in great profusion. He had improved greatly in the hospital under no treatment.

A CASE FOR DIAGNOSIS. Presented by Dr. Beeson.

A boy, aged 14, presented the following lesions: Along the outer aspect of the right leg from just above the patella down to the lower third of the limb were a number of well defined, pinkish, infiltrated lesions covered with scanty adherent scales of a silvery hue. These efflorescences ranged in size from that of a pea to that of a quarter and one attained a length of 4 cm. and a width of 2 cm. The lesions were indolent but were apparently spreading slowly. They had been present for a year. Several similar spots were seen on the left knee and a single one was present near the occiput, where the disorder first appeared. This condition was presented as a possible atypical psoriasis. The mother had had that disorder for fourteen years and exhibited typical lesions over the knees, elbows and trunk. (N. B. The boy's lesions responded to a mild oil of cade and Lassar's paste.)

DISCUSSION

Dr. Pusey said that the mother had psoriasis and the boy had lesions on the leg like those of psoriasis; he believed the whole condition was psoriasis.

Dr. Mitchell said he thought the condition was a verrucous nevus coexisting with psoriasis.

Dr. Finnerud said the lesions on the leg were probably nevi in connection with psoriasis.

Dr. Ravitch said he thought the condition was familial psoriasis.

Dr. Beeson said he thought the condition was a case of atypical psoriasis.

A CASE FOR DIAGNOSIS. Presented by Drs. Stillians and Oliver.

A Russian laborer, aged 42 years, gave a history of a chancre two months previously. Ten days before presentation he developed papular lesions closely grouped about a central ulcer over the forehead and trunk. The Wassermann reaction was positive.

DISCUSSION

Dr. Senear said he thought the condition was an exceedingly good example of corymbose lesions.

Drs. Zeisler and Ravitch agreed.

Dr. Ormsby said that it was the first case with typically corymbose lesions that he had seen for a long time, and he was much interested in this fact. He thought a greater number of cutaneous lesions were being seen this year than for a long time previously, some of which were common several years ago.

Dr. Stillians said the question was whether it was an early or late manifestation—whether the penile sore was a chancre and the corymbose lesions were precocious, or whether it was just a late case in which the first lesion had accidentally appeared on the penis, followed by the others. He thought the penile lesion was not a chancre but a late secondary lesion.

Dr. Ravitch said the patient denied ever having any lesion on the genitalia. and his wife had no lesion and no other symptoms of syphilis. However, it seemed to be a case of syphilis.

Dr. Pusey said he thought there was no reason why there should not be a corymbose rupial lesion. Whether it was early or late was not the question in rupia. A corymbose syphilid meant secondary syphilis. a large. papular syphilid, not a tertiary lesion. The patient had recent syphilis.

Dr. Oliver said that when the large crust was pressed it felt as if there was an abscess underneath.

Dr. Mitchell agreed that it was a corymbose syphilid with a certain amount of abscess formation.

CONGENITAL ICHTHYOSIFORM ERYTHRODERMA. Presented by Dr. Zeisler.

The patient was a child, aged almost 2 years. The condition had been present since birth, the scalp, face and body being scaly and red at birth, which was premature—seven and a half months. The child weighed 7 pounds (3.1 kg.) at birth and had remained underdeveloped.

At presentation there was a universal erythroderma with scaliness of the scalp and face, hands, forearms and legs below the knee. The child looked like an undernourished 6 months old infant.

DISCUSSION

Dr. Pusey said he did not like the term "ichthyosiform erythroderma," although it was an accepted term. The condition was essentially ichthyosis and happened to be one of those in which the epithelium over the body was translucent. Most of the horn was either not present or was rubbed off so that the color of blood showed through. He considered the condition a variant of ichthyosis.

Dr. Ormsby said he thought it was the most marked redness that had been seen and it was absolutely universal—the flexors, scalp and soles were all involved. He believed all would agree that the prognosis was hopeless. It was not a "collodion baby," as someone had suggested, for those babies look as if they were oiled and after slight scaling they usually die. The mother of this child said that when the baby was born it had crusts on the scalp.

Dr. Zeisler said he had never seen ichthyosis that showed such intense redness, and he thought the case fitted in with MacKee's description of ichthyosiform erythroderma. The child had received a little thyroid substance and an oily lotion had been used locally. She had improved somewhat under treatment.

PRURITUS IN SYPHILIS. Presented by Dr. Mitchell.

A man, aged 32 years, presenting itching lesions, gave a history of syphilis which did not respond to treatment. There was a primary intra-urethral chancre in December, 1920. This was treated as gonorrhea and sounds were passed. Later he received the usual series of arsphenamin and mercury treatment, and during the mercurial medication the secondary lesions persisted and increased to such an extent that the treatment had to be discontinued. He was then given a series of five arsphenamin injections, and the lesions were controlled. He did not come again for treatment until the summer of 1921, when he received eight injections of arsphenamin. He reported again in November, 1921, with mucous patches on the tongue and cheek. At that time the Wassermann reaction was negative and these lesions cleared up, but there were pruritic papules on the forearm. He was given more arsphenamin, but the lesions persisted. The lesions were vesicular and closely simulated dermatitis herpetiformis with intense itching. The lesions had recently become more psoriasiform.

DR. SENEAR said he thought it was a puzzling case and his impression was that the condition was lichen planus. The lesions were definitely annular, some were arranged in lines, and the general appearance suggested lichen planus.

DR. ZEISLER said he thought the condition was annular hypertrophic lichen planus.

DR. PUSEY said that although the history was not consistent with that view, the condition suggested to him nothing but an annular lichen planus. If it was not that, he did not know what it was. It might be one of the lichenoid eruptions following arsphenamin that have been reported.

DR. ORMSBY said that he saw the patient in the clinic and was undecided as to the nature of the eruption. Early it was vesicular and later it suggested lichen planus. It is well known that arsphenamin delays and modifies eruptions in syphilis, and that this was probably a syphilitic eruption modified by treatment.

DR. MITCHELL said he thought that no one who had seen the case three months previously would have called it lichen planus. The interesting thing to him was the decided resistance to mercuric medication. The lesions persisted in spite of mercury and they had to go back to arsphenamin medication because the lesions recurred. He saw the man shortly after he had received a series of arsphenamin injections, at which time he had typical mucous patches, and Dr. Ormsby demonstrated the lesions in the clinic. These cleared up under arsphenamin after which the vesicopapules appeared. Within the last ten days these lesions had flattened out and changed markedly. They were much more shiny, and he was satisfied that they were undergoing involution; within two more weeks the skin would probably be clear. He believed they were atypical syphilitic lesions with itching.

A CASE FOR DIAGNOSIS. Presented by DR. ZEISLER.

A woman, aged 35, presented lesions on the back of the right hand, which had been present for several days. Subsequently lesions developed on the arm and one on the shoulder. The lesions were elevated papules and some itching was complained of.

DR. ORMSBY did not believe that it was possible to arrive at any conclusion as to what the condition might be. It was only two days since the last lesions appeared, and the condition might develop into psoriasis or any one of a number of things.

DR. PUSEY said that the lesions were small patches of papular dermatitis, and any diagnosis beyond that was speculation at this presentation.

DR. MITCHELL said there was a history of taking some drug and that the condition might be a drug eruption.

DR. ZEISLER said he had felt chagrined when he had to tell the patient that he could not say what the trouble was, but he was much consoled to find that others did not know. He had considered a drug eruption and would make an effort to ascertain what the condition was.

LUPUS VULGARIS. Presented by Dr. Zeisler.

A negress, aged 25 years, had lesions on the right side of the face, over the eyelids, bridge of the nose and cheek, which had been present for seven years. The Wassermann reaction was four plus. No improvement had occurred under antisyphilitic treatment. She had received three injections of arsphenamin, ammoniated mercury locally and potassium iodid internally.

The lesions consisted of crusted, elevated papules, with superficial ulceration under the crust. The color changed to yellowish-brown under glass pressure.

DISCUSSION

Dr. Senear said that under glass pressure there was distinctly brown infiltration of the lesion on the bridge of the nose, and he thought the condition was lupus vulgaris.

Dr. Stillians said that he had seen the patient some time ago and thought the lesions were those of syphilis, but since they refused to yield to treatment and on account of the yellowish discoloration under pressure, he was inclined to change his diagnosis to lupus vulgaris. The arrangement of discrete lesions in a large circle was to him a striking feature.

Dr. Pusey said he thought the condition was lupus vulgaris.

Drs. Mitchell and Finnerud said that they agreed with this view.

LUPUS VULGARIS (SYMMETRICAL). Presented by Dr. Stillians.

A woman, aged 60 years, presented lesions of lupus vulgaris on the lower part of both ears and the adjacent portion of the neck in an area about 4 inches (10.16 cm.) long and 1½ inches (3.8 cm.) wide. The patient said that the condition was caused by piercing the ears at the age of 15.

DISCUSSION

Dr. Pusey said that the angle below the ear was not an uncommon location for lupus vulgaris, but this case was interesting because the condition had occurred there symmetrically without having developed on the nose.

Dr. Ormsby said that he saw lupus vulgaris on the ear rather frequently, and it produced a deformity which was characteristic. In the preceding case the infiltration was diffuse and not limited in nodules, such as occurs in the major portion of cases of nodular lupus vulgaris.

LINEAR ERUPTION. Presented by Dr. Stillians.

An American, 25 years old, a medical student, six weeks previously had noticed an itching eruption on the left shoulder. Subsequently an eruption appeared on the abdomen.

At the time of presentation a patch of brownish yellow lichenification about 7 inches (17.7 cm.) long and 1 inch (2.54 cm.) wide in the widest part was seen on the left scapular region, extending onto the posterior surface of the arm. Over the shoulder was a linear red stain 3 inches (7.62 cm.) long and about one-sixteenth inch (1.58 mm.) wide. On the abdomen was observed a patch of bluish-red macules from 1 to 3 mm. in diameter, not confluent. One or two of these had cleared in the center and become circinate. The linear eruption had itched. The new macular one did not itch.

Dr. Lieberthal said he thought the possibility of dermatitis herpetiformis should not be overlooked.

Dr. McEwen said he was impressed with the possibility of lichen planus.

Dr. Senear said that he presented a patient four or five years ago with lesions arranged similar to these with the lesions running down over the arm, and the Society was unable to make a diagnosis. He thought this condition looked as if it might be much the same sort of thing.

Dr. Stillians said that when he first saw the patient he had nothing but the linear eruption, the present lesions having appeared since that time. He had nothing definite to offer in the way of diagnosis.

NEW YORK DERMATOLOGICAL SOCIETY

Regular Meeting, April 25, 1922

Fred Wise, M.D., *President*

ADENOMA SEBACEUM TREATED WITH THE KROMAYER LAMP.
Presented by Dr. Highman for Dr. Rulison.

N. L., aged 31, single, an American, a clerk, shortly after birth had typical lesions of adenoma sebaceum. These lesions were readily irritated, and when cut a hemorrhage difficult to control resulted. The patient had had von Recklinghausen's disease since infancy. He left school at the age of 14 when in the seventh grade. He began treatment by electrolysis and trichloracetic acid, in the summer of 1919, at the Vanderbilt Clinic. Dr. Hays, early in January, 1922, instituted Kromayer lamp treatment at 4 inches (10.16 cm.) distance for four minutes, unscreened, and without pressure. There was a severe reaction after the first treatment, and a severer one after the second. The third and fourth treatments, on March 23 and April 20, produced only moderate reactions. His condition had markedly improved under the treatment given at the Vanderbilt Clinic, but the improvement following the use of the Kromayer lamp was so striking that Dr. Highman thought it of interest.

Dr. Trimble said he was not surprised at the result of the Kromayer light treatment, and cited the case of a young girl treated similarly with marked benefit, which he had presented about two or three years ago.

Dr. Howard Fox said he thought the result was excellent, especially in view of the fact that the usual methods of treatment were unsatisfactory. For this reason many cases were left untreated.

Dr. Highman said that Dr. Wise's experience with ultraviolet rays in angioma serpiginosum suggested to Dr. Rulison the use of this therapeutic agent.

Dr. Rulison said he had nothing to add except that perhaps the chairman would remember this case at the Vanderbilt Clinic. Not too much credit should be claimed for the improvement, for a good deal had been done for the patient before he came under private treatment.

LYMPHOCYTOMA TREATED WITH THE ROENTGEN RAY. Presented by Dr. Howard Fox.

D. P., aged 5, previously presented at the March meeting of the New York Dermatological Society, on the day following the last presentation was seen in consultation by Dr. Robert T. Morris, who considered the disease some type of sarcoma from the clinical standpoint, and advised radiation. He thought that surgery was contraindicated. The patient was treated with roentgen rays on March 29, receiving only a single dose of two filtered units (5 milliamperes, specific gravity 9, time 2 minutes 41 seconds, at 10 inch [25.4 cm.] distance [anode to skin], filtered through 3 mm. of aluminum). Four days later the patient was again observed, and the lesion had entirely flattened and disappeared except for moderate brownish pigmentation. At this time there was still an ulceration of one-fourth inch (6.35 mm.) in length at the point where the biopsy had been taken, and where the ulcer had not healed by first intention. In addition to the tumor the enlarged preauricular glands could no longer be palpated. The biopsy wound healed at the end of about five weeks.

DISCUSSION

Dr. Trimble congratulated Dr. Fox on the result. When the case was first presented he had thought it was malignant, and would have made a clinical diagnosis of sarcoma of a malignant type.

Dr. Kingsbury said that it was the most spectacular result that he had ever seen from the employment of the roentgen rays. In his opinion no other known therapeutic agent was capable of producing so rapid and so wonderful a change.

Dr. Highman said that the amazing feature of this case was the speed with which the tumor was absorbed. He recalled the fact that Dr. Symmers called the tumor a lymphocytoma, and the fact that he gave it that name must indicate that the cells were of a more primitive type even than those ordinarily seen in sarcoma, and that perhaps that was the reason the condition responded so much more rapidly to roentgen rays than was ordinarily the case. The case proved again that radiotherapy was the thing to emphasize in such conditions. Dr. Fox was certainly to be congratulated on the excellent result achieved.

NEVUS FIBROMATOSUS. Presented by Dr. Bechet.

R. A., a girl aged 2 years, born in the United States, had a lesion on the back of the scalp which had existed since birth. It was minute at first, but increased in size rapidly during the past year. The child was under observation in Dr. Sayre's clinic at the University and Bellevue Medical College, and was presented through his and Dr. Trimble's courtesy. A roentgenogram showed no connection with the brain. The lesion was about 2 inches (5.08 cm.) high, and 3 inches (7.62 cm.) in diameter, and situated near the posterior fontanel. It was rather dense and fibrous to the touch. There were a number of small lesions of apparently a similar nature, immediately adjacent to the larger one.

DISCUSSION

Dr. Trimble asked whether any one disagreed with the diagnosis of nevus.

Dr. Highman said he thought the lesion was a nevus, and said that we had no definite ideas as to the time limit when a lesion ceased to be a nevus and became something else. In the broadest sense this was a nevus, even though it was undergoing further alterations, but a microscopic study should be made, and it would not be surprising if it proved to be a fibrosarcoma or a kindred growth.

QUININ ERUPTION. Presented by Dr. WISE.

J. N., aged 50, a private patient, was the father of a druggist who had been giving him a tonic containing cinchona for several months, and the case was shown with the idea of its being an unusual form of quinin eruption. The eruption was almost generalized and was most marked on the trunk and lower portion of the back; it consisted of various erythematous plaques and macular, papular and urticarial lesions, diffused and isolated, somewhat resembling pityriasis rosea. Some of the lesions appeared to be hemorrhagic.

DISCUSSION

Dr. POTTER agreed with Dr. Fox, and said that he had seen several cases of giant urticaria caused by oxyl-iodid, a cinchona derivative.

SARCOID OF BOECK. Presented by Dr. WISE.

Mrs. I. W., aged 50, a widow, came to the clinic for the treatment of an epithelioma at the inner canthus of the right eye. She also had scattered lesions on the trunk and extremities. She was presented for diagnosis of the condition before one of the other societies by Dr. Rosen. The duration of the lesions was seven years. They consisted of atrophic brownish placques with scalloped border and central cup-shaped depressions. The microscopic finding was typical of the sarcoid of Boeck.

DISCUSSION

Dr. POTTER said it was a very interesting case.

Dr. HOWARD Fox congratulated the chairman on having made the diagnosis from the clinical appearance.

PAPULONECROTIC TUBERCULID ASSOCIATED WITH TUBER-CULOUS GLANDS. Presented by Dr. HOWARD Fox.

L. P., aged 28, a vocational student, was referred by the United States Public Health Service. About five years ago, for a period of a year, he had suffered from recurring attacks of sore throat. A tonsillectomy was then performed followed later by enlargement of the cervical glands of both sides. These were excised three years ago at the Walter Reed Hospital, where the patient was serving as an enlisted man in the Medical Department. He said that the histologic report of a section of one of the glands revealed the presence of tuberculosis. He had never exhibited any signs of pulmonary or other forms of tuberculosis, and the family history was negative. The eruption had existed for three years, and was situated in a symmetrical manner on the elbows and knees and backs of the hands and fingers. There were active lesions on the hands and fingers in various stages of evolution, while the elbows and knees showed only the result of former lesions in the form of pitted scars. The lesions showed no grouping suggestive of syphilis.

DUHRING'S DISEASE.   Presented by Dr. Wise.

J. H., aged 50, married, born in the United States, a painter, presented himself with an eruption on the trunk and extremities said to have been present at varying intervals for eighteen years. The patient was referred from the Presbyterian Hospital with a diagnosis of aneurysm of the aorta. In both axillae there were erythematous, scaling, dime-sized patches, with pigmentary remains of old lesions. In the antecubital regions there were erythematous patches, clean in the center, with slightly raised infiltrated borders. On the abdomen and in the groins were pigmentary remains of old lesions, and scaly, erythematous dime sized to palm sized plaques. The buccal mucosa was free from lesions.

DISCUSSION

Dr. Bechet said he thought that the grouping of the remains of what were probably vesiculobullous lesions and the erythematous plaques certainly resembled dermatitis herpetiformis. He could not explain the absence of itching, but did not think this symptom of sufficient importance to affect the diagnosis.

Dr. Howard Fox thought it the most puzzling and interesting case presented. The lesion on the arm suggested a very superficial nodular syphilid, but the history of the recurring attacks ruled out such a possibility. Some of the other lesions looked as if they might later develop into pemphigus. A diagnosis seemed impossible without further study.

Dr. Lane agreed with the diagnosis. The large lesion on the arm was peculiar. He had never seen such a lesion in Duhring's disease, and he wondered whether that might not be interpreted as some other condition.

Dr. Highman said that the striking feature was occurrence of the lesions every spring for nineteen years. This did not suggest the behavior of syphilis or dermatitis herpetiformis, but rather that there was something in the climatic or other conditions, that might be described as vernal. The surface temperature and moisture, on account of the relative heaviness of winter underclothes in spring, might favor the development of this condition—possibly a tinea. Studies should be made with this idea in mind.

Dr. Wise said that against the eruption being one of syphilis was the fact that the man had a chancre thirty-five years ago. He had never had a positive Wassermann reaction, and it was again negative five days ago. The points in favor of Duhring's disease were the axillary pigmentation and the fact that the lesions that looked like syphilis cleared up in five days under treatment with calamin lotion only; also the fact that there was one small blister on the leg. The point mentioned by Dr. Highman was worth considering. Dr. Hartzell had described a case resembling this, in which he found fungi. An attempt would be made to find a fungus here.

A CASE FOR DIAGNOSIS.   Presented by Dr. Bechet.

J. R., a Russian, aged 28, was shown because of a peculiar lesion on the glans penis, present for fourteen years without change. There was no history of traumatism. He had not noted any inflammatory lesion on the glans, almost half of which was covered by a sharply defined, rather depigmented circular patch, with the meatus near the center. Its surface was not depressed, and the line of demarcation between the lesion and the surrounding healthy skin was extremely sharp. There were no subjective symptoms.

POSSIBLE HODGKIN'S DISEASE OF THE SKIN. Presented by Dr. A. Schuyler Clark.

F. S., an Austrian, aged 45, a laborer, had had a severe itching eruption for the last six months, beginning in the crotch and gradually spreading symmetrically over large areas, finally involving most of the skin. On examination a week ago, the patient showed a markedly thick, infiltrated, exfoliation of the skin, with enlargement of the glands in the femoral, inguinal, axillary and cervical regions. This patient was in good general health, but complained of excruciating itching which had been considerably ameliorated during the last week by lanolin ointment and large amounts of alkalis given internally. The blood count was: white cells, 10,000; differential count: polymorphonuclears, 66 per cent.; small lymphocytes, 21 per cent.; large lymphocytes, 12 per cent., and eosinophils, 1 per cent.

THROMBO-ANGIITIS OBLITERANS. Presented by Dr. A. Schuyler Clark.

B. N., was a Russian Jewish painter, aged 37. He denied any illness prior to October, 1921, when he began to notice that his right foot was constantly cold and painful. Early in February, 1922 (three months ago), the first ulceration appeared on the toes. The great toe presented a darkened nail, a skin that appeared devitalized and an area of erythema about the base of the nail. The nail of the first toe was nearly destroyed, and the nail bed was ulcerated; there was also a shallow ulcer on the tip of this toe. The little toe also had a small ulcer on the tip. The foot and ankle were cold to the touch, with a clear line of demarcation between the cold foot and the warm leg. This line was at the lower edge of an old bruise at about the center of the leg when the patient was first observed, but had now receded to about 3 inches (7.62 cm.) above the internal malleolus, and seemed to vary slightly from time to time. There was entire absence of arterial pulsation in the foot. The blood Wassermann test was negative. Treatment since entering the hospital, April 20, 1922, had consisted of placing the foot in water for from one-half to three-quarters of an hour four times daily, and in the interim keeping the toes covered with unguentum ichthyol, 3 per cent. The patient was on a full diet and was receiving a saturated solution of potassium iodid, 45 minims, three times daily, the dosage being gradually increased.

A CASE FOR DIAGNOSIS (TUBERCULOSIS OR SYPHILIS). Presented by Dr. Wise.

M. R., 25 years old, married, gave a history of having been infected with syphilis by her husband, a year ago. She had a four plus Wassermann reaction and was treated for syphilis; when she came to the Clinic some weeks ago the Wassermann test was negative. The lesion on the ala nasi had been present since January. The diagnosis seemed to lie between tuberculosis and syphilis, though one of the men thought it might be the result of maldigestion of some drug.

DISCUSSION

Dr. Howard Fox said he felt that from its appearance the eruption might either be tuberculosis or syphilis. Its unilateral distribution, he thought favored syphilis. The diagnosis was one that could easily be settled by a therapeutic test.

Dr. Lane said he felt doubtful about the case; the fact of its being unilateral should not be emphasized too much. Tuberculosis might be unilateral, as well as syphilis.

Dr. Trimble said he was at first inclined to believe it a syphilitic lesion, regardless of the negative Wassermann test, but after further consideration he was more inclined to consider it a lesion of tuberculosis. He had seen a number of patients with tuberculosis of the margin of the nose which started in the mucosa.

Dr. Highman said he agreed with Dr. Kingsbury; he thought that the practical point was to continue the therapy.

SYCOSIS CURED BY THE ROENTGEN RAY: RESULT AT END OF FIFTEEN YEARS. Presented by Dr. Howard Fox.

A. S., a man aged 45, a manufacturer, born in Russia, had been treated for sycosis of the beard fifteen years previously by the roentgen ray. At that time Dr. Fox employed the usual unmeasured, fractional dose method, followed by complete epilation and subsequent return of the beard without ill effects. The patient had recently called in regard to another member of the family. He was presented with accompanying photographs, taken before and after treatment, to show that at the end of fifteen years there was no sign of radiodermatitis or abnormality of the skin.

DISCUSSION

Dr. Howard Fox said he felt that it was simply good fortune that the patient showed no ill effects from the old fashioned unmeasured dosage that had been used.

DARIER'S DISEASE. Presented by Dr. Wise.

J. D., aged 26, had suffered from hyperkeratotic lesions since the summer of 1921. The eruption was abundant over the shoulders, back of the neck and upper part of the back, consisting of closely set follicular papules with keratotic summits and occasional pustules and fawn-colored pigmented areas between them. A few lesions were present at the hairline of scalp.

DISCUSSION

Drs. Kingsbury and Trimble said that they agreed with the diagnosis.

Dr. Howard Fox said that he thought it was a classical case.

Dr. Lane said, in regard to the rapid growth of the lesions, that he had recently presented a case at the Academy (about three months ago) in which the lesions were so small that the diagnosis was not clear to some of the members; but that within three or four weeks they had developed rapidly, so that many of them were nearly as prominent as those in the present case.

Dr. Bechet asked Dr. Wise whether the roentgen rays were of real benefit in the treatment of this condition. The disease responded so slowly to the local application of keratolytics, and the results were so disappointing, that it would be of great value to know the real worth of radiotherapy in this disease.

Dr. Wise said he had employed roentgen rays with good results in mild cases, and little result in severe cases. In fact, he had in mind several cases which were entirely uninfluenced by roentgen-ray treatment.

Dr. Howard Fox said he had treated for many years the patient (an Italian girl) of whom Dr. Wise had spoken. She had received a large amount of treatment with both roentgen rays and radium, and considerable radio-dermatitis had resulted. On some of the areas showing radiodermatitis new crops of lesions had even developed. He felt that in such cases a permanent cure could not be obtained.

PRURIGO NODULARIS. Presented by Dr. Wise.

C. K., a man, aged 56, unmarried, a laborer, presented himself at the Vander-bilt Clinic, January, 1921, with an eruption on both legs of two weeks' duration. The lesions were erythematous papules, varying in size from that of a pinhead to that of a split pea, and were found practically only on the anterior surfaces of the legs. At that time a diagnosis of occupational dermatitis was made, and the patient was treated with Lassar's paste. The patient also gave a his-tory of a penile sore twenty years ago. His Wassermann reaction was reported four plus. The patient was given mercuric salicylate intramuscularly, and mixed treatment. The local condition, however, did not improve at all. Further observation of the case led to the diagnosis of prurigo nodularis, although some of the lesions on the legs had the appearance of lichen planus of the hyper-trophic type. At present he had numerous erythematous and somewhat violaceous-colored papules, which were confined mostly to the anterior surface of both legs. The lesions itched. There was no evidence of lichen planus in the mouth or elsewhere. The patient was given fractional doses of roentgen rays with some relief from itching.

DISCUSSION

Dr. Lane said that he agreed with the diagnosis, and noted the striking resemblance to lichen hypertrophicans.

Dr. Howard Fox considered prurigo nodularis the most probable diagnosis.

Dr. Bechet agreed with the diagnosis of prurigo nodularis despite the fact that a few of the lesions bore some resemblance to lichen planus hypertrophicus.

Dr. Highman said that the term prurigo nodularis meant nothing to him. He had known nothing about the case clinically when he examined the specimen and had seen in it the changes that occur in syphilis. On investigation of the history at the clinic a positive Wassermann test was reported. Whether or not this was merely coincidence, and the man had two conditions, he could not say; but the lesion that was examined was characteristic of syphilis, and he could not explain the clinical findings on the basis of the microscope. He had reported a case of itching syphilis which resembled granuloma annulare at the last meeting of the American Dermatological Association which did not suggest syphilis any more than this did, but it proved not to be granuloma annulare, and this case was not what was called prurigo nodularis.

Dr. Wise said the case would be studied further and reported on later; but be wished to emphasize the fact that no signs of lichen hypertrophicus were present when examined in daylight.

TUBERCULOSIS CUTIS PENIS. Presented by Dr. A. Schuyler Clark.

B. C., aged 35, a negro elevator man, from Santa Domingo, who had live' in New York since 15 years of age, married, whose wife had never been pregnant, had one brother, aged 37, living and well; one brother died in an acc:-

dent; two sisters were dead, one of typhoid fever and one from an unknown cause at 25. The cause of his parents' death was unknown. The patient had always been well until a crack appeared on the foreskin in March, 1921; this fissure gradually enlarged until in July of the same year, when circumcision was performed, but all of the diseased tissue was not removed. The wound never completely healed, and from that time until the present the process had been advancing. Bacterial findings for Vincent's angina and granuloma inguinale were negative. The Wassermann test was negative. Microscopic examination showed numerous miliary tubercles.

PITTSBURGH DERMATOLOGICAL SOCIETY

Annual Meeting, April 27, 1922

J. G. BURKE, M.D., *Presiding*

FAVUS IN AMERICAN BORN CHILDREN.   Presented by DRS. GUY and JACOB.

Two children, aged 3 and 7 years, respectively, with an extensive alopecia of two years' duration, were presented. At the edges there was an erythematous scaling area more or less sharply marginated, suggestive of ringworm. At the center atrophic scarring was noted. No sulphur yellow crusts or scales were present probably because the conditions had been treated with salves of various kinds during the past year. Direct examination and cultural studies revealed the presence of the achorion. The children were being depilated by the Adamson Kienbock technic.

DR. WERTHEIMER said that these children were members of a family all of whom had favus. He had successfully treated two older boys with the roentgen ray. These cases were particularly interesting to him because of the lack of yellow crusts which were typically present in all the other cases.

DR. HOWARD FOX mentioned a procedure used at Ellis Island to demonstrate the fungus when it was difficult to find by ordinary means. This consisted of excluding the air from the scalp by means of a rubber "sweat cap" which was worn for a week, at the end of which time the microscopic examination was made. Before a patient was judged to be permanently cured this procedure was performed three times.

POIKILODERMA VASCULARIS ATROPHICANS.   Presented by DR. WERTHEIMER.

An American, aged 46, had a diffuse, wrinkled, atrophic, shining skin on the lower extremities from the dorsal surface of the feet to the abdomen and from the dorsal surfaces of the hands up over the sides of the chest and mammary regions, the lower part of the abdomen and over the entire back. The color varied from pinkish red on the back to bluish red on the thighs and brownish on the legs. Over the arms marked scaliness resembling an exfoliating dermatitis was noted. Just below the elbows were palm sized thickened areas. On the thighs the veins were prominent. Numerous telangiectatic vessels were noted in the involved areas. The condition began twenty-five years ago on the legs, gradually extending upward symmetrically. No subjective symptoms were present.

Dr. Wise said that the case was very similar to one reported by Dr. Lane in the Archives of Dermatology and Syphilology, November, 1921, under the title of "Poikiloderma Atrophicans Vasculare." The principle point indicating such a diagnosis in contradistinction to atrophoderma diffusum was the appearance of the eruption simulating chronic roentgen-ray burns which were typically present in this case.

Dr. Howard Fox said that while at first glance a diagnosis of atrophoderma diffusum suggested itself to him, on closer examination he was led to agree with the diagnosis offered by Dr. Wise. He suggested the use of the Alpine lamp in the treatment of the condition.

Dr. Wertheimer agreed with Drs. Wise and Fox that poikiloderma vascularis atrophicans was probably the proper name for the condition.

BAZIN'S DISEASE. Presented by Dr. Crawford.

A woman, aged 23, during the past six years had had deeply seated infiltrations of the lower third of both legs. The overlying skin was a dusky red except over the ulcerated parts. One or two lesions had healed leaving an atrophic scar. The condition had always been diagnosed as syphilis, according to the patient's physician, though the blood Wassermann test (October, 1921) was negative. The condition improved with rest in bed, cod-liver oil and roentgenotherapy.

DISCUSSION

Dr. Wertheimer said that he had seen the case about three years ago, at which time a diagnosis of Bazin's disease was made. At that time the Wassermann reaction was four plus and on antisyphilitic treatment the entire condition had cleared up: this fact, however, had not changed his diagnosis.

NEVUS LIPOMATODES. Presented by Dr. Crawford.

A man, aged 23, since birth had had a huge, soft, fatty, flabby nevus of a pinkish yellow color, spreading over the left side of his face and neck. over the left shoulder and left side of the chest, anteriorly and posteriorly. The surface was papillated and lobulated, some of the fatty masses being pendulated. Scattered over the rest of the body surface were sacklike projections and small islands of pigmentation of von Recklinghausen's disease. (This case was previously reported in December, 1921, issue, p. 854.)

DISCUSSION

Dr. Wise said that no doubt nevus lipomatodes was the correct diagnosis for the neck lesion but that this only represented a part of the entire picture. which was that of von Recklinghausen's disease.

Dr. Ravogli said that in view of the presence of numerous soft tumors with some pigmentation scattered over the entire body. the diagnosis should be von Recklinghausen's disease. instead of nevus lipomatodes.

DERMATITIS DUE TO METOL. Presented by Dr. Hollander.

A photographer presented himself in October. 1920. with an acute dermatitis involving the hands, face, ears and one spot on the toe. which resisted all forms of treatment. After cleansing and a palliative treatment, and four ⅛ unit roentgen-ray treatments, the patient recovered with the exception of one small area about the wrist. He had developed the eruption after handling metol.

EPITHELIOMA OF THE LEG.   Presented by Dr. Burke.

A man, aged 41, fifteen years before had had his leg burned by hot sand. The wound healed leaving a cicatrix from the knee to the ankle. Last November after a slight injury he noticed a sore which became larger, and when presented at the January meeting it measured 3 inches (7.62 cm.) by 1½ inches (3.81 cm.). On account of the soft nodular individual masses, the condition was presented with a tentative diagnosis of tuberculosis. Since then a section had been taken and the mass removed by cautery. It had recurred and electrocoagulation was used, but it had again recurred, and he was now receiving heavy doses of the roentgen ray. The pathologic report was that of an infiltrating carcinoma with necrosis and infection of tumor tissue.

DISCUSSION

Dr. Hollander said that this was the third of similar cases in which a diagnosis of malignancy had finally been made.

Dr. Guy called attention to the fact that the glands in the groin were enlarged and that in view of the fact that the bone was evidently involved the prognosis was bad. He felt that the man's best chance for recovery was through operation followed by intensive radiation to the gland bearing areas. He suggested that when biopsy was performed it be preceded by treatment with the roentgen rays or radium to devitalize cells that might undergo metastasis as the result of trauma.

Dr. Crawford raised the question of the advisability of biopsy in such cases on account of the possibility of leading to early metastases. He favored intensive radiotherapy or amputation.

Dr. Wise suggested that it might be possible to remove the glands from the groin and to cure the growth by a combination of local surgery and radiotherapy, thus saving the man's leg. This was a particularly interesting condition.

Dr. Highman said that his procedure in this case would be ablation of the tumor locally, curetting down as far as possible and following up with intensive roentgen ray or radium therapy locally and to the gland bearing area rather than sacrificing the man's leg.

Dr. Cameron said that the first thing that should be done in this case was to make a roentgenogram to determine whether or not the bone was involved. He felt that biopsies should be made on all cases, otherwise we would receive innumerable reports of cured cancers in cases that never were malignant. He agreed with Dr. Guy that radiation preliminary to biopsy was advisable. In such cases as the present one radium had given good results in the hands of different men over the country. He would prefer the use of the needle where it was possible, remembering that where the bone is involved results are not so certain.

Dr. Jacob said that he favored local treatment of the lesion followed by intensive roentgen ray and radium therapy to the glands.

LUPUS VULGARIS. Presented by Dr. Burke.

A woman, aged 50. was first seen last November when she presented a silver dollar sized area of dark brown papules on the anterior surface of the right foot. The condition had existed for ten years. The area had been getting larger, but the patient would not permit any treatment that would produce a reaction as she was compelled to work in a printing office which required her to be on her feet continually. She was advised to apply Biers hyperemic treatment.

DISCUSSION

Dr. Howard Fox said that he did not see anything characteristic of lupus. There was a delicate raised border that suggested a superficial epithelioma. He urged that a biopsy be performed.

Dr. Wise said that he agreed with Dr. Fox.

EPIDERMOLYSIS BULLOSA. Presented by Dr. Wertheimer.

A girl, aged 2 years, had pea sized blebs, some of which were hemorrhagic, located particularly at points of pressure. Five months before when first seen, there were dirty yellowish crusts, superficial abrasions and pustules present. At this time a diagnosis of impetigo contagiosa bullosa was made, although a bromid or iodid eruption was considered. The nails had been shed from time to time. The skin had been sensitive since she was 6 or 8 weeks of age, slight rubbing causing abrasions.

A CASE FOR DIAGNOSIS (AN ENDOCRINOGENOUS OR METABOLIC ERYTHRODERMA). Presented by Dr. Crawford.

A woman, aged 43, born in England, had had a skin eruption since the age of 3 months, which, she said, was generalized until she had passed childhood, when the trunk became free of the eruption. The face and upper and lower extremities were involved constantly, the face alone showing improvement in recent years. The face at present has a smooth, drawn, slight atrophic appearance. The arms and legs, including the hands and feet, are thickened. lichenified, slightly swollen, red, feel hot and itchy, and present numerous small ruptured vesicles which work their way from the deeper portions of the skin. The thyroid is not enlarged. Basal metabolism is plus 13. A slight improvement had been noted under thyroid therapy.

DISCUSSION

Dr. Driver said it looked to him like a case of neurodermite.

Dr. Wise said that this was an exceedingly common condition and one that might be classed as a chronic neurodermatitis with lichenification. He questioned the direct relationship of the thyroid to the eruption.

Dr. Hollander said that he felt that there was a direct relationship between the internal secretory apparatus and such cases as this: that with rest in bed many of them would clear up without further treatment.

Dr. Fox agreed with Dr. Wise.

Dr. Crawford said that he quite agreed with the diagnosis of eczema for this group of cases, but that in view of the long standing of the condition and the positive findings, he felt the diagnosis as presented was justifiable.

NODULES DEVELOPING ON THE FACE OF A COLORED WOMAN WITH LUPUS ERYTHEMATOSUS (SARCOID?). Presented by Dr. BURKE.

A colored woman, aged 38, five years ago developed an eruption on the nose and cheek which had been diagnosed as lupus erythematosus and treated by freezing with carbon dioxid snow and the Kromayer lamp. Two months before she noticed a nodule on the left cheek and since then two nodules have appeared on the upper lip, and the lower border of the lupus area on the right cheek has become indurated. Wassermann tests made in 1917, 1920 and two weeks ago have all been negative, but the patient has been put on specific treatment. The nodules had been considered syphilitic or possibly sarcoid.

LUPUS ERYTHEMATOSUS. Presented by Dr. GUY and Dr. JACOB.

A man, 52 years of age, had an eruption of twelve years' duration, limited to the face and hands. On the bridge of the nose there was a dollar sized patch and on each cheek was a patch half the size of the palm. On the fingers were atrophic scars and these were active lesions over the knuckles. All lesions were erythematous, sharply marginated, covered with fine scales and had numerous telangiectatic vessels. His general health was good. His lungs were normal. His teeth were in exceedingly bad condition.

DISCUSSION

DR. McEWEN said this case was interesting to him because of the possible connection of the skin condition with the evident focus in the man's mouth; and that this was a fair example of the group of cases of lupus erythematosus which could not be associated with tuberculosis. He called attention to the work of the English dermatologists in isolating, in these cases, *Streptococcus longus* from various sources, and in using in treatment with distinct results an autogenous vaccine prepared from that organism.

NEUROTIC EXCORIATIONS. Presented by Dr. WERTHEIMER.

A woman, aged 55, showed on the extremities and neck, many split pea sized white atrophic scars. On the back of the neck were split pea sized, red, elevated and excoriated lesions. The sites of former lesions were marked by reddish stains. The patient said that each lesion started with a pricking sensation causing her to pick the lesion until a glass particle had been removed, which she thought entered while stringing glass beads.

KERATOSIS PILARIS WITH THICK CHALKY SCALES. Presented by Dr. BURKE.

A girl, aged 10, was first seen April 19 when she had pea to half dollar sized chalky scales on both lges. Psoriasis was considered, but on close inspection the scales could be removed with the fingers and were friable and also not greasy. The skin under the scales looked normal and lacked the bleeding points of psoriasis but showed plugged follicles. The areas on the legs and arms not covered by scales showed numerous plugged follicles. A salve was given her with instructions not to apply it to the right leg, so that the original condition could be shown.

Dr. Wise considered the diagnosis of psoriasis ostracea as probable.

Dr. Howard Fox considered this a most unusual case. The appearance of the scaling was certainly suggestive of psoriasis though that of the underlying lesions did not suggest this disease. The scaling patches and grouped follicular lesions might have represented two distinct diseases. He was at a loss to make a diagnosis.

ROENTGEN-RAY DERMATITIS. Presented by Dr. Hollander.

A woman, aged 32 years, about eight years ago received roentgen-ray treatment for a toxic goiter, which resulted in a burn. The case was presented to show marked improvement following unipolar desiccating treatment.

HYPERKERATOTIC PALMAR AND PLANTAR SYPHILID IN HEREDITARY SYPHILIS. Presented by Dr. Crawford.

A boy, aged 12, an Italian, presented markedly thickened and keratotic lesions on both palms and the heel of the right foot, of three years' duration. Those on the palms were near the wrist and were 2.5 cm. in diameter. The one on the sole of the right foot near the heel was about 6 by 4 cm. The border of each of the lesions was a rounded elevation of slightly red waxy appearance. The patient said a similar lesion had been on left sole two years ago. but had disappeared entirely. Both elbows presented papulosquamous lesions which were a dull red waxy color and covered with thin (greasy) scales. The scalp showed a rather moth-eaten alopecia. There was an epitrochlear adenitis on both sides. The upper incisor teeth were suggestive of 'Hutchinson's teeth.

Dr. Wise said that he could see no definite evidence of hereditary syphilis. The teeth were not typically Hutchinsonian and the alopecia to him was not suggestive. He felt that the palmar and plantar lesions were examples of keratosis palmaris and plantaris and not of syphilitic origin.

Dr. Scheer said that he agreed with Dr. Wise and suggested that a therapeutic test be made.

Dr. Crawford said that he felt the diagnosis as presented was justified. that he would institute antisyphilitic treatment and report his results in the near future.

(The patient was placed on specific treatment, the palmar lesions disappeared entirely and the heel lesion is decidedly smaller and less keratotic.)

LUPUS VULGARIS. Presented by Dr. Crawford.

A woman, aged 54, an American, presented on the right side of the neck a large ring consisting of lupus tubercles. Two years previously she had burned her neck with hot grease, and said the burn became infected. resulting in her present condition. The disease spread eccentrically forming a continuous ring extending from the midanterior line of the neck to the midposterior line: its upper margin laterally was at the lobe of the right ear and its lower margin at the base of the neck. It had progressed 4 cm. during the past five months. The enclosed portion was mostly scar tissue with scattered groups of tubercles. Over the right shoulder was a solid patch of tubercles forming an area 3 by

5 cm. and of only three months' duration. In the mid-portion of the upper lip, just above the vermilion border, was another patch of tubercles 1.5 cm. in width and of only two months' duration. The patient was healthy and the mother of fourteen healthy children. She had had no miscarriages. The Wassermann (blood) test was negative.

LICHENOID ERUPTION FOLLOWING ARSPHENAMIN INJECTED INTRAVENOUSLY. Presented by Dr. CRAWFORD.

A woman, aged 28, had been under treatment for syphilis. After the third intravenous injection of arsphenamin, 0.4 gm. (Metz), she developed a pinkish-red lichen-like papular eruption on extensor surfaces of both forearms. A week later a fourth injection was given and the eruption increased on both forearms and also developed on the lower anterior surfaces of both legs.

DISCUSSION

Dr. HIGHMAN said that similar cases had been recently reported in Germany and the United States.

MULTIPLE LIPOMAS. Presented by Dr. CRAWFORD.

A woman, aged 70, during the last twelve years, had been gradually developing soft, rounded nut sized masses in the deep tissues of the anterior surfaces of both arms. There was one in the left epitrochlear region and another larger one (3 by 3 cm.) over the right triceps muscle, also one in the left popliteal space (about 4 by 5 cm.). None of the masses were attached to the skin. They were painless. It is probable they are forming along the deeper veins.

SCLERODERMA FOLLOWED BY ATROPHY. Presented by Dr. CRAWFORD.

A woman, aged 34, presented diffuse areas of scleroderma, which had been followed in many places by atrophy, over the trunk, anteriorly and posteriorly and the upper portions of the arms and legs. The thyroid was not palpable and all teeth had been extracted. She was mentally defective.

KERATODERMA PALMARIS. Presented by Dr. CRAWFORD.

A boy, aged 10, presented palms which were markedly hyperkeratotic, in some places reaching a depth of almost 1 cm. The keratosed portion was in small block-like segments separated by deep clefts—quadrillated. The process extended only half way up the first phalangeal portion of each finger. The condition first appeared at 2 years of age. The feet are normal. A brother is similarly affected though not so markedly.

Index to Current Literature

DERMATOLOGY

Adhesive-Plaster Dermatitis. H. W. Siemens, München. med. Wchnschr. **69**: 506 (April 7) 1922.

Aleppo Boil: Also Called Delphi Boil, Kandahar Sore, Oriental Sore. A. K. Yoosuf, Boston M. & S. J. **186**:675 (May 18) 1922.

Anthrax, Paralysis Consecutive to. R. Onorato, Arch. ital scienze med. coloniali **3**:1 (Jan.-Feb.) 1922.

Blastomycosis. J. F. Langdon, Nebraska M. J. **7**:172 (May) 1922.

Blastomycosis: Clinical Pathology and Therapeusis. B. F. Davies, Minnesota Med. **5**:311 (May) 1922.

Bothriocephalus Carriers, Sachs-Georgi Reaction in. G. Becker, Acta med. Scandinav. **56**:453 (April 22) 1922.

Brain and Ear Lesions in Fatal Measles. M. Renaud, Bull. Soc. méd. d. hôp., Paris **46**:693 (April 28) 1922.

Cancer of Lip, Modern Treatment (Radiotherapy) of. H. K. Pancoas, Surg., Gynec. & Obst. **34**:589 (May) 1922.

Caterpillar, Texan. Pathology of Dermatitis Caused by Megalopyge Opercularis. N. C. Foot, J. Exper. Med. **35**:737 (May) 1922.

Chenopodium, Toxicity of. Areobaldo Lellis, Brazil-med. **1**:157 (April 1) 1922.

Cutaneous Effects of Dental Sepsis. H. C. Semon, Lancet **1**:889 (May 6) 1922.

Delphi Boil: Also Called Aleppo Boil, Kandahar Sore, Oriental Sore. A. K. Yoosuf, Boston M. & S. J. **186**:675 (May 18) 1922.

Dental Sepsis, Cutaneous Effects of. H. C. Semon, Lancet **1**:889 (May 16) 1922.

Dermal Leishmaniasis (Brahmacharii). J. W. D. Megaw, Indian M. Gaz. **57**: 128 (April) 1922.

Dermal Leishmanoid: New Form of Cutaneous Leishmaniasis. U. N. Brahmachari, Indian M. Gaz. **57**:125 (April) 1922.

Dermatitis, Adhesive-Plaster. H. W. Siemens, München. med. Wchnschr. **69**: 506 (April 7) 1922.

Dermatitis Caused by Megalopyge Opercularis, Texan Caterpillar, Pathology of. N. C. Foot, J. Exper. Med. **35**:737 (May) 1922.

Dermatitis, Oak, Caused by Rhus Diversiloba, Treatment of. H. E. Alderson. Calif. State J. M. **20**:153 (May) 1922.

Dermatologic Technic. M. Joseph, Deutsch. med. Wchnschr. **48**:361 (March 17) 1922.

Dermatologic Technic, Course in. II. M. Joseph, Deutsch. med. Wchnschr. **48**:391 (March 24) 1922.

Dermatology, Value of Roentgenotherapy in. G. M. Mackee and G. C. Andrews. Am. J. Roentgenol. **9**:241 (April) 1922.

Ear and Brain Lesions in Fatal Measles. M. Renaud. Bull. Soc. méd. d. hôp., Paris **46**:693 (April 28) 1922.

Ear and Face, Epithelioma of. W. J. Young. Kentucky M. J. **20**:367 (May) 1922.

Eczema in Breast-Fed Infants as Result of Sensitization to Foods in Mother's Dietary. W. R. Shannon, Am. J. Dis. Child. **23**:392 (May) 1922.

Eczema, Seborrheic, and Psoriasis. H. Sieben, Deutsch. med. Wchnschr. **48**: 357 (March 17) 1922.

Epithelioma of Face and Ear. W. J. Young, Kentucky M. J. **20**:367 (May) 1922.

Epithelioma, Roentgen, Cured by Diathermy. H. Bordier. Bull. de l'Acad. de méd., Paris **87**:526 (May 9) 1922.

Erysipelas, Metabolism in. W. Coleman, D. P. Barr and E. F. Du Bois. Arch. Int. Med. **29**:567 (May) 1922.

Face and Ear, Epithelioma of. W. J. Young, Kentucky M. J. **20**:367 (May) 1922.

Gonorrheal Affections of the Skin. A. Weill, Klin. Wchnschr. **1**:374 (Feb. 18) 1922.

Gonorrheal Keratosis or Keratosis Blenorrhagica. J. E. McDowell, New York M. J. & Med. Rec. **115**:518 (May 3) 1922.

Hand, Nodosities of. A. Léri, Bull. méd., Paris **36**:337 (April 29) 1922.

Heliotherapy and the Skin. Leuba, Arch. españ. de tisiolog. **2**:84 (Jan.) 1922.

Herpes, Experimental Research on. R. Vegni, Riforma med. **38**:270 (March 20) 1922.

Herpes Zoster and Varicella. Dumoutet, Arch. de méd. d. enf. **25**:97 (Feb.) 1922.

Itch, Grain, Epidemic of. E. de Longis, Riforma med. **38**:320 (April 3) 1922.

Kandahar Sore: Also Called Delphi Boil, Aleppo Boil, Oriental Sore. A. K. Yoosuf, Boston M. & S. J. **186**:675 (May 18) 1922.

Keratosis Blenorrhagica or Gonorrheal Keratosis. J. E. McDowell, New York M. J. & Med. Rec. **115**:518 (May 3) 1922.

Keratosis, Gonorrheal, or Keratosis Blenorrhagica. J. E. McDowell, New York M. J. & Med. Rec. **115**:518 (May 3) 1922.

Keratosis Tonsillaris. E. Gäbert, München. med. Wchnschr. **69**:431 (March 24) 1922.

Leishmaniasis, Cutaneous, New Form of Dermal Leishmanoid. U. N. Brahmachari, Indian M. Gaz. **57**:125 (April) 1922.

Leprosy, Case of. A. Wallace, Southwestern Med. **6**:193 (May) 1922.

Lip Cancer, Modern Treatment (Radiotherapy) of. H. K. Pancoast, Surg., Gynec. & Obst. **34**:589 (May) 1922.

Lupus, Intradermal Reaction in. Kusan, Wien. klin. Wchnschr. **35**:248; Reply, Busacca, ibid. **35**:250 (March 16) 1922.

Lymphogranulomatosis. H. Stahr and I. Synwoldt, Med. Klin. **18**:404 (March 26) 1922.

Malignancies, Superficial. C. F. Bowen, Am. J. Roentgenol. **9**:255 (April) 1922.

Measles, Fatal, Brain and Ear Lesions in. M. Renaud, Bull. Soc. méd. d. hôp., Paris **46**:693 (April 28) 1922.

Metabolism in Erysipelas. W. Coleman, D. P. Barr and E. F. Du Bois, Arch. Int. Med. **29**:567 (May) 1922.

Nematode Infection, Cutaneous, in Monkeys. H. F. Swift, R. H. Boots and C. P. Miller, Jr., J. Exper. Med. **35**:599 (May) 1922.

Nodosities of the Hand. A. Léri, Bull. méd., Paris **36**:337 (April 29) 1922.

Oak Dermatitis Caused by Rhus Diversiloba, Treatment of. H. E. Alderson, California State J. M. **20**:153 (May) 1922.

Oriental Sore: Also Called Kandahar Sore, Delphi Boil, Aleppo Boil. A. K. Yoosuf, Boston M. & S. J. **186**:675 (May 18) 1922.

Paraffinoma. H. Lefèvre, A. Bonnard and P. Piéchaud, J. de méd. de Bordeaux **94**:234 (April 25) 1922.

Paralysis Consecutive to Anthrax. R. Onorato, Arch. ital. scienze med. coloniali **3**:1 (Jan.-Feb.) 1922.

Pregnancy and Psoriasis. S. P. Impey, South African Med. Rec. **20**:156 (April 22) 1922.

Psoriasis and Pregnancy. S. P. Impey, South African Med. Rec. **20**:156 (April 22) 1922.

Psoriasis and Seborrheic Eczema. H. Sieben, Deutsch. med. Wchnschr. **48**: 357 (March 17) 1922.

Rhus Diversiloba. Treatment of Oak Dermatitis Caused by Rhus Diversiloba. H. E. Alderson, California State J. M. **20**:153 (May) 1922.

Roentgenotherapy. Value of, in Dermatology. G. M. Mackee and G. C. Andrews, Am. J. Roentgenol. **9**:241 (April) 1922.

Roentgen-Ray Epithelioma Cured by Diathermy. H. Bordier, Bull. de l'Acad. de méd., Paris **87**:526 (May 9) 1922.

Roentgen-Ray Treatment of Diseases of Skin. H. H. Hazen, Am. J. Roentgenol. **9**:247 (April) 1922.

Scabies, Diagnosis of. E. Baümer, Med. Klin. **18**:471 (April 9) 1922.

Scrofula, Tuberculin Test in Relation to. Landenberger, Klin. Wchnschr. **1**: 322 (Feb. 11) 1922.

Scurvy, Etiology of. IV. Observations Concerning Physiologic Action of Antiscorbutic Vitaliment. E. B. Vedder, Mil. Surgeon **50**:534 (May) 1922.

Scurvy, Infantile, Vascular Changes in. T. Ide, Ztschr. f. Kinderh. **32**:165 (April 12) 1922.

Skin and Heliotherapy. Leuba, Arch. españ. de tisiolog. **2**:84 (Jan.) 1922.

Skin. Congenital Marble Skin. C. H. J. van Lohuizen, Nederlandsch Tijdschr. v. Geneesk. **1**:1259 (April 1) 1922.

Skin. Cutaneous Nematode Infection in Monkeys. H. F. Swift, R. H. Boots and C. P. Miller, Jr., J. Exper. Med. **35**:599 (May) 1922.

Skin Diseases Commonly Seen by Industrial Physician. E. L. Oliver, J. Indust. Hygiene **4**:21 (May) 1922.

Skin, Gonorrheal Affections of. A. Weill, Klin. Wchnschr. **1**:374 (Feb. 18) 1922.

Skin, New Form of Cutaneous Leishmaniasis: Dermal Leishmanoid. U. N. Brahmachari, Indian M. Gaz. **57**:125 (April) 1922.

Skin, Roentgen-Ray Treatment of Diseases of. H. H. Hazen, Am. J. Roentgenol. **9**:247 (April) 1922.

Skin, Treatment of Tuberculosis of. J. Schweig, Med. Klin. **18**:470 (April 9) 1922.

Tuberculin Test in Relation to Scrofula. Landenberger. Klin. Wchnschr. **1**:322 (Feb. 11) 1922.

Tuberculosis of the Skin, Treatment of. J. Schweig, Med. Klin. **18**:470 (April 9) 1922.

Urticaria, Giant. Treated by Autogenous Streptococcus Vaccine. W. E. M. Armstrong, Lancet **1**:994 (May 20) 1922.

Varicella and Herpes Zoster. Dumoutet, Arch. de méd. d. enf. **25**:97 (Feb.) 1922.

Varicella, Vaccination Against. Thomas and Arnold, München. med. Wchnschr. **69**:464 (March 31) 1922.

Xanthoma Diabeticorum, Case of. G. R. Hamilton, Med. J. Australia **1**:385 (April 8) 1922.

SYPHILOLOGY

Antisyphilitic Treatments, Rural Administration of. H. R. Hays, South. M. J. **15**:387 (May) 1922.

Aortitis, Syphilitic, and Endocarditis. J. C. Lindsay, Canad. M. A. J. **12**:335 (May) 1922.

Arsenicals, Intolerance for. Gougerot and Blamoutier, Bull. Soc. méd. d. hôp., Paris **46**:598 (April 7) 1922.

Arsphenamin, Action of, on the Eye. C. Pava, Repert. de med. y cirug. **13**:193 (Jan.) 1922.

Arsphenamin and Mercury, Mixtures of. S. Rothman, München. med. Wchnschr. **69**:427 (March 24) 1922.

Arsphenamin Brain Fatalities, Present Status of. C. Hart, Med. Klin. **18**:411 (March 26) 1922.

Arsphenamin. Effect of Serial Administration of Silver Arsphenamin on Kidney. D. M. Sidlick and M. L. Mallas. New York M. J. & Med. Rec. **115**: 540 (May 3) 1922.

Arsphenamin, Idiosyncrasy to. Babalian, Paris méd. **12**:195 (March 4) 1922.

Arsphenamin Mishaps, Factors in. F. Jacobsohn and E. Sklarz, Med. Klin. **18**:567 (April 30) 1922.

Arsphenamin Questions. J. Citron, Med. Klin. **18**:459 (April 9) 1922.

Bismuth in Treatment of Syphilis. C. Ducrey, Policlinico, Rome **29**:473 (April 10) 1922.

Bismuth Salts in Treatment of Syphilis. G. Milian, Paris méd. **12**:189 (March 4) 1922.

Diabetes, Syphilitic. F. Rathery and Fernet, Bull. Soc. méd. d. hôp., Paris **46**:661 (April 28) 1922.

Digestion in Hereditary Syphilis in Nurslings. J. Vergely, J. de méd. de Bordeaux **94**:206 (April 10) 1922.

Endocarditis and Syphilitic Aortitis. J. C. Lindsay, Canad. M. A. J. **12**:335 (May) 1922.

Feeding Problems with Congenital Syphilis. E. Stransky, Ztschr. f. Kinderh. **32**:199 (April 12) 1922.

Formol and Wassermann Reactions. M. Armangue and P. Gonzales, J. Infec. Dis. **30**:443 (May) 1922.

Intestine, Case of Syphilis of. G. O. Scott and G. H. J. Pearson, Am. J. Syphilis **6**:269 (April) 1922.

Kidney. Effect of Serial Administration of Silver Arsphenamin on Kidney. D. M. Sidlick and M. L. Mallas, New York M. J. & Med. Rec. **115**:540 (May 3) 1922.

Lupus. Diagnosis of Late Hereditary Syphilis and Lupus in Otorhinolaryngology. G. Portmann, New York M. J. & Med. Rec. **115**:508 (May 3) 1922.

Malformations, Fetal, and Syphilis. J. Henrotay, Gynéc. et Obst., Paris **5**:287 (April) 1922.

Mental Deficiency and Syphilis. G. J. Key and A. Pijper, South African Med. Rec. **20**:142 (April 22) 1922.

Mercurial Treatment of Syphilis. J. Callico, Rev. españ. de med. y cirug. **5**:126 (March) 1922.

Mercury and Arsphenamin, Mixtures of. S. Rothman, München. med. Wchnschr. **69**:427 (March 24) 1922.

Mercury in Syphilis, Curative Action of. L. Cheinisse, Presse méd. **30**:346 (April 22) 1922.

Neo-Arsphenamin and Neosalvarsan, Action of, on Phagocytic Activity of Leukocytes. R. Tunnicliff, J. Infec. Dis. **30**:545 (May) 1922.

Neo-Arsphenamin, Experimental and Clinical Comparison of Therapeutic Properties of Different Preparations of. H. H. Dale and C. F. White, Lancet **1**:779 (April 22) 1922.

Neosalvarsan and Neo-Arsphenamin, Action of, on Phagocytic Activity of Leukocytes. R. Tunnicliff, J. Infect. Dis. **30**:545 (May) 1922.

Nervous System, Comparative Clinical Observations on Involvement of, in Various Phases of Syphilis. J. H. Stokes and A. R. McFarland, Am. J. Syphilis **6**:169 (April) 1922.

Neurosyphilis, Diagnosis of. I. H. Pardee, New York M. J. & Med. Rec. **115**:507 (May 3) 1922.

Neurosyphilis, Intraspinal Therapy in. J. A. Fordyce, Am. J. Syphilis **6**:198 (April) 1922.

Neurosyphilitic Patients, Serologic Changes in, During a Period of Nontreatment. H. Omar and P. H. Carroll, Arch. Neurol. & Psychiat. **7**:733 (June) 1922.

Ophthalmologist's Relation to Syphilis. S. R. Gifford, Nebraska M. J. **7**:167 (May) 1922.

Wassermann Reaction After Anesthesia. L. Domenici, Policlinico, Rome, **00:** 92 (March 20) 1922.

Wassermann Reactions and Formol. M. Armangue and P. Gonzales, J. Infec. Dis. **30:**443 (May) 1922.

Wassermann Reaction, Clinical Interpretation of. H. C. Solomon, Rhode Island M. J. **5:**242 (May) 1922.

Wassermann Reaction, Estimation of. H. Hecht, Med. Klin. **18:**537 (April 23) 1922.

Wassermann Reaction, Graphic Explanation of. F. Herb, Illinois M. J. **41:**354 (May) 1922.

Wassermann Reaction in Parturients, Unreliability of. K. Brünner, Monatschr. f. Geburtsh. u. Gynäk. **57:**42 (Feb.) 1922.

Wassermann Reaction in Relapsing Fever. Brit. J. Exper. Path. **3:**59 (Feb.) 1922.

Wassermann Reaction, Interpretation of. S. Wallenstein, New York M. J. & Med. Rec. **115:**514 (May 3) 1922.

Wassermann Reaction, Nonspecific, and Meinicke Reactions. K. Bauer, Wien. klin. Wchnschr. **35:**173 (Feb. 23) 1922.

Wassermann Reaction, Significance of. L. K. Baldauf, Kentucky M. J. **20:**225 (April) 1922.

Wassermann Reaction, Studies in Standardization of, XXIV. Comparative Study of Tissue Extracts (Antigens) and Methods of Preparation. J. A. Kolmer and M. E. Trist, Am. J. Syphilis **6:**289 (April) 1922.

Wassermann Reaction, Studies in Standardization of, XXVI. J. A. Kolmer and E. M. Yagle, Am. J. Syphilis **6:**319 (April) 1922.

Wassermann Test. L. B. Bull. M. J. Australia **1:**172 (Feb. 18) 1922.

Wassermann Test, Another Technic of. E. H. Buttles, Am. J. Syphilis **6:**280 (April) 1922.

Wassermann Test at Missouri School for Blind. H. D. Lamb, J. Missouri M. A. **19:**124 (March) 1922.

Wassermann Test, Basis and Value of. E. Lorentz, Rev. Asoc. méd. argent. **34:**1579 (Dec.) 1921.

Wassermann Test, Modification of. R. E. Houke, Mil. Surgeon **50:**278 (March) 1922.

Wassermann Test, Source of Error in. K. Meyer, Med. Klin. **18:**566 (April 30) 1922.

Archives of Dermatology and Syphilology

VOLUME 6   SEPTEMBER, 1922   NUMBER 3

YAWS: ITS MANIFESTATIONS AND TREATMENT BY NEO-ARSPHENAMIN *

PERPETUO D. GUTIERREZ, M.D.

MANILA, P. I.

In Parañaque, a small village 6 kilometers south of Manila, composed of six barrios, all of which border the eastern coast of Manila Bay, with the exception of the barrio of Ibays, which is on the eastern side of the Parañaque estero, yaws has been known to exist for a long time. Any one interested in the disease is sure to find cases in this village. It is endemic in the poorer class, and before the advent of modern treatment, parents practiced vaccination on their children so as to prevent severe infections. Of the six barrios, San Dionisio is the most heavily infected, 134 patients from this locality being treated by us out of 275 treated altogether; or, 48.72 per cent. of the patients came from this locality.

PREVALENCE AND TRANSMISSION OF THE DISEASE

The figures given herewith convey a false impression as to the prevalence of the disease, as we treated only patients in the infectious stage; those with latent and tertiary lesions, with the exception of a few, were refused treatment. The sanitary commission,[1] headed by Dr. Bantug, in 1915, reports, however, that the prevailing disease is yaws.

The disease prevails among the poor. Among our cases, only two families of the better class were infected. The disease is transmitted by direct contact; of 258 cases in which the mode of infection was recorded, in 132 the disease was contracted from relatives and playmates. A close personal contact, therefore, seems necessary. Many of the

---

* Part of the material used in this article is taken from the records of patients treated at Parañaque in connection with the campaign for the extermination of the disease in that locality by the Philippine Health Service. Material from unreported cases at the Philippine General Hospital was also used, permission having been granted by the director of the Philippine Health Service.

1. Report of the Sanitary Commission of Parañaque. Rizal. privately published by the Philippine Health Service **13**, 1915.

patients coming to the clinic were infected with scabies and not a few of the mothers insisted that the infection started from one of these lesions.

Whether the fact that this village is located along the seashore has anything to do with the prevalence of the disease in this locality will

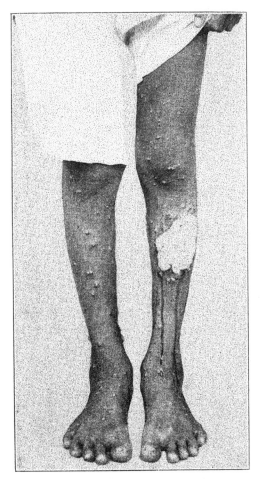

Fig. 1.—Frambesiform type of primary yaws. Note also papular and frambesiform eruption.

have to be investigated further. It is my impression that inhabitants of towns bordering on salt water, or towns reached by the ebb of the tide, harbor the disease; while inhabitants of interior towns are free from it, except such persons as are infected by contact with inhabitants of these seacoast towns. This has also been the observation of

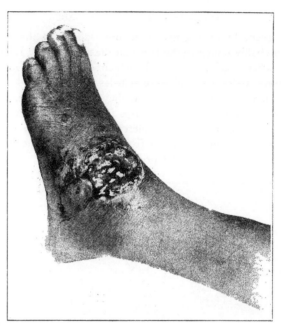

Fig. 2 (Case 53).—Frambesiform primary lesions of three weeks' duration. with no secondary lesions, in a patient 9 years of age.

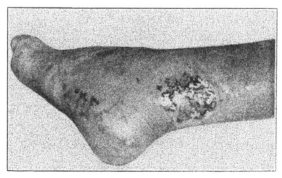

Fig. 3 (Case 59).—Primary lesions of three years' duration. in a girl of 10 years.

McCarthy [2] in the Chindwin District, Upper Burma; but he attributes it to the accessibility of these towns rather than to an inherent factor.

INCIDENCE OF SEX AND AGE

Males seem to be slightly more predisposed to the disease than females, probably owing to the fact that the former play rougher games than the latter. Of 271 cases in which the sex was recorded, 144 patients were males and 127 were females.

In the majority of the cases, in the infectious stage, the patients were children. Thus, of the 257 cases in which the age was recorded, 226 occurred in children and adolescents, or 87.93 per cent. If the census of those persons suffering from the disease in the tertiary stage were taken, the reverse would probably be found.

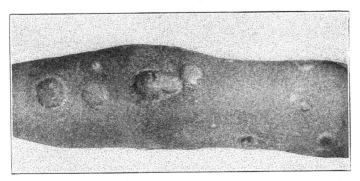

Fig. 4 (Case 66).—Lesions in a boy, aged 8 years, in whom the mother-yaw had persisted for three months. The secondary lesions appeared two weeks after the primary lesions.

TABLE 1.—AGE INCIDENCE OF THE DISEASE

Ages	No. of Cases	Percentages
12 months	9	3.89
13 to 24 months	24	9.33
25 months to 5 years	54	21.01
6 to 10 years	84	48.4
11 to 15 years	48	18.67
16 to 20 years	7	2.72
Over 21 years	31	12.06
Total	257*	

* Of the 275 patients treated, in four the age was not recorded; and of the forty-five adults, fourteen were in the tertiary noninfectious stage.

From Table 1, it will be seen that the incidence increases in direct proportion to the age, up to between the age of 6 and 10 years; however, the number of cases occurring between the ages of 25 months and

2. McCarthy, P. A.: Indian M. Gaz. **41**:53, 1906.

5 years is already considerable, as is the number occurring between the ages of 11 and 15 years; so the infection occurs before the victims reach adult age.

Forty-five adults were treated, but of these, only thirty-one presented lesions in the infectious stage; the other fourteen showed lesions in the tertiary stage. These were treated only that these lesions may be studied. They are not included in our table of age incidence.

THE COURSE OF THE DISEASE

The disease has been arbitrarily divided into three stages: the primary, the secondary and the tertiary. Up to the present time, Harper[3] is the only one who has reported a presumptive quaternary stage of the disease. He does not give confirmatory evidence, such as undoubted yaws infection or absence of syphilis.

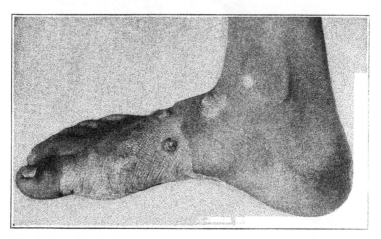

Fig. 5.—Frambesiform eruption. Note the verrucous appearance of the surface of the frambesiform lesion.

THE PRIMARY LESION

The incubation period lasts from two to four weeks, at the end of which time the primary lesion appears. The primary lesions may develop on any ulceration or abrasion of the skin. These are usually extragenital and on exposed surfaces. The lesion is manifested, according to Castellani,[4] as a papule, which becomes moist after one week and is then covered by a yellow secretion. This secretion dries up, forming a crust. If the crust is now removed, an ulcer will be found

3. Harper, P.: Lancet **2**:678 (Oct. 14) 1916.

4. Castellani and Chalmers: A Manual of Tropical Medicine. Ed. 3. New York, William Wood & Co., p. 1535.

with granulating fundus and clean cut edges. This lesion is often painful, and through secondary infections with pyogenic organisms, the neighboring glands may be enlarged and painful. The different types of primary lesions have been observed by us. The frambesiform type

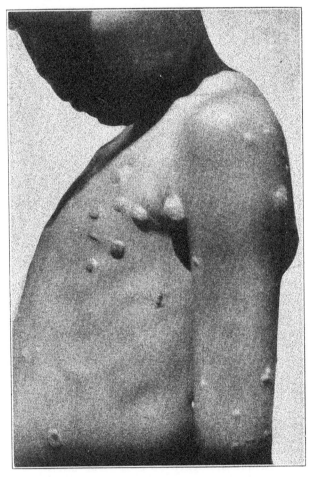

Fig. 6 (Case 66).—Same patient as in Figure 4. Note size of lesions and verrucous appearance of the surface.

is illustrated in Figure 1. The ulcers, after the scab is taken off, may be seen in Figures 2 and 3.

The primary lesion may heal before the secondary eruptions appear; but as a rule it is still present when the latter are observed. On the other hand, the primary sore may last for several months.

The primary lesion was observed to be still present in the majority of our cases when the secondary eruptions made their appearance. The time of healing of the primary lesions varied from one month to one year and a half. In the majority of these cases, however, the primary lesion healed in one year. In one case in which the primary

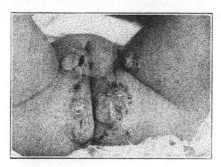

Fig. 7 (Case 102).—Frambesiform primary lesion of eight months' duration: secondary lesions of four months' duration. Moist papules about the genitals.

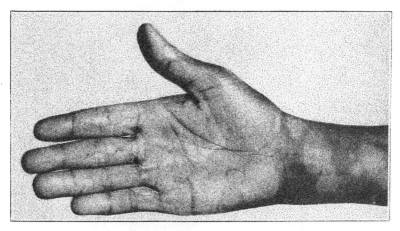

Fig. 8 (Case 54).—Palmar secondary lesions of three months' duration: primary of five months' duration. The macular eruption appeared three months after the primary lesions. There were numerous lesions on the face. forearms and trunk. Some may be seen on the wrist.

lesion was still present, it was noted six years after the development of the infection, at the time we gave the patient treatment.

There were six primary lesions in which all signs of the secondary lesions had entirely disappeared, and yet the primary lesions were still active. The disease in these cases was then of from two to six years' duration. In these cases, the lesions did not heal readily when treated with neo-arsphenamin; that is, they required more than one injection of the drug before healing.

THE SECONDARY LESIONS

As has been mentioned, the prime object of the campaign was to eradicate the focus of infection. There was, therefore, not sufficient

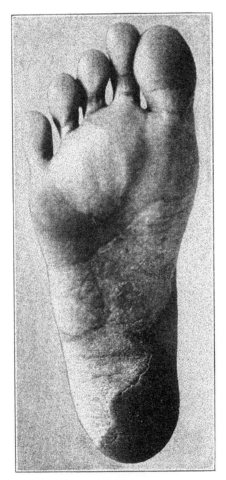

Fig. 9.—Plantar secondary lesions.

time to inquire minutely into the histories of the cases; moreover, even had we the time to do so, it would have been futile to try to determine just when the secondary eruptions first appeared in the class of patients we dealt with in the clinic. In many cases, the secondary eruptions had been resent for some time. The atients could not recall when they first appeared. In the cases in which this information could be obtained the usual time for their appearance was observed; that is, from one month to three months after the primary sore was first observed. The secondary eruptions are preceded by symptoms of general invasion of the system. These symptoms are malaise, fever, and pain in the muscles, joints and bones.

According to the generally accepted view, the secondary eruptions are of two forms—the papules and the nodules. Either of these may appear independent of the other. When, however, they occur together, the papules usually precede the nodules. Our observations, however, lead us to believe that there are more than these two types of eruptions found in the secondary stage of the disease.

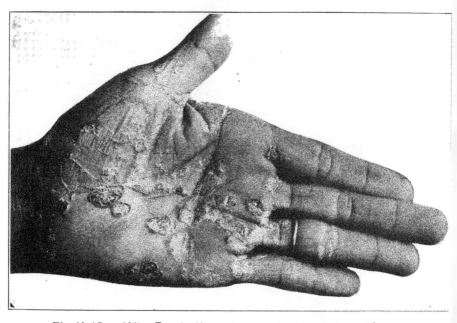

Fig. 10 (Case 126).—Frambesiform plantar and palmar lesions. There were also primary lesions of the right breast, secondary macular and a few frambesiform lesions.

THE NODULAR OR FRAMBESIFORM LESIONS

The frambesiform eruption is the most commonly observed in the secondary stage of the disease. As may be seen from Table 2, it was observed 159 times in 196 cases studied, or in 81.12 per cent. This type of eruption is so well known and has been so well described that little can be added (Figs. 4' 5 and 6). It may develop from the papular eruption (Fig. 1), or may appear as such from the beginning. When fully developed, the lesions vary in size from that of a pea to that of a quarter or larger (Fig. 6). They are raised from the surface of the skin. The surface of the lesions is studded with verrucous-like projections and is covered with an iodoform-like scab. If the scab is taken off, the surface is red and raw, and in some places minute bleeding points may be seen. These lesions may appear anywhere on the body. They are, however, less common on the head. They may remain the same size for months, after which the secretion dries up and the lesions finally disappear, in from three months to a year. We have seen these

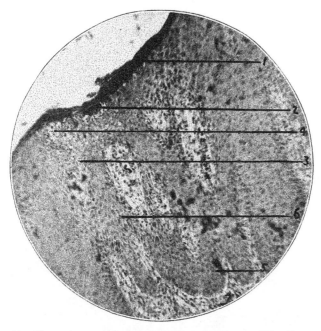

Fig. 11.—Photomicrograph of frambesiform lesions; × 110. Part of crust has been taken off: 1, hyperkeratosis and parakeratosis; 2, miliary abscess; 3, separation of nuclei from protoplasm; 4, degeneration of epithelial cells; 5, acanthosis; 6, infiltration with leukocytes and plasma cells; 7, edema and infiltration of corium.

lesions appear in crops, each crop healing in the time indicated; but they may be succeeded by another; and in this way two, three or four crops may appear before the lesions finally disappear. In one of our cases, these frambesiform lesions appeared and disappeared up to the time of treatment, twenty years after the appearance of the primary lesion; and these secondary lesions were accompanied by tertiary manifestations of the palms and soles. The secondary eruptions were found on the forearm and leg, having appeared one month and three months previously.

MOIST PAPULES

When the frambesiform eruptions are located on moist surfaces, such as that of the genitals, anus or axillae, or under the mammae, the yellow scab is taken off through maceration and rubbing of the opposed surfaces. The lesions then assume the character of a moist papule, which is not unlike the syphilitic moist papule (Fig. 7). As may be seen from Table 2, this type of lesion is not so uncommon.

PALMAR AND PLANTAR LESIONS

Palmar and plantar secondary lesions were observed thirteen times in 196 cases, or in 6.63 per cent. As illustrated in Figures 8, 9 and 10, they are not unlike palmar and plantar syphilis. A curious manner, but probably only one way, in which they are produced is illustrated in Figure 10.

TABLE 2.—CHARACTER OF SECONDARY ERUPTIONS

	No. of Cases	Percentages
Frambesiform	159	81.12
Papular	3	1.54
Macular	6	3.06
Frambesiform papular	15	7.65
Macular papular	2	3.92
Frambesiform macular	2	3.92
Frambesiform papular macular	6	3.06
Icbthyotic shins	1	0.51
Lesions found with other secondary eruptions		
Palmar plantar secondary	2	3.92
Total	196*	
Ichthyotic shins	2	1.54
Palmar plantar secondary	11	6.03
Moist papular	2	3.92

* In seventy-nine cases, we have not been able to study the lesion for lack of time.

HISTOPATHOLOGY OF FRAMBESIFORM LESIONS

The histopathology of the frambesiform type of secondary lesions has been described by Unna,[5] MacLeod,[6] Jeanselme [7] and Phlen [8] and more recently by Schuffner,[9] Marshall,[10] Seibert,[11] Ashburn and Craig.[12] White and Tyzzer [13] and lately by Schamberg and Klauder.[14]

5. Unna: The Histopathology of the Diseases of the Skin. New York. Macmillan & Co., p. 504.

6. MacLeod: Brit. M. J., 1902.

7. Jeanselme: Dermatologie Exotique, 1903.

8. Phlen: Mense's Handbuch der Tropenkrankheiten.

9. Schuffner: München. med. Wchnschr. 54:1364. 1907.

10. Marshall: Philippine J. Sc. 2:107, Sec. B.

11. Seibert: Arch. f. Schiffs- u. Tropen-Hyg., 1908.

12. Ashburn and Craig: Philippine J. Sc., 1908, Sec. B.

13. White and Tyzzer: J. Cutan. Dis. 29:138, 1915.

14. Schamberg, J. F., and Klauder, J. V.: Study of a Case of Yaws Contracted by an American Soldier in France. Arch. Dermat. & Syph. 3:40 (Jan.) 1921.

In brief, the histologic findings are: 1. A thick crust composed of necrotic material, leukocytes and bacteria. There is also hyperkeratosis and parakeratosis. 2. A marked proliferation of the rete, especially of the pegs, which dip down into the papillary layer. The suprapapillary rete is also increased in thickness. 3. Swelling and vacuolation of the

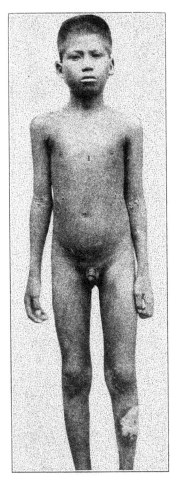

Fig. 12.—Papular type of eruptions.

epithelial cells. The nuclei in places are separated from the protoplasm by clear spaces. In places, these epithelial cells are changed; they do not take the stain well. 4. Infiltration of the intercellular spaces, in places, with leukocytes, chiefly of the polymorphonuclear type. Sharply circumscribed areas in the epidermis contain these leukocytes and detritus—the miliary abscesses. 5. A marked edema of the corium in the papillary and subpapillary layer. 6. An infiltration of the polymorphonuclear leukocytes and a few plasma cells. This infiltration is limited to an area below the rete pegs. In older nodules, the infiltration is made up chiefly of plasma cells. 7. No perivascular cell infiltration nor endothelial proliferation. There are no giant cells.

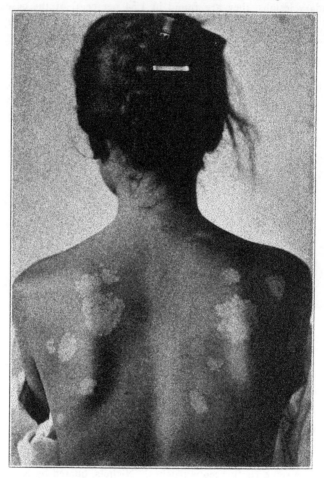

Fig. 13.—Macular eruptions of yaws. Note white patches. follicular heaping of scales and coalescence of lesions.

PAPULAR LESIONS

The papular form of secondary lesions occurs oftener than the macular, as is indicated in Table 2. This type of eruption is a flat papule. varying in size from that of a pinhead to that of a small pea. The apex is red when first formed. but later it is covered with the typical iodoform-yellow scab (Figs. 1 and 12). The lesions are discrete; they may remain the same size for weeks, and finally disappear or later develop into the typical frambesiform eruptions, as shown in Figures 1 and 12. As may be seen from Table 2, they are not so rare. Occurring as primary lesions, without the intermixture of other secondary lesions, they are found in 1.54 per cent. of the cases.; but when found together with other lesions, as is usually the case, they occur in 12.25 per cent. of the cases.

THE MACULAR ERUPTIONS

Those who have studied the disease do not always accede the occurrence of this type of eruption. A few believe that it occurs before any other type of eruption, while others are of the opinion that it

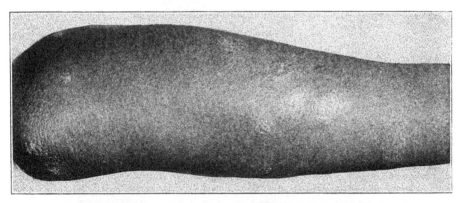

Fig. 14 (Case 94).—Primary lesion of more than three months' duration; healed after two months, when the patient was given an injection of neoarsphenamin. Frambetic secondary lesions appeared three weeks after the appearance of the mother-yaw; healed after injection. The present eruption was macular, of two weeks' duration. There was follicular heaping of scales, giving the appearance of pinpoint papular eruptions.

follows the disappearance of papular lesions. Castellani [4] merely states that other lesions besides the frambesial granulomatous lesions appear. Again, he says that when the papular eruptions disappear they occasionally leave some furfuraceous patches. Nichols, quoted by Rat,[15] denies the existence of this type of lesion. Maxwell [16] describes a scaly eruption in yaws "not unlike pityriasis versicolor" as one of the precursive eruptions. He is of the opinion that there is undoubtedly a "papulosquamous eruption which sometimes persists long after the disappearance of the general eruption, especially about the elbows and knees

15. Rat, N.: J. Trop. M. **5**:209, 1902.
16. Maxwell: J. Trop. M. **8**:82, 1905.

where they simulate psoriasis." Bowerbank, also quoted by Rat,[15] says that "These patches or blotches are of a brownish or dark red efflorescence. . . . From these patches small, pimple-like bodies, of a dark color, arise and project above the cuticle." Schuffner[9]

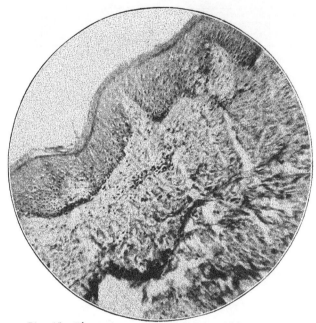

Fig. 15.—Photomicrograph of macular lesion; ✕ 110.

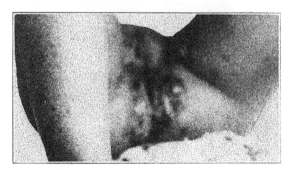

Fig. 16 (Case 102).—Ichthyosis shins; same case as in Figure 7.

describes macular lesions surrounded by minute papules, often becoming vesicular.

In our experience, these macular eruptions are not preceded by other secondary eruptions, nor are they always precursive to other frambesial eruptions; but they are a primary and distinct type of secondary eruption, similar to the macular eruptions of the secondary stage of syphilis (Fig. 13). They are discrete, macular, lighter in color than the surrounding skin, and vary in size from that of the head

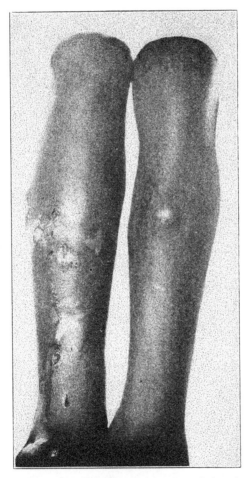

Fig. 17 (Case 209).—Primary lesions of two years' duration, still present; secondary lesions of two months' duration, still active; bone lesions of one year's duration.

of a match to that of a lima bean or larger. They are covered by fine furfuraceous white scales. These scales are easily detached and when a case is seen in the clinic only a few of the lesions are present on the surface. Around the follicles, however, they are closely packed, giving the appearance of a follicular lesion (Fig. 14). Two or more of these lesions may coalesce, forming bigger patches, as shown in Figure 13. These lesions remain for weeks as such, finally disappearing and leaving a white patch of skin. In other lesions, papular or frambesiform lesions eventually develop on the surface. This is not common, however; and, in our opinion, the lesions that grow on the surface develop accidentally on these macular patches. With reference to the

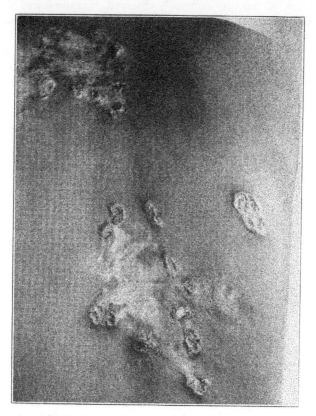

Fig. 18 (Case 76).—Primary lesions of three years' duration, healed in three months; secondary lesions, healed in four months; tertiary lesions about elbows, external malleolus and back.

time of their appearance, we have not observed any definite time, though most of them appear before other eruptions; still in not a few they come out after the frambesiform secondary eruptions have disappeared, or after insufficient treatment of the disease with arsphenamin.

This type of lesion must not be confused with another macular eruption sometimes observed in the later stages of the disease. This lesion is really papular. The papules are bright red, pinhead in size and discrete, and form circular patches. The eruption advances peripherally, leaving the center clear but covered with fine furfuraceous white scales. These are probably tertiary lesions. I have observed them in only two private cases, appearing in both later than the usual appearance of the secondary eruptions.

As may be seen from Table 2, these macular secondary lesions are not rare, nor are they commonly observed. Inexperienced observers might easily mistake them for some form of fungus infection, which abounds in this climate.

Another patient was seen (Case 165), who presented an erythematous, macular eruption of the body. The patient had a typical primary eruption of the frambesiform type soon followed by the

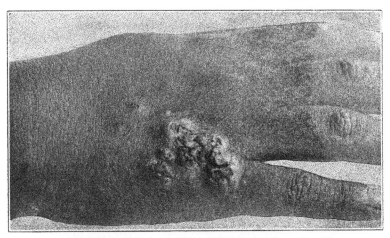

Fig. 19 (Case 116).—Primary lesions of three years' duration; tertiary lesions of five months' duration; on right hand, external aspect; flexor aspect of wrist; bend of elbows. Nodular type, from split-pea to lima bean size, covered with yellowish-brown scab.

erythematous eruption, rose-red, without any induration. The eruptions simulated those of macular syphilids, so that we were, for a time, in doubt as to the true nature of the case. The eruption, however, did not develop into the indurated copper colored papules of syphilis, and some of the lesions began to fade in two weeks, while the patient was under observation.

HISTOPATHOLOGY OF MACULAR LESIONS

The histologic description of the lesions is not dissimilar to that of frambesiform lesions (Fig. 15). 1. There is hyperkeratosis and parakeratosis. Around the hair follicles and in the opening of the sweat pores, the horny cells are heaped. 2. There is proliferation of the rete to about three times its normal depth. The pegs also proliferate in the same proportion. In places, the basal cells seem to be disintegrated, the protoplasm and nuclei are wanting. 3. The leukocytic infiltration in the epithelium is scanty and is scarcely discoverable in places. There are no miliary abscesses. 4. Some of the epithelial cells are edematous, and the nuclei of some are separated from the protoplasm by a clear space. 5. There is an infiltration of polymorphonuclear and small lymphocytes just below the pegs. 6. There is a marked edema of the papillary layer of the corium.

Closely related to this type of eruption is an eruption which we have termed, for want of a better name, ichthyosis-like shins. This is a diffuse mild keratosis not dissimilar to the skin found in persons

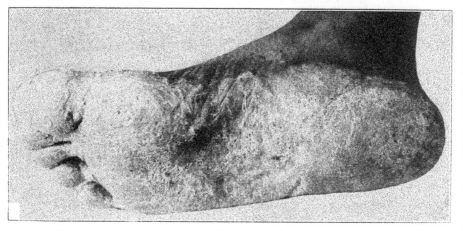

Fig. 20 (Case 217).—Keratosis of eight years' duration in a patient aged 25 years. The primary lesions appeared at the age of 10. Note the peculiar pitting.

suffering from xerodermia. The whole anterior portion of the tibia is affected, being covered with firm branny scales, white or grayish white (Fig. 16). The scales are more adherent than the scales found in the preceding type of eruption. Scattered over the surface at times are small papules. This type of eruption is not common, being found only three times in 196 cases, or in 1.53 per cent. of cases. It may be found in association with the macular, papular or nodular eruptions. We have observed it only in children.

The disease may end with the disappearance of the secondary eruptions. In some cases, however, the disease continues, and tertiary eruptions may be manifested soon after the secondary eruptions have dried; or the tertiary lesions may appear years after the disease is thought to have been cured. This is especially the case in keratosis of the palms and soles.

THE TERTIARY LESIONS

It was soon observed in our cases that the intermingling of secondary and tertiary lesions was frequent, the bone lesions often appearing with the secondary eruptions. In a few, the primary lesion was still present when the tertiary lesions made their appearance; thus there were present primary, secondary and tertiary lesions.

TABLE 3.—THE RELATION BETWEEN THE APPEARANCE OF THE PRIMARY, SECONDARY AND TERTIARY LESIONS

	No. of Cases	Percentages
Primary	10	4.63
Secondary	90	39.30
Tertiary	24	10.48
Combined Lesions:		
Primary, secondary	52	22.70
Secondary, tertiary	39	17.03
Primary, secondary, tertiary	14	6.11
Total cases	229	

In one of our cases (Case 47), the soft palate, which had been paining the child for one week, was red and arched. This case, if the patient is left untreated, may form one of the type called rhinopharyngitis mutilans by Leys.[17]

The distribution of the tertiary lesions is presented in Table 4.

The tertiary lesions described in the literature are bone lesions, gummas and plantar lesions or foot yaws.[18]

THE BONE LESIONS

The bone lesions are chronic periostitis or nodules under the periosteum, altering the size and shape of the bone in diverse forms, but

TABLE 4.—DISTRIBUTION OF PRIMARY LESIONS *

	No. of Cases	Percentages
Periostitis	7	29.16
Gumma	3	12.50
Keratosis	10	41.66
Periostitis ulcer	2	8.33
Periostitis, keratosis	1	4.16

* This table presents only the cases treated by us, the number of which is far below the actual number in Parañaque.

usually increasing the diameter. Long bones seem to be more prone to develop the lesions. Thus, the tarsals, metatarsals, radius, ulna, tibia and fibula are often affected; while other bones are not immune to attack. The lesions are painful, disabling and incapacitating. An example of this type of lesion is shown in Figure 17.

17. Leys: J. Trop. M. **9**:47, 1906.
18. Howard: J. Trop. M. **18**:25, 1915.

The gummas simulate gummatous formation due to syphilis and may be difficult to differentiate from the latter (Figs. 18 and 19). They are indolent ulcers, covered with yellowish-brown scabs, and involving the subcutaneous tissue. The edges are clear cut; if the scab is taken off, the fundus will be found granulating. Both of these cases yielded to a single injection of neo-arsphenamin.

KERATOSIS

This is the commonest tertiary lesion found in yaws, and yet it is the least known. It is sometimes called clavus; by Castellani[4] it is called "peculiar pitted appearance of the hands," by Howard[18] "foot yaws." There is no question that this lesion follows yaws and that it is a tertiary manifestation of the disease. It may, however, appear during the latter phase of the secondary eruptions, as observed by Castellani. On the other hand, it may appear years after all signs

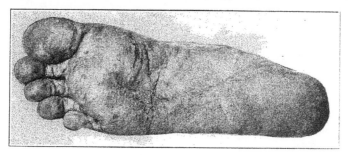

Fig. 21 (Case 213).—Keratosis of ten years' duration in a patient aged 45, who had yaws when about 12 years of age. The palms and soles are affected.

of the disease have disappeared, so that the patients have forgotten or do not see the relation between it and the yaws they had in childhood. In some of our cases, a history of yaws occurring during childhood was obtained, and this type of lesion did not appear until from ten to twenty years after the infection.[19] Examples of this type of lesion are shown in Figures 20 and 21. As may be seen from Table 4, these types of lesion are common, but because our object was to treat only the infectious cases, many of those suffering from keratosis were refused treatment.

TREATMENT

Soon after Ehrlich announced his discovery of arsphenamin for the treatment of syphilis and sent the drug to different parts of the globe.

19. A paper devoted to the manifestation and treatment of this particular form of tertiary eruption is under preparation.

Strong,[20] working in the Philippines, reported four cases of yaws successfully treated with the drug. At the same time, Nichols[21] also reported cures by the same drug in experimental animals. Ehrlich's ambition, "therapia sterilisans magna," applies more to yaws than to syphilis. The disease yields readily to the drug and secondary lesions require much less of the drug and heal in less time than do syphilitic eruptions.

DOSAGE

We employed a dosage somewhat larger than that employed in syphilis. To adults we gave as much as 0.6 gm. of neo-arsphenamin and for children we used an even proportionally higher dosage. We employed neo-arsphenamin exclusively, as it is easier to handle in the field than arsphenamin. The usual precautions observed prior to the administration of the drug in syphilis were carried out, and we have not observed any serious reactions. There were no Herxheimer nor nitritoid reactions.

EFFECT OF THE DRUG ON THE LESIONS

The efficacy of the drug in treatment of the lesions may be seen in Table 5.

TABLE 5.—Effect of Treatment

	No. of Cases	Percentages
Clinically cured	259	94.52
Improved	7	2.55
Not improved or Recurred	8	2.91
Total	275*	

* One duplication.

With the exception of eighty-six cases, a single injection was given in these cases. Of the eighty-six cases in which two injections were made, in about twenty-five the injection was repeated because the blood reactions were being studied. Three months after, the eighty-six patients were again seen, and it was found that three patients had not improved, while two were improved.

Table 5 does not take into account the type of lesions treated. We observed early in the course of the treatment that ulcers and primary lesions did not improve as was expected; while tertiary lesions required more than a single injection. Irrespective of the type of lesions or the stage of the disease, there was a clinical cure in 94.52 per cent. of the cases. This observation was made one and a half months after the last injection and three months after the first injections. In Table 3, the different types of lesions encountered are shown. The

20. Strong: Philippine J. Sc. **5**:433, Sec. B.

21. Nichols: J. Exper. M. **12**:161; Preliminary Note on the Action of Ehrlich's Substance 606 on Spirochaeta Pertenuis in Animals, J. A. M. A. **55**: 216 (July 16) 1910.

lesions that did not improve with the drug were tertiary, with the exception of two early secondary lesions, in one of which the dose was too small. These cases have not been controlled by blood reactions, with the exception of about twenty-five cases. The serum reactions in these twenty-five cases have been studied by Drs. Sellards and Good-pasture, whose observations will be published in a separate article.

SUMMARY AND CONCLUSIONS

1. Yaws is prevalent in the village of Parañaque, affecting the poor for the most part, particularly children.

2. The disease is transmitted by direct contact. We found many of the children in this locality affected with scabies, and we believe that it is responsible for the transmission of the disease.

3. There are three types of secondary eruptions: the frambesiform, the papular and the macular. The macular eruption is described herewith in detail.

4. A new lesion associated with secondary eruptions is described as ichthyotic shins.

5. Three tertiary lesions are described.

6. The disease yields readily to neo-arsphenamin therapy. In 275 patients treated, there was a clinical cure in 94.52 per cent. The observations in these cases extended from one and a half to three months. The secondary eruptions yielded best to the drug, the macular forms best of all. The primary lesions and tertiary keratotic lesions of the palms and soles did not do well.

LEUKODERMA IN PITYRIASIS LICHENOIDES CHRONICA

HENRY E. MICHELSON, M.D.

Assistant Professor in Dermatology, University of Minnesota

MINNEAPOLIS

Leukoderma may occur in the course of syphilis, leprosy, seborrheic eczema and psoriasis; a few cases have been observed in pityriasis lichenoides chronica.

CASES IN THE LITERATURE

Arndt,[1] in 1910, in his classical monograph on Brocq's disease, while discussing the great similarity of pityriasis lichenoides chronica to papulosquamous syphilids, described a case which he had observed in a 24-year old girl. The eruption had been present for eighteen months. A typical leukoderma had developed at the nape of the neck. Arndt remarked that, to his knowledge, this condition heretofore had been observed only in syphilis and psoriasis.

Oppenheim,[2] in 1913, demonstrated a case of pityriasis lichenoides chronica before the Vienna Dermatological Society, in which there was a leukoderma in the nuchal region.

Scherber,[3] in 1916, presented before the Vienna Dermatological Society a 17-year old patient having pityriasis lichenoides chronica, with an associated leukoderma.

Kren,[4] in 1917, before the same society, exhibited a case of pityriasis lichenoides chronica, with leukoderma, in a 32-year old woman.

Sachs,[5] in 1918, reported a case of leukoderma, occurring in the course of pityriasis lichenoides chronica, which he had observed in an 8-year old boy, who had shown a characteristic salmon-red macular and lichenoid papular eruption which had been present on the trunk and extremities. A marked leukoderma had been present on the neck. The Wassermann reaction was negative. The mucous membranes did not

1. Arndt, G.: Ueber Brocqsche Krankheit (erythrodermie pityriasique en plaques disseminées) nebst einigen Bemerkungen zur Frage der Parapsoriasis. Arch. f. Dermat. u. Syph. **100**:89, 1910.

2. Oppenheim, M., quoted by Sachs: Wien. med. Wchnschr., 1920, No. 30-31, p. 1376.

3. Scherber: Fall von Pityriasis Lichenoides Chronica, Meeting Vienna Dermat. Soc., Dec. 14, 1916; Arch. f. Dermat. u. Syph. **125**:30, 1917.

4. Kren, Otto: Schafferin mit Pityriasis Lichenoides Chronica, Meeting Vienna Dermat. Soc., May 24, 1917; Arch. f. Dermat. u. Syph. **125**:173, 1917.

5. Sachs, Otto: Zur Pathologic und Therapie der Pityriasis Lichenoides Chronica, Wien. med. Wchnschr., 1920, No. 30-31, p. 1376.

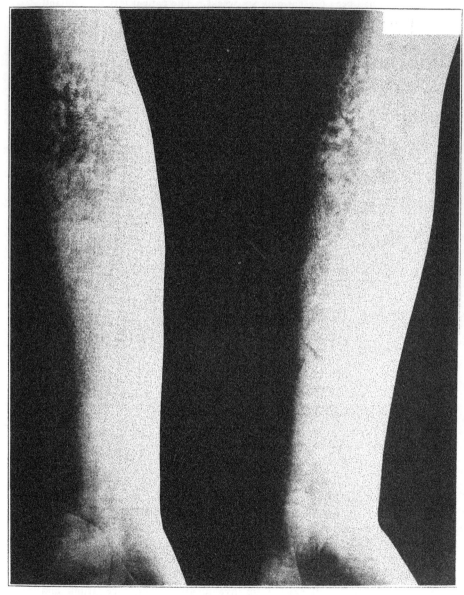

Fig. 1—View of arms showing leukodermic areas enmeshed in a retiform papular eruption.

show any lesions, and there had been no glandular enlargement. The eruption had been present only six weeks. The patient left for Holland before Sachs could make further observations.

Sachs not only described the foregoing cases of leukoderma, but also referred to cases of pityriasis lichenoides chronica, described or demonstrated by Mucha, Rusch and Oppenheim, as well as a case of his own, in which there were papulonecrotic lesions. He warned against the

Fig. 2.—Close view of arm.

danger of confusing cases of pityriasis lichenoides chronica, in which leukoderma or papulonecrotic lesions are present, with similar syphilitic manifestations.

Sato,[6] in 1921, reported a case of leukoderma in parapsoriasis which he had observed in the clinic of Professor Bruno Bloch in Zurich. This case occurred in a 17-year old patient who had a squamous papular eruption which had existed for five months. The face, trunk and extremities were involved. A typical syphilis-like leukoderma was

6. Sato, K.: Ueber Leukoderma bei Parapsoriasis, Dermat. Wchnschr. **73**:71 (Sept.) 1921.

present on the neck, upper part of the back and sides of the
The usual tests and investigations for syphilis were negative. His
examinations of an excised papule revealed only the slight path
changes which are commonly observed in pityriasis lichenoides ch

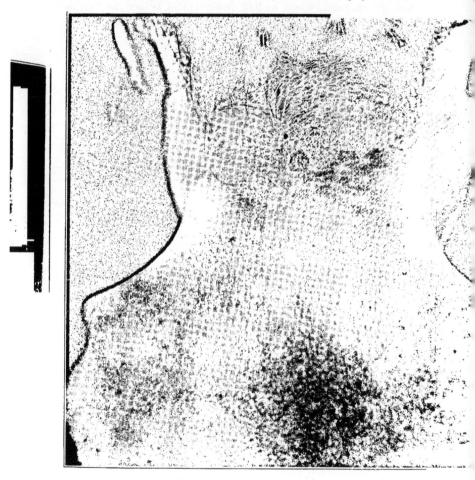

Fig. 3.—Leukoderma in nuchal region with biopsy scar.

J. Strandberg,[7] in 1921, presented, before a meeting of the
holm Dermatological Society, a 7-year old girl, who for two
had shown symptoms of parapsoriasis. Pigment changes, reser
closely syphilitic leukoderma, had gradually developed on the nec
shoulders. There was no evidence of syphilis in either the litt

7. Strandberg, J.: Case of Parapsoriasis. Meeting Stockholm Derma
Nov. 17, 1920; Acta dermat. ven. **2**:281, 1921.

or her parents. Almkvist discussed this case and admitted the close resemblance to a syphilitic leukoderma. He impressed the members of the society with the great significance of this fact.

Almkvist,[8] in 1922, reported a case of leukoderma in pityriasis lichenoides chronica, which he had demonstrated before the Stockholm Dermatological Society.[9]

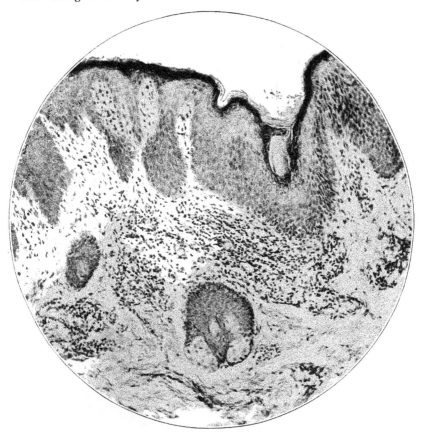

Fig. 4.—Low power ($\times$ 150) showing distribution of infiltrate in corium in area of eruption.

The patient was a 26-year old bookbinder, who had appeared before Professor Almkvist to be treated for syphilis. He had a generalized

8. Almkvist, J.: Ein Fall von Leukoderma bei Pityriasis Lichenoides Chronica, Dermat. Wchnschr. **74:** No. 9 (March) 1922.

9. Almkvist, J.: A Case of Pityriasis Lichenoides Chronica with Pigmented Spots After the Papules, Meeting Stockholm Dermat. Soc., Oct. 13, 1920; Acta dermat. ven. **1:**475 (Dec.) 1921.

papular eruption of four months' standing. A lay friend had diagnosed the condition as syphilis. The eruption consisted of reddish-
brown, sharply outlined, more or less scaly papules, varying in size
from that of the head of a match to that of a pea; scattered among
the papules were more diffusely marginated yellowish-red scaly macules.
The eruption was confined to the trunk. The head, neck, genitals

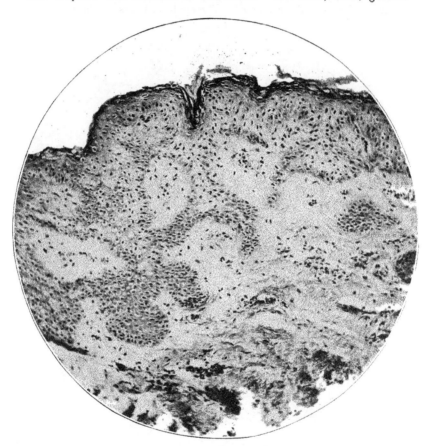

Fig. 5.—Low power (× 150) showing changes in epidermis.

and lower portions of the extremities were free from manifestations.
nor were the mucous membranes affected. There was no history or
scar of a chancre; nor was there general glandular enlargement. The
blood Wassermann test, repeatedly performed, was negative. There
was no mention of a spinal fluid examination. Subjective symptoms
were entirely absent. At first glance, Almkvist was inclined to agree
with the patient's diagnosis of his own case, that is, that it was syphilis.

He, however, withheld his decision until the serologic and histologic reports were completed. As stated, the Wassermann reaction was negative. A medium sized, apparently fresh, papule was excised. The findings were: A small degree of infiltration of small round cells in the cutis, less than is usually found in syphilis. There was a complete absence of plasma cells. A few polymorphonuclear leukocytes and an occasional mast cell were noted. The epidermis was not flattened as in

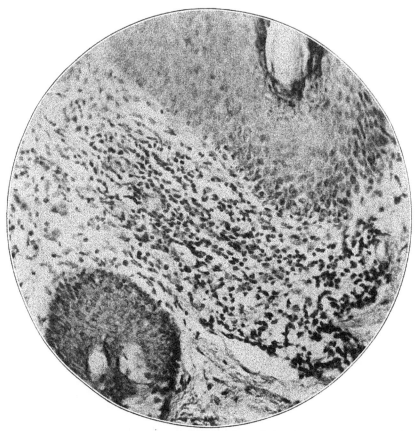

Fig. 6.—High power (× 300) of infiltrate.

syphilitic papules, but, on the other hand, there was a lengthening of the interpapillary projections, and the malpighian rete showed a degree of spongiosis. In certain areas, the cornified layer of the epidermis showed nuclei-bearing cells. There was some edema and a slight proliferation of the connective tissue.

The chronic appearance and the clinical aspect, together with the histologic and serologic findings, led Almkvist to make a diagnosis of pityriasis lichenoides chronica. Treatment with naphthol and sulphur ointments over a period of three months gave no favorable result. The patient was not seen again for two months, when he reported that he had been taking sun baths of long duration and that the eruption had gradually faded from the parts exposed. A month after he ceased taking sun baths, new eruptions appeared here and there, but more sparingly than previously. Examination at this time showed a marked

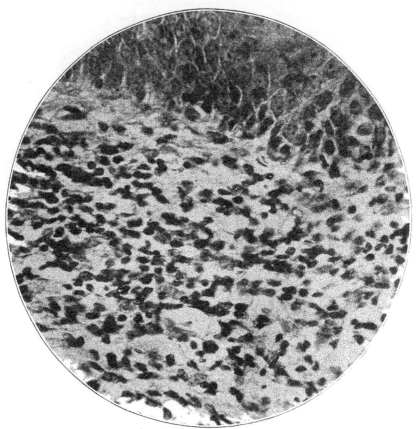

Fig. 7.—High power (× 600) of infiltrate.

diminution in the amount of eruption. The entire skin was tanned from exposure to the sun's rays. Diffusely scattered throughout the brown skin of the trunk were depigmented spots of various sizes. They were more clearly noted on the trunk where the skin was more intensely tanned. Besides these white spots, eruptions precisely like those observed four months previously were present. Almkvist came to the conclusion that the leukodermic spots occupied the areas previously covered with the papular eruption. He wished to excise a portion of a white area, but the patient refused to allow him to do so. Almkvist remarked that the previous cases of leukoderma in pityriasis lichenoides chronica were described as closely simulating the leukoderma of syphilis, while his case more closely resembled the leukoderma occasionally observed in psoriasis after chrysarobin treatment. He agreed with the

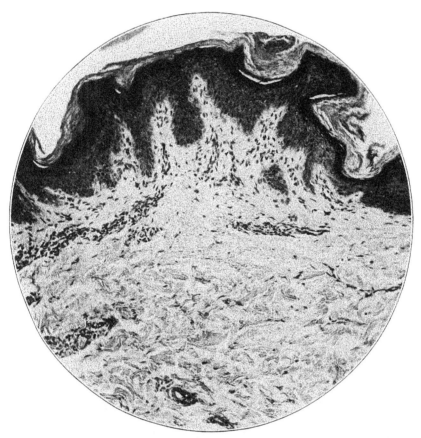

Fig. 8.—Low power (× 150) showing remnants of infiltrate in leukodermic area.

conclusions of Scherber and Kren that the leukodermic areas were the result of the preexisting lichenoid eruption. His observations that the sun's rays brought about a regression of the eruption agreed with the results of Klausner, who recommended Quartz lamp therapy in parapsoriasis.

In October, 1921, Professor Oppenheim brought to my attention a case of extensive leukoderma in pityriasis lichenoides chronica in his service at the Wilhelminénspital. The patient was a woman, aged 27, with a profuse, scaly, macular and papular eruption which enclosed white areas. The mucous membranes were free from manifestations. There were no glandular enlargements. The blood and spinal fluid Wassermann reactions were negative. The leukodermic spots were located on the neck and back, and were especially profuse on the lower extremities. The patient, when observed from a distance, presented a sort of a retiform appearance, such as is noted in erythema ab igne. She was exhibited before the Vienna Dermatological Society,[10] when the diagnosis of syphilis, acrodermatitis atrophicans and pityriasis lichenoides chronica were proposed and discussed. The consensus of opinion, however, favored the diagnosis of pityriasis lichenoides chronica with associated leukoderma and idiopathic atrophy of the skin. A biopsy was, I believe, not performed.

In October, 1921, Professor Kren also brought to my attention a case in his division at the Jubiläums-Spitals of marked leukoderma occurring in pityriasis lichenoides chronica. The patient was a little girl, aged 6. She had a scaling maculopapular eruption on the face. trunk and arms. The leukoderma was on the neck and cheeks. This case was exhibited before the Vienna Dermatological Society.[11]

REPORT OF CASE

History.—Evelyn L., an unmarried waitress, aged 20, presented herself for examination on Aug. 4, 1920. Her father was living and well at 53 years of age. Her mother died eight years previously of unknown cause. Two brothers and one sister were living and well. She said that her skin condition began in February, 1920. She first noticed a light brown eruption on the arms at the elbow region and near the axillae. Gradually the entire flexor surfaces became involved, and areas of eruption appeared on the chest and median surfaces of the thighs, also on the nape of the neck. After the eruption had been present about one month she went to a physician who took a specimen of her blood for a Wassermann test and reported it negative. There were no subjective symptoms. She did not lose weight or strength. nor did she suffer with headaches or general malaise. The eruption was not in solid areas. but made various lacelike figures. The color was at first a yellowish brown which gradually became much darker. At no time had she had any lesion that might have been diagnosed as a chancre, nor were the mucous membranes involved.

On examination one noticed a rather diffuse brownish lichenoid papular eruption at the nape of the neck. over the upper midscapular region. the antecubital areas, and the medium surface of the thighs. The papules were arranged in such a manner that one received the impression of a coarsely meshed net closely applied to the skin. The eruption was slightly scaly. some-

10. Oppenheim, M.: Lues recens oder Pityriasis Lichenoides Chronica mit Atrophica Cutis Idiopathica Progressiva. Meeting Vienna Dermat. Soc.. Oct. 20, 1921; Dermat. Wchnschr. **74**:25, 1922.

11. Kren, Otto: Pityriasis Lichenoides Chronica. Meeting Vienna Dermat. Soc., Oct. 20, 1921; Dermat. Wchnschr. **74**:25. 1922.

what resembling a marked tinea versicolor. A preliminary survey of the case was made, a blood Wassermann test was ordered and the patient dismissed. She was not seen again until February, 1922. The patient said that since the last observation, the eruption had gradually become more intense, but that white areas had developed which were especially noticeable at the back of the neck and at the antecubital spaces. The eruption was somewhat variable, at times being more profuse than at others. The fading was gradual while the reappearances were more sudden. There were no subjective symptoms. The mucous membranes and conjunctivae were entirely free, and there was no general adenopathy. Her general health was excellent. The scalp was free from manifestations.

The Face: The sides of the cheeks, especially the pre-auricular areas, were covered with minute, brownish tinted, flat-topped, scaly papules which were barely felt by the palpating finger. The papules were arranged in irregular lines, were not confluent and could not be removed by gently scraping with a scalpel blade. This irregular arrangement encircled areas of normal skin. The forehead was free.

The Neck: Here the striking feature was the leukodermic spots, which were numerous, varying in size from that of a dime to that of a five-cent piece, oval or round in contour, but with an irregular border, extending well up to the hairline; there was no associated alopecia, either diffuse or patchy. The color of the depigmented areas was lighter than that of her normal skin. The surface was smooth and showed normal texture. The skin between the areas was highly colored, of a dark brown tint, studded with minute, rather sharply demarcated, flat-topped, slightly scaly papules. The rest of the skin between the leukodermic spots appeared hyperpigmented. The picture was that of a pigmented network enclosing white areas in its irregularly sized meshes. At first inspection the aspect was that of a leukoderma syphiliticum.

The Trunk: Similar white areas surrounded by hyperpigmented skin, bearing dark brown minute papules arranged in a netlike formation were plainly noted at the midsternal and anterior abdominal areas.

The Upper Extremities: A striking leukoderma syphiliticum-like picture was present in both antecubital regions. The involved areas extended well up to the midbiceps and nearly down to the wrist. Similar lesions were present in the axillae. The hands were free.

The Lower Extremities: The median thigh regions alone were involved. There was no variation in the type of eruption.

The leukodermic areas were most plainly and strikingly noted at the nape of the neck and at the antecubital spaces. The predominating color was a smudgy seborrheic brown. The individual papules were about the size of the head of a match, slightly infiltrated, sharply demarcated and bore adherent scales which, when scraped off, were mere dustlike epidermic specks. There was no subsequent oozing of serum or pinpoint bleeding. There were no crusts present at any spot. Subjective symptoms were entirely lacking. There was no sclero-adenitis. No remnants or scars of initial lesions were detected.

The serologic study was rather extraordinary. The first Wassermann test, made on August 5, was frankly negative. The tests of August 12, 19 and 23, were positive. Wassermann tests were repeated on October 7 and November 21; both were negative. Five tests were made from February to April, 1922, all of which were frankly negative. No antisyphilitic therapy had been employed in the interim between the first and the second series of tests. Sachs also observed a patient who showed a positive Wassermann reaction which became negative after a single injection of arsphenamin and which remained negative. His case, clinically, showed no evidence of syphilis.

Histologic Study. — Three pieces of tissue were removed for microscopic study. Two of the pieces were from eruption areas, the third from the center of a leukodermic spot. The tissues were fixed in liquor formaldehydi and alcohol, imbedded in paraffin and serially sectioned and stained with hemotoxylin eosin, polychrome methylene blue, Weigert's resorcin-fuchsin and eosin.

The striking change was the edema of the epidermis with a distinct thinning of the stratum granulosum. Parakeratosis was present, and in a few areas some scaling was noted. In other areas the rete pegs were a bit broadened and slightly elongated, but there was no marked acanthosis. In other areas, the epidermal outline was irregular. Islands of corium were enclosed in a formation which resulted from a peculiar budding arrangement of the rete pegs with an apparent fusing of two or more pegs at their tips. The basal layer was somewhat blurred and edematous and at certain spots the infiltrate of the corium penetrated the epidermis.

The subpapillary layer showed a moderate degree of infiltration which was rather diffuse, but the degree was not constant. In certain areas the infiltrate was quite dense, in others only clumps of cells were noted. The papillary layers were less involved with the infiltrative process. There was no marked increase in the capillaries or proliferative changes in those present. The lymph spaces were dilated. The collagen bundles were edematous. The elastic fibers were clearly shown by Weigert's method. The infiltrate was composed almost entirely of lymphocytes. No plasma cells were noted. No changes were detected in the sudiferous or pilosebaceous glands or ducts. No changes were noted in the deeper tissues.

Treatment and Course. — The process was decidedly a chronic one. Little change was noted from month to month. The leukodermic areas became larger, and the eruption had the tendency to be more apparent at times; also a superficial scaling would appear and soon disappear. One arm was treated with ultraviolet rays. An intense erythema was produced, and, as exfoliation took place, the eruption faded decidedly. Five treatments brought about almost a complete disappearance. Because of the positive Wassermann tests of the previous year, the patient was given three injections of mercuric salicylate followed by an intravenous injection of neo-arsphenamin, 0.6 gm. This was done to note the effect on the areas not treated with the mercury vapor lamp. No appreciable change was noted. Sachs reported that neo-arsphenamin brought about a distinct regression in his case, which had shown a slightly positive Wassermann reaction. We did not deem it advisable to subject our patient to prolonged antisyphilitic therapy, for the clinical diagnosis was so decidedly against syphilis.

Diagnosis. — In this case one must consider leukoderma syphiliticum, psoriasis vulgaris, pityriasis versicolor and pityriasis lichenoides chronica.

Vitiligo, albinismus partialis, scars following acne vulgaris, variola and pediculi vestimenorum, the leukoderma following leprosy, seborrheic eczema, and the so-called pigmentary syphilid were considered, only to be hastily discarded.

Clinical Appearance of Eruption: There were no signs or history of sclerosis. The mucous membranes and glands were free from involvement. Stationary weight and general well being were decidedly against the diagnosis of syphilis, in spite of the positive Wassermann reactions which appeared during the period of observation, but which did not remain positive. The last five tests performed over a period of three months were all negative. I cannot account for the positive tests, but consider them of little significance. The leukodermic areas in our case were irregular in size and of a retiform appearance, while the individual leukodermic spots in syphilis are regular in outline and mostly of the same size; furthermore, the skin between the leukodermic areas in syphilis is normal, while in this case the skin surrounding the pale areas was covered with a minute pigmented eruption.

The absence of typical psoriatic lesions in the usual locations, the complete freedom of the scalp, inability to produce dew drops bleeding, conclusively ruled out psoriasis vulgaris.

Pityriasis versicolor can at times closely simulate a leukoderma syphiliticum. The yellowish brown scaling encloses areas of normal skin. Repeated examinations of the scales in our case revealed no fungi.

COMMENT

In conclusion, I may say that this case presents features which make the diagnosis of pityriasis lichenoides chronica with leukodermic areas quite certain. The chronic course, the character of the eruption and the histologic examination are positive evidences in favor of such a diagnosis.

The question arises whether we are dealing with a leukoderma due to pigment disturbance or to an apparent leukoderma due to enmeshing of areas of normal skin in the retiform eruption. There is no doubt that the leukodermic areas enlarged during the period of observation, and in the tissue removed from a leukodermic area, remnants of infiltrate were easily shown. I, therefore, believe that the leukodermic areas were, at least in part, due to a previously existing eruption, while the irregular outline of these areas could be accounted for by the retiform arrangement of the eruption.

Leukoderma has been looked on as a specific manifestation of syphilis, but a review of the literature shows the possibility of its occurring in other conditions.

A STUDY OF RINGED HAIR *[1]

LEE D. CADY, A.M., M.D. and MILDRED TROTTER, A.B. M.S.

ST. LOUIS

An unusual banded appearance of the hair was described by Karsch, in 1846, under the name of Pili annulati.[1] Such "ringed hairs" have proved to be of rare occurrence, and the few cases thus far reported have not afforded material for an entirely satisfactory account of the nature and genesis of the condition. Because of the apparent infrequency of the anomaly and some uncertainty as to its exact nature it seems desirable to report briefly on some cases that have recently been examined. These cases have all appeared in three families, one of which was being studied by the writers when the second was called to their attention by Dr. P. W. Whiting, of the University of Iowa, who generously supplied samples of hair for study. Dr. Whiting will take up elsewhere the heredity of this interesting condition. The third family has been in the practice of Dr. Martin F. Engman, Washington University, for about twenty years.

So far as we have been able to find, only eighteen cases are recorded in the literature. Since there has been no comprehensive review of this subject and no systematic microscopic study of hairs presenting this condition, it was thought desirable to review the literature up to date and to add such facts relating to the structure of ringed hairs as have been made out by a more detailed study than has previously been attempted.

REVIEW OF LITERATURE

The first case, described by Karsch in 1846 (quoted by Landois, 1866), appeared in the hair of a boy 19 years old. Some of the hairs were half dark brown and half white, others had short alternate rings of dark brown and white. Karsch concluded that the portions which appeared dark when seen under the microscope by transmitted light were the normal segments. Landois,[1] however, showed that it was the light segments of the hairs that appeared dark by transmitted light, and vice versa. Karsch believed a white pigment to be present in the white segments, but according to Landois, Speiss in 1859 attributed the whiteness to the presence of air bubbles.

---

* From the Department of Anatomy, Washington University School of Medicine, St. Louis.

1. Landois, L.: Das ploetzliche Ergrauen der Haupthaare. Arch. f. path. Anat. u. Physiol. **35**:575, 1866.

Wilson (1867) [2] noted the condition in a boy 7½ years old. In this case it was observed to become more general during the next two years. The hair shafts were uniform and presented alternate brown (1/50 inch [0.5 mm.]) and white (1/100 inch [0.25 mm.]) segments. He thought the whiteness was due to the presence of globules of air which sometimes communicated by short irregular canals. There were also air globules in the medullae.

Frazer [3] (1875) described some hair (about 13 inches [33.02 cm.] long) from an Italian woman procured from a hair dresser. Every hair had marked uniform alternate white and dark-brown bands (three brown and two white bands to an eighth of an inch [3.17 mm.]). The hair was moderately coarse, and in both the gross and the microscopic examination presented the characteristics of otherwise normal human hair.

Crocker [4] (1893) reported the case of an 8 year old girl whose hair had been natural and silky previous to the onset, two years before, of a condition considered to be a sequel to influenza and ophthalmia. The hair had a greater optical diameter opposite the light segments, which sometimes filled the entire diameter of the shaft, and were frequently four times as long as the pigmented segments. This infiltration commenced in the shaft just above the hair root and extended throughout the entire length of the hair. The condition was more marked on the left side of the scalp than on the right.

Unna [5] (1894) gave the condition the name leukotrichia annularis. His patient was a man, 26 years old, in whom part of the hairs of the scalp were affected. Those hairs in which the condition was present were dry, fragile and gray in appearance. The segments varied in length from mere points to 2 or 3 mm. Microscopically the white segments seemed normal with the exception of an unusually large number of interstices. This infiltration was most marked in the medullas, but air-containing cavities extended irregularly toward the cortex. He believed that the air streaks were due to an alternate increasing and decreasing functional activity of the matrix of the hair causing alternate harder and softer segments. When the softer parts became dried, they developed air spaces within them causing the white segments in a manner similar to the production of leukonychia, as explained by Unna. Leukonychia was found associated in this case.

2. Wilson, E.: On a Remarkable Alteration of Appearance and Structure of the Human Hair, Proc. Roy. Soc. of London **15**:406, 1867.

3. Frazer: Human Hair Presenting a Remarkable Alternate Transverse Dark and White Mottling, Quart. J. of Microscop. Sc. **15**:100, 1875.

4. Crocker, H. R.: Ringed Hair, Brit. J. Dermat. 5:175, 1893.

5. Unna, P. G., in J. Orth.: Lehrbuch der Specielien Pathologischen Anatomie, Erganzungsband 2, Berlin, A. Hirschwald, 1894, p. 1061.

Prew's case (quoted by McCall Anderson,[6] 1894) was that of a girl 9½ years old. The condition was of short duration and disappeared under treatment.

Kiwull[7] (1895) reported the case of a girl 20 years old with alopecia praematura universalis of three years' duration. The hair was all gone except about 50 thin hairs 1 or 2 cm. long. Microscopically several hairs showed spindle-shaped areas which appeared dark by transmitted light and white by reflected light. He thought the white streaks were due to the presence of air.

Galloway's[8] cases (1896) were those of two brothers, 8 and 10 years of age. The bands were of almost equal length, slightly less than 1 mm. The hair had a peculiar lusterless appearance. This is the first report that indicates that the condition may be hereditary.

Brayton's[9] case (1897) was noticed when the patient, a boy, was 2 years old, and the condition had persisted for fourteen years thereafter. The alternate light and brown segments gave the hair a "sandy" appearance. There were from 20 to 30 of the segments to an inch of hair shaft. The hair was becoming darker as the boy grew older. Two of the mother's brothers had similar hair, but four brothers and a sister of the boy had normal hair.

Meachen's[10] case (1902) was that of a boy 8 years old. The white and the dark segments averaged 0.2 and 0.3 mm., respectively. The infiltration of air was said to be confined to the medulla, there being always a narrow strip of normal cortical substance exterior to the abnormal segments. Melanoderma, syndactylia and polydactylism had been present from birth. Meachen was unsuccessful in establishing a bacterial origin for the condition.

Crocker's[11] second case (1903) of ringed hair occurred in the mustache of a man 39 years old and was associated with trichorrhexis nodosa. Some hairs showed air bubbles in stellate heaps around the medulla at regular intervals. The dark segments were much longer than the light ones. This is the only case in which the condition is reported in hair other than that of the scalp.

Fox's[12] case (1906) was associated with almost complete alopecia of two months' duration in a woman 25 years of age. The few remaining hairs had a "dusty" appearance due to alternate dark ($\frac{1}{50}$ [0.5 mm.]

6. Anderson, McC.: Diseases of the Skin, 1894, p. 64.

7. Kiwull, E.: Defluvium capillorum universale. Pili annulati. Arch. f Dermat. u. Syph. **32-33**:173, 1895.

8. Galloway, J.: Ringed Hair. Brit. J. Dermat. **8**:437, 1896.

9. Brayton, A. W.: A Case of Ringed Hair. Ind. M. J. **16**:10, 1897.

10. Meachen, F. N.: A Case of Leucotrichia annularis. Brit. J. Dermat. **16**:86, 1902.

11. Crocker, H. R.: Diseases of the Skin, 1903, p. 1196.

12. Fox, C.: A Case of Ringed Hair. Brit. J. Dermat. **18**:321, 1906.

inch) and light ($\frac{1}{75}$ inch [0.33 mm.]) segments. The woman subsequently had normal hair. Fox referred to another case of ringed hair but gave no description of it.

Haxthausen's [13] case (1917) was that of a girl 18 years old in whom the condition had been present as long as she could remember. The segments were about 1 mm. apart and were found in all the hairs of the scalp. Microscopic study, after removal of the pigment with sodium hydroxid, showed that the white segments were due to air bubbles.

Hoepke's [14] case (1921) was that of a man, 23 years old, in whom ringed hair was said to have been present since puberty. The hair was coarse and ringed and was said to have seasonal variations in color, being light blond in summer and dark blond in winter. The rings appeared and disappeared in much the same manner as the supposed pigmentary changes. When these hairs were boiled in glycerol the light segments disappeared. Boiling in alcohol, ether, benzol and oil apparently caused no changes. The tensile strength of these hairs averaged from 80 to 90 per cent. more than average hairs. These hairs when under tension always broke between the light segments. Attempts to exhaust the gas from the light segments in vacuo were unsuccessful.

MATERIAL STUDIED

The hair specimens available to us came from two families, the N family and the S family.

The N family, disregarding persons with normal hair who have married into it, consists of the maternal grandmother, N_1; her three daughters, N_{21}, N_{22} and N_{23}; her two sons N_{24} and N_{25}; and her three grandsons, N_{31} and N_{32}, children of N_{21}; and N_{33}, the child of N_{23}. Samples of hair were obtained from all members of this family except N_1, N_{25} and N_{32}.

The S family consists of the father, S_1; his son, S_{21} and daughter, S_{22}; and two grand-children, S_{31} and S_{32}, twin daughters of S_{21}. All members of this family contributed specimens of hair. Ten additional samples of hair from cousins of the S family have been subsequently received from Dr. Whiting.

The K family consists of the grandmother, K_1; three daughters, K_{21}, K_{22} and K_{23}; K_{31}, K_{32}, and K_{33}, the two sons and daughter, respectively, of K_{21}; K_{34} and K_{35}, daughters of K_{22}; K_{36} and K_{37}, the daughter and son, respectively, of K_{23}.

13. Haxthausen, H.: Pili Annulati, Dermat. Ztschr. **24**:298, 1917.

14. Hoepke, H.: Ueber Veränderungen des Pigments und Luftgehaetes im Haar, Verhandl. der Anat. Gesellsch. **30**:127, 1921.

The following description of "ringed hairs" refers only to those taken from the scalp. Hairs from other parts of the body were examined, but showed no evidence of this condition. Before describing the individual cases we may summarize briefly the general characteristics common to all the specimens we have examined.

To the unaided eye ringed hair shows alternating light and dark segments varying in length in different persons. The ends of the segments appear to be sharply defined. Other macroscopic points vary with the subject and will be described.

Microscopically the hair preserves a uniform diameter throughout its length, tapering toward the tips no more than in normal hairs. No variations, real or apparent, in the diameter of the hairs at the site of the bands of light and dark could be made out by careful examination and rotation of the hair shaft. By transmitted light, the macroscopically light segments appear as long irregular dark splotches, while the dark segments of the hair appear as of more or less homogeneous structure with fine pigment granules normally distributed throughout the cortex. These macroscopically dark segments may consequently be regarded as essentially normal in structure. In order to avoid confusion in terminology those portions of the hair which appear white macroscopically and by reflected light under the microscope, but dark by transmitted light, are referred to as the aberrant segments while those parts which in all lights have the appearance of ordinary hair are called normal. Frequently the aberrant portions in the hair appear to extend almost to the cuticle of the shaft. In such cases, if the hair is rotated from 90 to 180 degrees about its long axis, this area shows variation in the configuration of what at first appeared to be its boundaries. This shows that the aberrant areas are not symmetrical with respect to all diameters of the hair shaft. The ends of the dark and light segments, though sharply defined, are not regular. The aberrant segments are surrounded by a layer of normal, pigment-bearing cortex varying in thickness as the shape and size of these segments permit. In many hairs the medulla is not to be made out with certainty and bears no definite relation to the aberrant segments, while in others it is wide and conspicuous throughout most of the length of the shaft. In these hairs the segments which are dark in transmitted light appear to be due to widening of the dark part representing the medulla. Where the medulla thus widens to form the dark segment of the hair, no qualitative changes can be made out. In other hairs having no medulla the aberrant segments occur just as regularly and definitely and bear the same general relations to the rest of the hair shafts as in hair in which the medulla is conspicuous. When the hairs are viewed by reflected light the segments which were dark appear light, and the former light segments appear dark.

Although hair from N_1 was not available for study, it is stated by her relatives that in early life she had the same banded type that characterizes many other members of the family, so it may be presumed that hers was a typical case of ringed hair.

The hair of N_{21} (Plate 1, N_{21}) is of dark blond color. It is fine and soft, of normal length and thickness and, collectively, does not present the appearance of ringed hair. However, when examining the individual hairs without the aid of a glass, one can see that about one-fifth of the hairs have a segmented appearance in some portion of the shafts and about one-fifth more of the hairs are doubtfully segmented. The rest of the hairs would not be classed as abnormal. Microscopically, the segmentation does not extend throughout the entire hair shaft, but hairs are found that have the condition at the tips while 2 or 3 cm. further back the appearance is very much that of the nonsegmented hairs. That the segmentation is not confined to that part of the shaft already outside the follicle is plainly shown by a hair which had the condition in the basal 3 mm. of its shaft. The root of this hair showed segmentation with the same interval of spacing that the portion above the skin showed. The whiteness appears in the shaft some time after it is well cornified, but still within the hair follicle. Those hairs that to the unaided eye have a doubtfully segmented appearance show slight microscopic indications of segmentation. The so-called air infiltration appears dark by transmitted light and occurs for the most part only in traces, but at more or less regular intervals.

The hair of N_{22}, aged 49, is mostly gray. Some of the hairs appear more white than others and occasionally one finds a short segment whiter in appearance than the rest of the hair. The few pigmented hairs are medium brown. No macroscopic segmentation is present. The white segments in the gray hairs and the hairs that look especially white have conspicuous medullas. There is no segmentation in the cortex.

The hair of N_{23}, aged 33, is reddish-brown, or auburn, and is normal.

N_{24}, aged 36, has dark hair with an occasional gray hair. Approximately one-half of the hairs show macroscopic segmentation. About one-half of the remaining hairs show microscopic segmentation (Fig. 1, N_{24}).

The hair of N_{31}, aged 25, is of normal growth and presents a rather peculiar light leaden appearance which on closer inspection resolves itself into alternate bands of gray and dark blond. All of the hairs have the segmentation, but occasionally one is found that is not uniformly segmented. Microscopically the hairs are quite typical of ringed hair (Plate 1, N_{31}, upper hair). Examination of these hairs within one-half hour after pulling them out of their follicles does not show any difference in the position of the dark segments with reference to the hair bulb from that observed when the same hairs are examined several days later.

No specimen is available from N_{32}, but his hair is said to be of normal growth but similar in appearance to that of N_{31}.

We were unable to secure a satisfactory number of hair specimens from N_{33}, aged 19, for study. In the specimens available no macroscopic evidence of segmentation is visible until the hairs are mounted in balsam when segments of irregular length appear lighter in color.

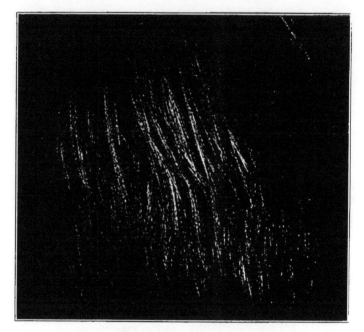

Fig. 1.—Photograph of back of head of N_{31}.

These lighter segments (by reflected light) correspond in position to segments of the medullas which are dark by transmitted light. There is no evidence of segmentation of the cortex.

In the S family, the hairs from the head of S_1, aged 58, are iron gray and brown. All of the gray hairs show segmentation into alternate opaque and rather translucent portions of the hair shafts, while approximately only one-half of the pigmented hairs are segmented. The segmentation is much more conspicuous in the gray hairs than in the pigmented hairs. As a whole, the segments are of uniform dimensions, but occasionally a hair is found that is not uniformly segmented. Microscopically the gray hairs are remarkably transparent (Fig. 1, S.).

There are slight indications of pigmentation in the cortical substance of these hairs. One can get a glimpse of light penetrating through the optically dark segments that cannot be seen in the pigmented specimens of ringed hair. Under a higher magnification the supposedly normal segments are seen to be rather diffusely sprinkled with small dark areas.

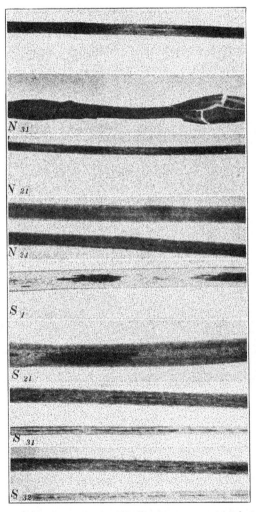

Fig. 2.—N_{31}, the upper part ($\times 40$) illustrates a typical hair of N_{31}; the lower part ($\times 40$) a hair of N_{31} boiled in liquid petrolatum. N_{21}, photograph ($\times 40$) of typical ringed hair of N_{21}. N_{24}, upper part illustrates ringed hair, lower, normal hair from N_{24} ($\times 73$). S_1, typical ringed gray hair of S_1 ($\times 73$). S_{21}, typical ringed hair of S_{21} ($\times 73$). S_{31}, ringed hair and normal hair with large medulla from S_{31} ($\times 73$). S_{32}, ringed hair and normal hair with large medulla from S_{32} ($\times 73$).

Where the ends of the hairs have been cut, there is no predominance of one type of segment cut through over the other. By reflected light the macroscopically white sections show up as clean-cut silvery areas. The same may be said of the small dark points between the white segments.

The hair of S_{21}, aged 30, is rich brown in color with an occasional gray hair, and it is only by careful examination of the individual hairs over a dark background that segmentation becomes apparent in about one-third of the hairs. Some of the hairs show the segmentation at the tip and others show it near the base, while still others show it throughout the entire length (Fig. 1, S_{21}). Microscopically many of the aberrant segments seem to be expansions of the medulla and show only inconspicuous medullary connections with each other. Smaller infiltration areas are no doubt an important factor in making the segmentation macroscopically less conspicuous in S_{21} than in N_{31} where the condition is typical. Many of the hairs that show marked segmentation also show large conspicuous medullas which extend almost uninterruptedly throughout the entire hair shafts.

The hair of S_{22}, aged 21, is of medium dark color. None of the hairs shows macroscopic or microscopic segmentation.

S_{31} and S_{32}, aged 13 months, have fine silky light brown hair with no macroscopic indications of any abnormalities. Microscopically the medulla is quite conspicuous, extending throughout the entire hair shaft as a relatively wide dark streak (by transmitted light). There are many interruptions of the continuity of the air-containing portions of the medulla which occasionally has a regularity that suggests segmentation. Portions of a hair that show unmistakable traces of cortical segmentation can be found (Fig. 1, S_{31} and S_{32}).

As this paper was being finished Dr. Whiting kindly sent us samples of hair from ten relatives of the S family. Of these, five showed unmistakably the ringed form. Two of the latter were for the most part gray and resembled the hairs from S_1. The other three presented nothing calling for special mention except that in at least one of them the banding became much less conspicuous after thirty minutes in thin balsam. This suggests the desirability of always examining hairs fresh or immediately after mounting.

K_1, at the age of 70, applied to Dr. Engman, about twenty years ago, for treatment for a gradually increasing bald spot in the center of the occiput. The patient's hair had never been abundant in growth and was at that time very coarse, sparse and gray. The ringed condition was conspicuous.

K_{21}, K_{22} and K_{23}, daughters of K_1, all have unmistakable ringed hair.

K_{31}, a man of 21 when seen by Dr. Engman, was almost entirely bald. Such hair as did grow was very fine and fragile and showed the ringed condition. Eventually he became entirely bald. The eyebrows were patchy.

K_{32} had a rather heavy growth of ringed hair and like his older brother was becoming bald on the occiput. His sister, K_{33}, had exceedingly tenuous, rich brown hair of normal growth. It was markedly ringed.

K_{34} and K_{35}, daughters of K_{22}, had fine, rich brown hair. The ringed condition was present in both. There was no tendency toward falling out or breaking off of the hair.

K_{36}, the daughter of K_{23}, had hair of more than average length and normal in every respect except that it was ringed. Her brother, K_{37}, is now 30 years old, has ringed hair, but shows no other abnormal tendencies.

EXPERIMENTAL DATA

The problem of determining the physical and chemical factors which cause the unusual appearance of these hairs presents itself, but it is outside the scope of this investigation to determine whether or not the condition can be produced experimentally. The following laboratory tests were made on representative speciments of ringed hairs in order to better establish or to disprove previous ideas about the presence of air in the hair substance as the cause for the white appearance of what otherwise seemed to be normal hair of a different color.

It is commonly recognized that the medulla of a hair often appears as a dark streak by transmitted light, due to the refraction of light by the walls of its air-containing spaces (MacLeod,[15] 1903). When normal hairs are soaked in oil and then viewed by transmitted light, the medullas no longer show up as dark streaks because of the light transmitting power of the oil which finds its way into the air spaces. When ringed hairs are put into liquid petrolatum and kept at about 70 C. for six or seven days, the aberrant segments are represented only by the outlines and traces of their former configuration. When the hairs were boiled in liquid petrolatum or kerosene for from ten to fifteen minutes, they became bright reddish brown, probably due to the yellowing effect of the oil within them and to a slight charring of the hair. Some of the hairs ruptured and appeared lighter in color than others. In these all traces of the white segmentation were gone. The hairs that retained their continuity still showed traces of their former banded appearance which was manifested by slight nodosity where the white segments had previously been located. Under the microscope the ruptured hairs showed large bubbles throughout their cortices and the medullas had enlarged so that the hairs had irregular central canals which connected

---

15. MacLeod, H. M. H.: Handbook of the Pathology of the Skin, London, Lewis, 1903, p. 213.

with almost every line of fracture in the cortex. Where the normal segments had previously been located only a smaller collection of bubbles remained. When pressure was exerted on the coverslip the hair was easily crushed leaving many fragments of hair and a line of bubbles, the largest of which were in positions corresponding to the former aberrant segment and subsequent nodosities mentioned in the foregoing.

Those hairs that had retained their integrity no longer showed the segments after they had been boiled enough to cause the appearance of the bubbles within them. Instead of the white segments there appeared to be relatively large cavities which were usually of sufficient size to cause the outlines of the hair to bulge opposite them, thus giving a beaded appearance suggestive of monilothrix (Fig. 1, N_{31}). Sometimes these cavities had ruptured and were filled with clear oil which permitted their walls to show up as normally pigmented hair cortex. Those portions of the medulla which after slight treatment appeared to be

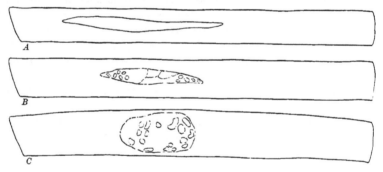

Fig. 3.—*A*, a camera lucida sketch including the outline of an aberrant segment (dark by transmitted light). *B*, the same segment after boiling in kerosene for five minutes; *C*, the same segment after boiling in kerosene for ten minutes ($\times$ 135).

patent and the small dark spots in the normal segments had likewise become frank cavities. These cavities had the appearance of globular gas bubbles. Unfortunately they could not be made to show in photographs, but the sketches (Fig. 3) are camera lucida outline drawings of the changes that take place while boiling in kerosene. The particular aberrant segment selected was not associated with a continuous medulla. Fig. 3 *A* shows the outline of the aberrant portion before boiling in oil. Figures 3 *B* and 3 *C* show the same hair segment after several minutes in boiling oil.

When hairs were subjected to the oxidizing action of nascent chlorin for forty-eight hours, they lost all their pigment and took on the appearance of normal, gray hair, but microscopically they presented an appearance suggestive of that in the untreated gray hairs of S...

The cortex was the same throughout. The medulla was clearly discernible with regular enlargements and constrictions corresponding in position to the light and dark segments, and extending throughout the length of the hair shafts. This observation furnishes an additional proof that the banding of the hair is not dependent on variations in pigment.

There are some indications that the gas globules in the hair are composed of carbon dioxid. If one of these hairs is immersed in a 5 per cent. solution of sodium hydroxid which has been thoroughly saturated with all the elements of air which obey the physical laws of partial pressures for gases in such a solution, the segmented appearance nevertheless disappears. This would not be expected if the gas were ordinary air, for the solution of sodium hydroxid would only be capable of chemically absorbing the very small percentage of carbon dioxid found in the air, and not the nitrogen, oxygen, etc. Since all the gas is absorbed by the sodium hydroxid, it is fair to assume that it may be carbon dioxid. Hairs treated in this manner swell and become softened but when thoroughly washed and dried they return to their normal size and recover their usual stiffness, seeming to be no more brittle than before treatment. But the segmented appearance does not return. Normal hairs with large medullae were treated with sodium hydroxid, but in these the medullae did not disappear so long as the hairs remained intact.

One of the segments was photographed at various stages of its disappearance in a 5 per cent. solution of sodium hydroxid at room temperature (Fig. 4). From the photographs it can be seen that the hair swelled to almost twice its normal size. During the course of such treatment the white segment is soon replaced by several globules which gradually grow in size until they occupy the space of practically the whole segment. In Fig. 4 B, taken nine and one-half minutes after the chemical treatment was begun, the bubbles have already begun to decrease in size. Finally they disappear entirely (Fig. 4 D). One would expect just this sort of reaction to occur if the white segments were caused by the aggregation of many very small interstices filled with carbon dioxid. Apparently as the hair substance becomes softened and swells by the action of the sodium hydroxid, the interstices enlarge and many of their very delicate walls break down letting the gas in them coalesce, thereby gradually forming appreciable globules. As the reaction proceeds there comes a time when the sodium hydroxid reaches what we assume to be carbon dioxid and absorbs it. This causes the gradual disappearance of the globules. It is possible to observe the formation and disappearance of the globules only under the high power lens, for under a low power lens the bubbles are not apparent and the dark segments merely appear gradually to fade away leaving the hair shaft homogeneous in appearance throughout.

Considerable difficulty was encountered when attempts were made to make serial transverse sections of these hairs. After many trials some success was attained by first putting a coating of thin pyroxylin over the hair and quickly following this by another coat of thick pyroxylin. This was hardened in chloroform for about twenty minutes and then

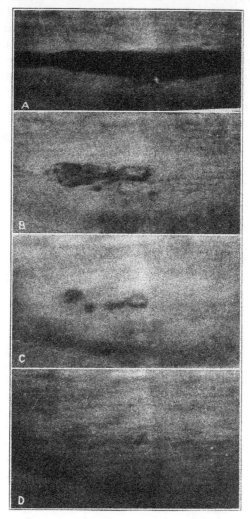

Fig. 4.—*A*, representative white segment (by transmitted light) of a hair from N₃₁ ($\times$ 355); *B*, same segment after nine and one-half minutes' treatment with 5 per cent. sodium hydroxid ($\times$ 355); C. same segment after fourteen minutes' treatment with 5 per cent. sodium hydroxid ($\times$ 355); *D*. same segment after eighteen minutes' treatment with 5 per cent. sodium hydroxid ($\times$ 355).

imbedded in hard paraffin and sectioned with a rotary microtome. By this method satisfactory sections from 15 to 20 microns thick were obtained. It was found convenient to dip the pyroxylin coated hair in an eosin solution before imbedding. This made the sections more conspicuous and saved a great deal of time in locating them on the slide. The paraffin ribbons were mounted on albumin coated slides and as soon as they were dry the paraffin was carefully dissolved off. To prevent the loss of sections it was necessary to exercise extreme care to maintain the slide almost level and to drop the xylol on the slide carefully. By following this technic, it was found to be unnecessary to let the ribbons dry on the slide. As soon as the xylol had evaporated off the slide, locations of the sections were marked by drawing rings around them with ink. A cover-glass was then put on in balsam.

A study of sections prepared in this manner showed that the dark areas were somewhat smaller than they had appeared to be in the intact

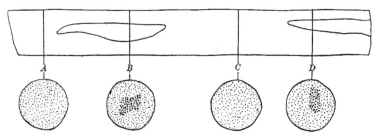

Fig. 5.—Camera lucida sketch of ringed hair and transverse sections of the same at the levels indicated by *A, B,* C and D ($\times$ 135).

hair, a fact no doubt to be attributed to the magnification concomitant to their centrally placed position in the shaft. The upper portion of Figure 5 is a camera lucida sketch of a hair before sectioning, and the lower portion is made up of sketches of the transverse sections at the places indicated by the lines across in the upper part of the sketch. It will be seen that where the aberrant segments are sectioned there is also a darker portion (by transmitted light) in the transverse sections. Where the sections were cut thinner than 15 microns, it was difficult to make out this area with definiteness. The sections between the aberrant segments show a more or less homogeneous hair cortex, and in the hair figured no medulla. These sections failed to reveal any apparent open spaces among the cells, but as well as could be made out these dark areas were made up of the keratin walls of very small interstices which reflected some of the transmitted light out of the field. Examination of the sections under the high power lens has added nothing to what could be seen under the low power.

DISCUSSION

If one is to judge the frequency with which ringed hair is to be observed in the white race by the number of references in the literature, it is a rare condition. From the summary it may be seen that only eighteen cases have been mentioned and that of these only fourteen have been described. Six of these cases were in females. There is no reference in the literature to any cases in which the condition has been transmitted directly from one generation to the next, but there is one case in which it occurred in a brother of the subject and another case in which it occurred in two maternal uncles. There is no effective attempt to assign to it a reasonable etiologic factor except heredity.

REVIEW OF CASES IN THE LITERATURE

Author	Date	Sex	Age, Years	Duration, Years	Family History	Associated Condition and Remarks
Karsch............	1846	M	19	?	None	None
Wilson...........	1867	M	7½	2	None	None
Frazer...........	1875	F (?)	?	?	?	?
Crocker..........	1893	F	8	2	None	Noticed following influenza and contagious ophthalmia
Unna..............	1894	M	26	?	?	Leukonychia
Frew............. (McCall Anderson)	1894	F	9½	1	None	Condition disappeared
Kiwull............	1895	F	20	3	None	Alopecia prematura universalis (neurotica ?)
Galloway..........	1896	{M / {M	8 / 10	8} / 10}	Brothers	Hair had peculiar lusterless appearance
Brayton..........	1897	M	16	14	2 uncles	"Sandy" appearance
Meachen..........	1902	M	8	8	None	Syndactylia, polydactylism and melanoderma
Crocker..........	1903	M	39	?	None	Trichorrhexis nodosa
Fox..............	1906	F / M	25 / ?	1 / ?	None / ?	"Dusty" appearance / Student
Haxthausen.......	1917	F	18	18	None	Present in all the hairs of the head
Hoepke...........	1921	M	23	10(?)	?	Hair said to show seasonal variations

We do not believe that any of the associated conditions mentioned by previous writers can be proved to have been responsible for the hair condition described in these persons.

The condition occurs in various degrees and no doubt there have been many unreported instances of it in the families of the patients previously described. Two of the families in which we have found it to occur do not seem to attach any particular importance to it nor to be very much interested in it even though they are above the average in intelligence. For instance, N_{31} knew that his maternal grandmother and his mother had the condition in their early life and that it is present in his only brother, but he did not know that it is still present macroscopically in his mother and present to a greater extent in his maternal uncle. Our three families have members in whom only normal hair is found. It occurs in females in more than the reported ratio as gathered from the literature. It obviously may be an inherited condition, and not an acquired condition, for none of the members of these two families have undergone experiences that could be held responsible for it. The mere fact that it has been found in persons who have had other abnormal conditions does not indicate that any one of the diseases named in the literature as associated with it can be an etiologic factor. Indeed, their diversity is entirely too great, and conversely, thousands of people have had the same diseases without having ringed hair. The cases of Galloway and Brayton, respectively, show that the condition occurs in families, and our three families show that it may be directly transmitted from one generation to another.

As to the cause of the whiteness in the white segments, we can simply state that it is caused by the presence of very minute spaces filled with gas. The walls of these spaces reflect the light incident to them thereby causing segments of the hair to appear white by reflected light as seen under ordinary conditions. For this reason the white segments of the hairs are not true gray in the accepted sense. In a hair of S_1 et al. there are both truly gray hair and hair that appears white on account of the presence of gas cavities within them. The segmented condition is more conspicuous in hairs gray by senescence than it is in pigmented hair. In the latter we have shown that the same kind and amount of pigment exists in the white segments as in the dark segments, and there is no question of a pigmentary atrophic condition as suggested by Meachen.

Kaposi [16] (1895) does not think that the presence of air bubbles in the hair can cause graying of hair. Strong [17] (1921) states that hair is white for the same reason that any transparent substance in a finely divided state is white. He looks on hair as being made of numerous cornified epithelial cells more or less completely fused. These cells furnish many reflecting surfaces and the amount of undispersed light reflected depends on the number of the internal reflecting surfaces not screened by pigment. We agree with this view, but it seems that in addition to this kind of whiteness another slightly different kind occurs as in the condition under discussion in which the reflecting surfaces are relatively farther apart than in the normal hair, thereby allowing less screening by pigment. We feel that there can no longer be any doubt that hair may appear white as a result of the presence of gas spaces in its substance.

CONCLUSIONS

The appearance of pili annulati is caused by gas-filled interstices in the cortex and medulla of the hair.

---

16. Kaposi, M.: Pathology and Treatment of Diseases of the Skin. English Trans., 1895, p. 486.

17. Strong, R. M.: The Causes of Whiteness of Hair and Feathers. Science **54**:356, 1921.

The condition occurs in normally pigmented hair and in hair turned gray as a process of senescence. It is not due to a lack of pigment or to pigment atrophy.

There is no evidence that the condition is caused by any known pathologic process.

It may vary in the degree to which it affects an individual hair, and may vary widely in the number of hairs it affects in different persons.

The condition is compatible with the normal growth of hair.

It may be transmitted by heredity directly from one generation to the next.

IS SYPHILIS CURABLE AND CAN IT BE ERADICATED?*

VICTOR G. VECKI, M.D.

SAN FRANCISCO

If ever proof were needed that animal experimentation is necessary, we need only point to the enormous services that science has rendered to the human race by numerous discoveries in regard to proper understanding of the character, behavior and treatment of syphilis. Experiments continue incessantly in the many laboratories of the various countries. We are anxiously awaiting reports on new discoveries which will lead to further perfection of our weapons in the fight against this most dangerous, this incredibly common and so frequently treacherous, disease.

It is due to animal experimentation by many thousands of tireless, and scarcely ever mentioned, scientists, that the assertion may be made that syphilis is curable, that it is comparatively easily curable, and that when the situation is understood by those in power, the scourge can be suppressed.

In order to cure syphilis one must first discard all rules for dosage and the number of injections to be given in the various stages of the disease. There is, and there can be, no schedule of any value to direct the physician in the treatment of syphilis. Every patient must be treated after careful study of his case. To tell a patient as soon as one is sure of the diagnosis, or even before, that he should receive a certain number of treatments at certain intervals is surely wrong. The patient's history and his physical condition, not the condition of the blood alone, must be clearly understood, and even then the physician is obliged to feel his ground before he can tell what kind and how long a treatment may in all probability be necessary to accomplish a cure.

The objection may be raised that all this takes too much time, and we must acknowledge that, at present, enough time is not given to the treatment of most cases of syphilis, because this seems impossible. In private practice, however, this excuse is not valid, because the best and most painstaking attention is not too good, and the man who has not time enough to devote to the proper treatment of a patient should not accept a case. Even in institutions, with real understanding and the necessary endowments, everything can be done, and in some is done.

---

*Read before the Fifty-First Annual Meeting of the Medical Society of the State of California, at Yosemite, May 16, 1922.

Efficient treatment can be given only after a correct diagnosis is made. For this one cannot depend entirely on the Wassermann reaction; one must be familiar with the various clinical symptoms; and must not rely on the personal history of the patient.

ABORTION OF SYPHILIS IN ITS PRIMARY STAGES

Most can be accomplished in the early primary stages when the chancre first appears, and, unfortunately, at that time there may be some doubt about the diagnosis. The experienced eye will be able to recognize a beginning syphilitic chancre before there is any induration or adenitis. Of course search for the spirochete must be instituted in any kind of a lesion on the genitals. Even when the most experienced physician may not be certain of the diagnosis the patient should be given the benefit of the slightest doubt. There is such a thing as therapeutic diagnosis. We now have remedies which, if used properly, do not damage the system and there is no excuse for allowing an infection to advance to a stage where the required treatment is more complicated and cure is more difficult.

Every case of early syphilis can and must be aborted. The way depends entirely on the bodily condition of the patient and his toleration for the remdies to be used. It is imperative before any treatment is instituted in any case, and at any stage of syphilis, to know the patient in every respect; therefore, a minute examination is indispensable. While we know that every patient must be treated, we must also known whether the patient is tuberculous, epileptic, has heart disease. and the condition of his digestive organs, liver, and kidneys; the patient's skin must be inspected for all, even seemingly trivial, skin eruptions. It is important to distinguish a syphilitic kidney. liver or circulatory system affection from a nonsyphilitic one.

When trying to abort syphilis, the stronger, the younger. the healthier the patient, the bolder the physician may be. but even in seemingly perfect cases there may be an oversensitiveness to the chosen remedy.

The doses must be regulated by the patient's bodily condition. by the reaction following each injection, and to a certain extent also by the weight, excluding obesity, which is not a sign of resisting power.

INTRAVENOUS INJECTION

Whoever becomes familiar with the method of intravenous injection of the various arsenical preparations surely will have no contempt. but only a sound respect. for this treatment. A conscientious physician will always fear untoward results, be apprenhensive of accidents. and take no risks. Therefore. the apparatus itself must he of the best and the technic perfect. It may be contrary to the routine of most clinicians and thus also contrary to their opinions, but it is nevertheless true that intravenous injections of the various arsphenamin preparations are, as a rule, best given by the gravitation method under all possible precautions. When one has to deal with large veins the hand syringe may be used, and by drawing sufficient quantities of blood into the syringe before and after the injection and by injecting slowly, accidents and the damage to the vein itself can be avoided. I must, however, warn against the busy man's injection, the negligent, the lazy man's injection and mainly against the ignorant man's injection. Too many patients are seen who, after having suffered a few intravenous injections, have no available veins left. Too often we hear that accidents, such as paravenous injection, seldom happen and one may read the boast of a clinician that he seldom has any infiltration and only once has he had a necrosis. The physician who cannot eventually give the complete, necessary course of treatments into one and the same vein should know that something is wrong with his apparatus or with his technic.

The most important arguments in favor of the gravitation method are that not a drop of the medicine is given before one is positively in the receiving vein, and that the vein after receiving all of the intended dose is being flushed with normal salt solution.

There are a number of small details that, in spite of their apparent insignificance, have an important bearing on the ultimate result, and the observation of every one of the precautions which may seem trivial, and for which the busy man says he has no time, will repay the physician by the absence of angioneurotic and other by-effects of the treatment.

This is the proper method of giving an intravenous injection: The patient, whose condition is well known to the physician, and who was instructed to eat a very light dairy meal at least three hours before the treatment, after his urine has been examined and the blood pressure taken, is placed on the operating table. All tightly fitting clothing, chiefly the collar, having been removed or unfastened, the proper vein is selected; the patient's arm is placed at right angle to the shoulder on a cushion so that the elbow is perfectly straight and at the same height as the shoulder; a blood pressure band is put around the arm, well above the elbow; then the skin over the vein is cleaned and partly anesthetized with a solution of alcohol and ether. When the blood pressure band is pumped up to 110, the vein shows at its best, and the needle can easily be plunged in.

The apparatus must previously be sterilized in an enameled sterilizer and in fresh boiling water.

Every ampule should be closely inspected for cracks after the label is washed off, and then immersed for a further test and with the purpose of sterilizing into alcohol. The one who handles the ampule, prepares the solution or handles the apparatus, should wear sterile gloves; the solution should be made with freshly distilled and redistilled water. If the patient has a clean intestinal tract, it is hardly ever necessary to use epinephrin, caffein, ether or camphorated oil, which, however, should always be available; nor is it ever necessary to use artificial respiration.

After the injection, the patient is instructed to hold his arm straight and elevated for a few minutes; if necessary, a drop of collodion is placed on the small puncture hole; then he is allowed to rest for about five minutes.

It is best to give the injections in the afternoon or evening after the patient's day's work is done. The patient is allowed to eat a light meal about three hours after the injection, and should keep as quiet as possible. Automobile, street-car, steamboat, and railroad trips home may be permitted; and when the proper dose has been properly injected, patients may attend theaters, concerts and banquets without any injurious effects.

Every patient should be treated as if he were supersensitive and even when all precautions are taken, he should be watched during the whole time of the injection. In the thousands of intravenous injections of arsphenamin, neo-arsphenamin, silver arsphenamin, and neo-silver arsphenamin given at my office during the last twelve years, only twice were symptoms observed of what was apparently an attack of angioneurosis. During the first nine years of our experience with arsphenamin and neo-arsphenamin, as a rule, only maximal doses were given. The possibility of complication must never be disregarded; the patient must be watched for reddening of the face and ears, reddening and bulging of the eyes, paleness of the nose, beating of the carotids, coughing, dyspnea, a feeling of oppression, nausea, vomiting, a high pulse rate—all symptoms which are so vividly described by many authors and which are never seen by men of experience who use careful methods.

It may be that the glorious San Francisco climate with its absence of hot days explains the absence of angioneurosis; or is it that sometimes a small undissolved particle of the medicament is overlooked and causes havoc in the circulatory system?

Any alarm signal given by the patient's organs must be watched for and never disregarded. Future treatment depends greatly on the proper interpretation of these signs. It is most important to know how the patient feels after each injection. The dosage of subsequent injections should depend entirely on the tolerance shown by the system for the preceding dose. Fever following an intravenous injection of an arsphenamin preparation requires careful watching and proper interpretation, so that the spirochetal fever may be differentiated from a fever that appears after a number of injections, when it may mean the development of intolerance. Even the fever following a first injection in cases of florid syphilis should never exceed 39 degrees. To avoid high fever the first dose given should be very small, or the arsenic treatment should be preceded by several doses of mercury. Should fever appear after several injections of arsphenamin have been given, it is imperative to use a smaller dose and to lengthen the intervals between injections. The possibility that the arsenic is not being properly eliminated and therefore is causing a cumulative action must always be apprehended.

Any reaction following an injection should pass before another dose is given. The patient's skin, examined before treatment is instituted, must be examined before each injection, and the patient instructed to report any unusual feeling, such as dryness, itching, or burning. Dangerous, even fatal dermatitis, may follow if slight alarm signals are disregarded. Many symptoms are explained by the Herxheimer reaction, but even this calls for care in future dosage.

TREATMENT OF SYPHILITIC PATIENTS

The ideal treatment would be to examine regularly all excretions and secretions, thus controlling the elimination of arsenic in every case. This is, unfortunately, not possible in the great majority of cases; therefore close watching and interpreting of symptoms is necessary. The urine must be examined for albumin and urobilin before each treatment. The total output of urine during the twenty-four hours preceding an injection should be measured, because a reduction in the output is a signal of an impairment of the kidney function that should not be overlooked.

Icterus, of which we read so much, I have seen only in some European hospitals; it surely can and must be avoided. Every syphilitic patient under treatment must be instructed in general hygiene, because all the resources that the patient can muster must be mobilized in the fight against the disease. The fight may be long; therefore regular habits, proper feeding, exercise and the promotion of a healthy skin function are absolutely necessary. Strict cleanliness of the mouth and all other orifices is imperative. The skin, this important partner of the kidneys, must never be forgotten. Turkish and similar baths are indicated in most cases. Proper functioning of the bowels is of great importance.

In general, the physician should endeavor to have the patient feel well. Fortunately, the remedies now at our disposal, when properly used, do not weaken the patient, but build him up.

It can never be emphasized enough that treatment of a syphilitic patient requires a great deal of care, consequently also of time, and that wholesale treatment produces poor results and cures only by accident, except in places in which even the treatment en masse is thoroughly systematized, as it is in a few clinics.

When beginning the treatment of a patient with syphilis, the physician is confronted with the question of preparing the patient for the treatment; this depends entirely on the patient's physical condition. Then come the questions of initial dose, of frequency of single treatments, and of length of the whole treatment. Plans may be made, but modifications of such plans are frequently necessary on account of subsequent indications. There must and there can be no fixed rules, no schedules, no stated time for any phase of the disease.

One may use large doses at short intervals in all patients with primary infection that come under treatment before there is any positive blood reaction. Twelve injections of silver arsphenamin, or better of neo-silver arsphenamin, given within one month may abort the disease and cure the patient. Success is almost certain in robust people who can be given at first a small dose of neo-silver arsphenamin and the next day a maximal dose. This usually causes quite a reaction, but after twenty-four hours spirochetes invariably cannot be found. Four or five days later, and in cases in which there is not much reaction, another full dose is injected. On week later the entire procedure is repeated, and if altogether twelve injections are given within the shortest possible time, the patient should be cured. In a primary infection after the blood reaction has become positive, eight intravenous injections of mercuric oxycyanid followed by twelve injections of silver arsphenamin or neo-silver arsphenamin may be sufficient to cure the disease, but one should remember that when an infection is over three weeks old the prospects of aborting it are not good.

Nothing must be taken for granted, and even those patients in whom an aborting of the disease is almost sure must remain under observation, and their blood frequently examined.

It must be emphasized that whenever there is any degree of a positive reaction, or when clinical symptoms reappear, the subsequent treatment must be more intensive than the preceding one which failed. Sometimes the remedy itself must be changed.

Late and latent active and inactive so-called tertiary syphilis requires long and persistent treatment, regulated by the blood reaction and the condition of the glands. It must not be forgotten that the glands are at least as important a pathognomonic symptom and guide for further treatment as any kind of blood test.

Neurosyphilis demands slowly increasing doses, especially small first doses wherever vital parts may be involved, while so-called para-syphilitic diseases, chiefly tabes dorsalis, yield only to long, regular, persistent and proper treatment.

As Vernes teaches, it is the rhythmic, not the desultory and jerky treatment that accomplishes a cure. At all the numerous treating stations under his direction at Paris, prospective patients are given a leaflet telling them that if they do not intend to be regular in their appointments, not to waste their and the physician's time. That is what every physician should tell every syphilitic patient.

The intermittent treatment has failed; it must be abandoned and replaced by the continuous treatment—by treatment until the patient is cured.

Medication.—An important question confronting the physician is that of the remedy to use. At the time when much was expected from one or a few injections of arsphenamin, it was the consensus of opinion, forced on syphilologists by numerous disappointments, that mercury is indispensable in all cases, and that only a combined treatment with arsphenamin and mercury may lead to a cure. Even at present, few syphilologists are willing to abandon mercury entirely; but we can see plainly the handwriting on the wall for mercury. Experience with the newer arsenical preparations, chiefly those combined with silver, causes less frequent use of mercury, which is a poison only, and which invariably, after prolonged use, causes chronic poisoning. At present it appears that mercury should be used only for patients who are hypersensitive to arsenical preparations, and as an introduction to the arsphenamin treatment in florid syphilis and in cases of brain involvement in which a Herxheimer reaction might be too dangerous. Recent experiences with the use of very small doses of arsphenamin eliminate more and more the necessity of returning to mercury. Kolle's experiments on animals have demonstrated that mercury is active against the spirochete only in almost fatal doses. Kolle was apparently surprised that syphilitic rabbits tolerate larger doses than nonsyphilitic rabbits. Sigmund taught the same thing about man more than forty years ago.

When mercury must be used, the choice of the preparation is of great importance. Many European clinics are returning to the use of intramuscular injections of insoluble salts and apparently also to the old idea that an almost toxic dose must be used. It may be that Kolle's experiments on animals have something to do with the adoption of such treatment that, as some clinicians confess, it disturbs them greatly, but it cures them. Every experienced physician remembers cases in which accidental mercurial poisoning in the course of some antisyphilitic treatment almost brought the patient's life to an untimely end; but the syphilis was cured. The severe stomatitis, intestinal inflammation, albuminuria and cylindruria caused by almost toxic doses, the terrible suffering and extreme emaciation combined with the danger of losing the patient's life, are too great a risk to take, even though the syphilis is cured. Therefore, one must always be sure to use the proper dose. One can never be sure of the dose brought into activity when using intramuscular injections of insoluble mercurial salts, when using the inunctions. Risks are easily avoided by using intravenous injections of mercuric oxycyanid, proper dilution of which even prevents damage to the vein.

The literature on the newer arsenic preparations is already enormous. In Europe, the reports on silver arsphenamin, for a time made almost daily, are becoming rare; therefore, we hear more about neo-silver arsphenamin. After almost two years' experience with the silver arsphenamin preparations—ever since my associate, Dr. Ottinger, brought a large amount of silver arsphenamin from Europe, and on the basis of my observations at many European clinics, I am glad that I can join the large majority of syphilologists who are so highly pleased with silver arsphenamin and neo-silver arsphenamin. The latter positively is the best arsenic preparation at our disposal; it is easy of solution, very slow to oxydize, and is the most parasitotrope and the least organotrope of all antisyphilitic remedies. We know that silver itself is an antisyphilitic, and experience teaches that the addition of silver to the arsenic has not increased the toxicity, but it has increased the effectiveness, of the remedy. It seems that the silver molecule activates the arsphenamin molecule. The arsenic being the spirillicide, the silver takes the place of mercury as the agent to make conditions in the tissues unfavorable to the multiplication of the spirochete, without being as toxic as mercury. There is no real evidence that the use of silver arsphenamin and neo-silver arsphenamin is dangerous— no case of fatal encephalitis has been reported. It is asserted that when silver arsphenamin is used the arsenic remains longer in the system. Interesting experiments by the Swedish chemist Engleson, seemed to demonstrate that the bulk of the arsenic remained in the patient's body up to the sixteenth day. If this were true, we should have more cases of cumulative action; it is, however, a warning against carelessness in its use, and a plea for the frequent use of small doses in preference to massive ones.

Again it should be emphasized that it is imperative to ascertain the tolerance in every case. There are instances of idiosyncrasy in which it is dangerous to persist, though in experienced hands such intolerance may be overcome by the tentative use of very small doses. Vernes is right when he asserts that the intolerants, when finally induced into enduring the remedy to a certain extent, profit by it considerably more than those that can stand any reasonable dose without reaction.

Kolle has demonstrated on rabbits that a very small injection immunizes the animal, so that the day after, even otherwise lethal doses are tolerated. It is a fact that if in some hypersensitive people a very small dose is given one day, a medium dose may be given with impunity the day after. Some authors recommend, also as a result of Kolle's animal experiments, one or more preliminary injections of collargol to immunize the patient for doses of silver arsphenamin.

The desire is expressed frequently to have an arsenic preparation that could be used for intramuscular injections without causing much pain and local reaction, as it would be desirable to have a deposit in the body; results would then be obtained similar to those obtained with the early intramuscular injections of arsphenamin. Considering that we would then again be placed in the position of never knowing the real dose the patient is utilizing in a given time, there may be some doubt that such a preparation would be of great advantage. The present preparations of arsenic cause too much pain, infiltration, and what is worse, too much local destruction; and so one must agree with Kreibich of Prague, who recommends the intramuscular route only for cases in which life itself is in danger.

It has been proved that silver arsphenamin and more so neo-silver arsphenamin, even when used intravenously, form deposits of silver and deposits of arsenic in the liver, spleen, kidneys, lungs, heart, bones and muscles. This is a further argument for small doses. Lenzman, for instance, demonstrated that an intravenous injection of 0.1 gm. silver arsphenamin had a good influence on condylomas, but that when two daily doses of half the quantity were injected the effect was considerably better.

In consequence of the lower toxicity of neo-silver arsphenamin, the total dose in any given case can be reached more quickly and safely, and therefore, with persistent, regular, rhythmic treatment our prognosis is better.

Neurorecidives.—While physicians who give sufficient treatment seldom see a neurorecidive, those who use the silver arsphenamin preparations in proper doses do not see them at all. Some authors recommend that in order to avoid a neurorecidive, a preliminary mercury treatment should be given in all cases in which an aborting of the disease may not be expected. For various reasons it is surely better to give mercury before arsphenamin in all such cases.

It is a question whether we now see cases of neurorecidive more frequently than in the pre-arsphenamin era, when we used to consider headache as one of the regular symptoms of syphilis. At present there are different methods of examination and different methods of interpretation of symptoms. Insufficient treatment and haphazard methods will always be responsible for neurorecidives, no matter what remedies may be used. It is important to know that neurorecidives are more frequent in cases of primary infection in the face and mouth, also in cases in which there are early syphilitic manifestations on the scalp.

Personally, I have seen cases of neurorecidive only in persons who refused sufficient treatment. I have never seen any damaging effect from arsphenamin medication on the opticus or acousticus, not even when treating persons belonging to professions in which hypersensitiveness of the acoustic system could be expected, such as musicians, blacksmiths and even artillerymen. Recently some Vienna clinicians claimed that damage was done to the cochlear and vestibular parts of the ear by treatment with silver arsphenamin.

Syphilis of the large blood vessels and gumma of the brain should be treated with very small doses, and it is best to give a preliminary mercurial treatment. Even a mild Herxheimer reaction might be too dangerous. Very small doses of arsphenamin may be given twice a day.

The treatment of patients with neurosyphilis also requires a great deal of precaution. Most of the patients are older people, worn out by various treatments, structural changes, impaired functions, suffering and mental worry. The treatment of an old person evidently must be different from that of a vigorous, young person. Whenever we touch the subject we are confronted with the imperative demand for individualization. Tabes is influenced more by silver arsphenamin preparations than by any other remedy, but tabetic patients generally tolerate small doses only. Leredde, however, reports good results in tabetic patients in whom the heart and kidneys are in good condition from weekly injections of neo-arsphenamin in gradually increasing doses, from 0.1 gm. up to 1.2 gm.

A rather severe Herxheimer reaction sometimes follows injections of silver arsphenamin preparations in tabetic patients. No amount of medication will relieve the unbearable pain, but draining of the spinal canal invariably does so. Tabes is most decidedly influenced if immediately after about every third or fourth weekly injection of neo-silver arsphenamin the spinal canal is drained almost dry. Treatments of this kind must be given at the hospital; proper rest is necessary and careful watching of the patient as a guide for future treatments. Although I have seen surprisingly good results from intraspinal injections of arsphenamized and mercurialized serum, I am now convinced that equally good results may be obtained from intravenous injections of silver arsphenamin preparations, at times followed by draining of the spinal canal. Such treatment is never dangerous and causes the patient little discomfort. It is very interesting and instructive to watch the progress made by having the spinal fluid obtained at each draining examined.

Reports on results obtained in paretic patients are not encouraging, though the remissions after treatments with silver arsphenamin seem to be somewhat too frequent to be accidental. It speaks well for the low toxicity of silver arsphenamin when it is reported that paralytic patients were given total doses up to 10 gm., and even in the cases in which it did no good, it did no harm.

Even in patients with no neurosyphilitic symptoms, the spinal fluid must be examined.

When it was made possible by Plaut's method of obtaining blood-less spinal fluid from rabbits, Mulzer's experiments with two kinds of spirochetal strains demonstrated that there are, as Ravogli expresses himself, strains that seem to be dermatropic while others must be neurotropic. The one, a strain obtained from an Italian source, caused an increase of the cells in the spinal fluid before any other symptom of a successful inoculation became visible. Then, we must ask ourselves, when does the neurorecidive appear? Surely we must not forget that there are also individual differences and great inequalities of the resisting power.

A great number of modern authors seem to ignore the iodid completely. Probably the neglecting of this remedy is responsible for many failures. It may have no direct spirochetal-destroying power; its chief action seems to be softening of the syphilitic foci. It has an affinity for diseased tissues, as these attract and retain it. Loeb, for instance, found about six times as much iodid in affected glands as in normal ones. Iodid should be given even in the early stages between arsphenamin or mercurial treatments, but its use is imperative in the late stages when one deals with gumma, bone involvement and sclerotic processes In neurosyphilis, when given before any other treatment is instituted. it often prevents a Herzheimer reaction.

Iodid may be injected intravenously and is then most effective. Klemperer injects 5, 10 and even 20 gm. of a 10 per cent. solution two or three times a week.

In patients who are weakened by too strenuous treatment, especially with mercury, the combination of iodid with iron in the form of syrup of ferrous iodid renders invaluable service.

WHEN MAY A SYPHILITIC PATIENT BE CONSIDERED CURED?

The question most difficult to answer that confronts the syphilologist is: When is a patient cured? A persistent negative Wassermann reaction of the blood and the spinal fluid, other negative findings in the latter, chiefly a normal cell count, and absence of all clinical symptoms and adenopathy, are considered proofs of a cure. There is great diversity of opinion as to how long the all-around negative findings must be established before the patient can be declared cured.

It is to be regretted that the colorimetric reaction of Vernes is being ignored by the medical profession at large, although its correctness is endorsed by the highest French, Belgian, German, and Swiss authorities, and even Carrel of the Rockefeller Institute authorized the publication of his judgment that at present the only places in the world where syphilis is treated scientifically are the Vernes' institutions.

Cornwall, who is investigating the Vernes reaction at Columbia University and the New York City Hospital, recently published a comprehensive report, and therefore it may be sufficient to say that according to Vernes: 1. All syphilitic infection is accompanied by a pathognomonic modification in the stability of the blood serum and spinal fluid. 2. This pathognomonic alteration disappears under the influence of arsenical treatment, but each time that the treatment has been insufficient it reappears from the second to the fifth month, rarely from the fifth to the seventh. 3. When, following arsenical treatment, this pathognomonic alteration remains absent for eight months after the discontinuance of treatment, and the spinal fluid is negative, reappearance has not been noted.

From personal investigation at Vernes' therapeutic, or as they are called, prophylactic, stations, and information gained from Parisian medical authorities not very friendly to Vernes, I am convinced that his assertions are in accordance with the truth and facts. We must also value Vernes' reaction because it permits a quantitative diagnosis, a periodic measuring of the poison left in the system.

We have learned that the most dangerous cases are those in which the patient fails to produce antibodies, and therefore his blood shows a negative Wassermann reaction. This is not possible with Vernes' reaction. The Vernes reaction will soon be available everywhere: under its control patients can be treated until a cure is accomplished.

The dangerous condition of destroying almost all spirochetes and then stopping treatment so as to give the surviving spirochetal clusters more favorable conditions for their pernicious activities must be avoided at any cost. We agree with Vernes' teachings, that one must do too much in order to do enough, but one must add that even the "too much" done shall be done so that it causes no damage to the patient's system.

CONCLUSIONS

We must hail with a certain enthusiasm neo-silver arsphenamin on account of its roborant action on the patient's entire system, and because with it one can with impunity follow Vernes' advice that each subsequent treatment must be more energetic and more powerful than the preceding one which failed to cure.

Neo-silver arsphenamin is prompt in its action on primary symptoms. The induration disappears promptly; secondary skin lesions, papules and condylomata lata, which are generally very stubborn, invariably disappear after six or eight injections, and one is always able to obtain a negative Wassermann reaction in from six to eight weeks, and by using a total of 3 to 6 gm. of the remedy.

Late syphilis seems to be easier to influence whenever the Wassermann reaction is positive, more difficult in the rare cases in which the blood reaction is negative, although clinical symptoms allow no doubt about the diagnosis. It will take years of experience to learn about the duration of the Wassermann negative period, even though the blood be tested every month. Personally, I have never seen any disagreeable by-effects from the use of neo-silver arsphenamin. Twice I thought it best to interrupt the treatment for about ten days on account of warning symptoms on the patient's skin; I suspect that in these cases I was a little too eager in the medication.

So far, I am sure that even energetic, although cautious use of neo-silver arsphenamin could not provoke albuminuria and cylindruria in originally intact kidneys.

Vernes refuses to try the silver arsphenamin preparations because, he told me, he obtains good results with neo-arsphenamin and galyl. While this is true, I suspect that the German origin of the new preparations is the real reason. One must agree with him when he teaches that a syphilitic patient properly treated under proper control has nothing to fear; he will not be undertreated or overtreated, he will not be damaged by the treatment, and he can be cured. In cases in which irreparable damage has been done to any kind of tissues, the progress of the disease and its further destructive action can be arrested.

The statement that syphilis is a comparatively easily curable disease is no exaggeration; we may insist that all patients can be cured, but we must consider no case easy; in fact, we must approach each case as a rebellious one.

It will be a great step toward the eradication of syphilis when the bulk of the medical profession becomes quite familiar with the character, and especially with the proper treatment, of syphilis. No doubt, we are progressing almost rapidly.

We must understand that syphilis is not a vice disease—just an infectious disease like any other. Again, we must give the patient the benefit of the doubt when he says he does not know, or when he tries to explain when and where he acquired the disease.

Compulsory reporting of the disease to the health authorities would be a calamity—another slap at justice, another assault on the professional secret, and, while the mollycoddles may not care, another unconstitutional assault on personal liberty.

When those in power will have been taught by the physicians of the country what syphilis does to humanity, then the city, state and national authorities will provide the necessary funds to fight the scourage. When the cost of insuring safety for every person, syphilitic or nonsyphilitic, is considered, also the cost of free, proper and kind treatment for the syphilitic person who cannot afford to pay his own way, it may be huge, but it still is quite insignificant when compared with the cost of maintenance of hospitals, asylums, prisons and orphanages populated by syphilitic persons and their tainted offspring, besides the amounts spent by persons who cannot afford it, in loss of time, medicine and treatment.

In our country the depopulating influences of syphilis may not be of the same importance as in countries in which food for cannons must be raised, but the degenerating influence of the disease on the race is of more consequence.

Progress in stamping out syphilis will be made when proper treatment shall be easy of access and easy to take, and when it will be made easy for every one to find out whether he has syphilis or not.

We know that syphilis is a curable disease in the hands of an experienced syphilologist, but in order to abolish it antisyphilitic remedies must cease to be dangerous weapons in the hands of the majority employing them.

516 Sutter Street.

A SIMPLE QUANTITATIVE PRECIPITATION REACTION FOR SYPHILIS

THIRD COMMUNICATION *

R. L. KAHN, Sc.D.

LANSING, MICH.

Further studies on the precipitation reaction for syphilis proposed by the author [1] suggested several changes in the procedure which appeared to enhance considerably the value of the test. It will be recalled that in the original method a cholesterinized antigen was employed, and because of its high sensitiveness the test was completed after four hours' incubation. In the new procedure a noncholesterinized antigen is also employed. The same alcoholic extract of heart muscle is used with and without the addition of cholesterin. When employing the noncholesterinized antigen, however, it was observed that the rapidity of precipitation is not as marked as in the case of the cholesterinized one. It was necessary to incubate the tests with the former antigen over night in order to elicit complete precipitation in most cases. On the basis of this finding, and because of another consideration to be discussed presently, it was deemed best to employ overnight incubation also with the cholesterinized antigen. Finally, it seemed advisable to adopt the plus sign as a basis for recording results of this test. Since a heavy and complete precipitation undoubtedly corresponds with complete fixation of complement in the Wassermann test, it seemed best to employ the nomenclature widely used by workers in connection with the older test.

Although the final reading of results is taken after overnight incubation, this test does not lose its spontaneous character with strongly positive serums. This is particularly true when employing the cholesterinized antigen. In close to 80 per cent. of serums giving a $+ + + +$ reaction in the Wassermann test, a definite precipitate will be seen within five minutes when employing this antigen. This spontaneous phase of the reaction should prove a valuable aid in corroborating an immediate diagnosis of syphilis. Yet, this phase appears to us only of relative importance, since most patients giving strong serologic reac-

*From the Bureau of Laboratories, Michigan Department of Health, Lansing, Mich.

1. Kahn, R. L.: A Simple Quantitative Precipitation Reaction for Syphilis. Preliminary Communication, Arch. Dermat. & Syph. **5**:570 (May) 1922. A Simple Quantitative Precipitation Reaction for Syphilis. Second Communication, ibid. **5**:734 (June) 1922.

tions show clinical evidence of syphilis. In this disease a specific test of such high sensitiveness that it will give helpful data to clinicians in cases in which clinical evidence is often lacking is particularly desirable. It was this consideration largely which led us to render the results with the cholesterinized antigen as sensitive as possible by extending the incubation period.

It should be remembered, however, that any biologic test, if highly sensitive, will occasionally give a slight nonspecific reaction. There are no sharp lines of demarcation in biology, and a test which is capable of detecting minute pathologic lesions will occasionally go beyond the realm of specificity. This explains why weak reactions obtained with the Wassermann test carried out with a cholesterinized antigen and prolonged fixation are considered of little value unless corroborated by clinical evidence. In this precipitation test, also, we believe that a weak reaction obtained with the cholesterinized antigen alone is not by itself to be taken as a symptom of syphilis.

There is this important difference between the precipitation and Wassermann reactions: Whereas the latter has numerous widely accepted sources of error, the precipitation reaction is practically free from them. The several factors essential for correct results can be readily mastered, and judging from the simplicity and ease with which this test can be carried out we are inclined to believe that it will become an important aid in the diagnosis of syphilis.

An important advantage of this precipitation test lies in the fact that one does not have to employ set quantities of serum and antigen in order to obtain the same results. A study of the quantitative relation between serum and antigen has revealed that one may vary the amount of serum provided the proper proportion of antigen is employed. Thus, instead of using 0.3 c.c. of serum and 0.05 c.c. of antigen, one may employ 1.5 c.c. of serum and 0.025 c.c. of antigen. or so-called microquantities, such as 0.03 c.c. of serum and 0.005 c.c. of antigen. This factor should be of help in cases in which it is difficult or impossible to obtain sufficient amounts of blood for regular tests.

PREPARATION AND DILUTION OF ANTIGENS FOR TESTS

An attempt was made to determine the effect of the temperature employed in extracting the heart muscle on the sensitiveness of the antigen when mixed with syphilitic serum. It was observed that when the alcoholic extraction of the heart muscle was carried out for ten days at room temperature, the sensitiveness of the antigen was slightly decreased compared with icebox extraction (6 to 10 C.). If the heart muscle was extracted at incubator temperature (37.5 C.). the antigen potency was considerably decreased. This was found to be true particularly in the case of the cholesterinized antigen.

It appears from these findings that the greater the content of heart-muscle lipoids of the cholesterinized antigen, the less sensitive it is when mixed with syphilitic serum. This is explained by the probability that the greater the lipoid content of a given alcoholic antigen, the more stable it is after the addition of cholesterin. The comparatively large amount of lipoids contained in the alcoholic antigen after incubator extraction holds the cholesterin in solution in a stable form, so that on addition of salt solution there is no tendency for precipitation even at low temperatures. The comparative stability of this antigen solution explains, in our opinion, its lesser sensitiveness when mixed with syphilitic serum; for, assuming that there exists a specific affinity between the combining molecules of the serum and antigen, the rapidity of this union is likely to be lessened when the antigen molecules are in a stable form.

When, on the other hand, the alcoholic extraction is carried out in the icebox, the antigen contains less lipoid material and is proportionally less stable after addition of cholesterin. The lesser stability of this antigen is demonstrated by the fact that it shows a marked tendency for precipitation after being mixed with physiologic salt solution. Thus. the mixing must be carried out rapidly and the antigen must be kept in the incubator to hold it in solution. This apparent instability of the cholesterinized antigen helps to explain its marked sensitiveness when added to syphilitic serum. The antigen molecules, being in an unstable form, attach themselves readily to the combining molecules of the serum.

The tendency of the cholesterinized antigen to precipitate when mixed with physiologic salt solution is an important criterion in judging the sensitiveness of a given antigen. Thus, an antigen-salt solution mixture which will not precipitate within half an hour when placed in the icebox will be considerably less sensitive than a mixture which will precipitate readily at that temperature. Now and then, however, an antigen possesses such marked precipitating properties as to necessitate the utmost care in its dilution with salt solution. This has occasionally been true with antigens prepared by extracting the heart muscle for ten days in the icebox. Attempts have thereupon been made to combine icebox and room temperature extraction of the heart muscle, in order to raise somewhat the lipoid content of the antigen and thereby lessen its precipitating tendency after being mixed with salt solution. It has been found that nine days' extraction at icebox temperature combined with one day's extraction at room temperature gives antigens of somewhat lesser precipitating tendencies, without noticeably affecting their sensitiveness when added to syphilitic serum. On the basis of this observation, we employ the following procedure in the preparation of antigens:

After freeing the dried heart muscle from ether extractives, 5 c.c. of a 95 per cent. or absolute alcohol is added per gram of dried material and extracted for nine days at icebox and one day at room temperature. The alcohol is then filtered off and a given amount cholesterinized by adding 4 mg of cholesterin per cubic centimeter. The second alcoholic extraction with the same dried muscle discussed in the previous papers has in some cases given inconstant results. At present, therefore, we would recommend the employment of the first alcoholic extract only.

The alcoholic antigen is diluted for the tests in the proportion of 1:2 with physiologic salt solution (0.85 per cent. sodium chlorid). The cholesterinized antigen is diluted in the proportion of 1:3. These proportions of salt solution represent approximately the smallest amounts which will hold the antigens in solution. Pipet 1 c.c. of alcoholic antigen into a small test tube (inner diameter about ⅜ inch [10.5 mm.]) or to a 10 c.c. cylinder of about the same inner diameter, and add 2 c.c. of salt solution from another cylinder; mix rapidly by inverting back and forth. The resulting mixture is opalescent and has no tendency to precipitate at room temperature. The advantage of employing a cylinder is that the gradations serve as a check on the amounts of antigen and salt solution employed. One may also use the same cylinder for mixing 0.5, 1.5, 2 c.c. or any intermediary quantity of antigen with proportional amounts of salt solution. This antigen-salt solution mixture is ready for use.

The cholesterinized antigen is diluted in essentially the same way as the alcoholic one except that 3 c.c. of salt solution per cubic centimeter of antigen is employed. This antigen has a tendency to precipitate if improperly mixed with salt solution. To overcome this tendency, delay must not be permitted in mixing after the salt solution has been added to the antigen. The following simple procedure will be found helpful in preventing precipitation of the final mixture: The test tube or cylinder containing the antigen is held between the thumb and third finger of the left hand. The salt solution is added with reasonable rapidity from another cylinder held in the right hand, and the opening of the antigen tube is immediately covered with the index finger of the left hand and shaken by inverting back and forth several times. This mode of shaking is sufficient for complete mixing. Vigorous shaking is not necessary. This mixture may precipitate at low room temperature and is best kept in the incubator when not in use. Sterile precautions are not necessary, but the employment of chemically clean glassware is of utmost importance.

The question whether the potency of the diluted alcoholic and cholesterinized antigens increases or decreases with age is now being investigated in this laboratory. We have employed antigens immediately after dilution with physiologic salt solution as well as two weeks after dilution, with approximately the same results. Now and then, however, serums have been observed which react somewhat more strongly with freshly diluted antigen as compared with those diluted one or two weeks before. On the basis of this observation, we employ at present in our routine tests antigen mixtures from one-half hour to several hours after dilution. It is best to wait about one-half hour because a diluted cholesterinized antigen is frequently clear immediately after dilution and becomes cloudy a short time later.

THE TESTS PROPER

In the preceding paper it was shown that a 4 : 1 proportion of serum to antigen appears to give good results. This finding was obtained by employing strongly positive serums. It was subsequently observed that when employing weak serums, proportionally smaller amounts of antigen give better results. On the basis of this observation a 6 : 1 serum-antigen proportion is employed. With regard to the serum, one may safely vary the amount in accordance with the quantity available. For routine tests, however, 0.3 c.c. of serum is recommended because the proportional amount of serum which is likely to evaporate during the incubation period is practically insignificant when this amount is employed.

Measure with a 1 c.c. pipet graduated in tenths, two 0.3 c.c. quantities of clear inactivated serum (one-half hour at 56 C.) into two small test tubes. Add 0.05 c.c. of alcoholic antigen mixture to one and the same amount of the cholesterinized mixture to the other. For this purpose a 0.2 c.c. pipet graduated in hundredths is best employed. Shake the rack vigorously from two to three minutes. Shaking is of importance because colloidal solutions, such as the serum and diluted antigens, will not mix readily by themselves. The strongly positive serums will, in most cases, show spontaneous precipitations with the cholesterinized antigens and in many cases also with the alcoholic antigens.

In this connection it should be stated that it is of the utmost importance properly to clear the serum by centrifugation, since the presence of red blood cells as well as dust particles will often give the impression of false precipitation. It is also well to mix the serum and antigen as soon as possible after addition of the latter. This is of particular importance when working at low room temperature, since there is a possibility of slight precipitation of the cholesterinized antigen layer covering the serum. At such temperature, also, it is well to keep this antigen in a glass of warm water to prevent its precipitation. The vigorous shaking of the racks can best be carried out after all tubes have received antigen. Finally, when adding antigen to serum with a 1 c.c. pipet graduated in 0.05 c.c., each serum tube should receive the proper amount of antigen. It was observed that such a pipet will occasionally not deliver the 0.05 c.c. of antigen into a given serum tube, the small amount of fluid encircling the tip of the pipet.

After properly mixing the antigen with the serum, the racks are placed in the incubator (37.5 C.) and permitted to remain over night. When employing 0.3 or 0.2 c.c. quantities of serum, it is not necessary to keep the tubes stoppered during the incubation period. It might be added that a temperature of 37.5 C. is not essential for the entire period of incubation. We have, in some cases, incubated our tests for four hours in the water bath, followed by overnight incubation in the icebox, with equally good results.

The results are read after about eighteen hours' incubation. The tubes should not be shaken again before the first reading. The specific precipitates are lipoidal in character and are suspended in the medium. The strongly positive will be recognized without difficulty. The four plus reactions will show either one or several clumps. The three plus reactions will show comparatively large flocculi or granules. The two plus reactions will show clumps or granules of a lesser size but large enough to be unmistakable. The +

and ± reactions are best seen by slanting the tubes and observing the upper point of contact between the fluid and tube wall. The slanted tube should be several inches above the level of the eye and held in front of a window, focusing on some dark object, such as a window shade or frame. One will then see, by looking up, a thin layer of fluid with a precipitate floating in it.

When working with comparatively old serums, as is true in a public health laboratory where specimens are received through the mails, it will be found that a considerable number of tubes have a fine whitish precipitate settled on the bottom. This is the chief reason why it is important not to shake the tubes before the first reading of the results. In many cases, however, these nonspecific precipitates go back into solution on shaking. The questionable tubes, therefore, after the first reading, are given a vigorous shaking for one minute, and the reading is repeated preferably after about one hour. At the end of this period the very weak specific precipitations will be found also to have become somewhat more pronounced.

The extremely fine serum precipitates discussed in the previous papers give no difficulty in reading this test. The specific precipitates after this period of incubation are so marked that even the + and ± reactions should be recognized with comparative ease. If the particles are so fine that there is a question as to whether or not they represent a specific reaction, the test may be safely considered negative.

Some workers may prefer to employ the cholesterin antigen alone in this precipitation reaction. Such workers, we believe, may safely shorten the incubation period to from six to eight hours, provided the racks are shaken for about one minute at the end of each hour's incubation until the total shaking period is no less than five minutes. We believe that the bringing of the reacting serum and antigen substances into closest possible contact with one another is of the utmost importance in this reaction. We have elicited by means of shaking, not only strong precipitation reactions, but weak ones as well. According to our findings, centrifugation will not do this, although it will help to coalesce the flocculi after they have been formed. The construction of a shaking machine is now being contemplated in this laboratory with a view to finding whether sufficient shaking may eliminate the element of incubation in this test.

Clear serums showing a tendency to absorb large amounts of complement (anticomplementary) in the Wassermann test do not react differently from other serums in this precipitation test. They are either positive or negative, depending on whether they have specific reagin.

In the case of spinal fluids, 1 c.c. amounts are employed with 0.05 c.c. quantities of antigen. Although precipitates frequently become visible immediately after shaking when employing strongly positive fluids, we nevertheless find, as a whole, that the reactions with these fluids are somewhat less sensitive than with serums.

In the earlier communications the employment of "strongly positive," "positive" and "weakly positive" as a reading scale was suggested. For the sake of simplicity, however, and because of the widely accepted reading scale of the Wassermann test, the employment of the plus sign was adopted in accordance with the following scheme: (1) A precipitate consisting of one or several large clumps, $+ + + +$; (2) a large flocculent precipitate, $+ + +$; (3) moderate-sized flocculi or

TABLE 1.— RELATIVE SENSITIVENESS OF CHOLESTERINIZED AND ALCOHOLIC ANTIGENS IN PRECIPITATION TEST AS COMPARED WITH WASSERMANN TEST IN TWENTY-FIVE CASES OF SYPHILIS IN VARIOUS STAGES OF TREATMENT

Case Number	Wassermann Test	Results with	
		Precipitation Test	
		Cholesterinized	Alcoholic
1	++++	++++	++++
2	++	++++	±
3	+±+	++++	+
4	—	++	—
5	++++	+++	+++
6	+++	+++	+
7	+	++	—
8	±	++	—
9	±	++++	+
10	++	++++	+++
11	+	++	+
12	++	+++	++
13	+	++	—
14	+	++++	++
15	+++	++++	++++
16	+	+++	—
17	+	+++	+
18	+	++	—
19	++	—	—
20	++	++++	+++
21	±	++	—
22	+	++++	+++
23	++++	+++	+
24	+	+++	—
25	+++	++++	++

granules, $+ +$; (4) small-sized flocculi or granules, $+$; (5) fine flocculi or granules, $\pm$, and (6) negative precipitation, $—$.

With regard to the comparative sensitiveness of the two antigens, the cholesterinized antigen will be found to be considerably more sensitive than the alcoholic. The former antigen appears to retain its sensitiveness in many cases after administration of antisyphilitic treatment. The alcoholic antigen, on the other hand, loses its sensitiveness in a large number of cases after treatment. In our experience, the tests carried out with the cholesterinized antigen give results considerably more sensitive than the Wassermann test performed with the same antigen. In the daily routine precipitation tests carried out in this laboratory, it is a common occurrence to find $+ + + +$ and

+ + + reactions in treated patients, with corresponding Wassermann tests giving only + or ±, and in a small number of cases, negative reactions. And yet, occasional specimens are encountered which give somewhat stronger reactions in the Wassermann than in the precipitation test.

Table 1 indicates the comparative sensitiveness of the two tests in a small group of treated cases of syphilis.

THE SPONTANEOUS REACTION

This reaction is elicited in about 80 per cent. of serums giving a + + + + reaction with the Wassermann test as carried out in this laboratory. After adding antigen to the serum and shaking vigorously for several minutes, a distinct precipitate suspended in a clear serum will be observed. This precipitate will show a tendency to coalesce on standing so that if observed again within from fifteen to thirty minutes, the particles will be found to be considerably larger. Most of these spontaneous reactions are obtained with the cholesterinized antigen, although occasionally such a reaction is obtained with the alcoholic antigen and not with the cholesterinized one.

This spontaneous reaction will not be brought about in most cases unless the tubes are vigorously shaken for several minutes. Shaking is necessary because colloidal solutions such as the serum and the diluted antigen mixture do not readily mix by themselves. Mechanical mixing brings the antigen and reagin substances in close contact enabling them to react rapidly with one another.

When employing improperly centrifuged serums, particularly those which are several days old, one will occasionally obtain cloudiness on shaking the tubes with the production of a faint precipitate. This precipitate is distinguished from the true one by the turbid appearance of the medium. The typical precipitiate consists of distinct whitish particles floating in a clear medium and is unmistakable.

In order to distinguish further true from false spontaneous precipitates, the tubes are centrifuged for a few minutes. The true precipitate will coalesce into one or several clumps and remain suspended, whereas the false one will go to the bottom of the tube. A simpler way is to permit the tube to remain from fifteen to thirty minutes at room temperature or in the incubator, as indicated in the foregoing. The true precipitate will become still more distinct, due to the coalescing of the particles, whereas the false one will become somewhat less distinct due to the settling of the particles. The presence of red blood cells in the serum will also give a false impression of precipitation. The reddish character of this precipitate, however, will distinguish it readily from the true one.

We find it best, in this laboratory, to glance over the serums before adding the antigen and make note of those serums showing clouding either because of contamination or red cells. By this means, the factor of false precipitation is reduced to a minimum.

THE MICROPROCEDURE

It was shown in the preceding paper that there exists a definite quantitative relation between serum and antigen. Thus, when employing a 6 : 1 proportion of serum to antigen, for example, one may vary the serum from 0.6 c.c. to microscopic quantities and obtain comparable results, provided the amount of antigen employed is one-sixth that of serum in every case. This suggested the development of a

TABLE 2.—COMPARISON OF RESULTS OF MICRO (0.03 C.c. SERUM, 0.005 C.c. ANTIGEN) WITH REGULAR (0.3 C.c. SERUM, 0.05 C.c. ANTIGEN) PRECIPITATION AND WASSERMANN TESTS

Serum No.	Wassermann Results	Precipitation Results			
		Regular		Micro	
		Cholesterinized Antigen	Alcoholic Antigen	Cholesterinized Antigen	Alcoholic Antigen
1	+ +	+ + +	+	+ +	+
2	±	+ + + +	+ + + +	+ + + +	+ + +
3	−	±	−	±	−
4	+	+ + + +	±	+ +	−
5	+	+ + +	+	+ +	±
6	+ +	+ + + +	+ +	+ + +	+ +
7	+ + + +	+ + + +	+ + + +	+ + + +	+ + +
8	+	+ + +	±	+ +	−
9	±	+ + +	+	+ +	+
10	−	+	−	±	−
11	+ + + +	+ + + +	+ + + +	+ + + +	+ + + +
12	−	+	−	±	−
13	+ + + +	+ + +	−	+	−
14	+ + + +	+ + + +	+ + + +	+ + + +	+ + + +
15	+ + + +	+ + + +	+ + + +	+ + + +	+ + + +
16	+ + + +	+ + +	+ + +	+ + +	+ + +
17	+ + + +	+ + + +	+ + + +	+ + + +	+ + + +
18	+ + + +	+ + + +	+ + +	+ + + +	+ +
19	+ +	+ + + +	+ + + +	+ +	+
20	+ + + +	+ + +	+	+ + +	+

microscopic procedure with the hope that it may prove helpful in those cases in which regular quantities of serum are not available. Hanging drop preparations were prepared with minute amounts of serum measured with a capillary pipet and approximately one-sixth the amount of antigen measured with a pipet of similar size, employing the usual procedure. After given periods of incubation, the positive serums showed under the microscope clumps of minute globules, whereas in the case of negative serums the mixture appeared homogeneous.

It was observed, however, that this method gave considerably weaker results than the regular one. large numbers of weak serums giving no precipitation reactions with these microscopic quantities. This was found to be due, not to the relatively minute serum and antigen quantities, but to improper agitation of these two substances. For successful precipitation reactions, the serum and antigen must be thoroughly mixed. We have, therefore, found it more dependable to employ small agglutination tubes for this microprocedure and thus to enable proper mixing of the serum and antigen by shaking.

The Method.—Measure with a 0.1 or 0.2 c.c. pipet graduated in hundredths cubic centimeter, two 0.03 c.c. quantities of serum into two agglutination tubes. With a similar pipet measure approximately 0.005 c.c. of diluted alcoholic antigen into one tube and the same amount of cholesterinized antigen into the other. The minute amounts of antigen should reach the serum in each case. Shake the racks vigorously for several minutes and incubate in the usual manner. The tubes should be properly corked to prevent evaporation. The results will be found to approximate closely those obtained with regular quantities. Table 2 gives a summary of findings with a small number of serums.

GRANULOMA INGUINALE WITH LESION ON THE LOWER LIP

REPORT OF A CASE

B. BARKER BEESON, M.D.

CHICAGO

In connection with the paper of Drs. Parounagian and Goodman, which appeared in the May number of the ARCHIVES OF DERMATOLOGY AND SYPHILOLOGY, the following case report seems worthy of attention:

CASE REPORT

A negro affected with granuloma inguinale was seen by Dr. Fernando Terra, professor of dermatology at the University of Rio de Janeiro. The patient first exhibited ulcers of the groin and later an ulcer on the lower lip, from which, as well as from the inguinal lesion, the characteristic organisms were recovered. He found only seven cases with this combination of symptoms in the literature. This is of interest because of the statement by Drs. Parounagian and Goodman: "As far as we know there has been but one other case with lesions about the lip, reported by Sequeira." Terra's patient was cured by intravenous injections of tartar emetic. He exhibited this case before the Brazilian Dermatological Society in 1917, and also reported it in extenso in the *Annals of the Faculty of Medicine of Rio de Janeiro* for that year.

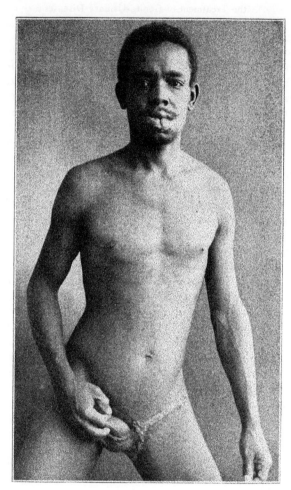

Granuloma inguinale with lesion on lower lip. Dr. Terra's patient.

THE CLINICAL VALUE OF THE KOLMER COMPLEMENT-FIXATION TEST FOR SYPHILIS *

CHARLES H. DE T. SHIVERS, M.D.

Assistant Professor of Syphilology, Graduate School of Medicine, University of Pennsylvania; Chief of the U. S. Public Health Service for the Treatment of Genito-Urinary Diseases

ATLANTIC CITY, N. J.

The complement-fixation reaction has proved of great value in the diagnosis of syphilis and as a guide to specific therapy. Unfortunately, the original method of Wassermann and his co-workers lacks sufficient sensitiveness; and, as a result of attempts to improve the technic, a large number of modifications have come into use. These different methods vary in sensitiveness and practical specificity; for that reason portions of the blood of the same person examined in different laboratories may yield varying results, lead to considerable confusion, and result in undetermining the fundamental and high values of the complement-fixation test in syphilis.

For these and additional reasons a demand for standardization of the Wassermann reaction has arisen, and a good start in this direction has been made by the exhaustive investigations of Kolmer and his colleagues.[1] These studies have resulted in the elaboration of a new antigen[2] and a new technic[3] which Kolmer believes may fulfil the aims of increased sensitiveness and practical specificity, as well as yield a true quantitative reaction of greater value as a serologic guide to treatment than afforded by present methods. The new method has been employed by Kolmer in the Polyclinic Laboratories of the Graduate School of Medicine of the University of Pennsylvania for the last two years, and recently Schamberg and Klauder[4] have published the results observed by them in about 2,000 tests. These authors found the new Kolmer method distinctly more sensitive than the older method and highly specific, inasmuch as false positive reactions in non-syphilitic subjects were not observed. The new method was found to harmonize better with the clinical findings, and its quantitative character

---

* Read before the Philadelphia Urological Society, April 24, 1922.

1. Series of thirty-two papers being published in the Am. J. Syphilis, beginning **3**:1, 1919.

2. Am. J. Syphilis **6**:74, 1922.

3. Am. J. Syphilis **6**:82, 1922.

4. Medical Clinics of North America, Philadelphia, W. B. Saunders Company, 1921, p. 667.

permitted a better gage of the effects of antisyphilitic treatment than yielded by older methods.

AUTHOR'S INVESTIGATIONS

I have had 320 tests made by Dr. Kolmer with the serums of private patients, whom he was able to study clinically with particular care. Each serum was examined by the new method and likewise by Dr. Kolmer's older three antigen method. All serums yielding a positive reaction with the new method either had a previous history of syphilitic infection or presented clinical evidences of the disease. In no instance were falsely positive reactions observed.

The new test was frequently positive early in the primary stages when the old method reacted negatively even with cholesterolized antigens. The new test likewise was the first to detect a relapsing case and the last to give a negative reaction during treatment.

REPORT OF CASES

CASE 1.—H. L., a man, aged 51, had had a primary lesion twenty years ago. He was under treatment for six months at that time with mercury and iodids. Two years ago a Wassermann test was made and found to be four plus. Following this examination he received four injections of arsphenamin, 0.6 gm. each. At present there is no clinical evidence of syphilis. The Kolmer method gave a moderately positive reaction, while the old method was negative. This illustrates the value of the new test in detecting reagin[5] in the blood of a patient with latent asymptomatic syphilis.

CASE 2.—F. C., a man, aged 22, gave no history of a primary infection. He had had one attack of gonorrhea with many recurrences. Following his first Neisserian infection, he noticed falling of the hair. A Wassermann test was made at that time and found to be four plus. He was then given twenty-four injections of neo-arsphenamin. At present there are no symptoms except the loss of hair. Examination was negative. The Wassermann reaction made on Aug. 30, 1920, was weakly positive with the Kolmer method, and negative with the old method. After ten injections consisting of 0.6 gm. each of arsphenamin, at weekly intervals, combined with inunctions of mercury, 1 dram (3.9 gm.) four times a week, the Wassermann test was again made and showed negative in both tests. Without further treatment a third Wassermann test was made on Feb. 25, 1921, which was weakly positive with the new method and negative with the old. The Kolmer method, as illustrated in this case, is the last to show a negative reaction while the patient is under treatment, and the first to detect a relapsing positive.

CASE 3.—A. J., a man, aged 52, gave a history of a primary lesion thirty-two years ago. Secondary symptoms followed. No treatment was received by the patient at this time. The only symptoms complained of when the patient reported were severe frontal and occipital headaches. This man had been treated previously for sinus infection. Examination showed the pupils to be slightly irregular, with a sluggish reaction to light. The Kolmer method

---

5. Term designated by Neisser for the reacting substance in the blood serum.

showed a moderately positive reaction; the old test was weakly positive. This patient was entirely relieved of his head symptoms after a few injections of neo-arsphenamin. In this case the test gave one more assurance of the correctness of the clinical diagnosis. A spinal Wassermann test was not made.

CASE 4.—M. S., a woman, aged 45, gave no history of any infection. The first Wassermann test made by the health department of another city showed a three plus reaction with all three antigens. This patient had received twelve injections before the Kolmer technic was used. The Wassermann test made on Oct. 15, 1920, showed a moderately positive reaction with the Kolmer method and a weakly to moderately positive reaction with the old method. Fifteen injections of neo-arsphenamin were then given at irregular intervals, and the Wassermann test on Nov. 3, 1921, was weakly positive with the Kolmer method and negative with the old. This persistent positive reaction with the new test indicates the necessity for more treatment, at the same time showing improvement in the higher dilutions of the patient's serum.

CASE 5.—S. R., a man, aged 23, reported for treatment on Aug. 24, 1919, with a positive previous history of syphilis. The only symptom he complained of was general weakness. The physical examination was negative. The Wassermann test made at this time showed a four plus reaction with all three antigens with the old test. Twenty-four injections of arsphenamin, 0.6 gm. each, were given, together with mercury by inunctions and potassium iodid. The Wassermann test made on Nov. 9, 1920, showed a moderately positive reaction with Kolmer's new method, and a negative reaction with the old. Several more injections of arsphenamin were then given; the blood examination following these treatments was negative with both tests. This case also showed the slowness of the new method to become negative while the patient is under treatment.

CASE 6.—S. M., a man, aged 28, had a primary lesion in June, 1917, or three years before he first reported to me for treatment. He had received six injections of arsphenamin at that time; there was no history of secondary symptoms. One year ago he noticed that the vision was blurred in his left eye. The oculist reported retinal hemorrhages in the macular region. At this time he received twelve injections of neo-arsphenamin at weekly intervals. Spinal fluid and blood Wassermann tests on Nov. 30, 1920, showed a weakly positive reaction with the new method and a negative reaction with the old. In addition, in the spinal fluid examination the colloidal gold test showed the syphilitic curve; the cell count was normal. This is a case of neurosyphilis of the vascular type, in which immediate and intensive treatment was essential; yet the blood and spinal fluid reactions were negative with the old method.

CASE 7.—W. H. Mc., a man, aged 20, denied all venereal infections. He consulted a physician on account of enlargement of the inguinal glands. Examination disclosed a poorly nourished man with general glandular enlargement. No other signs of the disease were present. Blood was taken for a Wassermann test on April 4, 1921. The Kolmer method showed a weakly positive reaction; the old method was negative. It was later discovered that the father of this boy contracted syphilis two years before the patient was born, and that he had received insufficient treatment. This is a case of congenital syphilis in which the old method was negative with all three antigens, and in which the clinical findings were not sufficient to make a diagnosis.

CASE 8.—F. H., a man, aged 28, had a primary lesion of two weeks' duration; the dark field was positive. The blood for a Wassermann test was taken on the fifteenth day, and the result obtained is very interesting. The Kolmer method showed a strongly positive reaction, while the old method was weakly positive, giving evidence of the earlier positives with the new method. After giving seventeen injections of neo-arsphenamin, 0.9 gm. each, with a course of mercury, the Wassermann test was again made and showed a weakly positive reaction with the Kolmer method, and a negative reaction with the old method. The new test later became negative after the patient had received more treatments.

CASE 9.—J. S., a man, aged 28, had a primary lesion during the early part of September, 1921. Diagnosis was made by dark-field examination. Seventeen injections of neo-arsphenamin, 0.9 gm. each, were given at stated intervals. Treatment was instituted about two weeks after the appearance of the sore. The Wassermann test made by the new method was strongly positive and by the old method moderately positive. Mercury was given by inunctions together with potassium iodid. The blood Wassermann test was made again on Dec. 6, 1921, and was negative with both tests. Up to this time twelve of the seventeen injections had been given. On Jan. 17, 1922, the patient, while walking along the street, had a convulsion, followed by a period of unconsciousness lasting several hours. Another attack similar to the first occurred on Feb. 4, 1922. The blood continued negative with both tests. On Feb. 10, 1922, spinal fluid was withdrawn for an examination. The fluid came out with considerable pressure but was clear. The report showed a cell count of 40 per cubic millimeter. The colloidal gold reaction was negative. The Kolmer method showed a one plus, or weakly positive reaction, while the old test was negative. Treatment was again started with weekly injections of neo-arsphenamin, 0.9 gm. each, followed every other week by spinal drainage. The patient has shown wonderful improvement as to nervousness, mentality and strength. This case is of special interest because it shows that Dr. Kolmer's new method is even more sensitive than the colloidal gold reaction in a case of clinical neurosyphilis of the meningeal type.

The accompanying table briefly summarizes cases from this series in which the two methods yielded different reactions; in every instance the results of the new tests have proved correct and consistently indicative of superior sensitiveness and specificity.

SUMMARY

From the standpoint of the practitioner, the complement-fixation test for syphilis should be as sensitive as is consistent with specificity. There can be no difference of opinion in regard to the absolute necessity for practical specificity, that is, extreme sensitiveness is undesirable if it means the possibility of securing falsely positive reactions. This point has been kept clearly in mind by Dr. Kolmer, and his efforts to improve the sensitiveness of the reaction without at the same time running the risk of falsely positive reactions has evidently been realized in my experience. This is due in large part to the remarkable antigen being employed which in a dose of 10 units is forty or more times less than the anticomplementary unit.

In my experience this increased sensitiveness of the complement-fixation reaction for syphilis is highly desirable for the early diagnosis

THE RELATIVE EFFICIENCY OF THE KOLMER COMPLEMENT-FIXATION TEST FOR SYPHILIS

Case No.	History	Clinical Findings	State of the Disease	Date	Amount of Treatment to Date	Kolmer's Method	Old Method
1	+	—	Latent	8/24/20	4 injections of arsphenamin 0.6 gm.	Blood $0.1 = +++$ $0.02 = ++$ $0.004 = -$ $0.002 = -$ $0.001 = -$	Blood Antigen 1 — Antigen 2 — Antigen 3 —
2	—	Loss of hair	Latent	8/30/20	24 injections of neo-arsphenamin 0.9 gm.	Blood $0.1 = +$ $0.02 = -$ $0.004 = -$ $0.002 = -$ $0.001 = -$	Blood Antigen 1 — Antigen 2 — Antigen 3 —
3	+	+	Neuro-syphilis	10/22/20	....	Blood $0.1 = ++++$ $0.02 = ++$ $0.004 = -$ $0.002 = -$ $0.001 = -$	Blood Antigen 1 + Antigen 2 — Antigen 3 —
4	—	—	Latent	10/15/21	12 injections of neo-arsphenamin	Blood $0.1 = ++++$ $0.02 = ++$ $0.004 = \pm$ $0.002 =$ $0.001 =$	Blood Antigen 1[3] + Antigen 2[1] + Antigen 3[2] +
4	—	—	Latent	11/ 3/21	27 injections of neo-arsphenamin 0.9 gm.	Blood $0.1 = +$ $0.02 =$ $0.003 =$ $0.002 =$ $0.001 =$	Blood Antigen 1 — Antigen 2 — Antigen 3 —
5	+	—	Latent	11/ 9/21	24 injections of arsphenamin 0.6 gm. mercury	Blood $0.1 = +++$ $0.02 = +$ $0.004 = -$ $0.002 = -$ $0.001 = -$	Blood Antigen 1 — Antigen 2 — Antigen 3 —
6	+	+	Neuro-syphilis, arterial type	11/30/21	18 injections of arsphenamin 0.6 gm. mercury	Spinal fluid $0.1 = +$ $0.02 = -$ $0.004 = -$ $0.002 = -$ $0.001 = -$	Spinal fluid Antigen 1 — Antigen 2 — Antigen 3 —
6	+	+	Neuro-syphilis, arterial type	11/30/21	18 injections of arsphenamin 0.6 gm. mercury	Blood $0.1 = +$ $0.02 = -$ $0.004 = -$ $0.002 = -$ $0.001 = -$	Blood Antigen 1 — Antigen 2 — Antigen 3 —
10	+	—	Latent	12/ 3/20	9 injections of arsphenamin 0.6 gm.	Blood $0.1 = +$ $0.02 = -$ $0.004 = -$ $0.002 = -$ $0.001 = -$	Blood Antigen 1 — Antigen 2 — Antigen 3 —
11	+	—	Latent	12/ 3/20	....	Blood $0.1 = +$ $0.02 = -$ $0.004 = -$ $0.002 = -$ $0.001 = -$	Blood Antigen 1 — Antigen 2 — Antigen 3 —
12	+	—	Latent	8/ 3/21	....	Blood $0.1 = ++$ $0.02 = -$ $0.004 = -$ $0.002 = -$ $0.001 = -$	Blood Antigen 1 — Antigen 2 — Antigen 3 —
8	+	Multiple chancres, 15 days' duration	Primary	8/12/21	....	Blood $0.1 = ++++$ $0.02 = ++++$ $0.004 = ++$ $0.002 = -$ $0.001 = -$	Blood Antigen 1[2] + Antigen 2 — Antigen 3 —

THE RELATIVE EFFICIENCY OF THE KOLMER COMPLEMENT-FIXATION
TEST FOR SYPHILIS—(*Continued*)

Case No.	History	Clinical Findings	State of the Disease	Date	Amount of Treatment to Date	Kolmer's Method	Old Method
14	+	—	Latent	5/5/21	Mercury + potassium iodid, many	Blood 0.1 = +++, 0.02 = +, 0.004 = —, 0.002 = —, 0.001 = —	Blood Antigen 1 —, Antigen 2 —, Antigen 3 —
7	—	—	Congenital	4/4/21	....	Blood 0.1 = +, 0.02 = —, 0.004 = —, 0.002 = —, 0.001 = —	Blood Antigen 1 —, Antigen 2 —, Antigen 3 —
9	+	+	Neurosyphilis	2/10/22	12 injections of neo-arsphenamin 0.9 gm.	Spinal fluid 0.1 = +, 0.02 = —, 0.004 = —, 0.002 = —, 0.001 = —	Spinal fluid Antigen 1 —, Antigen 2 —, Antigen 3 —
13	+	—	Latent	7/29/21	....	Blood 0.1 = ÷+, 0.02 = —, 0.004 = —, 0.002 = —, 0.001 = —	Blood Antigen 1 —, Antigen 2 —, Antigen 3 —
14	+	Multiple chancres, 21 days' duration	Primary	7/29/21	....	Blood 0.1 = ++++, 0.02 = ++++, 0.004 = —, 0.002 = —, 0.001 = —	Blood Antigen 1[2] +, Antigen 2[1] +, Antigen 3[1] +
15	+	+	Paresis	8/20/21	10 injections of arsphenamin	Blood 0.1 = ++++, 0.02 = ++, 0.004 = —, 0.002 = —, 0.001 = —	Blood Antigen 1[3] ÷, Antigen 2[1] ÷, Antigen 3[1] ÷
16	+	—	Latent 2d	1/6/22	30 injections of neo-arsphenamin 0.9 gm.	Blood 0.1 = +, 0.02 = —, 0.004 = —, 0.002 = —, 0.001 = —	Blood Antigen 1 —, Antigen 2 —, Antigen 3 —

of syphilis, and more especially for diagnosis in the latent and tertiary stages and in congenital syphilis. Furthermore, this sensitive method requires more thorough treatment for the eradication of positive reactions, and I regard this as an important point in view of the tendency to undertreat this disease. Negative reactions with the new test have been secured by treatment, but considerably more treatment is required for this result by the new method than by older methods.

In my opinion the complement-fixation reaction in syphilis is not too delicate, but not delicate enough; as pointed out by Kolmer,[6] the reaction may yield falsely negative reactions in cases of syphilis in which the spirochetes are present in such few numbers or in such a condition of latency or quiescence that sufficient amounts of "reagin" are not being produced in the blood and spinal fluid to yield positive reactions. For this reason the complement-fixation reaction for syphilis

6. Kolmer, John A.: Standardization of the Wassermann Reaction. J. A. M. A. **77**:776 (Sept. 3) 1921.

is still apt to err on the negative side and is worthy of further efforts toward rendering the test even more sensitive, providing, always that it is safely kept within the bounds of practical specificity.

The quantitative feature of the new test secured by testing each serum in varying amounts had likewise proved useful in my experience. Of course the question of whether a serum or spinal fluid does or does not yield a positive reaction is of primary importance, and treatment aims to render the reaction negative. But during the course of treatment an accurate gage of the progress of reduction of "reagin" in the blood is of value and offers distinct encouragement to both physician and patient.

The new method has likewise proved of superior sensitiveness and reliability for the examination of spinal fluids, and in a number of cases it has yielded true positive reactions with fluids from cases of early neurosyphilis when the older method has yielded negative reactions.

CONCLUSIONS

1. The writer has employed the Kolmer complement-fixation test for syphilis in 320 cases—some with a definite history of specific infection and presenting clinical evidences of syphilis, others with negative histories and presenting no signs or symptoms of syphilis.

2. The new method has proved a very sensitive and reliable test, much more so than the old method, being frequently positive while the latter is negative.

3. The new method has yielded earlier positive reactions in primary syphilis than other methods, and is much slower in becoming negative when the patient is under treatment than the old method.

4. A negative reaction with the Kolmer method is of more value when giving a prognosis.

5. The new Kolmer method has not yielded falsely positive reactions in nonsyphilitic persons.

6. The method has been proved more valuable in aiding a diagnosis of congenital syphilis in obscure cases than the old method.

7. The new method marks a distinct and valuable advance in the serum diagnosis of syphilis, being much more sensitive and at the same time yielding no falsely positive reactions.

A NAIL TUMOR OF UNUSUAL TYPE *

RICHARD L. SUTTON, M.D.

KANSAS CITY, MO.

In January, 1921, while delivering a clinical lecture before the Douglas County Medical Society, at Lawrence, Kansas, I encountered a case of nail disorder which was entirely new to me.

REPORT OF CASES

CASE 1.—The patient was a young woman, under the care of my friend. Dr. H. L. Chambers, and the affection, which involved the nail of the left thumb, had been present for about one year.

There was no history of injury, and, in so far as could be demonstrated. the patient was free from syphilis and tuberculosis.

The earliest noticeable manifestation was a small, hard, rounded, painless tumor at the base of the nail. The growth had increased gradually in size until it was about 0.5 cm. in height, and 0.7 cm. in width. Coincident with its development, a V-shaped groove had appeared in the nail, extending from the matrix to the free margin, and gradually becoming broader and shallower as it passed outward. The sides of the groove were smooth and glossy, and no signs of atrophy or similar change were present. The little tumor was pinkish, smooth and hard, insensitive to pain, and free from capillary dilatation.

The possibility of trauma as an etiologic factor was of course the first suggestion, but this was positively denied by the patient, who was an exceptionally intelligent woman.

Owing to the character of the lesion, and its location. Dr. Chambers proposed to excise it, and he promised to forward the specimen to me following the operation. He was kind enough to do this, and the accompanying photomicrographs are made from the material supplied by him.

CASE 2.—On April 4, 1921, Dr. H. H. Lane, of this city, referred to me a young woman with an identically similar lesion, which involved the nail of the right forefinger. In this case, also, no history of trauma could be elicited. The presence of the growth had first been noted in July, 1920, and the tumor had changed little during the last four months.

The patient was willing to follow any plan of treatment that might be suggested, although she objected to surgical intervention because of the associated pain and inconvenience. Consequently, a small, circular, unscreened radium plaque was applied directly to the lesion for a period of one-half hour, on three successive days. When the ensuing reaction had subsided, the tumor had practically disappeared, and no other treatment was required. Figure 1 B shows the condition of the nail seven months later.

HISTOPATHOLOGY

The original specimen had been hardened, mounted in paraffin, sectioned, and stained before it reached me, but owing to the strong affinity for eosin, the differentiation was very poor.

* Read at the Forty-Fifth Annual Meeting of the American Dermatological Association, Washington, D. C., May 2-4, 1922.

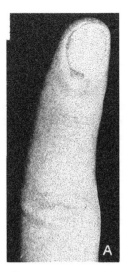

Fig. 1.—*A*, character and location of lesion in Case 2; *B*, result of radium treatment.

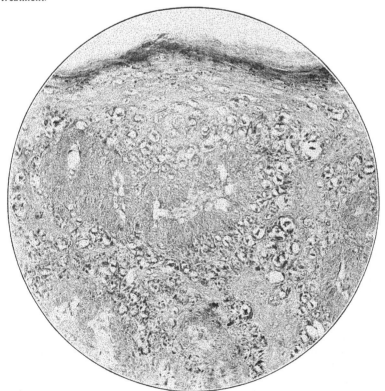

Fig. 2.—Photomicrograph of upper portion of tumor. Note slight hyperkeratosis, parakeratosis, dilated lymph spaces and hypertrophic nuclei. (100 diameters.)

I have submitted the slides to a number of more experienced dermatologists and pathologists than myself in this country, but, even with their assistance, no definite conclusion regarding the exact nature of the growth has yet been reached.

Description of the Specimen.—The corneous layer was somewhat thickened, and there was marked parakeratosis. At many points, the epidermis was lifted from the surface of the papillae. This may have been a result of injuries incurred during the cutting, or restaining processes, but it was more likely due

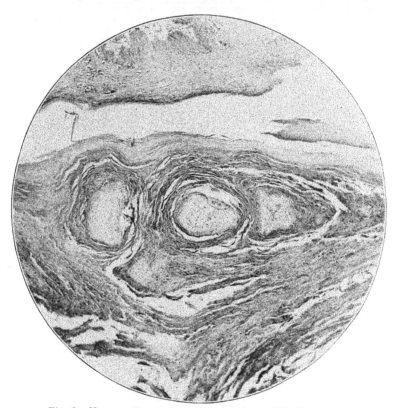

Fig. 3.—Horny cell nests at base of lesion. (200 diameters.)

to the condition of the upper portions of the papillary bodies. In this locality, and at many other points in the specimen, there were large collections of hypertrophic nuclei in the lymph spaces. The latter were dilated and greatly increased in number. Apparently, the blood vessels were little affected, if at all.

Owing to the direction in which the specimen was sectioned, some of the papillary bodies presented an unusual appearance, but this was readily explained when the various tissue interrelationships were deciphered. Near the base of the nail proper, the corneous material was arranged in peculiar, irregularly oval nests. Dr. Fordyce suggested their resemblance to the little horny cysts sometimes seen in healed lesions of pemphigus and in epidermolysis bullosa. Dr. William Allen Pusey, who was kind enough to look over the sections, suggested a resemblance to granuloma pyogenicum. Unfortunately, we did not have an opportunity to examine them together, but to me they do not simulate granuloma pyogenicum in the least.

I at first thought that these pearl-like bodies were the most characteristic tissue change in the tumor, and for that reason would have placed the growth in the keratoma group, but since studying the restained sections, I have concluded that the lymphatic and nuclear alterations probably are the most representative, and that the corneous changes are simply a result of irregular pressure, with ensuing disarrangement and malformation of the immature horn cells.

COMMENT

The only disorder that I have found described which at all resembles the condition in the present case is Polland's fibromatosis subunguinalis,[1] but judging from a comparison of the illustrations, and from Polland's description of the histopathology, the similarity is only a superficial one.

DISCUSSION

Dr. H. H. Hazen, Washington: I have been interested in this paper of Dr. Sutton's because I think we have had a similar case under observation during the last winter. This opinion was derived from conversation with Dr. Sutton rather than from the talk we have just listened to. In our case the patient had two of the lesions, one at the base of the nail, the other at the middle phalanx of the finger. This was similar to the digital lesions, except that after they appeared they became markedly hardened and keratosed. We used the roentgen ray and the lesions disappeared entirely, only to reappear within a few months. The lesions were cured by applications of the cautery. No section was made for the patient would not permit it.

It is a question to me whether this is a disease of the nail or of the skin. The lesion on the middle phalanx apparently indicates that the disease is not associated with the nail.

Dr. Walter J. Highman, New York: I wish Dr. Sutton would reinterpret the pathologic and histologic findings in connection with the clinical findings. I, frankly, do not understand them. I have looked at the photograph and at the section and find nothing distinquishing in the composite picture. I do not understand what is new about it or why it is called a tumor.

Dr. Richard L. Sutton, Kansas City, Mo. (closing): These cases have been more or less of a puzzle to me and to a score or more of other dermatologists and pathologists who have seen the photographs and examined the sections. Dr. Pusey, who was so kind as to examine the slides, suggested that the disorder might belong in the granuloma pyogenicum group, but with this conclusion I cannot agree. I have done some research work on granuloma pyogenicum, and the sections from lesions of the two conditions do not in the least resemble each other.

---

1. Polland: Dermat. Ztschr. **23**:42-44, 1916.

Abstracts from Current Literature

RETICULATED ATROPHY OF THE CHEEKS WITHOUT APPARENT FOLLICULAR KERATOSIS AND ACCOMPANIED BY ERYTHEMA. PAUTRIER, Bull. Soc. franç. de dermat. et syph. **29:** R.S. 21, 1922.

There is given an illustrated report of a case of folliculitis ulerythematosa reticulata, without the usual follicular keratoses and especially remarkable on account of an erythematous border which extended onto the apparently normal skin. The condition, in a boy of 17 years, was of three years' duration. No biopsy had been made.

A NEW CASE OF CHRONIC CIRCUMSCRIBED NODULAR LICHENI-FICATION. PAUTRIER, Bull. Soc. franç. de dermat. et syph. **29:** R.S. 25, 1922.

This condition, generally known as lichen obtusus corné, had been present for twenty-two years in a woman, aged 40 years; only the extremities were affected. In a recent article by this author (*Ann. de dermat. et syph.*, Feb., 1922), the differences between this condition and lichen planus have been brought out, and this case further emphasizes them.

PARKHURST, Toledo, Ohio.

CONCERNING TUBERCULINS AND VACCINES OF COLD-BLOODED ANIMALS IN DERMATOLOGY, AND SOME THERAPEUTIC EXPERIENCES. HUBSCHMANN, Ceska dermat. **3:**115, 140, 177, 1922.

The author discusses all the known forms of tuberculins, various methods of application, the nature and types of tuberculin reactions and therapeutic methods used. From the diagnostic standpoint, the best results were obtained by a modification of the Pirquet-Petreoschky method: a double scarified cross was used; it gave a large percentage of positive, well pronounced reactions. In dermatology, vaccines and tuberculins play, therapeutically, an important rôle as accessory measures to medicinal and phototherapy. Good results are reported in tuberculosis of the mucous membranes, where subjective symptoms were promptly relieved. For ambulatory cases the author recommends Ponndorf's inunction method. Weleminsky's tuberculomucin given in injections was unsatisfactory; when used in form of compresses it usually stimulated an abundant growth of granulation tissue (in scrofuloderma).

Chelonin (turtle vaccine) was not found to be a specific. Its beneficial effect on skin tuberculosis cannot, however, be denied. It has an advantage over the old tuberculin as it causes a less severe reaction and has a longer period of activity.

INTRACUTANEOUS INJECTIONS OF A MILK PREPARATION. GAWALOWSKI, Ceska dermat. **3:**147, 1922.

A milk preparation for intracutaneous injections causes—like many other foreign proteins—an acute inflammatory reaction in chronically diseased areas, thus increasing their vitality. At the skin clinic in Prague a milk preparation was used in sixteen cases of deep parasitic sycosis with good results. I:

might be of value especially to a country practitioner to whom roentgen rays and specific trichophytin are inaccessible. From 0.2-0.5 c.c. doses were used to produce a local reaction. The dose was repeated after the first reaction subsided. From two to eight doses are necessary. Patients with chronic sycosis coccogenes were not benefited.

ETIOLOGY AND HISTOGENESIS OF NEVI. Kogoz, Ceska dermat. **3**:169, 1922.

An elaborate and painstaking review is given of all known theories on the subject which so far remains undecided.

SPINKA, St. Louis.

ACUTE LUPUS ERYTHEMATOSUS. L. GOERL and VOIGT, Dermat. Wchnschr. **74**:129 (Feb. 11) 1922.

The nosologic situation of lupus erythematosus is still disputed. The author divides the acute form into three types: lupus erythematodes disseminatus Kaposi, appearing without systemic disturbances and differentiated from chronic discoid lupus erythematosus by the greater number of circumscribed patches, the scaling tendency and its localization; lupus erythematodes discoides acutus Kaposi, an acute outbreak on a previously existing typical discoid lupus erythematosus, often accompanied by severe fever and a multiform exanthem of an erythematous, hemorrhagic, vesicular, bullous or crusted nature; true lupus erythematodes acutus, analogous to the preceding without the antecedent or subsequent appearance of chronic lupus erythematodes discoides. He suggests that the weight of evidence is against a tuberculous etiology of the disease, and favors a still unknown invader—possibly the streptococcus.

ANDREWS, New York.

CHROMATOPHORE QUESTION. B. BLOCH, Dermat. Ztschr. **34**:253 (Oct.) 1921.

One must differentiate two types of pigment containing cells in the cutis of man and other suckling animals. The first of these is represented by the ordinary chromatophores. They lie in the papillary body and in the upper cutis, and also lower in instances of deep pigmentation, although in fewer numbers. These cells never take the Dopa reaction, which acts as a differentiation with other epidermal cells, and with the second type of pigment containing cell.

The second type of pigment cell in the cutis is very different from the first type. In many of the apes, this second type dominates the pigment picture of the skin. In man, this type is seldom encountered (occasionally in the skin of the neighborhood of the sacrum, and as Jadassohn has said, in the "blue nevi"). On the other hand, this type is always found in the sacral region of the new-born, especially among Mongolians, in which cases they form the so-called "Mongolian spot" which is evidently an atavistic remainder of our ape family forebears. The Mongolian cells lie deep in the cutis, and are distinguished from the other cells and the chromatophore cells by their shape, and by the fact that they take the Dopa reaction; in other words, they are pigment builders.

CEREBROSPINAL FLUID FINDINGS IN PRIMARY SYPHILIS. R. FRÜHWALD, Dermat. Ztschr. **34**:263 (Oct.) 1921.

The cerebrospinal fluid of 140 seronegative primary syphilitic patients was examined. Pathologic changes were evident in fifteen, or 10.7 per cent. of these. Increase of cells was present in three cases; and in nine there was increase in globulin; two gave positive Wassermann reactions; and one showed increased number of cells and increase in globulin. The increase in globulin was the most marked finding. The cell increase was not so great and was a little above normal. The Wassermann reaction was never strongly positive, but was reported one or two plus.

The seropositive primary syphilitic patients examined numbered 283. Pathologic fluids were found 48 times, or in 17.3 per cent. There was increase in cells 15 times; increase in albumin, 16 times; 3 positive Wassermann reactions; increase in cells and albumin 12 times; increase in cells and a positive Wassermann reaction once; increased globulin and a positive Wassermann reaction once. The increased globulin again shows itself to be the most frequent change encountered.

A similar condition was found in a group in whom the serum Wassermann test was not performed.

The colloidal gold reaction was performed in twenty-four cases of seronegative primary syphilis; once there was a "trace"; twice a weak reaction; once a weakly positive reaction; and a negative reaction twenty times. Seventy-eight seropositive primary syphilitic patients were given the colloidal gold test, among whom twenty-four showed a "trace"; fifteen gave positive and thirty-nine negative reactions.

SILVER ARSPHENAMIN. H. PLANNER, Dermat. Ztschr. **34**:271 (Oct.) 1921.

Silver arsphenamin is undoubtedly an energetic arsphenamin preparation. Spirochetes disappear rapidly from serum procured by teasing lesions, and there is a prompt regression of the syphilitic manifestations. The influence on the Wassermann reaction is also satisfactory, although somewhat slower than following the combination of neo-arsphenamin and mercury. Although the number of cases observed was too small to enable the author to make definite statements it has appeared that the permanence of the effect on the serology was similar for the two drugs. The results of the so-called abortive cure of syphilis in Planner's hands have not been as favorable as results reported by others. By-effects have been more frequent than following the injection of neo-arsphenamin, almost harmless, and most often expressed by fever, a feeling of malaise, angioneurotic syndromes and erythema. Still, severe by-effects have also been noted which do not differ from similar severe reactions of the other arsphenamins. The technic is a complicated one, much more so than with neo-arsphenamin. It should be a consideration also in practice that a larger number of injections of silver arsphenamin are required than with neo-arsphenamin. Further study is needed before one can state the optimum dosage and interval of injections. It is not known either whether mercury in combination with silver arsphenamin would improve the results obtained.

A PEMPHIGOID PYOCYANEOUS INFECTION RESEMBLING SMALL-POX IN AN INFANT. E. ZURHELLE, Dermat. Ztschr. **34**:300 (Oct.) 1921.

A pure culture of the *B. pyocyaneous* was grown from lesions in the skin of a 3 month old child, who had a rise in temperature and skin lesions of the abdomen when it came under observation. The primary lesion was a papule, with development into pustules. There were no mucous membrane lesions. Necropsy was refused so that the pathogenesis was not revealed.

ARSPHENAMIN ERUPTION. A. STÜHMER, Dermat. Ztschr. **34**:304 (Oct.) 1921.

Every by-effect of the injection of arsphenamin, including the skin eruptions, is due not to the arsphenamin itself but to some product formed during the manufacture or solution, or in the injected organism. Stühmer classifies the conditions of the skin following the injection of arsphenamin as: 1. Acute vasotoxic arsphenamin dermatitis. This type appears within a few hours or at most one or two days after the injection. All types of acute urticarial and erythematous lesions are classified with this group. 2. Subacute anaphylactoid arsphenamin dermatitis. This type appears from six to twelve days after the first arsphenamin injection. That the eruption appears between the second and third injection is only apparent, and there is no connection between these and the dermatitis. Stühmer believes that this is due to the formation of arsphenamin-oxid-protein bodies (oxytoxin). 3. Chronic arsphenamin dermatitis. This type is divided into (*a*) early form, and (*b*) late form. The early form may appear toward the end of the arsphenamin course, perhaps at the fifth or sixth injection, and the late form may appear from several weeks to two or three months after the end of the arsphenamin course. These forms represent the most severe skin injuries due to arsphenamin. They may appear as apparently benign erythematous eruptions, possibly follicular, often urticarial. The eruption is quickly transformed into the ordinary dermatitis, "erythrodermia," scale formation, hyperkeratosis, changes of the nails and hair, and finally pyodermic processes which give rise to grave disease pictures.

EPINEPHRIN IN DERMATOLOGY. J. K. MAYR, Dermat. Ztschr. **34**:317 (Oct.) 1921.

This is a preliminary report on the effect of epinephrin which gives the reaction of this drug on the normal skin. As is well known, subcutaneous injection calls forth a local, irregularly circumscribed area of goose flesh and anemia. The blood pressure rise and fall was also measured, and charted. The white blood cells are increased in the first few hours with an absolute fall in the count of the polymorphonuclears. After an hour or two this increase decreases. The effect of epinephrin in seventy patients with dermatoses gave the normal reactions in only a third. The atypical reactions included both phases of the blood picture and modification of the blood pressure curve. Observations of the therapeutic action of epinephrin on dermatoses is reserved for further contributions.

EPIDERMAL BASAL MEMBRANE. S. BORN, Dermat. Ztschr. **34**:324 (Oct.) 1921.

The conclusion is reached that the so-called basal membrane exists between the epidermis and cutis formed of bundles of connective tissue. This membrane is connected to the cutis by innumerable little bundles, but no such connections are sent out to the epidermis.

TEN YEARS OF ARSPHENAMIN THERAPY AT THE SKIN CLINIC AT BONN. E. HOFFMANN and O. MERGELSBERG, Dermat. Ztschr. **35**:1 (Nov.) 1921.

This is a review of the results of treatment of the patients under observation for primary and secondary syphilis. Every effort was made to obtain the late results by consulting records of the clinic, hospital, private office, advisory clinic, investigation of births, health of children, stillbirths, Wassermann reactions and provocative procedures. The therapeutic procedures are outlined. In the consideration of abortive treatment of primary seronegative syphilis, only those cases were entered in which no Wassermann reaction ever changed to positive, although the serologic reaction was performed at every arsphenamin injection. There were 176 seronegative patients with primary syphilis, of whom ninety-one were followed for ten years. Of thirteen of these patients treated with old arsphenamin, seven had received the drug intramuscularly, and six had received intravenous injections. Mercury was also given. There was one clinical recurrence in this series (after 0.5 gm. arsphenamin intramuscularly and one mercury course). Sodium arsphenamin was used in sixty-six patients, with mercury rubs and by injection. There were two serologic remissions and one clinical recurrence. One of the patients with serologic remission was later found not to be an example of abortive treatment since the patient had received two previous courses with an initial positive Wassermann reaction. Silver arsphenamin was used without mercury in eleven patients, and after two years no recurrence or remission has been noted. Of the total ninety-one patients, recurrence could be said to have occurred in four, or 4.4 per cent. Reinfection was observed in four patients of this series.

There were 354 patients treated in the seropositive primary stage of syphilis, of whom 160 were followed. Thirty-nine had been treated with old arsphenamin, and nineteen of these had received only one or two intramuscular injections with a mercury course. Of the nineteen, four had had clinical recurrence, and of the twenty treated with intravenous arsphenamin, three had had clinical recurrences; but there were extenuating circumstances, such as prolonged intervals between injections. Few patients were treated with large doses of neo-arsphenamin, with one recurrence after four months. Sodium arsphenamin was injected into eighty-nine patients with thirteen serologic recurrences and seven clinical recurrences. In eight cases of recurrence, there had been prolonged intervals (over fourteen days) between injections, and in others the individual doses were too small (begun with 0.3 gm.), and the total dosage was less than 5 gm. However, there still remained three patients showing recurrence who had received the full course, including mercury. Silver arsphenamin had been used in nineteen patients with seropositive primary syphilis with records of two serologic and one clinical recurrence. The serologic recurrences followed 2.2 gm., and the clinical recurrence 1.3 gm. without mercury. Reinfection following intensive treatment of seropositive primary syphilis was recorded four times. Summing up seropositive primary syphilis, one finds recurrence thirty-one times in 160 patients, or 18.7 per cent., as compared with 4.4 per cent. for persons with seronegative primary syphilis. This led to the conclusion that such patients should receive two courses; experience showed the value of this if the second course was begun when the Wassermann test was still negative, but if the Wassermann test was positive, a second reversal of the Wassermann test to positive after the course was to be expected.

Of an immense number of patients with secondary syphilis treated with old arsphenamin, only twenty-five were followed for from six to ten years, and all were found to have a negative Wassermann reaction, and with no organic lesions of syphilis. Seventeen patients were treated with one course of old arsphenamin, from four to six injections, one patient with seven, and a good mercury course. In half the series the Wassermann reaction had been reversed, but no difference could be detected from six to ten years later. The same results were found for patients treated with neo-arsphenamin, and examined from eight to nine years later. On the other hand, patients who did not complete the course of treatment in the secondary stage gave numerous clinical and serologic recurrences. A number of patients have positive serologic reactions which cannot be influenced by treatment. The negative Wassermann reaction does not exclude possibilities of clinical lesions for recurrent secondary infections have been seen when the Wassermann test was negative. Silver arsphenamin has been used in fifty patients. Of eighteen seen later, eight had negative Wassermann reactions, four had serologic recurrence, and two had weakly positive Wassermann reactions; two other patients had had positive Wassermann reactions throughout the first series of treatments, and this positive Wassermann reaction was existent at the beginning of the second course. There was a clinical recurrence after six months (twelve silver arsphenamin, two mercury injections and ten rubs); also one neurorecidive two months after receiving fourteen silver arsphenamin injections (total of 3.35 gm.) but no mercury. Patients treated with two courses of silver arsphenamin have not yet appeared for reexamination.

There is much discussion of theoretical possibilities in treatment, many notes of historical interest, and observations of considerable value on reactions and difficulties of follow up work. There are numerous tables. The article is forty-three pages in length.

GOODMAN, New York.

ARTIFICIAL COMPLEMENT. LIEBERMANN, Deutsch med. Wchnschr. **47**: 43, 1921.

To prepare this complement 2 c.c. of a fresh mixture of 5 c.c. of a 0.1 per cent. methyl alcohol-sodium oleinate solution and 1 c.c. of a 0.1 per cent. methyl alcohol-calcium chlorid solution are added in drops to 3 c.c. of an inactivated 1:10 diluted normal rabbit serum. With this artificial complement hemolytic immune bodies are activated as with a natural complement.

SKIN ERUPTION DUE TO THE HAIRS OF THE CATERPILLAR. MARCOTTY, Deutsch. med. Wchnschr. **47**:1015, 1921.

The author discusses the formation of tubercle-like nodules around the os frontale of a boy who had rubbed caterpillar hairs into his eye. The hairs were found deep in the subcutaneous tissue. There was regression of the nodules in six months.

DISEASES OF THE SKIN FROM PUS COCCI (STAPHYLODERMA). UNNA, Deutsch. med. Wchnschr. **47**:1251, 1921.

The painfulness of perifolliculitis, furuncles and carbuncles is due to toxin tension in the hair follicles. In the abscesses of sucklings the pains are much less severe as the skin is soft and gives way. Staphylococci are found chiefly in the "reducing loci" (Reduktionsorte) of the skin. The reducing toxin which they produce kills the leukocytes by abstraction of oxygen.

THE ANTIGEN PROPERTIES OF ORGANOLIPOIDS. NIEDERHOFF, Deutsch. med. Wchnschr. **47**:1284, 1921.

Experiments proved that pure lipoids do not possess antigen properties in the sense of hemolysis and lipoid flocculation. This is contrary to the theory of Wassermann who believes that the antibodies in the serum of a syphilitic patient whose reaction is positive are of lipoid origin.

NONCONTAGIOUS ERUPTIVE FEVERS. KUDICKE, Fortschr. d. Med. **38**: 263, 1921.

This article contains a description of a new disease discovered in Portuguese East Africa. Chills, headache, conjunctivitis and swelling of the spleen are followed by the development of pea-sized reddish spots similar to the eruptions in measles. The patient's temperature is from 38 to 40 C. (100.4 to 104 F.). After the fifth day the eruptions begin to disappear. From the seventh to the tenth day there is a crisis or lysis. The prognosis is favorable. The author proposes the name "inuga fever."

AHLSWEDE, Hamburg, Germany.

A CASE OF ACNITIS. L. BUSSALAI, Gior. Ital. mal. ven. **58**:40 (Feb.) 1922.

The author reports a case of acnitis. He is in favor of the theory of the toxic origin of tuberculids.

A RARE CASE OF EXTRAGENITAL CHANCRE. G. NARDI, Gior. Ital. mal. ven. **58**:58 (Feb.) 1922.

The author reports a case of syphilitic chancre of the scalp. The patient had been bitten on the head during a fight with two other men.

PARDO-CASTELLO, Havana.

FOLLICULITIS DECALVANS PROFUNDA. S. HAGIWARA, Japan, Ztschr. f. Dermat. u. Urol. **21**: No. 6, 1921.

The usual pathology and bacteriology were reported in a case of folliculitis decalvans.

LUPOID SYCOSIS. K. NAKAGAWA, Japan. Ztschr. f. Dermat. u. Urol. **21**: No. 7, 1921.

The author reports a case of lupoid sycosis of thirteen years' duration involving the face and temporal regions of the scalp. Smears and cultures of pus from new lesions and from roots of hairs revealed *Staphylococcus pyogenes aureus*. Repeated histologic examinations revealed early degeneration of the collagen fibers with no changes in the elastic fibers in fresh inflammatory lesions. The reverse is true in sycosis vulgaris. He thinks that this is due to a specific action of the *Staphylococcus albus*. He agrees with Brocq and Arndt in calling lupoid sycosis a distinct clinical entity.

THE ACTION OF MERCURY IN SYPHILIS: ITS EFFECT ON ALBUMIN AND CASTS IN THE URINE. SHINZO ISHIHARA. Japan. Ztschr. f. Dermat. u. Urol. **21**: No. 7, 1921.

The author noticed fatigue in patients receiving mercury salicylate injections. The urine of many of these contained albumin and casts. He studied the effect of mercury in 138 patients with syphilis and found that male and female Japs of average weight showed no ill effects after ten injections of a

10 per cent. mercury salicylate emulsion. Albumin and casts were found after a course of twenty injections. He recommends small doses of mercury for the treatment of syphilis.

URTICARIA PERSTANS. S. Dohi, Japan. Ztschr. f. Dermat. u. Urol. **21:** No. 8, 1921.

A report is made of five cases of urticaria perstans. The author agrees with Kreibich in differentiating urticaria perstans papulosa from urticaria perstans verrucosa. The size of the lesions in the first condition varies from that of a lentil to that of a pea. The lesions are quite hard and are situated mostly on the trunk and extremities. The size of the lesions in the second condition vary from that of a pea to that of a hazelnut. These lesions are very hard and appear chiefly on the extensor surfaces of the extremities.

A SPECIAL FORM OF SEPTIC TOXICODERMA (ERYTHEMA SEPTICOTOXICUM). C. Tanimura, Japan. Ztschr. f. Dermat. u. Urol. **21:** No. 8, 1921.

In this condition the first lesions appear on the mucous membrane of the uvula, tonsils, soft and hard palate, pharynx and larynx. Later the mucous membranes of the cheeks, tongue and lips are involved. The skin of the ears, neck, scalp and extensor surfaces of the extremities are subsequently attacked. The trunk is usually spared.

On the mucous membranes the lesions consist of swollen red and white patches, erosions and small swellings. On the skin they are in the form of dark red, pea to walnut sized macules with small, hard papulopustules in the middle. At the onset there is a rise in temperature accompanied by malaise, headache, albuminuria and finally prostration. With amelioration of the general symptoms the macules and pustules fade leaving pigmented areas. Crops of the lesions may be noticed. The condition is a septicoderma resembling impetigo herpetiformis and erythema multiforme. The causative agent is unknown. Good results in treatment were obtained with calcium chlorid injections, a proprietary electric colloid silver solution and inunctions with soluble silver salves.

Levin, New York.

VINCENT'S ANGINA WITH SPECIAL REFERENCE TO THE BLOOD PICTURE. Tarnow, Med. Klin. **17:**34, 1921.

The disorder has not only a topical effect but also stimulates the activity of the bonemarrow.

THE GENERALIZATION OF CUTANEOUS VACCINATION WITH SPECIAL REFERENCE TO THE GONOCOCCAL CUTANEOUS VACCINATION. Schmidt-La Baume, Med. Klin. **17:**43, 1921.

The author applied the Ponndorf method to other infectious diseases, particularly to such as respond with difficulty to subcutaneous vaccination, such as gonorrhea. The skin was scratched and the gonococcal vaccine rubbed in with distinctly better therapeutic results than by intravenous or intramuscular administration.

APPLICATION OF FLAVICID IN DERMATOLOGY. KALLMANN, Med. Klin. **17**:49, 1921.

The acridinium dye flavicid (acriflavine) proved superior to tincture of iodin and equally as effective as cinnabar ointment in impetigo, pustular eczemas, furunculosis and sycosis parasitaria. The antipruritic and epithelizing effects were marked. Stains on linen were removed with hot soapy water.

SCLERODERMIC DYSTROPHIA. CURSCHMANN, Med. Klin. **17**:1223, 1921.

The author discusses the importance of pluriglandular insufficiency with regard to the general symptoms accompanying scleroderma, such as asthenia, asthma cachexia and anemia. Pluriglandular insufficiency is not the cause of scleroderma, but both are the coordinated consequence of a primary damage to the nutritive center and of the domination of the endocrine system by the sympathetic nerve. Scleroderma is a tropho-angio-neurosis of central origin.

TECHNIC OF INTRAVENOUS INJECTION AND MERCURIC CHLO-RID INJECTION TREATMENT OF VARICES. MODEL, Med. Klin. **17**:1292, 1921.

The best treatment of ulcus cruris varicosum is to obliterate the varices by injecting mercuric chlorid according to the method of Linser, and then apply-ing Unna's glycogelatin dressing. At one treatment not more than one injec-tion of 1 to 2 c.c. of a 1 per cent. solution of mercuric chlorid was given.

TREATMENT OF ERYSIPELAS WITH 16 PER CENT. SILVER NITRATE. HIRSCH, Med. Klin. **17**:1299, 1921.

The lesions are painted once well into the healthy surrounding part with 16 per cent silver nitrate. Slight pains are unavoidable. From six to eight days later desquamation occurs. There were only 3 per cent. of recurrences in 120 successfully treated patients.

SUCCESSFUL ABORTIVE TREATMENT OF SYPHILIS WITH SILVER ARSPHENAMIN BASED ON TWO YEARS' EXPERIENCE. ENGLESON, Med. Klin. **17**:1323, 1921.

Engleson administers silver arsphenamin without synchronous mercury medication. He injects at three or four day intervals, twice 0.15 gm. and twice 0.2 gm. Then he injects three times 0.25 gm. at five or six day intervals and finally three times 0.3 gm. also at five or six day intervals. Not less than 2 gm. are necessary for one "course." The injections should be made slowly, requiring at least two minutes.

THE EVALUATION OF THE LINSER METHOD IN THE TREAT-MENT OF SYPHILIS. EICKE and ROSE. München. med. Wchnschr. **68**:45. 1921.

Spirochetes do not disappear from lesions as quickly as in arsphenamin medication alone. The clinical symptoms were not influenced with more advantage than with arsphenamin alone.

PROTEIN BODY TREATMENT. Schittenhelm, München. med. Wchnschr. **68**:46, 1921.

The author advises protein treatment in chronic infectious disorders. The proteins gained from milk are particularly effective in the treatment of ophthalmic disorders. The dosage requires attention. The author has not seen anaphylactic reactions or disturbances. The proteins act by "activation of the protoplasm" (Weichardt).

THE NEW SIMPLIFIED SYPHILIS FLOCCULATION REACTION (TURBIDITY REACTION) AFTER DOLD. Poehlmann, München. med. Wchnschr. **68**:1350, 1921.

Dold asserts that his method gives macroscopically visible results as early as three or four hours after the reaction. Poehlmann tested the method and found that twenty-four hours are necessary, as well as the aid of an agglutinoscope to avoid mistakes. Otherwise the reaction is very exact and almost corresponds to the Sachs-Georgi method. Dold's reaction has the disadvantage of requiring more serum and nearly double the quantity of extract.

THE SPINAL FLUID CURRENT AND THE HOMOGENEITY OF THE CEREBROSPINAL FLUID. Walter, München. med. Wchnschr. **68**:1352, 1921.

Walter discusses the source of the spinal fluid. He believes it is a secretion of the meninges or of the medulla itself. The composition of the fluid is not homogeneous. There is consequently no active spinal fluid current. The fluid forms various layers as it were. This also explains some hitherto incomprehensible observations, such as the absence of lymphocytosis in some cases of progressive paralysis as well as a negative spinal fluid reaction in multiple sclerosis.

DEMONSTRATION AND ACTION OF EXTRACT LIPOIDS IN THE VARIOUS FLOCCULATION REACTIONS. Niederhoff, München. med. Wchnschr. **68**:1419, 1921.

Examination of the flocculae showed that only one eighth of the lipoid quantity consists of globulin. As to the theoretical explanation of the flocculation process, the author believes that the appearance of the flocculae is chiefly due to the desiccation of the extract lipoids through abstraction of water.

Ahlswede, Hamburg, Germany.

PROTEIN THERAPY IN DERMATOLOGY. G. A. Ambrosoli, Osp. magiore **9**:232 (Oct.) 1921.

The author has employed nonbacterial proteins in the treatment of several skin diseases. He has used intramuscular injections of peptone, deuteralbumose and sterile milk. The results have been favorable in Duhring's disease, eczema, pemphigus, lichen planus, furunculosis and dermatitis seborrheica. In psoriasis and parapsoriasis there was no improvement with this treatment.

CEREBELLAR ATAXIA IN JUVENILE HEREDITARY PARESIS. A. Dufour, Osp. magiore **9**:293 (Nov.) 1921.

The study of the author's case and the review of the literature suggest that early ataxic symptoms of cerebellar type are very frequent in juvenile paresis. According to Dufour, this may serve to make the differential diagnosis with general paresis of acquired syphilis.

ARTHRITIS IN THE AGED AS THE ONLY MANIFESTATION OF SYPHILIS. R. Ortega, Prensa med. Argentina **8**:277 (Jan.) 1922.

The author presents four cases of chronic arthritis which had lasted for several years, in patients from 60 to 84 years of age. All were cured by specific therapy. No other signs of syphilis could be detected.

Pardo-Castello, Havana.

FRENCH SOCIETY OF DERMATOLOGY AND SYPHILOLOGY. Presse méd. **6**:64 (Jan.) 1922.

Tuberculin Therapy.—Drs. Chevalier and Blamontier presented a woman who had consulted them about papulonecrotic tuberculid of the legs accompanied by two subcutaneous gummatous nodosities and chilblain ulcers of the toes. These lesions yielded in eight days to three injections of tuberculin.

Normal Number of Lymphocytes in the Spinal Fluid.—Dr. Leredde estimated that 3 lymphocytes per cubic millimeter, ordinarily admitted as pathologic, is too high, and that even one lymphocyte per cubic millimeter should be regarded as pathologic.

Application in Dermatology of Tar and of the Essence of Cedar of Marocain Atlas.—Drs. Lepinay and Massy presented some specimens of tar and of the essence of cedar. Liquid tar, as oil of cade, may be utilized in glyceroles or ointments, or be employed pure.

They believe that the essence of cedar is just about as good as oil of cade, without the objectionable odor of tar. It is indicated in any dermatosis that is scaly and infiltrated.

Bismuth Stomatitis.—Drs. Milian and Perin presented several patients who had been treated at close intervals with several injections of insoluble salts of bismuth. Some of these patients presented lesions of stomatitis analogous to those which Dr. Balzer had provoked experimentally in 1889 in the dog. There were three degrees of stomatitis: a simple gingivitis, gingivitis with complications and gingivitis with ulcerations. One occasionally saw some slate colored pigmented spots on the buccal mucosae, soft palate and tongue, suggesting Addison's disease. The pigment was deposited on the summit of the papillae and was bismuth as shown chemically. The urine was black and was proved to be due to bismuth.

Dr. Hudelo said that he had observed serious lesions of stomatitis in 30 per cent. of the cases. Bismuth stomatitis has less salivation than mercurial stomatitis.

Dr. Milian has observed some general symptoms occurring from injections of bismuth; general fatigue, anorexia, headache.

He employed bismuth in some patients who resisted arsenical and mercurial treatment and obtained some good results. In a patient who had a positive Wassermann reaction for two years, in spite of arsenic and mercury, seven injections of bismuth was sufficient to produce a negative Wassermann reaction

The Employment of Soluble Bismuth-Tartrate in the Treatment of Syphilis. —Drs. Jeanselme and his associates have employed a soluble preparation of potassium and sodium bismuth tartrate in glucose solution in the treatment of syphilis. The injections were made intragluteally, in a dose of 10 centigrams every two days. It is important not to inject the drug into a blood vessel. Experimentally, an injection of 10 centigrams intravenously in a rabbit will cause instant death. In man an attack of syncope is produced if only a small amount of the injection gets into the blood stream. The presence of bismuth is established in the urine, saliva and cerebrospinal fluid some hours later by the reaction of Leger.

The action of this drug on primary and secondary syphilis is very satis-factory; it is identical with the insoluble preparations. In a case of secondary syphilis, in poor general health and headache, the symptoms disappeared after the fifth injection. The Wassermann reaction has not been changed during the treatment, which has not been continued for longer than a month, in the thirty patients under treatment.

These injections are painless and give rise to no nodosities. In forty per cent. of the cases one notices slight buccal mucosae changes.

Dr. L. Fournier spoke very favorably of the insoluble salts of bismuth. He did not approve of the use of soluble salts of bismuth because of their extreme toxicity. He believed that the gingivitis could be controlled by smaller doses and well spaced. He has never observed albuminuria.

Transmission to Man of the Sarcoptic Itch of the Dog.—Dr. Thibierge points out that this itch is more frequent than one suspects. The lesions in man are characterized by localized nodules on the face, flexors of forearms, thorax and abdomen. One does not find furrows interdigitally nor scaling lesions. The finding of the sarcoptes in dog is quite difficult; it is necessary to scrape deeply to discover it.

McCAFFERTY, New York.

THE TREATMENT OF SYPHILIS WITH BISMUTH SALTS. J. CEBRIAN, Prog. Clin. **10**:320 (March) 1922.

The bismuth salts, introduced in syphilography by Levaditi and Sazerac, are powerful spirocheticides. The severe nitritoid reactions and the late accidents observed after arsenical therapy are not produced by the bismuth preparations. Another advantage is the fact that the latter permeate the meninges and therefore have a direct action on the nervous system. The com-pounds that have been used are the tartrobismuthate of sodium and potassium, the hydroxid of bismuth and the iodobismuthate of quinin. Bismuth injections produce severe stomatitis and sometimes marked asthenia. Dr. L. Fournier of the Hôpital Cochin in Paris is using iodobismuthate of quinin exclusively instead of the arsenical compounds.

EXPERIMENTAL STUDIES ON THE INFECTIOUS NATURE OF HERPES. R. VEGNI, Riforma med. **38**:270 (March) 1922.

The author succeeded in reproducing herpes by inoculating the contents of the vesicles of herpes labialis into the cornea of rabbits. He concludes that herpes may be transmitted indefinitely from rabbit to rabbit when inoculated into the cornea; that rabbits thus inoculated die from encephalitis in 83 per cent. of the cases; that brain material from infected rabbits may reproduce the disease when inoculated into the cornea; that the surviving animals are immune to a new inoculation; and finally that the virus of herpes is a filtrable germ which is destroyed at 50 C.

GHILARDUCCI'S METHOD FOR THE UTILIZATION OF SECONDARY ROENTGEN RAYS. C. Guarini, Riforma med. **38**:361 (April) 1922.

Ghilarducci's suggestion that secondary roentgen rays produced when the direct radiation strikes a metallic surface have a marked therapeutic action, has been tried by the author. He claims to have cured several persons of lupus vulgaris by irradiating the lesions, covered with lead foil.

PSEUDOGRANULOMA MAJOCCHI. G. Pini, Proc. Seventeenth Meeting. Soc. ital. derm., 1921, p. 80.

The author describes a peculiar form of folliculitis of the scalp very similar to trichophytic granuloma. The disease formed a thick, infiltrated, raised patch the size of a silver dollar, situated on the vertex and formed by the aggregation of numerous follicular papules and nodules which gave it a convoluted aspect. No fungus was found. The author discusses the differential diagnosis with cutis verticis gyrata, folliculitis and folliculitis decalvans. Roentgenotherapy effected a complete cure.

VALUE OF THE SACHS-GEORGI TEST IN THE DIAGNOSIS OF SYPHILIS. L. Morini, Proc. Seventeenth Meeting Soc. ital derm., 1921, p. 95.

According to Morini, the test is positive in 90 per cent. of the cases of syphilis. In 83 per cent. the results are in accord with the Wassermann test. The Sachs-Georgi test is positive earlier than the Wassermann and remains positive after syphilitic treatment even after the Wassermann test has become negative.

ON THE ETIOLOGY OF ECZEMA. Mario Copelli. Proc. Seventeenth Meeting Soc. ital. derm., 1921, p. 138.

The author has found a marked diminution of the coagulability of the blood in cases of eczema. He claims to have cured many patients with enemas of gelatin, 50 gm.; calcium chlorid, 10 gm.; laudanum. 2 gm., and water. 700 c.c. In cases of artificial eczema and in cases of dermatitis seborrheica, the coagulability is practically normal. The organic and mineral acidity of the blood of patients with eczema does not differ from that of normal persons.

HOMAGE TO PROFESSOR MAJOCCHI. Proc. Seventeenth Meeting Soc. ital. derm., 1921.

The proceedings of the seventeenth meeting of the Societa Italiana di Dermatologia e Sifiligrafia give the details of the homage paid Prof. Domenico Majocchi on the fortieth anniversary of his professorship. The eminent dermatologist was presented with a gold medal and a diploma by his admirers and disciples. Professor Majocchi is a prolific writer. having contributed to the dermatologic literature 128 original articles. His studies on purpura annularis telangiectodes and on trichophytosis have given him international fame.

CUTANEOUS LEISHMANIASIS IN SARDINIA. I. Righi, Sperimentale **76**:87, 1922.

This article contains the report of a case of oriental sore with an anatomopathologic study.

BISMUTH IN THE TREATMENT OF SYPHILIS. N. V. Greco and A. H. Muschietti, Semana méd., 1921, p. 51.

After a review of the results obtained with bismuth salts in the treatment of syphilis by Sazerac, Levaditi, Louis Fournier and L. Guenot, the authors go into the details of this new treatment and the results obtained by them. They conclude that the iodid of bismuth and the tartrobismuthate of potassium and sodium have a favorable influence on syphilitic lesions; the cutaneous and mucous lesions disappear rapidly, and the Wassermann test becomes negative. They are not, nevertheless, enthusiastic about this new form of therapy of syphilis, and they finally conclude that further studies are necessary to establish its true value.

Pardo-Castello, Havana.

RINGWORM OF THE NAILS OF THE HANDS. H. C. Semon, Proc. Roy. Soc. **15**:27 (May) 1922.

A man, aged 22, had had the condition since 1918, when he was in a camp at Wareham; before its commencement he had been in France ten months, and before going to France he was in America—he is an American subject. The American authorities refused to receive him back when he was repatriated, because of the nail disease, and they returned him to us. He was shown especially in order to discuss treatment. In view of his urgent desire to return home, the inclination was to remove all the nails of the hands, and to treat the bases with some caustic, such as pyrogallic acid, for some time after the operation. Ringworm of the nails is comparatively rare in England, and generally only one or two nails are affected. Usually the fungus which affects the nails is a trichophyton of animal origin.

Dr. MacLeod said that three months ago he had treated a man from Java with a similar condition. In his case all the nails of hands and feet·were affected. He obtained a trichophyton-like fungus from the scraping, which he thought might possibly have been *Epidermophyton inguinale*, but he had not succeeded in growing it. The patient had had tinea cruris previously. Numerous forms of treatment had been tried, without success, and it was decided to remove all the nails. This was done under an anesthetic. The nail bed was then scraped and iodin applied. The parts were subsequently dressed with mercurial ointment When last seen the nails were growing and appeared to be healthy

Guy, Pittsburgh.

SOME CASES OF MYIASIS IN INDIA AND PERSIA, WITH A DESCRIPTION OF THE LARVAE CAUSING THE LESIONS. J. A. Sinton, Indian J. M. Res. **9**:132 (July) 1921.

Six cases of larval infection are reported. The nose, gums and hand were affected in three persons; there were two infections in camels and one in a dog. Complete descriptions of the larvae accompany the article.

NOTE ON THE BEHAVIOR OF HERPETOMONAS TROPICA WRIGHT, THE PARASITE OF CUTANEOUS HERPETOMONAS (ORIENTAL SORE) IN THE BED BUG CIMEX HEMIPTERA FABRICIUS. W. S. PATTON, H. M. LA FRENAIS and SUNDARA RAO, Indian J. M. Res. 9:240 (Oct.) 1921.

Insects were allowed to feed on the blood of infected cases and later examined microscopically and cultured. It was found that the organism in question could live in the bed bug for from twenty-three to forty-four days and probably longer, depending on varying conditions. The writers believe that their experiments prove that the bed bug is the true invertebrate host of this parasite.

NOTE ON THE BEHAVIOR OF HERPETOMONAS DONOVANI LAVERAN AND MESNIL IN THE BED BUG, CIMEX HEMIPTERA FABRICIUS. W. S. PATTON, H. M. LA FRENAIS and SUNDARA RAO, Indian J. M. Res. 9:252 (Oct.) 1921.

Experiments similar to those in a preceding article are described and with similar conclusions.

SIGNIFICANCE AND VALUE OF A POSITIVE WASSERMANN REACTION IN TUBERCULOSIS. K. R. K. IYENGAR, Indian J. M. Res. 9:369 (Oct.) 1921.

Of seventy patients examined, 20 per cent. returned a positive reaction. As the author had obtained a similar percentage in an unselected, apparently healthy Indian population, he concludes that his results are due to latent syphilis and that tuberculosis does not produce a positive reaction.

SOME REFLECTIONS ON THE KALA-AZAR AND ORIENTAL SORE PROBLEMS. W. S. PATTON, Indian J. M. Res. 9:496 (Jan.) 1922.

This is an account of the work of the author and his associates in their search for the insects carrying the infection and the finding of the organism in the midgut of the bed bug. The length of life in the carrier has not yet been definitely determined, although a great deal of human experimentation was done but is not yet complete. An intracellular form of the parasites is now known to exist.

COIL GLAND NUCLEOLI. KREIBICH, Arch. f. Dermat. u. Syph. 124: No. 4, 1918.

Coil gland nucleoli contain nuclein and nucleolin, and therefore take their origin from the nuclei.

RELATION BETWEEN ERYTHEMA NODOSUM AND SYPHILIS. STUEMPKE, Arch. f. Dermat. u. Syph. 124: No. 4, 1918.

The author believes that a staphylococcus is the cause of erythema nodosum. while syphilis only forms the basis on which it develops its activity.

ETIOLOGY OF PEMPHIGUS VULGARIS. STUEMPKE. Arch. f. Dermat. u. Syph. 124: No. 4. 1918.

The author reports two cases of pemphigus which developed in connection with infected wounds.

A CONTRIBUTION TO THE STUDY OF KALA-AZAR (V). J. W. CORNWALL and H. M. LA FRENAIS, Indian J. M. Res. **9**:533 (Jan.) 1922.

This is a report of experimental work on the stomach and gut of bed bugs fed on infected material. The authors feel convinced that there is not an intracellular phase of the organism.

HISTOPATHOLOGY OF A NONULCERATED ORIENTAL SORE. J. W. CORNWALL, Indian J. M. Res. **9**:545 (Jan.) 1922.

No parasites were found in any cells of the epidermis itself, including the sweat and sebaceous glands and hair follicles, although the breeding place was the mononuclear endothelial cells of the papillary layer. Proliferation of the cells and organisms causes an interference with the blood and nerve supply with subsequent ulceration, which is said to occur as a curative process.

THE RELIABILITY OF GATÉ AND PAPACOSTAS' FORMOL-GEL TEST FOR SYPHILIS AS COMPARED WITH THE WASSERMANN REACTION. S. RAMA KRISHNAN, Indian J. M. Res. **9**:620 (Jan.) 1922.

In 539 cases the two reactions were compared and agreed in only two thirds of the cases. The former test is not considered reliable enough to displace the Wassermann.

CHEMICAL STUDIES OF THE BLOOD AND URINE OF SYPHILITIC PATIENTS UNDER ARSPHENAMIN TREATMENT, WITH A NOTE ON THE MECHANISM OF EARLY ARSPHENAMIN REACTIONS. C. WEISS and A. CORSON, Arch. Int. Med. **29**:428 (April) 1922.

Small increases in the nonprotein nitrogen of the blood were almost constantly observed three hours after 0.6 gm. doses of arsphenamin had been injected intravenously. Patients with the most severe reaction showed the greatest increase, and there were no significant increases except in those presenting pronounced reactions. Urea nitrogen increases did not parallel the nonprotein nitrogen, nor were the blood readings on discharge of the patient any higher than on admission. Impaired kidney function was not followed by arsphenamin reactions.

Variable increases in blood sugar were also noted, uric acid was normal as was phenolsulphonephthalein elimination and the carbon dioxid combining power of the plasma.

The authors suggest that early reactions may be due to a general tissue injury due to the toxic action of the drug or its products of oxidation or reduction in the tissues of hypersensitive patients.

JAMIESON, Detroit.

SYMMETRIC CYSTIC ENLARGEMENT OF THE LACRIMAL GLANDS DUE TO SYPHILIS. H. W. COWPER, Am. J. Ophth. **5**:125 (Feb.) 1922.

The author gives a case report. One arsphenamin injection resulted in a gradual disappearance of the swellings.

IS CANCER MORTALITY INCREASING? WENDELL M. STRONG, J. Cancer Res. **6**:251 (July) 1921.

The conclusion drawn from a study of reliable life insurance statistics for the period 1911-1921 is that there is no appreciable increase in cancer mortality. A decrease or slight fluctuation has been indicated for ages below 65, an increase for ages 65 and over. The latter is attributed to more careful diagnosis.

H. R. FOERSTER, Milwaukee.

THE PATHOGENESIS OF DYSHIDROSIS. KREIBICH, Arch. f. Dermat. u. Syph. **122:** No. 10, 1916.

The author reports a case of gunshot damage of a nerve with subsequent development of dyshidrosis on the corresponding skin surface.

SKIN LYMPHOGRANULOMATOSIS. DOSSECKER, Arch. f. Dermat. u. Syph. **124:** No. 2, 1918.

A woman, who carried heavy burdens on her head, developed a tumor of the scalp which macroscopically and microscopically proved to be a malign lymphogranuloma. From the course which the disease ran, the author concludes that the virus entered the system through the scalp. He therefore considers this case to be a genuine primary skin granulomatosis.

EXPERIMENTS CONCERNING VIRULENT TUBERCLE BACILLI IN THE BLOOD AFTER DIAGNOSTIC APPLICATION OF TUBER-CULIN IN A CASE OF TUBERCULOSIS CUTIS. SCHOENFELD. Arch. f. Dermat. u. Syph. **124:** No. 2, 1918.

In tuberculosis cutis, the bacilli are found in the circulating blood far more seldom than in tuberculous disorders of the internal organs. It was not possible to decide whether diagnostic administration of tuberculin or intravenous injections of gold potassium cyanid can mobilize the bacilli.

A POSITIVE WASSERMANN REACTION IN TUBERCULOSIS CUTIS AND TUBERCULIDS. SCHOENFELD. Arch. f. Dermat. u. Syph. **124** No. 2, 1918.

In all of the cases tested the Wassermann reaction was negative.

EROSIO INTERDIGITALIS BLASTOMYCETICA. BERENDSEN. Arch. f. Dermat. u. Syph. **124:** No. 2, 1918.

Bacteriologic examination revealed a certain species of myces (Hefe) which the author assumes to be the cause of the disorder.

THE TYPHUS EXANTHEM. LIPSCHÜTZ. Arch. f. Dermat. u. Syph. **124:** No. 2, 1918.

The author reports seventeen cases in which the various symptoms and types of typhus exanthems are exemplified. The circulatory disturbances in the skin and the hemorrhagic constituent of the exanthem need special attention. The diagnosis and differential diagnosis, also typhus sine exanthemate. are discussed.

GROUPED PAPULAR TUBERCULIDS. SCHERBER. Arch. f. Dermat. u. Syph. **124:** No. 2, 1918.

This is the report of a case in which acnitis-like eruptions developed along the side of the neck. The clinical symptoms, swollen glands and doubtful condition of the lungs pointed to a tuberculous organ. Injections of old tuberculin effected a cure.

EPIDERMOLYSIS BULLOSA CONGENITA. Stühmer, Arch. f. Dermat. u. Syph. **124:** No. 2, 1918.

The author ascribes the cause of this disorder to a disturbed function of the thyroid gland and the suprarenals. An abnormal irritation of certain nerve centers accounts for the symptoms on the skin (vesicles, etc.) and the vessels. The normal vasomotor regulations being disturbed, a permanent irregular inhibition of the tissue follows. Histologically, the elastica and other elements become atrophic. The disorder is therefore a dystrophia cutis spinalis congenita.

VACCINATION EXPERIMENTS WITH VENEREAL WARTS. Wülser, Arch. f. Dermat. u. Syph. **124:** No. 4, 1918.

In all three cases vaccination was positive after an incubation period of two and one-half to nine months. Small flat warts developed on the skin at the site of vaccination. The author believes their development was due to implantation.

THE PATHOGENESIS OF PSORIASIS. Kreibich, Arch. f. Dermat. u. Syph. **124:** No. 4, 1918.

The author reports a case which supports the neuropathic hypothesis. A psoriasis disappeared on one side after a gunshot wound of the shoulder.

SKIN INFLAMMATIONS AND WAR EXPERIENCES IN SKIN DISEASES. Hammer, Arch. f. Dermat. u. Syph. **124:** No. 4, 1918.

The author discusses the inflammations of the skin from a new point of view. He classifies the disorders into two groups: (1) acute eliminating processes, (2) secluding or enclosing processes.

MERCURY ADMINISTRATION IN SYPHILIS AND ALBUMINURIA. Forstmann, Arch. f. Dermat. u. Syph. **124:** No. 4, 1918.

Albuminuria is caused by stomatitis and only in exceptional cases by mercury itself. Mouth washes and disinfection of the gums prevent albuminuria.

CAUSE OF MISSING LOCAL REACTIONS. Karl and Koch, Arch. f. Dermat. u. Syph. **124:** No. 4, 1918.

Eruptions which are in a rising stage of development do not show local reactions.

TREATMENT OF PARAPSORIASIS (BROCQ). Wiesmann, Arch. f. Dermat. u. Syph. **124:** No. 4, 1918.

The author reports therapeutic success with the use of pilocarpin.

MACULAR EXANTHEM IN DIABETES MELLITUS. Koch, Arch. f. Dermat. u. Syph. **124:** No. 4, 1918.

In nine cases of diabetes, the author observed bluish macular eruptions with central reddening.

A CASE OF EPIDERMOLYSIS BULLOSA HEREDITARIA. Zweig, Arch. f. Dermat. u. Syph. **125:** No. 1, 1918.

The disorder was traced through three generations in twelve members of a family.

LYMPHOGRANULOMATOSIS. KREN, Arch. f. Dermat. u. Syph. **125:** No. 4-5, 1919.

The tuberculous origin of the disorder is by no means certain.

FREQUENCY, DIAGNOSIS AND TREATMENT OF SYPHILITIC AORTITIS. SCHRUMPF, Arch. f. Dermat. u. Syph. **125:** No. 4-5, 1919.

Suprasigmoidea aortitis is most frequent; abdominal aortitis comparatively rare. Syphilis of the arteria coronaria is rarely found alone, but is generally combined with other forms of aortitis. Treatment: 3 gm. iodid of potassium a day for six weeks, and 0.45 gm. neo-arsphenamin once a week.

BOECK'S MILIARY LUPOID. LUTZ, Arch. f. Dermat. u. Syph. **125:** No. 4-5, 1919.

The author reports two hereditary cases. In one the hypodermic injection of 2 mg. of tuberculin caused strong local reaction; in the other 1 mg. caused a reaction at the site of injection.

A CASE OF ESSENTIAL TELEANGIECTASIS. FUCHS, Arch. f. Dermat. u. Syph. **136:**325, 1921.

This is the report of a patient who developed teleangiectases on the face, arms and trunk after removal of the uterus. The author believes in a neurogenous origin of the affection.

MYCOTIC GENERAL INFECTIONS IN TRICHOPHYTOSES AND MICROSPOROSES. ARZT and FUHS, Arch. f. Dermat. u. Syph. **136:**333. 1921.

The authors distinguished between various kinds of mycotic general infection. Whether these are caused by antigens or fungi elements is not decided. They distinguish (1) the exanthematous, generally scarlatine form; (2) eczematous lichenoid or vesiculo-pustular form; (3) rheumatoid group (resembling erythema nodosum or erythema exudativum multiforme).

CHILBLAIN LUPUS, ITS PATHOGENESIS, HISTOLOGY AND TREATMENT. FISCHL, Arch. f. Dermat. u. Syph. **136:**345, 1921.

Chilblain lupus can be distinguished from lupus pernio by the regular development of papules with central necrosis. The relation of chilblain lupus to tuberculosis is proved by: (1) positive local tuberculin reaction. (2) histologic structure (giant cells, epithelioid cells), and (3) the success of specific therapy.

THE INFLUENCE OF ARSPHENAMIN ON THE PERCENTAGE OF BILIRUBIN IN THE BLOOD SERUM. WECHSELMAXX and HOHORST. Arch. f. Dermat. u. Syph. **136:**285, 1921.

The authors' investigations prove that arsphenamin has no toxic effect on a healthy liver. In latent icteric, preicteric and subicteric conditions, there is sometimes increase of bilirubin in the serum. This points to previously damaged liver cells which are inefficient and do not bind arsphenamin as they should. It follows that arsphenamin icterus generally develops in "hypersensitive" patients the condition which is expressed by a preicteric hyperbilirubinemia.

PATHOGENESIS OF LIVEDO IN TUBERCULOSIS. Fischl, Arch. f. Dermat. u. Syph. **136**:362, 1921.

Tuberculous patients occasionally develop a livedo lenticularis which resembles the livedo racemosa of Ehrmann. The author describes two of these cases histologically. Adamson described this livedo lenticularis in six cases of erythema Bazin. The disorder represents an incompletely developed erythema induratum.

A CASE OF UNILATERAL ZOSTERIFORM LEUKOPATHY. Randak, Arch. f. Dermat. u. Syph. **136**:368, 1921.

The location of the skin disorders in the case described points to a disturbance of the central nervous system. As albinos are known to develop a circumscribed aplasia in the region of the central nervous system, the author assumes for his case an hypoplasia of the corresponding central apparatus. Cases of vitiligo are probably based on the hypoplasia.

ATYPICAL FORMS OF COLLIQUATIVE TUBERCULOSIS CUTIS. Arzt and Kumer, Arch. f. Dermat. u. Syph. **136**:377, 1921.

The authors describe a case in which the therapeutic injections of bacilli emulsion caused the development, at the site of injection, of a lesion resembling scrofuloderma. They propose to call this an atypical colliquative skin tuberculosis.

PATHOGENESIS OF THE TRICHOPHYTIDS. Jessner, Arch. f. Dermat. u. Syph. **136**:416, 1921.

The author succeeded in cultivating from the blood the fungus which caused the skin lesions of two patients suffering from lichen trichophyticus. This proves the possibility of a hematogenous origin of the lichen. In one of the cases the author also found the fungus in a lichen exanthem.

URTICARIA. Hahn and Kraupa, Arch. f. Dermat. u. Syph. **136**:425, 1921.

The authors report a curious case of urticarial eruption in a patient having mitral stenosis and synchronous hypoplasia of the whole heart-vessel apparatus. Good results were obtained with papaverin injected intravenously. The authors ascribe the urticaria to vessel crises.

CALCIFIED EPITHELIOMAS OF THE SKIN AND OSSIFICATION THEREIN. Bilke, Virchows Arch. f. path. Anat. **236**:177, 1922.

In four cases of ossified epitheliomas, histologic investigation showed that these new formations histogenetically take their origin from scattered epidermis germs. In their histologic structure, they very much resemble cholesteatomas. As to the calcium contained, the calcified epitheliomas do not essentially differ from the benign noncalcified epitheliomas, and should not be considered as a special species of tumor.

SALICYLIC ACID POISONING AFTER CUTANEOUS APPLICATION. Kiess, Therap. Halbmonatsh. **35**:433 (July 15) 1921.

The treatment of scabies with a salicylic acid tar tincture (10 per cent. salicylic acid and 15 per cent. oil of cade) caused death in two children by salicylic acid poisoning. The author and others believe in an idiosyncrasy toward salicylic acid.

RESEARCH ON TUBERCULIN. SELTER and TANCRÉ, Ztschr. f. Tuberk. **35**:171 (Nov.) 1921.

Protein body and tuberculin reactions are essentially different; from 100 to 200 times the quantity of the former is necessary to provoke a reaction. Tuberculin is very resistant to temperatures up to 150 C., a fact which speaks against its antigen nature.

WOUND INFECTION WITH VACCINE VIRUS. SCHNEITER, Schweiz. med. Wchnschr. **51**:1071 (Nov. 17) 1921.

A girl aged 10, who had never been vaccinated, happened to scratch her arm, and to come in contact with the vaccine virus of a school friend, who had just been vaccinated. Development of a large abnormal vaccination pustula followed. Subsequent vaccination with cow's lymph showed no reaction.

SKIN HEMORRHAGES IN UREMIA. KAULEN, Monatschr. f. Kinderh. **22**: 4, 1922.

This is the report of two cases, in a boy of 9 and a girl of 5. The author believes the hemorrhages are due to an inflammatory alteration of the vessels effected by a toxic damage. The increased blood pressure is also considered as an encouraging factor.

ANTIBODY FORMATION BY TRANSPLANTATION. OSHIKAWA, Ztschr. f. Immunitätsforsch. u. exper. Therap. **33**:297, 1921.

Transplantation of the skin of actively immunized rabbits on normal rabbits effects antibody formation in the latter.

DANGER OF ROENTGEN-RAY BURNS AFTER TAKING VARIOUS DRUGS. FRAENKEL, Fortschr. d. Med. **39**:28, 1921.

The author reports several cases of roentgen-ray burns in patients who had been given arsphenamin, iodids, and bromids. He concludes that drugs can increase the radiosensibility of the skin. A patient should always be asked whether he has taken drugs before being exposed to the rays.

HEXAMETHYLENTETRAMIN IN THE TREATMENT OF VINCENT'S ANGINA. PHILIPP, Deutsch. Monatschr. f. Zahnh. **40**:1, 1922.

The author reports a case successfully treated with four intravenous injections of 15 c.c. at a time, of a 40 per cent. solution of hexamethylentetramin.

CAPILLARY STUDIES IN VASONEUROSES. PARRISIUS, Deutsch. Ztschr. f. Nervenh. **72**:5, 1921.

The author emphasizes the fact that purely spastic and purely atonic conditions are just as rare in the vessels as in the digestive tract. A vessel neurosis therefore appears as a disharmony between vegetative and autonomic influence.

THE OCCURRENCES OF SKIN PIGMENT IN LYMPH GLANDS. LIGNAC, Zentralbl. f. allg. Path. u. path. Anat. **32**:8, 1921.

In seven cases, pigment was traced in the inguinal and subinguinal lymph glands. The pigment found gave a positive silver reaction, was bleached by hydrogen peroxid, and was therefore considered as skin pigment. The author believes that skin pigment can be carried away by the lymph vessels.

AHLSWEDE, Hamburg, Germany.

Society Transactions

NEW YORK ACADEMY OF MEDICINE, SECTION ON DERMATOLOGY AND SYPHILIS

Regular Meeting, May 8, 1922

Howard Fox, M.D., *Chairman*

FOR DIAGNOSIS (PURPURA ANNULARIS TELANGIECTODES?). Presented by Dr. Chargin.

M. S., a man, 50 years of age, a dishwasher, had an eruption which began about six years before, appearing first on the legs. Except for the scalp, face, hands and feet, the entire body was affected. The individual lesions varied in size from a few tiny loops to patches 3½ inches (8.89 cm.) in diameter, numerous lesions being 2 inches (5.08 cm.) by 1 inch (2.54 cm.) in size. Except for a series of linear lesions on the anterior aspect of the right shoulder and upper arm, the eruption was not raised above the skin. On the arm and shoulder area the eruption was slightly verrucous and somewhat raised above the level of the skin. Many of the lesions were perfectly smooth, while others showed a tiny amount of very fine scaliness. For the most part, the lesions were either round or oval, but many areas showed no definite configuration, the lesions being of various sizes and shapes. Many of them were quite indistinct, and in these areas the skin was mottled in appearance. What appeared to be the younger lesions were uniform. The older lesions, however, whether large or small, showed two distinct zones—a central brownish ecchymosis-like area and a peripheral zone made up of clearly aggregated bricked capillary loops. This zoning was not present in all the round areas, even some of the largest lesions (presumably the oldest) failing to show the two zones. The capillary border of the patches occupied about one-fourth of the area of the lesions.

The beginning lesion was evidently a tiny capillary loop, later becoming aggregated in small patches and the patches increasing in size by the formation of new loops at the periphery. As the lesions increased in size, the loops in the central portion of the patch became less and less distinct, finally losing their identity and producing the two zones described. Many of the central zones seemed to be atrophic; this was particularly noticeable in the lesions on the leg. Under the diascope the central portion of the lesions lost some color, but for the most part the dark brown stain was retained. It was impossible to obliterate entirely the capillary bodies, which showed pinpoints under even the strongest pressure. The general appearance of the eruption was strikingly brick-red in color. The patient suffered from no subjective symptoms, except occasionally a slight itching. The Wassermann reaction was negative. There were no areas of anesthesia. Response to heat and cold was normal. The mucous membranes were normal.

DISCUSSION

Dr. Ludwig Weiss said that the lesions, especially the purple ones, showed some characteristics of Majocchi's disease, but that the lack of central pigmentation and the absence of the cayenne pepper lesions were against that diagnosis. Its presence mostly on the upper part of the body and less on the lower part and extremities was also a point against Majocchi's disease. The condition could not well be confounded with erythema perstans, nor etiologically and clinically with the beginning premycotic type of mycosis fungoides, for which some corroborative symptoms were present, especially on the shoulders and chest. He rather leaned to the diagnosis of parapsoriasis of an atypical character.

Dr. Pollitzer said that the suggestion of parapsoriasis could be entertained only at the first glance. On observing it more closely it would be noted that the lesions on the upper chest and arms were made up of minute vascular points. That alone would rule out parakeratosis. Furthermore, parakeratosis was not suggested by the deep vascular lesions on various parts of the body. On the whole, the picture clearly seemed to be due to some form of vascular disease and was possibly an aberrant type of Majocchi's disease, but no diagnosis could be reached without a careful biopsy. The diagnosis of Majocchi's disease was strengthened by the evident atrophy in parts of the skin where the vascular lesions had been, and the case seemed to belong in that group rather than elsewhere.

Dr. Williams seconded everything said by Dr. Pollitzer, who had pointed out the various characteristic phases—hemorrhages, atrophy, telangiectases, all being present.

Dr. Chargin said that the capillary formation noted so markedly in the case was never observed in parapsoriasis, although in parapsoriasis there was a decided tendency in the lesion to respond by punctate hemorrhages on moderate trauma. In regard to atrophy, it seemed that there were many lesions, on the legs in particular, that showed central atrophy.

SYNOVIAL LESION OF THE SKIN. Presented by Dr. Rostenberg.

Mrs. A., 56 years old, an American, had always been well except for occasional attacks of gout. The trouble for which she was presented started about six months previously, when the patient first noticed a globular protrusion over the distal interphalangeal joint of the left little finger, on the dorsal surface. There was no pain except on severe pressure. The swelling gradually increased to the size of a small pea. The lesion was pinkish white and transparent, rather firm, but seemed to fluctuate on pressure. On being punctured, a whitish syrupy fluid exuded. Roentgen-ray examination disclosed the presence of arthritis involving the terminal phalangeal joint, being due to several exostoses about the articulating surfaces of both bones, some of them having been broken off.

DISCUSSION

Dr. Pollitzer said that the history of the gouty deposits in the skin afforded an etiologic factor for the production of the synovial cyst. The foreign body might injure the synovial membrane and produce a cyst. The lesion corresponded with the usual picture of synovial cyst.

Dr. Gilmour asked whether any of the members had had any experience with the treatment of such conditions, and, if so, what treatment had yielded the best results.

Dr. Andrews said that the lesion corresponded clinically with the cases that Dr. MacKee and he had described. In two of these cases there had been a history of rheumatism, and on some of the fingers there were rheumatic enlargements of the joints. Probably rheumatism or gout had something to do with the formation of some of the lesions.

Dr. Howard Fox said that he had had a patient under his charge whom he had treated successfully with electrolysis.

PSORIASIS AND LICHEN PLANUS. Presented by Dr. Rostenberg.

Mrs. K., 49 years old, born in Russia, had had psoriasis since her eighteenth year. Psoriatic lesions were present on the forearms and legs when the lichen planus appeared about three weeks previously, and spread with great rapidity over the entire body. The outlines of some of the psoriatic lesions were still recognizable, although greatly overshadowed by the lichen planus.

DISCUSSION

Dr. Rostenberg expressed regret that he could not have shown the case three weeks earlier, for neither the lichen nor the psoriasis showed up as well now as then. The woman had had psoriasis for eighteen years, and there were typical psoriatic lesions present when she developed the lichen planus. Dr. Rostenberg said it would be interesting to know whether any of the members had seen a coincidence of these two lesions before. The literature on the subject was very sparse. Graham Little mentioned two cases in which the psoriasis was implanted on lichen planus.

Dr. Abramowitz directed attention to the fact that although the psoriatic lesions on the body disappeared, one could still see the typical pinpoint lesions on the nails. He was inclined to agree with the diagnosis of psoriasis, although no lesions were present on the body, for the patient showed the characteristic pitting on the nails as seen in that disease. There was no question of the patient having lichen planus.

LINEAR PSORIASIS. Presented by Dr. Clark.

B. L., an American school girl, 15 years of age, presented a lesion which began six months before on the finger and gradually spread to the elbow. There were no subjective symptoms at any time, nor was there any history of a previous outbreak. As presented, the lesion extended in a line along the ulnar nerve from the elbow to the tips of the fingers; it was erythematous along the arms and was covered with thin white laminated scales. From the wrist to the finger tips the area was verrucous. A clinical diagnosis of tuberculosis verrucosa cutis was made; but the pathologic diagnosis was psoriasis. Microscopic examination revealed: Acanthosis, with lengthening of the dermal papillae, with small round cell infiltration of the pars papillaris of the derma. These cells are largely mononuclears. There was no parakeratosis or hyperkeratosis. There was also some inflammatory exudate in the substance of the horny layer. In the lower portions of the derma there were small groups of round cells but no changes suggesting tuberculosis.

DISCUSSION

Dr. Pollitzer said he did not like to question on clinical grounds the report of the pathologist who said the condition was psoriasis. If the microscopic diagnosis had not been so positive, he would regard the lesion as a nevus which had lost its verrucous character through treatment. A psoriasis with that localization would be unusual, and its peculiar distribution alone would militate strongly against psoriasis. He said that he believed in the evidence derived from microscopic examination, and while not all examiners were equally reliable, in the absence of any proof to the contrary he would accept the microscopic report; but he did so with a great deal of bewilderment in this case.

DR. WILLIAMS said he had seen the patient a week before at the Skin and Cancer Hospital, and thought the diagnosis was correct. He thought it was psoriasis clinically as well as histologically. There were two points against it: First, the distribution, and, second, the warty character of the lesions on the finger, which were not like the lesions in psoriasis. On the other hand, a case of linear psoriasis of the lower extremity was reported in the *Dermatologische Wochenschrift* (vol. 72, p. 193). The lesions on the elbow and arm, taken by themselves, had the appearance of psoriasis: there was the small amount of infiltration, the color was the dull color of psoriasis, the surface was not warty, the silvery scaling was increased by a slight irritation. The lesions on the forearm seemed to be those of psoriasis; the others were not so characteristic.

DR. RULISON asked whether there was any history of injury to the nerves.

DR. MELLON replied in the negative; the lesion began on the fingers and gradually spread upward. On looking up the case, Dr. Clark had seen a description of a case quoting some German authorities as to the nerves of the extremities.

DR. HOWARD FOX agreed that at first glance the eruption strongly suggested a linear nevus. Close inspection, however, showed plain evidence of psoriatic lesions. He was sure that psoriasis could present a linear configuration, and although he had no recollection of having seen a counterpart of this case he had a photograph of a distinct linear psoriasis on one leg.

A CASE FOR DIAGNOSIS (LESION ON CHEEK). Presented by DR. CLARK.

F. K., an American school girl, 15 years of age, presented on the right cheek, 1½ inches (3.81 cm.) below the eye, a lesion the size of a split pea, which had appeared four and a half years previously and had not apparently increased in size during that time. There were no subjective symptoms. The lesion was yellowish white, markedly infiltrated, and was depressed in the center. There were several typical milia in the lesion.

DISCUSSION

DR. POLLITZER directed attention to the distinct and unusual infiltration: on pinching it between the fingers the lesion felt hard, like a cork. Notwithstanding the absence of any border of dilated vesicles, he was inclined to think it was morphea. The mother was quite sure that it had increased in size during the last year, but she may have been mistaken.

DR. ROSTENBERG said he also thought the condition was morphea.

A CASE FOR DIAGNOSIS (LESION ON CHIN). Presented by DR. CLARK.

B. H., an American school girl, 15 years of age, presented a lesion on the chin the size of a small pea. It was yellowish, ivory white, slightly indurated, with a slightly elevated border and depressed center. The lesion was of about one year's duration, during which time no increase in size had been noticed. There were no subjective symptoms.

DISCUSSION

DR. ABRAMOWITZ said that he would call the lesion an epithelioma if the patient were much older. It might be a colloid milium or a hyaloma, somewhat similar to the case reported by Rudemann in the May issue of the ARCHIVES OF DERMATOLOGY AND SYPHILOLOGY. The same remarks might be applied to the other patient presented with a similar lesion.

A CASE FOR DIAGNOSIS (PIGMENTATION AND ATROPHY ON THE INNER SURFACE OF BOTH KNEES). Presented by DR. SCHEER.

(Previously presented before the Manhattan Dermatological Society.)

A CASE FOR DIAGNOSIS: LUPUS VULGARIS OR SYPHILIS? Presented by DR. WILLIAMS.

M. L., 20 years old, an American by birth, had an eruption which had been present for five years, increasing gradually, involving the extensor surface of the left forearm and the external and posterior aspect of the right thigh. In each region there was a large smooth atrophic scar, with active inflammatory nodules at parts of the periphery of each. Some of these nodules near the elbow resembled closely the apple jelly nodules of lupus vulgaris. Those on the thigh were firmer and more suggestive of syphilis. The Wassermann test was negative. Mild antisyphilitic treatment had been followed by slight improvement, but hardly as much as one would expect in untreated syphilis. The entire lesion suggested tuberculosis rather than syphilis, while the scarring was more like that of syphilis.

DISCUSSION

DR. POLLITZER said that against the diagnosis of tuberculosis was the fact that the lesions on the thigh, consisting of two or three elevated lesions manifestly infiltrated at the border, were the remains of an extensive lesion, twice the size of a hand, which was now atrophic and slightly pigmented. A syphilitic lesion might disappear in a short time, and a tuberculous one would not. Judging by the lesion on the thigh, he thought the condition was a syphiloderm and not tuberculosis. He admitted that some of the lesions on the arm showed brownish nodules under the diascope, but that was hardly enough to satisfy one that the picture was one of tuberculosis. Against the diagnosis of syphilis was the negative Wassermann reaction and the girl's general appearance of health. If it were a tertiary syphilid, she must have acquired it as a child. Hereditary syphilis was ruled out by her excellent appearance; she had unusually perfect teeth, and that alone might suffice to rule out hereditary syphilis. Syphilis contracted in childhood, never having been treated, would probably cause more serious general disturbance than was shown by this girl. The same thing might be said, however, about a tuberculous affection, for if she had such an extensive tuberculosis of the skin she would have a tuberculous focus inside. On the whole, he thought it was a case of syphilis.

DR. HOWARD FOX said that though from the clinical appearance the case might be either syphilis or tuberculosis, he was inclined to make the latter diagnosis. He felt sure that the superficial character of the scarring could not rule out tuberculosis.

Dr. WILLIAMS, referring to Dr. Pollitzer's remark about the spread of the disease being rather rapid for tuberculosis, said that the disease had been present for eight years, and that was sufficient time for tuberculosis to spread over the area involved. He was still in doubt as to the correct diagnosis.

BLASTOMYCOSIS. Presented. by Dr. OULMANN.

C. B., 9 years old, born in the United States, three weeks before had developed a lesion on the vertex capitis which grew larger and was raised to the size of a small apple, and discharged pus from numerous sinuses. The double contoured cells of blastomycosis were found in smears and cultures.

DISCUSSION

Dr. WILLIAMS said it was an interesting case. His first impression of it. and the one which he was still inclined to adhere to, was that it was a case of kerion. The rapid development was like that of a kerion. He did not know whether or not it was preceded by the ordinary superficial type of ring-worm, as the history was not given, and it was not certain that the parents could enlighten one on that point. The discharge of pus from many small foci was like kerion; the small mass just below and to the left of the main one. the big brownish crust, was such as one might see in a neighboring small kerion. He had seen few cases of blastomycosis, and pleaded ignorance about that condition, but his impression was that it did not spread so rapidly. He was not sure of the warty excrescence; that struck him as being rather masses of epidermal cells, serum matted on the surface. The culture would be the deciding factor; if blastomycetes were cultivated, he would, of course, accept the diagnosis. Both conditions subsided under simple antiseptic treatment. He had seen a blastomycosis cured with boric acid lotions, and a kerion could be cured with water.

Dr. POLLITZER said he did not see how any one could discuss the diagnosis in the face of the microscopic report and the fact that the culture showed blastomycetes. It was an unusual case because of its location. It would be interesting to know something about the environment of the child. Most of our cases of blastomycosis occurred in the Middle West; it was seen pre-dominantly in Chicago, Cleveland, Ann Arbor, Mich., and St. Louis: a case in New York was rather a rarity and the patient generally applied for medical attention. That was the purpose of his inquiry about the occupation of the parents.

LUPUS ERYTHEMATOSUS OF THE NOSE, SHOWING RESULT OF TREATMENT. By Dr. BECHET.

J. R., a man, aged 28, came to the New York Skin and Cancer Hospital on Oct. 13, 1921, with a typical lupus erythematosus, covering most of the front of the nose. The prominent patulous follicles, scales and atrophy were all present; the lesion was not, however, deeply infiltrated. It had been present for a year. From Oct. 13, 1921, to Jan. 25, 1922. it was painted with 95 per cent. phenol, the solution being thoroughly rubbed in with a cotton swab. Five or six applications in all were made. at intervals of two weeks: the acid was allowed to dry and was not neutralized. The last application was made on Jan. 5, 1922. At the time of presentation the nose seemed entirely well. with no evidence of scarring.

Dr. Pollitzer said there was a type of lupus erythematosus resembling erythema perstans that was a toxic eruption which disappeared under mild treatment and recurred from time to time. He had cured several such cases by injections of arsenic, some with injections of streptococcus vaccines. He thought one might expect a return, for no doubt the underlying condition had not been affected by the external treatment.

Dr. Bechet replied that he also had occasionally observed superficial lupus erythematosus of the erythema perstans type. As Dr. Pollitzer had observed, it frequently disappeared spontaneously; but the case under consideration was totally different and was typical of the chronic discoid type. It had been present for a year without change; it was scaly, covered with dilated follicular openings, more or less plugged with sebaceous matter, and was slightly atrophic in its center. The nose had remained well for several months, though of course there was always a possibility of a recurrence.

PAPULAR SYPHILID OF THE GLANS PENIS AFTER INTENSIVE SPECIFIC TREATMENT. Presented by Dr. Bechet.

P. J., a man, aged 34, born in Denmark, was presented at the previous meeting of the Section held on April 4. At that time, he said that the lesions had been present for four weeks. They consisted of several, rather discrete, raised, indurated, copper colored papules. They were not umbilicated, depressed, or violaceous colored. The patient said that fifteen years before he had had a primary lesion followed by secondary symptoms. He first came to the New York Skin and Cancer Hospital on April 6, 1920, complaining of vague general pains. His family history was negative. The spinal fluid findings were negative, but the blood Wassermann test was four plus. From April 6, 1920, to Aug. 18, 1921, he received thirty injections of arsphenamin, varying in dose from 0.2 to 0.4 gm., and thirty-four intramuscular injections of mercuric salicylate of 1 grain (0.06 gm.). The Wassermann test was negative in four tests made from Dec. 2, 1920, to March 3, 1922; but it was one plus at the time of the occurrence of the eruption, which appeared seven months after the cessation of the specific treatment. At the time of the first presentation, Dr. Parounagian agreed with the diagnosis of syphilis; Dr. Pollitzer was of the opinion that the case was one of lichen planus; Dr. Abramowitz agreed with Dr. Pollitzer, but stated his belief that the arsphenamin had been responsible for the appearance of the lesions; Dr. Wise said that he had noted five or six articles in the literature relating to lichen-planus-like lesions appearing as the result of arsphenamin injections. In the month that had elapsed since the presentation and discussion, the patient had received three arsphenamin injections within two weeks. The eruption practically disappeared after the first injection, and entirely so after the second. No local treatment was used. This would tend to prove the correctness of the diagnosis of syphilis. The arsphenamin could not be held responsible, for the eruption appeared seven months after its use.

EPITHELIOMA OF THE HARD PALATE . Presented by Dr. Scheer.

A CASE FOR DIAGNOSIS: PARAFFINOMA? Presented by Dr. Scheer.

C. C., aged 15, had had the present condition for thirteen years. At the age of 2, injections of some "medicine" had been made in the umbilical region.

for congenital umbilical hernia, and the father attributed the condition presented to these injections. In and around the umbilicus were about half a dozen hard subcutaneous painless nodules varying in size from that of a buckshot to that of a dime. The skin over them was normal in appearance and felt movable.

DR. POLLITZER said he thought there was no doubt that it was a case of paraffinoma; the fact that the lesions were spherical did not militate against that diagnosis. The injected paraffin (probably petrolatum) had gathered together in small droplets roundish in shape; where there was a single large mass it was not apt to be spherical because the tissue pressure on the large mass forced it into an irregular shape, but where there were so many small deposits it was in accordance with the simple physics of the condition that spherical masses would result.

DR. GILMOUR said he had once seen a spherical lesion the size of the end of the thumb on the cheek of a young man, which was due to the injection of paraffin. When it was dissected out, it came out in sago-like grains, although it felt like a single lump the size and shape of a marble.

A CASE FOR DIAGNOSIS: PREMYCOSIS? PARAPSORIASIS? Presented by Dr. WILLIAMS.

A. V., aged 45, born in the United States, a driver, first noticed an eruption, similar to the one presented, twenty years ago. Similar eruptions had been present in various locations since. The blood Wassermann test was negative. The white blood count was 8,400; the differential count showed no deviation from normal.

The biopsy report was as follows: "There is some thickening of the dermal papillae, and edema of a few cells in the malpighian layer of the epidermis. In the superficial derma, there is small round cell infiltration around the blood vessels. There is one feature which appears unusual, and that is a depression of the derma in the middle of the specimen over which the epidermis is thickened and nearly obliterated."

DR. ROSTENBERG remarked that while there was some resemblance to the picture of parapsoriasis, the condition seemed to him to have more the resemblance of a phenolphthalein eruption.

DR. ABRAMOWITZ said he had a case—which Dr. Pollitzer also saw—that of a woman who had a distinct brownish eruption arranged in linear plaques, which could almost be mistaken for pityriasis versicolor. They had concluded that it was parakeratosis variegata.

DR. POLLITZER said that the smooth round pigmented patches were characteristic of a phenolphthalein eruption; he had seen only the upper portion of the body, and that kind of lesion did not at all suggest parakeratosis or parapsoriasis.

LUPUS VULGARIS AND TUBERCULOUS ADENITIS IN A CHILD. Presented by Dr. ABRAMOWITZ.

DERMATITIS HERPETIFORMIS. Presented by Dr. WILLIAMS

MULTIPLE HEMORRHAGIC SARCOMA OF KAPOSI. Presented by Dr. WILLIAMS.

B. P., was an Italian, 34 years of age, an optician, had an eruption which had existed for twelve years, and which when presented consisted of purplish areas on both lower extremities, from some of which small nodules projected. The Wassermann test was negative. On biopsy, the derma showed groups of fibroblastic cells arranged in bundles, etc.

NEW YORK DERMATOLOGICAL SOCIETY

Regular Meeting, May 16, 1922

HOWARD FOX, M.D., *President*

FOR DIAGNOSIS. Presented by Dr. WILLIAMS.

C. B., a white girl, 7 years old, had an eruption which was first noticed about three years ago. It disappeared for a year and returned. It consisted of round, brownish-red spots, occurring on the face and chest, about 2 inches (5.08 cm.) in diameter, slightly scaly, slightly hyperkeratotic, with ill defined borders.

DISCUSSION

DR. WHITEHOUSE said it was not parapsoriasis, on account of the keratosis, but he could not make a diagnosis.

DR. HIGHMAN said he thought it was not parapsoriasis; it might be a neurodermite or one of the follicular seborrheids.

DR. WILLIAMS said the case at first suggested parapsoriasis, but on close inspection it seemed to belong rather to the neurodermite group.

VERRUCA PLANA JUVENILIS SUCCESSFULLY TREATED BY THE INTERNAL ADMINISTRATION OF MERCURY. Presented by Dr. HOWARD FOX.

S. W., 10 years of age, had suffered for two months from juvenile flat warts of the face, left hand and forearms. The lesions were moderately profuse on the face and few in number on the forearms and left hand. In the center of the right cheek they were closely aggregated in a patch an inch (2.54 cm.) in diameter. Some of the lesions on the hand presented a linear configuration. The patient was given tablets of mercurous iodid in doses of one-fourth of a grain (0.016 gm.) three times a day. At the end of seventeen days the eruption had entirely disappeared from the face, leaving a few ill-defined pinhead brownish pigmented spots in place of the former lesions. On the hand the eruption had not quite disappeared. Mercury was continued for another week and was followed by the disappearance of the eruption on the hand. No local treatment was administered at any time. A photograph before and after treatment was presented.

DR. BECHET remarked that the value of the mercurous iodid in the treatment of this condition had been demonstrated in a number of cases. He recalled a patient who recovered after a few weeks of treatment. It had to be given in fairly large doses.

Dr. Williams said that he became enthusiastic about mercurous iodid after reading Dr. White's article, and treated a number of cases; the first four patients made remarkable recoveries, in from ten days to four weeks, but the next patients did not seem to improve at all. There was a class of warts for which mercurous iodid seemed to be effective, but it was impossible to tell beforehand what the result would be.

Dr. Howard Fox said that in his experience with mercury for flat warts he had not been able to duplicate the results of Dr. C. J. White, who had first used this method. He had obtained brilliant results in the case of a young girl who presented large numbers of lesions on the face. After three weeks of treatment with mercurous iodid tablets the entire eruption had disappeared. In some other cases he had had complete failures. He felt that the treatment of flat warts was somewhat comparable to the treatment of warts in general, especially verruca vulgaris. The latter, for instance, would respond at one time to radiation in a striking manner, while at another they would be unaffected by such treatment.

Dr. Whitehouse said mercurous iodid was not effective in all cases and often failed. He had under observation a case which improved to a certain degree, but then stopped, and new lesions were constantly appearing.

Dr. Schwartz reported two cases which had cleared up entirely under treatment with mercurous iodid.

Dr. Winfield had not seen the case, but said he had treated a number of patients with mercurous iodid and, as Dr. Williams had said, it seemed to be a wonderful remedy in certain cases.

Dr. Williams said that in some of the patients he had treated successfully the lesions were flat and in some distinctly papillomatous. He could not tell which patients would recover and which would not.

RINGWORM OF THE SCALP TREATED INADVERTENTLY BY TWO EPILATING DOSES OF ROENTGEN RAY. Presented by Dr. Howard Fox.

L. M., a colored boy, 7 years old, applied at the Harlem Hospital for treatment of ringworm of the scalp. The disease was of the small spored type, and consisted of numerous patches scattered over the occiput and posterior portion of the parietal region. The disease had been present about three months. On July 21, 1921, he was treated with the roentgen ray by the Kienbock-Adamson method, receiving an epilating dose of 1 Holzknecht unit (skin distance) over each of the usual five areas. Two weeks later the patient was inadvertently given a second epilating dose, similar to the previous one. The mistake was discovered when the treatment was completed. At the suggestion of Dr. Sampson of the U. S. Public Health Service, the patient was irradiated by the mercury vapor quartz lamp on the same day, a well marked erythema being produced. This treatment was repeated on the following day, after which the patient refused to return for further treatment. The quartz lamp was used owing to the claim of Dr. Sampson that it was able to counteract the effect of even large overdoses of roentgen ray. The patient was seen six months later, at which time the hair had entirely returned, with a disappearance of the disease. The only ill effect of the double epilation had been a delay in the return of the hair. According to the mother's statement, the new hair had begun to make its appearance three months after treatment.

Dr. HIGHMAN said that there were three possibilities to be considered: first, that enough of the accumulated roentgen-ray dosage from the first treatment had disappeared, so that by the time the second treatment was given the sum total was still below the danger limit; second, that the patient had possibly not received an overdose; and third, that as sometimes double the ordinary epilating dose would not produce permanent epilation, so far as the scalp was concerned, this might be all the more true in the negro with his highly resistant scalp.

Dr. WILLIAMS remarked that Dr. Highman's first suggestion seemed the most likely: that the interval was enough to allow the last dose to wear off so that the boy never received enough to cause a permanent alopecia.

Dr. WISE referred to an interesting report in a German periodical in which a man experimentally exposed a patient to the rays of the sun and gave a certain dose of roentgen rays after a short interval, and exposed control patients to the roentgen ray without exposure to the sun. Those who were exposed to sunlight contracted radiodermatitis, and those who were not exposed did not, the results being exactly the opposite of those noted in a report recently made—that the actinic rays might prevent the ill effect of subsequent roentgen-ray exposure. This was an isolated report of roentgen-ray procedure.

A CASE FOR DIAGNOSIS.   Presented by Dr. WILLIAMS.

J. M., aged 14, an American boy who worked for an express company, presented himself at the Skin and Cancer Hospital with lesions on both legs, below the knee, which had been present for more than a year, the left leg was first affected for six months, after which the lesion appeared on the other leg. There were no subjective symptoms. The patient said that he had applied iodin locally for two weeks, and ammoniated mercury for the last week, but had received no other treatment. The lesions were plaques of minute capillary hemorrhages, from $\frac{1}{32}$ (0.79 mm.) to 2 inches (5.08 cm.) in diameter.

Dr. WHITEHOUSE said that Dr. Highman had suggested a possible phenolphthalein eruption. So few cases had been reported that he was not familiar with all the types this drug might produce. He was not prepared, however, to make a definite diagnosis.

Dr. HOWARD FOX said he thought a diagnosis of phenolphthalein rash was entirely possible, especially as the pigmentation sometimes lasted for years.

Dr. HIGHMAN said he did not know of anything else that seemed probable, unless it was idiopathic erythema perstans, in which these circular lesions were found; and in view of Dr. Wise's numerous and convincing contributions on the subject, it seemed that only phenolphthalein or antipyrin could have produced this picture. The boy said he had taken Ex-Lax.

Dr. WISE said he felt confident that the eruption was due to phenolphthalein or to antipyrin or antifebrin. The fact that it was limited to the legs did not militate against that diagnosis. A patient had been presented at the Academy of Medicine who had had only one lesion on the shoulder blade for months.

Dr. WILLIAMS said that in view of Dr. Wise's experience he accepted the diagnosis of phenolphthalein eruption. He inquired how long it might be expected to remain, and whether a marked reaction occurred after giving the drug.

DR. WISE replied that the eruption remained for different periods in different persons; it might remain for a year or six months, and might leave pigmented spots for years.

AN UNUSUALLY EXTENSIVE CASE OF LICHEN PLANUS. Presented by DR. WILLIAMS.

Mrs. M. P., 51 years of age, had suffered from an acute lichen planus eruption all over the body since the middle of March. The interesting features of the case were the great extent and confluence of the eruption—the lesions looking more like lichenification than lichen planus—and the bright red color.

DISCUSSION

DR. WHITEHOUSE inquired whether any of the members had noted the association of gallbladder disease—gallstones, obstruction of the common duct, etc. —with lichen planus. He had had two distinct cases in women with acute generalized lichen planus. Both patients were operated on, and in a week or ten days the eruption had entirely disappeared. Whether or not there was any connection between the two, he did not know. This woman had had a gallbladder operation two or three years previously, but said she did not have an attack of lichen planus at that time. It would be interesting to know whether she has any trouble of that kind now.

DR. WINFIELD said the woman had been a private patient of his since April. When he first saw her, she had one of the most severe cases of lichen planus he had ever seen. The skin was acutely inflamed, probably due to a strong sulphur ointment that had been prescribed by a physician who had mistaken the eruption for scabies. Under proper treatment the condition had rapidly improved. According to the history, the patient had had some sort of operation about the gallbladder, but she still complained of occasional attacks of pain in that region that simulated bilious colic. Dr. Winfield said he could bear out Dr. Whitehouse's remarks on the association of gallbladder trouble and lichen planus.

DR. STETSON (by invitation) said that Dr. Whitehouse's remarks about the gallbladder and this trouble were very interesting. All knew the profound effect arsphenamin had on lichen. At the Skin and Cancer Hospital it was found that many of these cases were markedly influenced by arsphenamin; not all patients were improved, but the majority of them were.

DR. HIGHMAN said he did not understand Dr. Stetson's statement, for it was in conflict with other reports, and so far as he knew in lichen planus arsphenamin did no good. Furthermore, there was a large amount of literature at present indicating that arsphenamin produced a rash so closely resembling lichen planus clinically and histologically that it was difficult to differentiate the arsenical and classic forms. If there was any relation between lichen planus and the gallbladder it might be due to diminished cholesterin metabolism, but not because of any affinity of arsphenamin for the liver.

DR. HOWARD FOX thought that any observations which might tend to throw light on the etiology of lichen planus were of value, as really nothing was known of its etiology. He himself had never observed any relationship between this condition and disease of the gallbladder. He had seen lichen planus follow overwork and mental strain.

Dr. Bechet, referring to Dr. Howard Fox's remark about mental strain as a causative factor, told of a man who had come to his office a few days previously suffering from an extensive lichen planus which began in January. At that time, shortly after giving birth to a child, his wife developed acute tuberculosis; his home life was broken up, and he and his children were living with his parents under disagreeable circumstances. There was also much financial worry.

Dr. Williams said he had obtained good results in lichen planus by giving mercuric chlorid wash externally and mercury internally.

A CASE FOR DIAGNOSIS.   Presented by Dr. Bechet.

F. P., 39 years of age, born in the United States, married, a metal grinder, said that the lesions presented had existed for nine months. They consisted of keratotic and pigmented areas, covering a large part of the arms and thighs. The keratosis minus the pigmentation was present on the flanks. The patches on the arms and legs were reticulated in appearance. There was marked hyperpigmentation on the temples, but no keratosis. For ten years the man had been exposed to metal dust, which flew off during the grinding process, together with a large quantity of oil; his overalls were always saturated with oil. He knew of no other metal workers with similar, or other lesions of the skin. The case had recently been presented at the Manhattan Dermatological Society, but would not appear in the minutes of that society. Most of the members at that time considered the eruption an occupational dermatosis.

DISCUSSION

Dr. Whitehouse said he could not give a definite opinion. The man had been a metal worker for six years, but had had the dermatosis for only six months. Stone cutters acquired a pigmentation from fragments of the chisels used, called siderosis; they were like gunpowder stains, of a bluish color, not at all like the condition exhibited in this case.

Dr. Highman said he thought the lesions on the hands and forearms looked like pityriasis rubra pilaris; on the thighs, a reticular atrophy; on the face, a hyperpigmentation. Was this Devergie's disease or pigmentation due to a sort of tattooing from absorption of pigment and its distribution through the blood stream?

Dr. Williams said the tarry constituent in the oil might account for the hyperkeratosis, the metal for the pigmentation, but how would one account for the atrophy?

Dr. Wise said that Dr. Pollitzer had treated a metal worker with an identical history and eruption, but no atrophy.

A CASE FOR DIAGNOSIS.   (LUPUS ERYTHEMATOSUS? SARCOID?)
Presented by Dr. Wise.

M. McK., aged 23, a colored man, single, born in the United States, a laborer, was referred by the medical department of the Vanderbilt Clinic on account of lesions on the cheeks and forearms which had been present for the last four months. The lesions on the left cheek were circinate, slightly infiltrated and had no papules in them. On the right malar region there was a bean sized lesion, slightly erythematous and scaling, raised about 0.5 mm.

above the surrounding skin. Both elbows showed scaly superficial lesions. The Wassermann reaction was negative. Examination for tinea was negative.

Dr. Bechet said he thought the condition was lupus erythematosus.

TUBERCULOSIS VERRUCOSA CUTIS. Presented by Dr. Williams.

J. F., aged 40, born in the United States, an ironworker, presented a rounded lesion on the center of the chin which he stated had been present for from three and one-half to four years. The lesion began as a small papule and gradually increased to its present size, with its slight encroachment on the vermilion border of the lower lip. The patient was being treated in a hospital for general tuberculosis.

Dr. Whitehouse said he agreed with the diagnosis.

Dr. Highman said he thought the condition was lupus due to inoculation from saliva.

Dr. Williams said he thought the condition was due to inoculation from sputum.

TUBERCULOSIS CUTIS (?). Presented by Dr. Williams.

S. A., aged 30, a Danish machinist, presented a lesion which he stated had been present since birth. It was located just below the crotch on the inner aspect of the left thigh. It was raised, indurated, purplish red, and measured 1 (2.54 cm.) by 2½ inches (6.35 cm.). Small crusts were present, covering what appeared to be multiple abscesses. The lesion was gradually increasing in size and was migratory, leaving scar formation in its wake. The Wassermann test was negative.

Dr. Howard Fox said he agreed with the diagnosis.

Dr. Highman said he thought possibly it was a self-inflicted lesion.

Dr. Whitehouse said he thought it was possibly a scrofuloderma, as there seemed to be no evidence of a sinus leading deeper into the tissues.

Dr. Wise said he thought that an irritated linear nevus would account for the whole story.

Dr. Williams said he thought Dr. Wise's suggestion the best—a nevus verrucosus with possibly superimposed tuberculosis.

LEPRA. Presented by Dr. Howard Fox.

J. W., 23 years of age, a mulatto, born in Turk's Island, West Indies, had emigrated to the United States three years previously. He presented a circumscribed patch on the right side of the forehead, which was yellowish red, smooth, infiltrated and moderately anesthetic. It measured about 2½ inches (6.35 cm.) in its longest dimension. There was a suggestion of wrinkling and pigmentation on the backs of the hands, and a questionable enlargement of the ulnar nerve. No one in his family had ever suffered from leprosy. He had been married for six months, his wife being said to show no evidence of the disease. A nasal smear failed to show lepra bacilli. A biopsy had been made which would be reported on subsequently.

DISCUSSION

Dr. Whitehouse said he thought the lesions on the forehead looked like lepra.

Drs. Williams and Kingsbury said they thought the case was suggestive of lepra.

TROPHIC CHANGE IN THE HANDS. Presented by Dr. Williams.

E. M., an Irish longshoreman, aged 60, presented himself at the clinic of the New York Skin and Cancer Hospital stating that ten years previously both hands and feet had been frozen. Recovery apparently was perfect, and for six years the patient remained in this condition. Four years previous to presentation the right hand began to swell and turned a purplish red during the winter or cold weather. Some improvement took place under local treatment, but the condition gradually returned and became worse. Two years previously the left hand and both feet became affected in a similar way. The condition had been growing markedly worse on the hands. The eczema present on all extremities had developed within the last three weeks and was identical. The Wassermann reaction was negative.

When presented, both hands were markedly deformed, the heads of the phalanges having slipped from the heads of the metatarsals, resting rather on the flexor surface of the ends of these bones. The small muscles of the hands were atrophied. The skin was cyanotic, rather cold. Roentgenograms showed no involvement of the bony structure. The condition seemed to be due to a trophic destruction caused by some disease of the central nervous system.

TRICHOPHYTID? Presented by Dr. Wise for Dr. Fordyce.

J. P., a negro boy, 9 years of age, was presented with a condition which might possibly be trichophytid. He was given roentgen-ray treatment for ringworm of the scalp, and later returned with a follicular rash which spread down to the waist. Examination failed to reveal any fungi, and no biopsy had been made.

Book Review

AN INTRODUCTION TO DERMATOLOGY. By Norman Walker, LL.D., M.D., F.R.C.P., Physician for Diseases of the Skin at the Royal Infirmary, Edinburgh. Seventh edition. Cloth. Price, $7. Pp. 366, with 164 illustrations. New York: William Wood & Co., 1922.

The seventh edition of Walker comes to us as evidence of the deserved popularity of this well-known work. The subjects have been brought up to date and the book enlarged by the addition of a number of colored plates, nearly all of which are excellent. Since the publication of the first edition, Walker's book has been recognized as one of the valuable treatises in dermatology. It is orthodox, but shows the characteristics of the strong personality of the author. It is a good book, and we congratulate the author on its continued success.

Index to Current Literature

DERMATOLOGY

Addison's Disease, Case of, Rapidly Fatal. C. M. Fleming, Brit. M. J. **1**:951 (June 17) 1922.

Anthrax, Analysis of 123 Cases of, in Pennsylvania Leather Industry. H. F. Smyth and E. Bricker, J. Indust. Hygiene **4**:53 (June) 1922.

Anthrax Bacillus, Mutation of. A. C. Marchisotti, Semana méd. **1**:622 (April 20) 1922.

Anthrax: Report of Case. M. G. Wohl and J. E. Pulver, Nebraska M. J. **7**:202 (June) 1922.

Anthrax Septicemia, Serum Treatment of. D. Symmers, Ann. Surg. **75**:663 (June) 1922.

Anthrax Spores in Shaving Brushes, Detection of. A. D. Stewart, Indian M. Gaz. **57**:204 (June) 1922.

Arc Light Treatment of Lupus, etc. A. Fried, Med. Klin. **18**:695 (May 28) 1922.

Ascaridiasis and Urticaria. O. Pentagna, Pediatria, Naples **30**:308 (April 1) 1922.

Baldness in the Twenties. R. Sabouraud, Presse méd. **30**:465 (May 31) 1922.

Burns and Their Treatment. A. Kotzareff, Rev. de chir. **60**:5, 1922.

Cancer of Lip Treated by Radiation or Combined with Electrocoagulation and Surgical Procedures. G. E. Pfahler, J. Radiol. **3**:213 (June) 1922.

Chaulmoogra Oil Derivatives in Treatment of Leprosy, Experiences with. H. Morrow, E. L. Walker and H. E. Miller, J. A. M. A. **79**:434 (Aug. 5) 1922.

Chickenpox, Epidemic Herpes Zoster Alternating with. Netter, Bull. de l'Acad. de méd., Paris **87**:535 (May 16) 1922.

Dermatitis During Treatment of Syphilis. J. Klaar, Wien. klin. Wchnschr. **35**:266 (March 23) 1922; concluded p. 297.

Dermatitis from Fur Dye. C. Rasch, Ugesk. f. Læger **84**:365 (April 13) 1922.

Dermatitis, Professional. Gougerot and Blamoutier, Bull. et mém. Soc. méd. d. hôp. de Paris **46**:739 (May 5) 1922.

Dermatologic Technic, Course in. M. Joseph, Deutsch. med. Wchnschr. **48**:426 (March 31) 1922; ibid. **48**:461 (April 7) 1922.

Dermatology, Needs and Duties of. D. Chipman, J. A. M. A. **79**:419 (Aug. 5) 1922.

Dermatoses, Common Parasitic, in Southern California. M. Scholtz, Calif. State J. M. **20**:190 (June) 1922.

Dermography, Yellow, in Icterus. J. Schürer, Deutsch. med. Wchnschr. **48**:593 (May 5) 1922.

Dye. Dermatitis from Fur Dye. C. Rasch, Ugesk. f. Læger **84**:365 (April 13) 1922.

Epitheliomà. F. L. Meleney, China M. J. **36**:93 (March) 1922.

Epithelioma, Squamous-Cell, of the Lip: Its Surgical Indications. J. H. Sheppard, Surg., Gynec. & Obst. **35**:107 (July) 1922.

Epithelium, Ciliary, Possible Hormone Action of. Scalinci, Riforma med. **38**:345 (April 10) 1922.

Eruption, Recurrent Vesicular, After Influenza. A. W. Panton, Brit. M. J. **1**:995 (June 24) 1922.

Eruptive Disease, Peculiar, Occurring in Infancy. J. H. Park, Jr., and J. C. Michael, Am. J. Dis. Child. **23**:521 (June) 1922.

Eruptive Fever, New, in Infancy. E. Tso, China M. J. **36**:130 (March) 1922.

Erysipelas, Abortive Treatment of. J. Kumaris, Zentralbl. f. Chir. **49**:368 March 18) 1922.

Erysipelas and Streptococcal Septicemia. A. Erian, Practitioner, London **108**:373 (May) 1922.

Erysipelas, Swine, in Man. Gestewitz. Med. Klin. **18**:729 (June 4) 1922.

Erythema Nodosum Associated with Acute Rheumatism. H. Wetherbee, Brit. M. J. **1**:995 (June 24) 1922.

Erythrocyanosis Cutis Symmetrica. F. Bolte, Klin. Wchnschr. **1**:578 (March 18) 1922.

Furunculosis, Local Vaccine Therapy in. A. von Wassermann, München. med. Wchnschr. **69**:596 (April 21) 1922.

Granuloma Inguinale. A. Randall, J. C. Small and W. P. Belk, Surg., Gynec. & Obst. **34**:717 (June) 1922.

Granuloma Inguinale. P. G. Morrissey, Tenn. State M. A. J. **15**:105 (June) 1922.

Herpes and Varicella. W. M. Elliott, Glasgow M. J. **97**:274 (May) 1922.

Herpes Zoster and Facial Paralysis. G. Worms and V. de Lavergne, Paris méd. **12**:481 (June 10) 1922.

Herpes Zoster, Epidemic, Alternating with Chickenpox. Netter, Bull. de l'Acad. de méd., Paris **87**:535 (May 16) 1922 .

Hodgkin's Disease in Which Endoscopy Led to Diagnosis. L. M. Hurd, New York M. J. & Med. Rec. **115**:746 (June 21) 1922.

Hyperhidrosis, Treatment of. M. Joseph, Deutsch. med. Wchnschr. **48**:557 (April 28) 1922.

Hypertrichosis, General, with Dog-Like Face. P. Pagniez and L. de Gannes, Bull. et mém. Soc. méd. d. hôp. de Paris **46**:773 (May 12) 1922.

Influenza, Recurrent Vesicular Eruption After. A. W. Panton, Brit. M. J. **1**:995 (June 24) 1922.

Irradiation in Malignant Disease. Possibilities of. L. J. Clendinnen, Med. J. Australia **1**:456 (April 29) 1922.

Larynx, Stenosis of, Following Smallpox. A. Flores, Crón. méd., Lima **39**:136 (April) 1922.

Leg Ulcers, Treatment of. L. Simon, München. med. Wchnschr. **69**:589 April 21) 1922.

Leprosy, Chaulmoogra Oil Derivatives in the Treatment of. H. Morrow, E. L. Walker and H. E. Miller, J. A. M. A. **79**:434 (Aug. 5) 1922.

Leprosy, Gaté-Papacostas Reaction in. D. A. Turkhud and C. R. Avari, Indian J. M. Res. **9**:850 (April) 1922.

Leprosy in Sumatra. L. Bodaan, Med. v. d. Burg. Geneesk. Dienst, Batavia **1**:1, 1922.

Leprosy. Is Rat Leprosy Transmissible to Man? E. Marchoux, Bull. de l'Acad. de méd., Paris **87**:545 (May 16) 1922.

Leprosy, Modern Treatment of. H. Fowler, China M. J. **36**:115 (March) 1922.

Leprosy. Spread, Probable Mode of Infection, and Prophylaxis of Leprosy. L. Rogers, Brit. M. J. **1**:987 (June 24) 1922.

Lip, Cancer of, Treated by Radiation and Combined with Electrocoagulation and Surgical Procedures. G. E. Pfahler, J. Radiol. **3**:213 (June) 1922.

Lip, Squamous-Cell Epithelioma of: Its Surgical Indications. J. H. Shephard, Surg., Gynec. & Obst. **35**:107 (July) 1922.

Lips, Ulcers of, and of the Mouth Cavity. Ledderhose. Deutsch. med. Wchnschr. **48**:527 (April 21) 1922.

Lupus, Arc Light Treatment of. A. Fried, Med. Klin. **18**:695 (May 28) 1922.

Lymphangitis of Arm Cured by Antigonococcus Vaccine. Matarasso, Ann. d. mal. vénériennes **17**:448 (June) 1922.

Lymphogranulomatosis. V. Hecker and Fischer, Deutsch. med. Wchnschr. **48**:520 (April 21) 1922.

Lymphogranulomatosis, Case of. H. Barbier et al. Arch. de méd. d. enf. **25**:338 (June) 1922.

Malignant Disease, Possibilities of Irradiation in. L. J. Clendinnen, Med. J Australia **1**:456 (April 29) 1922.

Measles, Columbus Barracks. H. H. Rutherford. Mil. Surgeon **50**:619 (June) 1922.

Measles, Prodromal Eruption in. F. J. Nöthen. Jahrb. f. Kinderh. **98**:211 (May) 1922.

Measles, Purpura Fulminans Following. E. H. Kelly, Brit. J. Child. Dis. **19**:86 (April-June) 1922.

Measles, Recent Research on. P. L. Marie, Presse méd. **30**:456 (May 27) 1922.

Melanoderma. Melancholia with Melanoderma of Exposed Parts. H. Damaye, Encéphale **17**:293 (May) 1922.

Mercury and Arsphenamin, Recovery Under; Encephalitis and Myelitis in Early Syphilis Under Arsphenamin. Werther, Deutsch. med. Wchnschr. **48**:443 (April 7) 1922.

Mongolian Blue Spot. E. Apert, Arch. de méd. d. enf. **25**:295 (May) 1922.

Mouth Cavity, Ulcers of, and of the Lips. Ledderhose, Deutsch. med. Wchnschr. **48**:527 (April 21) 1922.

Mycosis Fungoides and Noma. Rüsing and Schulte, Deutsch. med. Wchnschr. **48**:555 (April 28) 1922.

Neoplasms, Malignant, Value of Radium in Treatment of. R. H. Jackson, Wisconsin M. J. **20**:624 (May) 1922.

Noma and Mycosis Fungoides. Rüsing and Schulte, Deutsch. med. Wchnschr. **48**:555 (April 28) 1922.

Ochronosis; with Study of Additional Case. B. S. Oppenheimer and B. S. Kline, Arch. Int. Med. **29**:732 (June) 1922.

Paralysis, Facial, and Herpes Zoster. G. Worms and V. de Lavergne, Paris méd. **12**:481 (June 10) 1922.

Purpura Fulminans Following Measles. E. H. Kelly, Brit. J. Child. Dis. **19**:86 (April-June) 1922.

Quartz Lamp Irradiation, Effect on the Susceptibility of the Skin to Pain. F. von Gräer and W. von Jasinski, Klin. Wchnschr. **1**:683 (April 1) 1922.

Radium, Value of, in Treatment of Malignant Neoplasms. R. H. Jackson, Wisconsin M. J. **20**:624 (May) 1922.

Rheumatism, Acute, Associated with Erythema Nodosum. H. Wetherbee, Brit. M. J. **1**:995 (June 24) 1922.

Rhinopharyngitis Mutilans from Yaws. B. M. van Driel, Nederlandsch. Tijdschr. v. Geneesk. **1**:1604 (April 22) 1922.

Roentgen Ray in Dermatology. C. A. Simpson, Virginia M. Monthly **49**:122 (June) 1922.

Scalp, Diagnosis of Diseases of. R. Blosser, Rhode Island M. J. **5**:271 (July) 1922.

Scarlet Fever. Convalescent Human Serum in Treatment of Severe Cases of Scarlet Fever. B. Bernbaum, J. Mich. M. S. **21**:249 (June) 1922.

Scarlet Fever, Distribution of Leukocytes in. T. Mironesco and A. Codreano, Bull. et mém. Soc. méd. d. hôp. de Paris **46**:752 (May 5) 1922.

Septicemia, Streptococcal, and Erysipelas. A. Erian, Practitioner, London **108**:373 (May) 1922.

Skin and Subcutaneous Tissues, Hyperalgesia of, as Factor in Diagnosis of Lesions of Abdominal Viscera. G. F. Thompson, Wisconsin M. J. **21**:14 (June) 1922.

Skin Diseases, Indications from Analysis of Blood in. E. Pulay, Klin. Wchnschr. **1**:414 (Feb. 25) 1922.

Skin. Effect of Quartz Lamp Irradiation on the Susceptibility of the Skin to Pain. F. von Gröer and W. von Jasinski, Klin. Wchnschr. **1**:683 (April 1) 1922.

Skin of Children and Fetuses, Pigment in. M. Gonnella, Jahrb. f. Kinderh. **98**:123 (May) 1922.

Skin, Removal of Pigmentations of. G. Kromayer, Deutsch. med. Wchnschr. **48**:526 (April 21) 1922.

Smallpox, Stenosis of Larynx Following. A. Flores, Crón. méd., Lima **39**:136 (April) 1922.

Smallpox, Transmission of, by Flies. H. Hunziker and H. Reese, Schweiz. med. Wchnschr. **52**:469 (May 18) 1922.

Spirochetes, Staining of, in Cover Glass Smears by Silver-Agar Method. A. S. Warthin and A. C. Starry, J. Infec. Dis. **30**:592 (June) 1922.

Urticaria and Ascaridiasis. O. Pentagna, Pediatria, Naples **30**:308 (April 1) 1922.

Varicella and Herpes. W. M. Elliott, Glasgow M. J. **97**:274 (May) 1922.

Varicella, Ultraviolet Rays in. A. Sack, München. med. Wchnschr. **69**:591 (April 21) 1922.

Yaws in Malaya. A. Viswalingam, Indian M. Gaz. **57**:172 (May) 1922.

Yaws, Rhinopharyngitis Mutilans from. B. M. van Driel, Nederlandsch Tijdschr. v. Geneesk. **1**:1604 (April 8) 1922.

SYPHILOLOGY

Aneurysms, Syphilitic, of Arch of Aorta. Decrop and Salle, Ann. d. mal. vénériennes **17**:438 (June) 1922.

Aorta, Syphilis of. C. W. McGavran and E. Scott, Ohio State M. J. **18**:477 (July) 1922.

Aorta. Syphilitic Aneurysms of Arch of the Aorta. Decrop and Salle, Ann. d. mal. Vénériennes **17**:438 (June) 1922.

Arsphenamin and Mercury, Observations of Practitioner on. Kromayer, Deutsch. med. Wchnschr. **48**:686 (May 26) 1922.

Arsphenamin and Mercury, Recovery Under; Encephalitis and Myelitis in Early Syphilis Under Arsphenamin. Werther, Deutsch. med. Wchnschr. **48**:443 (April 7) 1922.

Arsphenamin, Hemolytic Properties of, and Fifteen Allied Compounds. G. P. Grabfield, J. Pharmacol. & Exper. Therap. **19**:343 (June) 1922.

Arsphenamin, Technic in Mixing and Administering Arsphenamin. J. J. Giesen, Virginia M. Monthly **49**:206 (July) 1922.

Ascites from Inherited Syphilis. M. Acuña and A. Casaubon, Arch. de méd. d. enf. **25**:257 (May) 1922.

Bladder. Another Case of Syphilis of the Bladder. A. Cosacesco, J. d'urol. **13**:365 (May) 1922.

Bone Growth in Nose of Old Syphilitic. E. Hopmann, Schweizer. med. Wchnschr. **52**:504 (May 25) 1922.

Bones. Recognition of Congenital Syphilitic Inflammation of Long Bones. H. M. Turnbull, Lancet **1**:1239 (June 24) 1922.

Calomel in Treatment of Inherited Syphilis. E. Müller, Med. Klin. **18**:694 (May 28) 1922.

Chancre, "Invisible," of the Vulva. G. Belgodere, Ann. d. mal. vénériennes **17**:442 (June) 1922.

Chancres, Primary Soft, on Tongue. G. Martini, Riforma med. **38**:490 (May 22) 1922.

Chancre, Soft, Treatment of. C. Bruck, Klin. Wchnschr. **1**:689 (April 1) 1922.

Cholesterin Content of Antigens; Bearing on Wassermann. Frank. Klin. Wchnschr. **1**:419 (Feb. 25) 1922.

Dermatitis During Treatment of Syphilis. J. Klaar. Wien. klin. Wchnschr. **35**:297 (March 30) 1922.

Ear. Syphilis of Inner Ear and of the Eighth Nerve. G. W. Mackenzie. Virginia M. Monthly **49**:120 (June) 1922.

Encephalitis and Myelitis in Early Syphilis Under Arsphenamin: Recovery Under Mercury and Arsphenamin. Werther. Deutsch. med. Wchnschr. **48**:443 (April 7) 1922.

Hydrocephalus, Syphilitic, in Children. Cassel, Deutsch. med. Wchnschr. **48**:655 (May 19) 1922.

Ileus with Yellow Atrophy of Liver in Syphilitic. F. Breuer, München. med. Wchnschr. **69**:666 (May 5) 1922.

Infancy and Childhood, Syphilis in, Review of Literature of. P. J. White. Am. J. Dis. Child. **23**:535 (June) 1922.

Joint Lesion, Tertiary Syphilitic. P. Lechelle. Bull. et mém. Soc. méd. d. hôp. de Paris **46**:756 (May 12) 1922.

Laryngeal Crisis, Severe, Neurosyphilis with: Tracheotomy. J. W. Leitch, Brit. M. J. **1**:949 (June 17) 1922.

Liver. Ileus with Yellow Atrophy of Liver in Syphilitic. F. Breuer, München. med. Wchnschr. **69**:666 (May 5) 1922.

Lung, Syphilis of. A. Friedlander and R. J. Erickson, J. A. M. A. **79**:291 (July 29) 1922.

Lungs, Syphilis of, Unrecognized for Fifteen Years. Winkler, München. med. Wchnschr. **69**:667 (May 5) 1922.

Mental Defect and Venereal Disease. F. E. Brown, Pub. Health J. **13**:222 (May) 1922.

Mercury and Arsphenamin, Observations of Practitioner on. Kromayer, Deutsch. med. Wchnschr. **48**:686 (May 26) 1922.

Mercury Not Only a Symptomatic Remedy, But One Affecting Favorably the Course of Syphilis. J. Heller, Klin. Wchnschr. **1**:519 (March 11) 1922.

Myelitis and Encephalitis in Early Syphilis Under Arsphenamin; Recovery Under Mercury and Arsphenamin. Werther, Deutsch. med. Wchnschr. **48**:443 (April 7) 1922.

Neo-Arsphenamin, a Filtering Adapter for the Administration of. J. F. Schamberg, J. A. M. A. **79**:216 (July 15) 1922.

Neo-Arsphenamin. Prevention of Toxic Manifestations (Fever, Cutaneous Inflammation) After Injections of Neo-Arsphenamin by Concomitant Administration of Calcium Bromid and Calcium Chlorid. D. Kennedy, Deutsch. med. Wchnschr. **48**:586 (May 5) 1922.

Neo-Arsphenamin, Staining Spirochetes with Aid of. Krantz, München. med. Wchnschr. **69**:586 (April 21) 1922.

Neo-Silver-Arsphenamin. K. Ullmann, Wien. klin. Wchnschr. **35**:316 (April 6) 1922.

Neo-Silver-Arsphenamin, Clinical Experiences with. A. Stühmer, Deutsch. med. Wchnschr. **48**:584 (May 5) 1922.

Neo-Silver-Arsphenamin in Treatment of Syphilis. Zeller, München. med. Wchnschr. **69**:737 (May 19) 1922.

Neo-Silver-Arsphenamin Sodium, Experiences with. Sternthal, Deutsch. med. Wchnschr. **48**:457 (April 7) 1922.

Neo-Silver-Salvarsan. F. Hanemann, Med. Klin. **18**:627 (May 14) 1922.

Nerve, Eighth, and Inner Ear, Syphilis of. G. W. Mackenzie, Virginia M. Monthly **49**:120 (June) 1922.

Nervous System, Central, Syphilis of. D. A. MacGregor, W. Virginia M. J. **16**:384 (April) 1922.

Neurosyphilis in Ex-Service Men. R. H. Prince, J. Nerv. & Ment. Dis. **55**:485 (June) 1922.

Neurosyphilis, Preventive Treatment of. G. Pellacani, Riforma med. **38**:491 (May 22) 1922.

Neurosyphilis, Spinal Fluid in. A. Terzani, Riv. crit. di clin. med. **23**:97 (March 25) 1922; concluded p. 109.

Neurosyphilis with Severe Laryngeal Crisis: Tracheotomy. J. W. Leitch, Brit. M. J. **1**:949 (June 17) 1922.

Prurigo in Inherited Syphilis. M. A. Guerrero, Arch. latino-amer. de pediat. **16**:284 (April) 1922.

Sachs-Georgi Versus Wassermann Reaction. D. E. Cohen, Nederlandsch Tijdschr. v. Geneesk. **1**:1698 (April 29) 1922.

Silver Arsphenamin, Old and New. Hübner and Marr, Deutsch. med. Wchnschr. **48**:624 (May 5) 1922.

Spirochaeta Pallida, Excretion of, Through Kidneys. A. S. Warthin, J. Infec. Dis. **30**:569 (June) 1922.

Spirochetes in Rabbits, Chemotherapeutic Differentiation of. W. Kolle and R. Ruppert, Med. Klin. **18**:620 (May 14) 1922.

Spirochetes, Staining, with Aid of Neo-Arsphenamin. Krantz, München. med. Wchnschr. **69**:586 (April 21) 1922.

Sulfoxylatsalvarsan in Treatment of Syphilis. F. Fabry, Med. Klin. **18**:690 (May 28) 1922.

Syphilis, Acute Malignant Degenerative. A. Pfeiffer, Deutsch. Arch. f. klin. Med. **139**:245 (May 5) 1922.

Syphilis of the Bladder, Another Case of. A. Cosacesco, J. d'urol. **13**:365 (May) 1922.

Syphilis of Inner Ear and Eighth Nerve. G. W. Mackenzie, ·Virginia M. Monthly **49**:120 (June) 1922.

Syphilis of Intestine, Case of. G. O. Scott and G. H. J. Pearson, Am. J. Syphilis **6**:269 (April) 1922.

Syphilis of the Lung. A. Friedlander and R. J. Erickson, J. A. M. A. **79**:291 (July 29) 1922.

Syphilis of Nervous System. S. I. Schwab, .South. M. J. **15**:254 (April) 1922.

Syphilis of the Spleen. A. Furno, Policlinico, Rome **29**:123 (March 1) 1922.

Syphilis of Stomach. J. W. McNee, Quart. J. Med., April, 1922, p. 215.

Syphilis, Ophthalmologist's Relation to. S. R. Gifford, Nebraska M. J. **7**:167 (May) 1922.

Syphilis. Physiognomic Signs of Congenital Syphilis in the Second and Third Generation. P. Kranz, Zentralbl. f. inn. med. **42**:977 (Dec. 24) 1921.

Syphilis, Practical Observations on. H. H. Hazen, Am. J. Syphilis **6**:204 (April) 1922.

Syphilis, Precipitation Reactions in. A. Sordelli and C. E. Pico, Rev. Asoc. méd. argent. **34**:1651 (Dec.) 1921.

Syphilis, Present Treatment of, with Especial Reference to Efficacy of Modern ⸱ Methods. W. M. Brunet, Kentucky M. J. **20**:229 (April) 1922.

Syphilis, Prevalence of, in China Expedition, 15th U. S. Infantry. R. E. Houke, Mil. Surgeon **50**:251 (March) 1922.

Syphilis, Primary, Absolute Diagnosis of. I. C. Sutton, Am. J. Syphilis **6**:283 (April) 1922.

Syphilis Problems. Fabry and Wolff, Med. Klin. **18**:106 (Jan. 22) 1922.

Syphilis, Prophylaxis and Cure of. L. Queyrat, Paris méd. **12**:177 (March 4) 1922.

Syphilis. Relation Between Syphilis and Cancer of Respiratory and Digestive Tracts. Lambert, Arch. méd. belge **74**:1132 (Dec.) 1921.

Syphilis. Reliability of Gate and Papacostas' Formol-Gel Test for Syphilis as Compared with Wassermann Reaction. S. Ramakrishnan, Indian J. M. Res. **9**:620 (Jan.) 1922.

Syphilis. Second Neurorelapse Following Combined Treatment of So-Called Seronegative Primary Syphilis. F. Krömeke, München. med. Wchnschr. **69**:668 (May 5) 1922.

Syphilis, Soft Soap as Adjuvant in. Hübner, Deutsch. med. Wchnschr. **48**:157 (Feb. 2) 1922.

Syphilis, Some Problems in. R. V. Hoffman, Indiana State M. A. J. **15**:152 (May) 1922.

Syphilis Spirochetes, Stain for. J. J. Puente, Rev. Asoc. méd. arg. **34**:1134 (Nov.) 1921.

Syphilis, Standard of Cure in. A. R. Fraser, South African Med. Rec. **20**:102 (March 25) 1922.

Syphilis, Sulfoxylatsalvarsan in Treatment of. F. Fabry, Med. Klin. **18**:690 (May 28) 1922.

Syphilis, Tabes Dorsalis Plus Tertiary Syphilis. B. Barker Beeson, J. A. M. A. **78**:1537 (May 20) 1922.

Syphilis, Temporary Natural Resistance to. R. Brandt, Wien. klin. Wchnschr. **35**:223 (March 9) 1922.

Syphilis, Transmission of, by a Bite. G. Martini, Riforma med. **38**:467 (May 15) 1922.

Syphilis, Treatment of. L. Brocq, Presse méd. **30**:421 (May 17) 1922.

Syphilis, Two Fundamental Forms of. F. X. Dercum, New York M. J. & Med. Rec. **115**:504 (May 3) 1922.

Syphilis, Urologist's Views on. C. H. Chetwood, New York M. J. & Med. Rec. **115**:501 (May 3) 1922.

Syphilis, Value of Neurological Examination in. R. Hoyt, Am. J. Syphilis **6**:273 (April) 1922.

Syphilis. When Does Parenchymatous Syphilis Develop? J. Calicó, Rev. españ. de méd. y cirug. **4**:683 (Dec.) 1921.

Syphilitic Aortitis and Endocarditis. J. C. Lindsay, Canad. M. A. J. **12**:335 (May) 1922.

Syphilitic Diabetes. F. Rathery and Fernet, Bull. Soc. méd. d. hôp., Paris **46**:661 (April 28) 1922.

Syphilitic Diabetes Insipidus. J. Lhermitte, Ann. de méd. **11**:89 (Feb.) 1922.

Syphilitic Disease of Heart. N. B. Koppang, Norsk Mag. f. Lægevidensk. **83**: 65 (Feb.) 1922.

Syphilitic Hydrocephalus in Children. Cassel, Deutsch. med. Wchnschr. **48**: 655 (May 19) 1922.

Syphilitic Infection, Body's Natural Means of Defense Against; How Affected by Mercury. S. Bergel, Klin. Wchnschr. **1**:204 (Jan. 28) 1922.

Syphilitic Inflammation of Long Bones, Congenital Recognition of. H. M. Turnbull, Lancet **1**:1239 (June 24) 1922.

Syphilitic Parotitis in Adolescent. J. P. Garraghan, Semana méd. **1**:172 (Feb. 2) 1922.

Syphilitic Serum, Formaldehyd Test of. M. Armangué and González, Rev. españ. de méd. y cirug. **4**:685 (Dec.) 1921.

Syphilitic Serum Reactions. K. Taoka, Japan Med. World **2**:126 (May 15) 1922.

"Syphilitics' Pater Noster," 1540. R. Barthélemy, Ann. d. mal. vénériennes. Paris **17**:298 (April) 1922.

Syphilitics, Pityriasis in, and Herxheimer Reaction. Feit, Med. Klin. **18**:209 (Feb. 12) 1922.

Syphilitics, Spermatozoa of. V. Widacowoch, Rev. Asoc. méd. argent. **34**:1564 (Dec.) 1921.

Syphiloma. Hypertrophic Ulcerative Form of Chronic Vulvitis (Elephantiasis. Esthiomene, Syphiloma). F. J. Taussig, Am. J. Obst. **3**:281 (March) 1922.

Tabes and Paget's Disease. H. Claude and P. Oury, Bull. et mém. Soc. méd. d. hôp. de Paris **46**:283 (Feb. 10) 1922.

Tabes and Paget's Disease. G. Guillain, Bull. et mém. Soc. méd. de hôp. de Paris **46**:291 (Feb. 10) 1922.

Tabes Dorsalis Plus Tertiary Cutaneous Syphilis. B. Barker Beeson. J. A. M. A. **78**:1537 (May 20) 1922.

Tartar Emetic in Venereal Disease, Freshly Dissolved. F. G. Cawston. J. Trop. M. **25**:126 (May 15) 1922.

Tongue, Primary Soft Chancres on. G. Martini, Riforma med. **38**:490 (May 22) 1922.

Urine. Chemical Studies of Blood and Urine of Syphilitic Patients Under Arsphenamin Treatment. C. Weiss and A. Corson, Arch. Int. Med. **29**:428 (April) 1922.

Veins, Hepatic. Obstruction of Hepatic Portion of Inferior Vena Cava and of Hepatic Veins Due to Syphilis. T. Kimura, Sei-i-Kwai M. J. **41**:1 (March) 1922.

Vena Cava. Obstruction of Hepatic Portion of Inferior Vena Cava and of Hepatic Veins Due to Syphilis. T. Kimura, Sei-i-Kwai M. J. **41**:1 (March) 1922.

Venereal Disease and Mental Defect. F. E. Brown, Pub. Health J. **13**:222 (May) 1922.

Venereal Disease Clinic of Maryland State Department of Health. A. G. Rytina. Am. J. Syphilis **6**:185 (April) 1922.

Venereal Diseases as We See Them Today. J. E. R. McDonagh. Practitioner **108**:172 (March) 1922.

Venereal Diseases, Florida's Program for Eradication or Control of. G. A. Dame, Florida M. A. J. **8**:178 (April) 1922.

Venereal Disease, Freshly Dissolved Tartar Emetic in. F. G. Cawston. J. Trop. M. **25**:126 (May 15) 1922.

Venereal Diseases from Army Standpoint. M. C. Sycle. Virginia M. Monthly **49**:155 (June) 1922.

Archives of Dermatology and Syphilology

VOLUME 6	OCTOBER, 1922	NUMBER 4

THE TISSUE REACTION IN MALIGNANT EPITHELIOMAS OF THE SKIN

ITS VALUE IN DIAGNOSIS AND IN PROGNOSIS [*]

HOWARD J. PARKHURST, M.D.

TOLEDO, OHIO

A survey of the literature dealing with this particular phase of the cancer problem indicates that surprisingly little investigation has been made in this direction. It was Borst's opinion [1] that the parenchyma of the epithelioma is often retarded by the new connective tissue development roundabout. According to Unna's rule,[2] "The cellular infiltration of the cutis increases with the activity of the epithelial growth, when the epithelial margin is the seat of marked proliferation."

Concerning the presence of plasma cells, Aschoff, Ribbert and Borst say little. In 1891, Jadassohn [3] referred to the "encircling wall of plasma cells and leukocytes," and Unna,[2] describing the plasmoma of Paget's disease, characterizes it as "a bulwark óf defense against cancer invasion." Reviewing a series of twenty-eight cases of epithelioma, Unna reports that fourteen contained many plasma cells, variously distributed, but often encircling the epithelioma. He also found numerous mast cells, usually in inverse ratio to the number of plasma cells present. The striking participation of the mast cell moved him to suggest that carcinoma should not be too widely separated from other chronic inflammatory processes. With Joannowicz,[1] he asserted that the rate of tumor growth is in inverse proportion to the number of plasma cells. Prytek [1] has studied a series of thirty-eight cases from Jadassohn's and other clinics, and he noted that the specimens with many mitoses often contained few plasma cells. However, he concludes that plasma cells, while not always present, "are often numerous, but bear no constant relationship to the type of neoplasm, nor to the presence

---

* Read before the Section on Dermatology and Syphilology at the Seventy-Third Annual Session of the American Medical Association, St. Louis. May, 1922.

* From the Laboratory of the Department of Dermatology, Vanderbilt Clinic, Columbia University, New York.

1. Prytek: The Plasma Cells in Epithelioma of the Skin. Arch. f. Dermat. u. Syph. 120:611, 1914.

2. Unna: Histopathology (Walker's translation). New York: Macmillan Co., 1896.

3. Jadassohn: Verhandl. d. deutsch. Dermat. Gesellsch., Leipzig. 1891.

Tumor	Growth	nvaded (¼, ½ or All)	Hyaline Type	Basophilic Type		(0, 1, 2, 3 or 4)	3 or 4				ascular	(0, 1, 3 or	Epithelioma Cells	Remarks
Early (?) prickle	Fairly rapid	All	2	2		—	—	1			No	—	Hardy	[illegible]
Late prickle	Slow	All	3	3	All	1	2	1			No	Few	Many hyaline	Acanthosis
Early (?) prickle	Slow	All	2	0	All	Very slight	1	0			No	Few	Faded	Slight acanthosis
1 year basal	Slow	½	Slight	1	All	—	1	1			Somewhat	1	Fairly hardy	Acanthosis
Early basal	Slow	¼	0	1	½	—	2	0			No	2	Hardy	Epidermis thin
Early prickle	Rapid	All	—	—	—	—	—	2			—	3	Hardy	Hyaline vessels; acantl
Late prickle	Rapid	All	4	4	All	2	2	1			No	1	Hardy hyaline	Hyaline vessels; acantl
Late basal†	Fairly slow	All	3	3 U‡	All	1	2	1			No	1	Hardy	Epidermis thin
Early basal	Fairly slow	Not ¼	1	1 U	½—	Slight	1	0			No	1	Hardy	Epidermis thin§
Early basal	Fairly slow	Not ¼	1	1 U	All	1	2	0			No	Few	Fairly hardy	Epidermis thin
Late prickle	Rapid	All	1 U ‡	1	All	3	2	0			Somewhat	2	Hardy	Acanthosis
Early basal	Slow	¼	1	1 U	All	1	2	0			No	Very few	Hardy	Epidermis thin
Early prickle	Rapid	¼	1	1	All	—	1	1			No	4	Hardy	Acanthosis
Early prickle	Rapid	¾	3	0	All	2	2	1			No	Few	Fairly hardy	No epidermis
Early prickle	Rapid	All	1	0	All	Slight	1	1			No	0	Fairly hardy	Slight acanthosis ?
Early basal	Slow	¼	0	1 U	¼—	1—	1	0	1	0	No	—	Fairly hardy	Epidermis thin§
Early prickle	Rapid	All	1	1	All	0	Few	1	2	1	No	0	Fairly hardy	Acanthosis
Early basal	Slow	½	Slight	1	All	Slight	1	1	2	0	No	1	Hardy	Epidermis thin
Early prickle	Fairly rapid	All	1	1	All	3	3	2	1	1—	No	1	Hardy hyaline	
Early prickle	Rapid	All	1	0	All	2	2	0	2	1	No	1	Hardy hyaline	Hyaline vessels; acantl
Early basal	Slow	½	1	1	All	1	2	0	3	0	No	Few	Hardy	Epidermis thin
Early prickle	Rapid	All	1	0	All	Slight	1	0	2	0	Somewhat	0	Hardy hyaline	Acanthosis
Late prickle	Fairly rapid	All	1	1	All	Slight	2	2	1	3	Yes	Few	Faded hyaline	Hyaline vessels; acantl
Early basal	Slow	Not ¼	1	1	¼	Slight	1	0	1	1—	No	1—	Fairly hardy	Epidermis thin
Late basal	Fairly slow	All	1	1	All	—	1	0	1	1—	No	1—	Hardy	
Late basal	Slow	All	2	2	All	Slight	1	1—	3	1	No	0	Variable	After 2 [illegible]gen ray (
Late basal	Slow	All	1	1	All	1	2	0	1	1—	No	2	Hardy	Epidermis thin
Early prickle	Rapid	Not ¼	1	1	¼	0	0	0	3	1	Yes	1	Fairly hardy	Slight acanthosis
Early basal	Slow	½	1	1	½	Slight	1—	2	2	1	No	1—	Fairly hardy	Epidermis thin
Early prickle	Rapid	½	2	2	All	Slight	2	2	1	3	No	1	Hardy	Acanthosis
Late basal	Fairly slow	All	2	2	All	1	3	2	1	0	No	2	Hardy	No epidermis
Late basal	Slow	½	1	1	All	Slight	1—	1—	2	1—	No	3	Hardy	Epidermis thin§
9 mo. (?) prickle	Fairly rapid	All	1	1	All	1	1—	1	1	1	Yes	1	Fairly hardy	Acanthosis
Early prickle	Fairly rapid	Not ¼	1	1—	¼	0	1—	1—	1	0	No	1—	Fairly hardy	Acanthosis
Early prickle	Rapid?	Not ¼	1	1—	¼	0	1—	1—	2	1—	No	1—	Fairly hardy	Vessels hyaline; acant
Early prickle	Rapid	All	1	1	All	1	1	1—	2	1—	No	1	Hardy	Acanthosis
Late basal	Fairly slow	All	1	1	All	Slight	1—	1	1	0	No	1	Hardy	Epidermis thin
Late basal	Fairly slow	All	1	1	All	0	2	1	1	1—	No	1	Hardy	Epidermis thin
Early basal	Fairly slow	½	1	1	All	Slight	1	1—	1	1—	No	1—	Hardy	Epidermis thin; ulcer
Late basal†	Fairly slow	All	1—	0	All	0	1—	0	1—	0	No	1—	Hardy	Epidermis thin; metas
Early basal	Fairly slow	¼	0	1—	¼	0	1—	0	1	1	Yes	1	Hardy	Epidermis thin
Early prickle	Fairly rapid	All	1	1	All	Slight	1—	2	1	1	Yes	1	Some hyaline	Vessels hyaline; acantl
Early basal	Slow	Not ¼	1	1	All	1	1	0	1	2	No	1—	Hardy	Epidermis thin
Early prickle	Fairly rapid	½	1	0	All	Slight	1—	0	1	0	Somewhat	1—	Fairly hardy	Hyaline vessels; acantl
Early prickle	Rapid	½	1	1—	All	Very slight	1—	1	3	1—	Yes	1	Hardy	Acanthosis
Early prickle	Rapid	½	1	0	All	Very slight	1—	0	2	0	Somewhat	1—	Fairly hardy	Acanthosis
Late basal	Slow	½	1—	1	All	Slight	1	1	1	2	No	2	Hardy	Epidermis thin
Late basal	Fairly rapid	All	1	1	All	0	1—	1	1	1—	Yes	2	Hardy	Epidermis thin
Late basal	Fairly rapid	All	1	1	All	Slight	1—	1	1	0	No	1	Hardy	Slight acanthosis ?
Late basal	Fairly slow	All	2	2	All	Slight	1	1	1	1—	No	2	Hardy	Slight acanthosis

Early basal	?	Not ¼	1	1	All								Hardy	Epidermis thin
Late prickle	Fairly slow	All	1	1	All		1	–	2	0			Hardy	[illegible]
Early prickle	Fairly rapid	Not ¼	1	1	All		1	1—	3	—			Fairly hardy	Pegs acanthotic; epiderm thin
Late basal	?	All	0	1	All	2	3	2	1	0			Hardy	Floor [illegible]
Late basal	Fairly slow	All	1	2	All	1	1	0	1	0			Fairly hardy	Epidermis thin
Late [illegible]	Fairly slow	All	1	0	All	1	1	0	1	0			Hardy	Epidermis thin
Early basal	Fairly slow	¼	1—	1—	¼	0	0	1—	2	1			Hardy	Epidermis thin
Late basal	Fairly rapid	¾	Stain poor			Slight	1—	0	1	0			Fairly hardy	Thickness of epiderm varies
Late prickle	Fairly rapid	All	1	1—	All	0	0	1	1				Fairly hardy	Vessels hyaline; acanthos
Late prickle	Fairly rapid	All	1	0	All	0	0	0	1	0			[illegible]	Acanthosis
Late basal	Fairly slow	All	0	2	All	0	0	0	1—	3			Variable	Epidermis thin
Early basal	Fairly slow	¼	1	1	¼	Slight	1—	0	2	1			Hardy	Epidermis thin
Late prickle	Fairly rapid	All	1	0	All	—	—	1	1—				Hardy	Vessels hyaline; acanthos[illegible]
Late basal	Fairly rapid	All	1—	1	All	Slight	1—	0	1—	0	No	1—	Hardy	Epidermis thin
Early prickle	Fairly rapid	All	1	Stain poor		2	1	1	1	0	No	1	Hardy	Vessels [illegible]; acanthos
Late prickle	Fairly rapid	All	1	1—	All	Very slight	1—	1	1	3	Yes	1	Hardy	Vessels hyaline; acanthos
Early basal	Fairly slow	¼	1—	2	All	Slight	1—	1—	1	2	No	1—	Variable	Roentgen rayed
Early prickle	Fairly rapid	All	2	1—	All	0	?	1	2	1	No	1	Hardy	Vessels hyaline; acanthos hyperkeratosis
Early prickle	Fairly rapid	All	2	1—	All	Very slight	1—	0	1	1	Somewhat	1—	Degenerative	Vessels hyaline; acanthos
Late prickle	Fairly rapid	All	1	1	All	Very slight	1	1	2	1—	Yes	1—	Fairly hardy	Slight acanthosis
Early prickle	Fairly rapid	Not ¼	2	2	¼	1	1	0	1	4	Yes	1—	Hardy	Acanthosis and hyperkeratosis
Early basal	Fairly rapid	¼	1	1	All	2	2	1—	1	3	No	1—	Hardy	Acanthosis
Early prickle?	Fairly rapid	½	1	1	All	Slight	1—	0	2	0	No	1—	Fairly hardy	Nevus ?; acanthosis
Early prickle	Fairly rapid	½	1—	1—	½	Slight	1—	1	2	1—	No	1	Hardy	Acanthosis
Early prickle	Fairly rapid	All	1	0	All	Very slight	1—	1	1	1	Yes	2	Hardy	Acanthosis and hyperkeratosis
Early basal	Fairly slow	¼	1—	2	¼	0	0	1—	1—	3	No	1	Hardy	Acanthosis, parakeratosis and hyperkeratosis
Early basal	Fairly rapid	½	2	3	All	0	0	2	1	0	Somewhat	1—	Hardy	Nevus [illegible]; acanthosis
Early prickle	Fairly rapid	½	3†	2	All	Very slight	1—	0	3	0	Yes	1—	Hardy	Vessels hyaline; acanthos
Early prickle	Very rapid	½	1	2	All	0	0	1—	1—	0	No	1—	Fairly hardy	Acanthosis and hyperkeratosis
Early prickle	Fairly rapid	½	1	1	All	Slight	1	1	1	2	Yes	1—	Fairly hardy	Acanthosis
Early prickle	Fairly rapid	¾	1	1	All	Very slight	1	2	2	1—	No	1—	Faded	Vessels hyaline; acanthos
Early basal	Fairly slow	¼	0	1	¼	1	1	0	1	0	No	1—	Fairly hardy	Epidermis thin
Early basal	Fairly rapid	½	1	1	All	1—	1	0	2	1—	No	1—	Fairly hardy	Pegs [illegible]; epidermis thin
Early prickle	Rapid	¼	1	0	All	0	0	0	1	3	Somewhat	1—	Fairly hardy	Paget's disease; vessels hyaline
Early prickle	Rapid	½	1	0	½	2	2	0	2	0	No	1—	Fairly hardy	Acanthosis and hyperkeratosis
Late basal	Slow	All	1	1	All	1	1	1	2	1	No	—	Hardy hyaline [illegible]	
Early basal	Slow	¼	1	1	All	On	1—	0	1	1—	No	1		Nevus papillomatosus acanthosis
Late prickle	Fairly rapid	All	1	0	All	1	2	1—	2	1—	No	1—	Fairly hardy	Acanthosis
Early basal	Fairly slow	½	1—	1	½	0	1—	0	1	0	No	1	Fairly hardy	Epidermis thin
Early basal	Fairly rapid	½	1—	1—	½	Slight	1	0	1	0	No	1—	Fairly hardy	Epidermis thin
Late basal	Slow	All	2	2	All	2	1	0	1	0	No	1—	[illegible] degen.	Slight acanthosis
Late basal	Fairly slow	¾	1	1	All	1	1	1—	1	1—	No	0	[illegible] degen.	Epidermis thin
Early prickle	Fairly rapid	All	1	0	All	Slight	1—	0	1	2	No	1	Fairly hardy	Vessels [illegible]; acanthos
Early prickle	Fairly rapid	¼	1	1	¼	0	0	0	1	1	Slightly	1—	Hardy	Slight acanthosis
Late prickle	Fairly rapid	All	1	0	All	0	0	2	2	0	No	1	Hyaline hardy	Ulcer
Late basal	Fairly slow	¾	1	1—	All	2	1	1	0	1	No	1—	Some degen.	Slight acanthosis
Late basal	Fairly slow	All	1	1—	All	3	2	0	2	0	No	2	[illegible] hardy	Epidermis thin
Early prickle	Rapid	¼	2	0	All	1	1	1	1	1	No	1—	Fairly hardy	Vessels hyaline; acanthos
Early prickle	Fairly slow	¾	1	0	All	2	2	1	1	1	Slightly	1	Hardy	Vessels hyaline
Early basal	Fairly slow	½	1—	1	All	Slight	1	0	1	0	No	1—	Fairly hardy	Epidermis fairly thin

or absence of ulceration, nor to the rate of tumor growth." From animal experiments, DaFano[4] has concluded that plasma cells as well as lymphocytes appear to be agents of the immunity process. McDonagh[5] believes that the plasma cell is present as an oxidizer of the deteriorating epithelioma cells.

Beginning in 1915, Murphy and his collaborators[6] of the Rockefeller Institute apparently showed the lymphocyte to be a bearer of tissue immunity against malignant invasion, upholding the views of DaFano in this respect. Itami[7] later claimed to have raised the immunity of animals against cancer by injecting lymph node extract. Mitoses have been reported as being very numerous in the spleen after tumor inoculation.[8] However, the work of Sittenfeld[9] and of Bullock and Rohdenburg,[10] the latter using splenectomized animals, tends to disprove the theories of DaFano and Murphy and to show that the lymphocyte, after all, is not necessarily the agent of immunity. Woglom[11] found that the spleens of immunized and inoculated rats were not enlarged; and Prime,[12] as the result of recent extensive observations, reaches the following conclusions: "Decreasing the circulating lymphocytes by small doses of roentgen ray does not render mice more susceptible to the inoculation of a spontaneous tumor from another mouse of the same strain. Mice with spontaneous lymphocytosis are not resistant to the implantation of a primary tumor from another mouse of the same strain." Thus far, animal experiments have been limited to work with epitheliomas of the prickle cell type, only one case of basal cell epithelioma, occurring in a rat, having been reported.[13]

Here and there throughout the literature, the apparent relationship between chronic inflammation and the development of epithelioma is alluded to, some authorities stating that, without previous chronic inflammation, cancer does not exist (Billroth's dictum). According to McDonagh,[5] the occurrence of epithelioma follows a chronic inflammation, which produces lipoid-globulin substances in the cells.

4. DaFano: Ztschr. f. Immunitätsforsch. u. exper. Therap., Orig. **5**:1, 1910.
5. McDonagh: The Epithelial Changes in Inflammation and Their Relationship to Malignant Epithelioma, Arch. f. Dermat. u. Syph. **120**:289, 1914.
6. Murphy, J. B.: J. Exper. M. **22**:204, 1915; **25**:609, 1917; **29**:25 (Jan.) 1919. Murphy, J. B., and Nakahara, W.: J. Exper. M. **31**:1 (Jan.) 1920.
7. Itami: J. Cancer Res. **4**:23 (Jan.) 1919.
8. Murphy, J. B., and Nakahara, W.: Footnote 6, fourth reference.
9. Sittenfeld, M. J.: J. Cancer Res. **2**:151 (April) 1917.
10. Bullock, F. D., and Rohdenburg, G. L.: J. Cancer Res. **2**:455, 465 (Oct.) 1917.
11. Woglom: J. Cancer Res. **4**:281 (July) 1919.
12. Prime, F.: J. Cancer Res. **6**:1 (Jan.) 1921.
13. Morris, D. H.: J. Cancer Res. **5**:147 (April) 1920.

With the purpose of further investigation, we have examined the slides from 100 human epitheliomas, noting the following points in each: the type of the tumor, whether basal or prickle cell; its apparent age and rate of growth; the depth of its extent into the underlying corium; the appearance of the cells of the tumor parenchyma and the number of mitotic figures observed; the state of the overlying epidermis, whether thinned or acanthotic; and the characteristics of the stroma, including the connective tissue degeneration, its degree, location and type (whether hyaline or basophilic), the growth of new connective tissue, and the types and relative numbers of the plasma cells, lymphocytes and polymorphonuclear leukocytes, their relation to the

TABLE 2.—An Analysis of the Findings in Fifty Prickle Cell and Fifty Basal Cell Epitheliomas

Findings	Basal Cell		Prickle Cell	
	Typical	Otherwise	Typical	Otherwise
Epithelioma arising from thin epidermis	24	..	..	..
Signs of a preceding inflammatory process	..	45	50	..
Noninflammatory	5	..	..	..
Epidermis acanthotic	..	8*	45	..
Epidermis thin	35	..	..	..
Infiltration of lymphocytes alone	21	..	..	17
Lymphocytes and plasma cells	..	27†	..	35‡
Infiltration of plasma cells alone	..	..	..	..
Cellular infiltration perivascular	..	4	19	..
Connective tissue degeneration basophilic only	5	..	..	..
Connective tissue degeneration basophilic and hyaline	..	41	..	34
Connective tissue degeneration hyaline only	..	2	15	..
Connective tissue degeneration in upper corium basophilic only	18	..	..	..
Connective tissue degeneration in upper corium basophilic and hyaline	..	20	..	20
Connective tissue degeneration in upper corium hyaline only	..	..	26	..
Hyaline changes in vessel walls	..	..	19	..
Fibrosis	..	44§	..	4•§
Mitoses in epithelioma cells	..	45¶	..	45¶
Epithelioma cells of hardy appearance	..	46	..	47
Epithelioma cells of faded appearance	..	2	..	3

* Cylindromas, nevi, etc.
† Plasma ++ in seventeen.
‡ Plasma ++ in twenty-one.
§ Fibrosis ++ in thirteen.
¶ Mitoses ++ in six.

blood vessels, and the condition of the vessel walls, especially as to the presence or absence of hyaline degeneration. The specimens had been fixed in Bouin's solution and stained with hematoxylin and eosin: a few were stained with hematoxylin orange and acid fuchsin. Fifty of the specimens were from basal cell epitheliomas, while the remaining fifty were of the prickle cell variety, all stages of development and various rates of growth being represented. The basophilic degeneration noted was of the so-called mucoid type, such as that occurring in senile atrophy of the skin, and the hyaline or acidophilic degeneration was that which accompanies chronic interstitial inflammation: its location in the derma was noted, and the locations in which each type of degeneration predominated, whether immediately beneath the epidermis or deeper. The stain did not permit an examination for mast cells, nor could the elastic tissue be studied. The results have been tabulated as shown in Table 1, presenting the findings in each case, and these findings have been summarized in Table 2.

RESULTS OF OBSERVATIONS

1. Neoplasms of the epidermis, associated with thinning of the remaining epidermis and not accompanied by a chronic inflammatory process, usually are basal cell epitheliomas (Fig. 1).

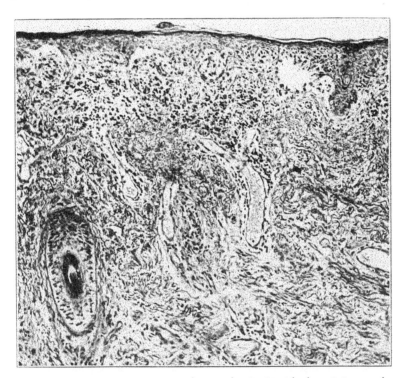

Fig. 1.—Neoplasms of the epidermis, associated with thinning of the remaining epidermis and not accompanied by a chronic inflammatory process, are usually basal cell epitheliomas; compare Slide 16.

2. If these basal cell epitheliomas are slow growing, they usually present slight inflammatory tissue reaction, with lymphocytes as the predominant cells (Fig. 2).

3. If a basal cell epithelioma is accompanied by much tissue reaction, we find a mixture of lymphocytes and plasma cells (Fig. 3).

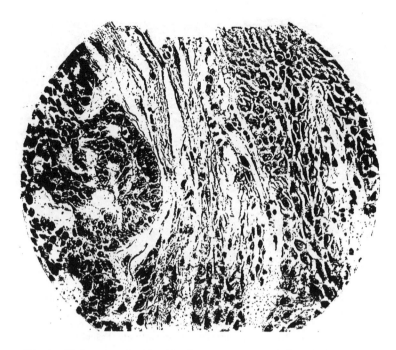

Fig. 2.—If these basal cell epitheliomas are slow growing, they usually present slight inflammatory tissue reaction, with lymphocytes as the predominant cells; compare Slide 18.

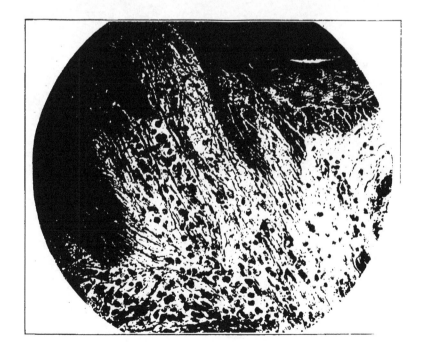

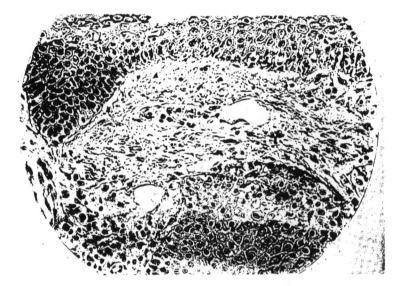

Fig. 4.—When a basal cell epithelioma is slow growing, as a rule we find little evidence of connective tissue degeneration, and vice versa; but there is always some connective tissue degeneration. In basal cell epitheliomas, the type of connective tissue degeneration is prevailingly basophilic rather than hyaline; compare Slide 5.

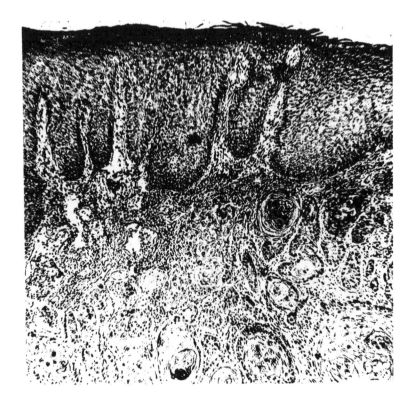

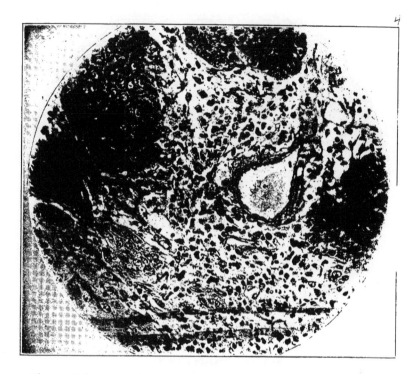

Fig. 6.—This chronic inflammatory process has ordinarily been present for a long time, so that the tissue has had time to develop a certain amount of resistance, as evidenced by the proliferation of connective tissue, by the presence of plasma cells, and by changes in the blood vessels; compare Slide 7.

The slow development of a prickle cell epithelioma is accompanied by the appearance of plasma cells (Slide 7).

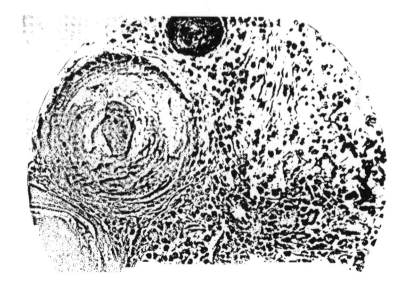

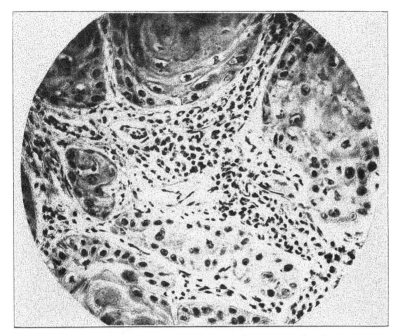

Fig. 8.—Connective tissue degeneration in prickle cell epitheliomas is more hyaline than basophilic, as a rule; compare Slide 98.

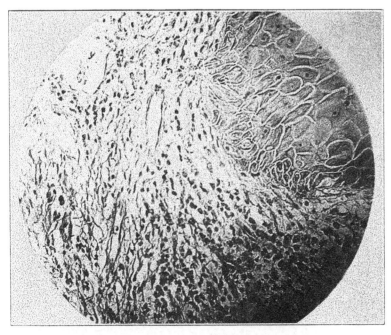

Fig. 9.—The rapid development of a prickle cell epithelioma is accompanied

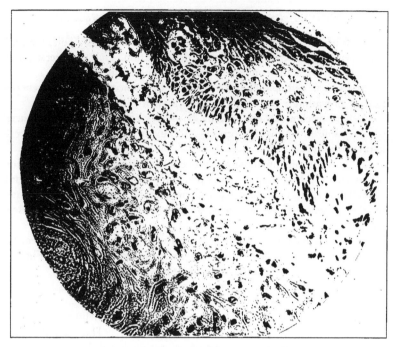

Fig. 10.—The number of plasma cells and, to a somewhat less extent, the number of lymphocytes, vary directly with the amount of hyaline degeneration of the connective tissue. Here it is slight.

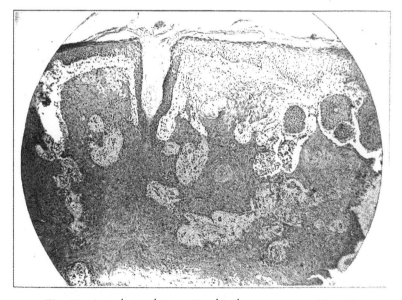

Fig. 11.—A typical prickle cell epithelioma: compare Slide 28.

4. When a basal cell epithelioma is slow growing, as a rule, we find little evidence of connective tissue degeneration, and vice versa; but there is always some connective tissue degeneration (Fig. 4).

5. In basal cell epitheliomas, the type of connective tissue degeneration is prevailingly basophilic rather than hyaline (Fig. 4).

6. The prickle cell epithelioma is always associated with evidences of a chronic inflammatory process; for example, acanthosis or hyperkeratosis (Fig. 5).

7. This chronic inflammatory process has ordinarily been present for a long time, so that the tissue has had time to develop a certain amount of resistance, as evidenced by the proliferation of connective tissue, by the presence of plasma cells, and by changes in the blood vessels (Fig. 6).

8. This preceding chronic inflammatory process is a complicating factor, according to the nature of its pathologic picture. (Fig. 7: prickle cell epithelioma in tissue affected by lupus vulgaris.)

9. Connective tissue degeneration in prickle cell epitheliomas is more hyaline than basophilic, as a rule (Fig. 8).

10. The rapid development of a prickle cell epithelioma is accompanied by the presence of lymphocytes (Fig. 9). The slow development of a prickle cell epithelioma is accompanied by plasma cells (Fig. 6).

GENERAL CONCLUSIONS

1. The number of plasma cells and, to a somewhat less extent, the number of lymphocytes, vary directly with the amount of hyaline degeneration of the connective tissue. (Compare Figure 10, showing a slight amount, and Figure 8, showing a great amount.)

2. The apparent strength of the cancer cells and the number of mitoses bear no constant relationship to any other feature, nor to each other.

3. Mitotic figures may be entirely lacking, and they are usually not so numerous as might be expected.

4. The number of plasma cells in prickle cell epitheliomas varies directly with the number of pearls, as a rule.

5. Plasma cells are never found in the absence of hyaline degeneration.

6. As the number of plasma cells is an indication of the degree of resistance (immunity) of the tissue (derma), the malignancy of the neoplasm varies inversely in proportion to the number of plasma cells. The more malignant the process, the less the number of plasma cells, showing that the neoplasm is developing so rapidly that the tissue has not the time to develop any resistance. (This is a note of prognostic value.) (Figure 4 represents a typical basal cell epithelioma, and Figure 11 a typical prickle cell epithelioma.)

EXPECTANCY IN ROENTGEN-RAY TREATMENT OF SKIN LESIONS FROM THE PATHOLOGIC STANDPOINT *

WALTER J. HIGHMAN, M.D., AND RAY H. RULISON, M.D.

NEW YORK

Skin lesions of the most diversified types, unrelated in causation and structure, respond to treatment with the roentgen rays. Conversely, lesions apparently related will often show varied responses to this peculiar agent. Nothing could be more completely unrelated than a basal cell epithelioma and a psoriasis lesion, and yet they resolve under irradiation. Psoriasis and parapsoriasis are apparently cousins under the microscope, but parapsoriasis is uninfluenced by the roentgen rays. Acne, with no apparent anatomic similarity to any of the foregoing conditions, affords one of the most brilliant examples of responsiveness to roentgenotherapy. What is there to reconcile the implied divergencies?

Reflection will reveal that there are a sufficient number of common denominators to relate these phenonema in nearly all instances. Certain effects of the roentgen rays are understood. It is known that in varying doses they either stimulate, inhibit or destroy the reproductive property of cells. This is particularly true of embryologic cells, reproductive cells, secretory cells and certain groups of abnormal cells, whether inflammatory or neoplastic. It is also known, as would follow from their effect on secretory cells, that the roentgen rays diminish or entirely destroy gland function.

In overdosage, the roentgen rays attack particularly elastic tissue, glands and the normal proliferative power of the skin. Through their effect on the elastic tissue, there are two distinct results; the arterioles lose their elasticity and the corium tends to atrophy. In a word, one of the striking morbid effects of the roentgen rays on the skin, is to produce artificially, from beginning to end, a series of events absolutely paralleling the picture of scleroderma. Should the destruction be slight, no permanent damage is done; should it be severe, even necrosis may take place. At the same time that these changes develop, the sweat glands, oil glands and hair papillae shrink or entirely disappear, the skin thus becoming dry and brittle. Pigmentation of the skin and keratoses, either due to the roentgen rays or byproducts of their effect, supervene, the keratoses at times terminating malignantly. We thus have artificially produced by the roentgen rays a second great skin picture closely paralleling that of xeroderma pigmentosum.

---

* Read before the Section on Dermatology and Syphilology, New York Academy of Medicine, Nov. 17, 1921.

For the practical student in this field, then, it is important to remember that overdosage with roentgen rays, according to its degree, will produce a simple picture of transitory erythema, mild atrophy, restricted or extensive necrosis, or one reminiscent of scleroderma, or, finally, of xeroderma.

DOSAGE

To prevent any of the foregoing disasters, sincere efforts have been made to determine the minimum quantity of radiation that will produce the maximum therapeutic effect. In the entire history of this subject, no one has done more to place roentgen-ray treatment of the skin on a firm, safe and intelligent foundation than MacKee. After Kienboeck had reestimated dosage by means of placing the Sabouraud pastil on the skin, instead of half way between the skin and the target, it was MacKee, working with modern apparatus, who elaborated a completely successful technic. At first, he did so by means of the Holzknecht radiometer, but later he was able to abandon this because it had been established that under known constant factors, namely, voltage, milliamperage, distance and time, definite quantities of roentgen rays could be applied.

It had been determined that from four to five of Holzknecht's units (4-5H) corresponded to the scalp depilating dose called Tint B on the Sabouraud scale. Since the intensity of the rays varies inversely as the square of the distance, it took four times as long to discolor the pastil placed on the skin, as by the half distance method. This was arbitrarily called the Holzknecht unit, skin distance (H.s.d.). As a result, the symbol 1 H in this country means four or five times the dose it represents abroad, and great confusion has been created. For all practical purposes, 1 H s.d. equals the erythema dose except on the scalp, where one and a quarter H s.d. are required to produce erythema. It would simplify matters to substitute the letter E. for H s.d., the E being an abbreviation for erythema. Since E might be an abbreviation for epilation as well, and since MacKee has been the greatest student of the subject under discussion, it seems that the symbol M should be adopted to represent the erythema dose, under the conditions included in the symbol 1 H s.d.

Thus one-quarter M would equal a fractional dose, 1 M a massive dose, etc., according to MacKee's terminology. It is a pity that MacKee used so many fanciful expressions in describing his dosage, instead of simply adhering to the numerical units of measure. The words hyperintensive, superintensive, intensive, fractional and the like, convey nothing uniform to different minds; whereas, the figures and symbols, which he uses synonymously, do. For this reason, it is to be hoped that in the future, whether the symbol of the erythema dose remains 1 H s.d., 1 M, or 1 E, the gradations will be expressed numerically and not verbally.

From this article, the method of determining dosage, a discussion of the different types of apparatus, the various radiometers, and all kindred topics will be omitted, partly because of lack of space and partly because the subjects are all well known, and are so thoroughly discussed in MacKee's work that a recapitulation would be presumptuous.

THERAPEUTIC AIMS AND SCOPE

The object of this article is to outline what the roentgen rays may be expected to accomplish with different skin lesions, regarded from the standpoint of morbid anatomy and normal or abnormal cutaneous function. In addition, their therapeutic value from the purely mechanical standpoint will be discussed.

In general, a lesion may be considered the result of the response of tissue to a pathogenic agent to which it is peculiarly susceptible. Cures, except in the domain of surgery, are produced either by eliminating or by destroying the pathogenic agent, or by so altering tissue as to render it unable to respond to the pathogenic factor or factors. In the treatment of epithelioma, probably the former mechanism is illustrated, because of the destruction of the malignant cells themselves, or of the destruction, primarily, of the conditions which favor their growth. In acne, on the other hand, the second state of affairs is illustrated: for acne is a disease of puberty. By irradiation, the skin is so altered that it can no longer respond in that abnormal manner, clinically designated as acne; whereas, the underlying forces, assembled in the mechanism designated as puberty, persist until adult life. Crude as this illustration is, it nicely elucidates the points. The mechanical use of the roentgen rays is illustrated in the cure of ringworm of the scalp by epilation. Here, the falling of the hair, with the resultant mechanical removal of the fungi, produces the cure, not the effect of the roentgen rays on the fungi themselves.

It will not be possible in all types of lesions so precisely to indicate the effect of the roentgen rays as in the foregoing examples. The groups of conditions in which the roentgen rays are efficacious are simple inflammations, infections, noninfectious granulomas, dystrophies, benign new growths, malignant new growths and certain nevi. In short, some lesions in the entire range of dermatoses are amenable to the roentgen rays. The factors are unknown which determine the susceptibility of one lesion and the insusceptibility of its nearest relative to this mode of treatment, even though anatomically there may be only the slightest difference between the two. For example, some forms of tuberculosis respond readily. Syphilis does not. Here the causative parasites are as wide asunder as the animal and vegetable kingdoms. But lepra does not either so far as we know, and the lepra bacillus and tubercle bacillus are remarkable for their similarity in appearance and staining properties. But further, not all forms of cutaneous tuberculosis respond equally readily. What determines these variations would be pure speculation if the answer were sought today.

As briefly as possibile, then, will be discussed the lesions that respond or do not respond to roentgen-ray treatment; the probable explanation of the phenomena, based on histology, and finally, in some instances, the best dosage for the given lesion. It is understood that the hypotheses advanced are merely tentative and that we are postulating no dogma, but will gladly welcome any evidence the future may unveil, either for or against our beliefs. The dosage will be given in terms of the letter M, following which will appear the symbol (H s.d.). It is hoped that this new symbol will find favor among Americans, partly in recognition of MacKee's work, and partly because it will remove confusion. It is further hoped that the views advanced will furnish a modest basis for an intelligent conception of roentgenotherapy of the skin.

GENERAL CONSIDERATIONS

It is not so important as one would imagine from the literature whether filtered or unfiltered rays are used, or whether several short or fewer long exposures are made. There are, of course, many specific instances in which this statement does not apply. But for the purposes of this article, the discussion involved would have to be too long. Thus, in subsequent paragraphs certain beliefs will be more or less arbitrarily stated. In general, however, not a single enthusiasm expressed by MacKee in his recent work, not a single one of his qualifications fails of corroboration in our experience. This indicates our views on the problems inherent in the foregoing.

We wish to disclaim the impression that we regard roentgenotherapy as the only way of treating disturbances of the skin. Today, however, it is undoubtedly the most important single method of managing such diseases. When the attempt to apply our gleanings from investigations in altered biochemistry or endocrine disbalance have failed to make a skin lesion disappear, roentgenotherapy often succeeds. It is admitted that our studies of the causation of skin diseases must continue and are of first importance; for no one claims that any other method of approach to the problem of curing disease is rational. But while our investigations proceed, and until they are fruitful, we must use the best available symptomatic methods for relieving the sick; and so far as the skin is concerned, as stated, roentgenotherapy affords the greatest possible hope.

As we particularize in the following paragraphs, in each condition discussed, when possible, its etiology will be given, its pathology, the volume of the lesion and the best method of administering irradiation, together with the prognosis under such treatment. Not every skin disease that has been successfully managed by the roentgen rays will be included. Unless there is a special reason, only the commoner ones will be mentioned.

SIMPLE INFLAMMATIONS

For want of a better term, under simple inflammations we classify those cutaneous catarrhal reactions of which the causation is unknown. The range of this group is from simple determatitis to lichen planus, and the primary and secondary lichenifications. The main groups to be discussed are simple dermatitis, implying eczema, the psoriasiform dermatoses and the lichens.

Dermatitis has so many causes that it is not astonishing that the condition, however constant in aspect, shows no uniform response to roentgenotherapy, any more than to any other form of treatment. In general, the disease is due to an interoperation between external and internal factors; but in spite of this the attempt to alter the reacting properties of the skin by means of the roentgen rays is not invariably successful. Pathologically, the condition is an exudative catarrh, acute, subacute or chronic. When the cause is known, as in dermatitis venenata, there is no object in using the roentgen rays, for the cure is obvious. In obscure cases, whether in the vesicular or in the scaling phase, the roentgen rays are valuable in doses of from one-eighth to one-quarter M (H s.d.), repeated at weekly intervals for from four to even ten exposures, with the normal surrounding skin screened. In extensive eruptions, different parts of the body should be irradiated on as many days as feasible without producing leukopenia; but the same area should not be exposed more than once a week. The lesions in question are superficial and in general show relatively slight alterations in the epidermis, edema, and not profound infiltration in the upper half of the corium. The dose mentioned is probably only sufficient to inhibit the tendency in the epidermis to hyperplasia, and to destroy the deeper inflammatory cells.

In the squamous form, the process is partly as outlined in the foregoing, but there is more marked hyperkeratosis and parakeratosis, with distinctly more fixed connective tissue cells in the infiltration, and hence the need for at least one quarter M per week to each area. Otherwise, the remarks in the preceding paragraphs also apply here.

In forms of dermatitis due to fungi, the radiation does very little good until after the organisms have been destroyed, although a slight degree of inhibition may be ascribed to the rays. In varieties due to excessive secretion of the sweat glands, and in those whose basis is seborrhea, the rays are of value in their effect on the lesions and in their inhibitory effect on gland function. In cases of undetermined etiology, the rays sometimes work and sometimes do not; but it is difficult to forecast the result. It is equally difficult always to state what the expectancy of success is; but in the vast majority of cases the lesions disappear and remain away for a variable period, in a striking number, apparently permanently. When they have disappeared, they return only either when the effect of the rays on the skin has worn off, or when, because of the interruption of general treatment, the original conditions determining the disease have been reestablished.

Other vesicular and bullous diseases do not respond encouragingly to the rays, although there are reports of cures of simple herpes in the literature.

PSORIASIFORM DERMATOSES

The type of this group is psoriasis. The cause of the disease is unknown. It is obviously due either to a metabolic disturbance or to an external infection. The lesions vary in size and shape, and under the microscope show distinct changes in the epidermis and corium. A psoriasis lesion may be from 1 millimeter to three eighths of an inch thick, and the latter is covered by a dense scale of hyperkeratotic and parakeratotic tissue. There are numerous mitoses. The infiltration consists mainly of small round cells of the lymphatic type, with a variable number of fibroblasts. The object of roentgen-ray treatment is to inhibit epidermal hyperplasia and promote resorption of the inflammatory deposit. The rationale of this is a direct attack on the multiplying cells of the rete and small round cells in the infiltration, which, probably by analogy with lymphocytes, are vulnerable to the rays. The main technical difficulty lies in the fact that the scale acts as a screen in direct ratio to its thickness. The majority of lesions disappear under intelligent treatment. Some are inexplicably obstinate and, if unresponsive after six exposures, the attempt to remove them by means of roentgen rays should cease. The management is precisely as in the squamous form of dermatitis. Acute early attacks are unfavorable for the roentgen rays. Coincident with irradiation, general treatment should be pressed, but local irritating applications are contraindicated.

Related dermatoses vary in their response. Seborrhea does particu-. larly well. Parapsoriasis. which is not as intense a process by one-twentieth as psoriasis, does not respond at all. No one can explain the reasons. Properly employed, the roentgen rays may be used in psoriasis and seborrhea of the scalp, but for not more than from four to six weekly exposures of one quarter M (H s.d.), employed by the regional method used in scalp epilation; epilation should never be produced. Obviously psoriasis recurs, although we have one case on record in which there was no relapse after seven years.

LICHENS AND LICHENIFICATION

Lesions in this group are characterized by profound infiltrations and marked epidermal changes. In lichen planus, the epidermal changes are relatively less intense than in lichenification, although the infiltrations are equally voluminous in the two groups. In acute lichen planus and in many of the chronic subvarieties, roentgen-ray therapy appears to be almost a specific, both as to the disappearance of the lesions and as to the control of itching. The infiltrating cells resemble lymphocytes, admixed with melanoblasts. The latter persist long after the papules have clinically disappeared, and the roentgen rays have no influence on the remaining pigmentation. The treatment is carried out as in universal psoriasis, or, for restricted lesions, one quarter M (H s.d.) is given weekly, although in hypertrophic forms higher doses must be employed. In nearly all generalized cases the patients recover more rapidly under this treatment than under any other, and at least 75 per cent. of the other types of lichen planus respond. When the mouth is involved, of course, the use of roentgen rays is inconvenient.

In lichenification, whether primary or secondary, small doses of roentgen rays cure three quarters of the cases, except when an underlying dermatosis not amenable to the roentgen rays exists. Under these circumstances, the main consideration is to eliminate the underlying state.

None of the other conditions bearing the name lichen seem amenable to the rays.

PRURIGO

Prurigo is probably papular urticaria. At times, it responds well to small repeated doses of roentgen rays. The lesions consist of infiltrations of round cells, below an epidermis which is slightly vesicular. The disease is metabolic, and the skin is not capable of change under the roentgen rays sufficient to render it irresponsive to the internal disturbance. The lesions disappear rapidly enough in favorable instances, but recur. There is a transient influence but nothing definite. Obviously, the agent would not be employed in the erythema and urticaria groups related to prurigo. Not even in erythema nodosum would there be any indication for its employment.

INFECTIONS

The roentgen rays are apparently of no use in skin diseases caused by animal parasites of any variety. Neither are they of value in superficial, bacterial or fungus infections. In fact, there seems to be no disease primarily due to pus cocci in which the use of roentgen rays has been successful. In acne, in which the pustulation is incidental, the roentgen rays are effective because they stop the formation of comedones. In ordinary sycosis, as well as in that due to fungi, the value of the roentgen rays resides in the removal of the germs by producing falling of the affected hairs. On the other hand, in bacillary diseases and even in those due to fungi, the roentgen rays are of great value when the lesions are granulomas, the one notable exception being lepra. Syphilis is not included because it is due to a protozoon, and in this condition there would be no particular reason for using the roentgen rays.

Infections Due to Cocci—Nonparasitic sycosis is treated by a depilatory dose and the cure is due to falling of the affected hairs. Acne is not essentially a pus disease. It is a manifestation of puberty, and is the result of follicular hyperkeratosis and overactivity of the sebaceous glands. If the functional disturbance can be controlled and the hyperkeratosis stopped, abscess formation will automatically cease. This can be accomplished by the roentgen rays, administered according to the MacKee technic, in at least 95 per cent. of all patients. In this article, acne has again been mentioned at this point, because its striking clinical feature is the presence of pustules. In general, pyodermas are not affected by the roentgen rays.

Infections Caused by Bacilli.—Lupus vulgaris, tuberculosis verrucosa cutis and many other forms of tuberculosis of the skin will disappear under from one to three irradiations of 1 M (H s.d.) at intervals of four weeks. The result is possibly due to some effect on the micro-organisms, but probably the correct explanation is that the granuloma is absorbed through the direct influence of the rays on the inflammatory cells.

Except in erythema induratum, the tuberculids are not often influenced by the roentgen rays. This is difficult to explain, for nearly all of this group of lesions are small granulomas. Erythema induratum yields to one quarter M (H s.d.) applied weekly, or larger doses applied at longer intervals. In England, lupus erythematosus is treated by this means. We have not attempted to verify the reports by test, because lupus erythematosus microscopically shows dilatation of the vessels and destruction of the elastic tissue, and ends in atrophy. Since these effects can all be produced by the roentgen rays, their use in this disease seems unsound. Next to the Finsen lamp, the roentgen rays afford the greatest promise in skin tuberculosis.

Why they are not effective in lepra, or whether not enough studies have been made, cannot be stated; nor have we any personal experience with sarcoid. In rhinoscleroma, the roentgen rays are invaluable, but we cannot speak from personal experience.

Fungus Infections.—In sporotrichosis, blastomycosis and actinomycosis, the roentgen rays are almost a specific, unless the systemic involvement is too great; and, even in this event, the lesions themselves often may be caused to disappear. The treatment is carried out as in tuberculosis. Resorption of the lesions is evidently due to the direct effect of the rays on the infiltrating cells.

In ringworm of the scalp, with and without kerion, and in favus, the value of the rays lies in their depilating action, when properly administered by the Kienboeck-Adamson method, with the MacKee system of dosage. This, perhaps, constitutes the only rational treatment for these diseases. In ringworm of the nails, in which the rays are often valuable, the way in which they work is not understood.

NONINFECTIOUS GRANULOMAS

This group of conditions includes mycosis, leukemia and Hodgkin's disease. The relation of these conditions to lymphosarcoma is not clearly understood; but the fact remains that their lesions are highly responsive to roentgen rays administered in doses of from one-half to three-quarters M (H s.d.), or even slightly more, at suitable intervals. To all intents and purposes, the lesions are new growths, and are probably subject to the laws governing the effect of roentgen rays' on young growing cells. Of course, treating the skin lesions successfully does not cure the disease, but merely temporarily removes its manifestations. No other method of attack affords so much promise, so far as symptomatic therapy is concerned.

NEW GROWTHS

In new growths, the roentgen rays are inconsistent in action. They are far more effective in malignant than in benign types. In benign connective tissue neoplasms, except at times in keloids, they are useless. In benign epithelial growths, except in the ordinary wart, of which about 60 per cent. are responsive, they are likewise useless, unless plantar warts are included. In malignant neoplasms, whether sarcoma or epithelioma, the roentgen rays are of extraordinary value. The majority of such lesions will disappear after one irradiation with from one and one-half to two M (H s.d.). Often further treatment is required, but it is not within the province of this article to enter into technical details. Nowhere is the value of roentgen-ray therapy better illustrated than in this field. The relative merits of roentgen rays and radium are not part of the subject under discussion, so they will not be mentioned. Nor do we wish to champion the roentgen rays to the exclusion of other recognized methods of treatment. To consummate a victory in battle, all forces are employed; and, in the war on malignant new growths, the roentgen rays constitute a valuable force. The attack is a direct one on the malignant cells, which, being young and rapidly reproductive, are far more vulnerable than the maturer, less rapidly growing cells of benign neoplasms.

Nevi, which might well be included under neoplasms, since they are growths due to intra-uterine anomalies, whether evidenced at birth or in later life, are so rarely amenable to roentgen-ray treatment as to require no discussion in this brief article. On the whole, they are highly organized and rather mature lesions. Some of them are capable of giving rise to malignancy, and if this occurs, the resultant growth can often be successfully treated by the roentgen rays.

The so-called precancerous dermatosis, xeroderma pigmentosum, Paget's disease, leukoplakia and roentgen-ray keratoses themselves, will not be discussed.

DYSTROPHIES

Dystrophies may be atrophies or hypertrophies. Obviously, atrophies afford none of the conditions under which the roentgen rays could be efficacious. Hypertrophies, except those mechanically produced by irritation, also are no particularly fruitful field for roentgen-ray therapy. Icthyosis, keratosis of the hair follicles, possibly Darier's disease and acanthosis nigricans, do not seem to respond often to the roentgen rays. Occasional favorable reports creep into the literature, but in our experience only follicular keratoses seem at all amenable. Some inflammatory hypertrophies, not properly belonging to this group, and perhaps better regarded as hyperplasias, respond with a certain degree of uniformity to the roentgen rays. These are clavus and callus, including the plantar wart. In a preponderance of cases, from two to five irradiations of 1 M (H s.d), at intervals of four weeks, will cause the lesions to disappear, if the underlying mechanical irritation is likewise removed.

FUNCTIONAL DISEASES: PRURITUS

Excessive function of skin glands is controllable by the roentgen rays under conditions mentioned in connection with acne. Hirsutes does not properly belong here, and the attempt to produce permanent alopecia by means of the roentgen rays is mentioned only to be condemned.

Pruritus, particularly of the vulva and anus, is amenable to small doses of the roentgen rays at frequent intervals, or larger doses at less frequent intervals, the maximum at each exposure, however, being one-half M (H s.d.). Three quarters of these cases can thus be cured, or at least relieved.

CONCLUSIONS

1. The therapeutic use of the roentgen rays covers a wide territory. All other methods of internal and external management should be pursued at the same time. What stands out most clearly is that voluminous infiltrations, whether neoplastic or inflammatory, and whether accompanied by epidermal changes or not, are most amenable. In addition to this, diseases depending on functional or productive overactivity, such as acne, are equally amenable. Further, the roentgen rays are of equal use in producing the mechanical removal of infected hair.

2. Neoplasms, including the noninfectious granulomas, are favorably affected through the influence of the rays on young, rapidly multiplying cells.

3. Acne is cured by an alteration of the skin through the inhibition of gland function, and of the reproductive ability of the follicular epidermis.

4. The infectious granulomas are cured partly through the mechanism outlined in connection with neoplasms, and possibly because the causative organisms themselves are slightly affected.

5. The simple inflammatory lesions are curable only when there is hyperplasia of the epidermis and a marked infiltration. The former is influenced by the inhibiting effect of the rays on the reproducing cells, and the latter by the destructive effect on the infiltrating cells, which are mainly of the lymphatic type, as well as on the reproducing fibroblasts.

6. Why the rays favorably influence pruritus is not known.

7. By understanding the type and volume of lesions and by realizing that conditions in themselves atrophic are unfavorable for roentgen-ray treatment, it can be determined, from an understanding of the simple histopathology of skin lesions, what the dose and what the intervals should be.

8. Without this knowledge, the use of roentgen rays is a purely arbitrary and mechanical procedure.

780 Madison Avenue.

CARCINOMA OF THE TONGUE AND ITS TREATMENT WITH RADIUM *

LAURENCE TAUSSIG. M.D.

SAN FRANCISCO

Cancer of the tongue is most often seen between the fourth and sixth decades and is much more common in men than in women. It occurs most frequently on the side of the tongue, but may occur any place. Pathologically, it is practically always of the squamous cell type of carcinoma. Among the etiologic factors, syphilis, and trauma produced by rough teeth and by the use of tobacco are of prime importance.

The variation in the reports of the frequency of syphilis in carcinoma of the tongue, (3.38 per cent., according to Meller, to 84.23 per cent., according to Fournier), is probably in proportion to the incidence of syphilis in the clinics from which the statistics are taken. It is certainly true that a syphilitic lesion may be a precancerous lesion. A gumma, leukoplakia, or chronic syphilitic glossitis may be the starting point of cancer, though the determining factor may be obscure. This determining factor is undoubtedly often a matter of time or of trauma, or of both. An untreated syphilitic lesion of the tongue should always be watched with suspicion, especially when subjected to the trauma of the excessive use of tobacco or of a rough tooth. In the nonsyphilitic patient, cancer may apparently be caused by the use of tobacco in any form. Also, in the nonsyphilitic, carcinoma may develop in a chronic ulcer caused by an untreated rough tooth. Nevertheless, cancer of the tongue does appear with startling frequency in nonsyphilitic nonsmokers, without the presence of a rough tooth. In addition to these factors, there is probably an inherent tendency toward cancer formation which is, after all, the chief factor. The recognition and proper treatment of syphilis of the mouth, and proper dentistry, will undoubtedly lessen the frequency of cancer of the tongue.

Leukoplakia should be treated by stopping smoking, by specific treatment if indicated, and by the use of a mouth wash, such as sodium thiosulphate (hyposulphite). If these measures fail, radium should be applied. It is usually curative and is far more satisfactory than surgery or cauterization. The treatment of a chronic ulcer, due to a smoker's burn or the irritation of a ragged tooth, is the removal of the apparent

---

* Read before the Section on Dermatology and Syphilology at the Seventy-Third Annual Session of the American Medical Association, St. Louis, May, 1922.

cause, and, if this is not sufficient, surgery, cauterization with the actual cautery, electrocoagulation or the galvanic cautery, or radiation, should be invoked.

The diagnosis of carcinoma of the tongue is frequently difficult. It is often impossible to differentiate positively syphilis, tuberculous ulcer and carcinoma, clinically. As a rule, the syphilitic lesion is not so hard as carcinoma, develops more rapidly, and occurs most frequently on the dorsum of the tongue, while carcinoma is most common on the sides. These criteria are, however, not final. The blood Wasserman test should be made in every case and, though it is negative, a therapeutic test consisting of two or more arsphenamin injections should be given, if there is still some doubt. The Wassermann reaction here, as elsewhere, should be regarded as only one piece of evidence. Even the therapeutic test may be misinterpreted at first, because we often see syphilis and carcinoma in the same lesion, with the result that the lesion clears rapidly for a time under antisyphilitic medication, giving us a false sense of security. Tuberculous ulcers simulating broken down gummas, though rare, may be found on any portion of the tongue and are usually seen in persons with chronic tuberculosis. Although these tuberculous lesions are usually irregular, undermined and soft, it is occasionally impossible to make a positive clinical diagnosis, and a biopsy, as well as therapeutic tests, should be resorted to. There is still much controversy as to the danger of doing a biopsy, but probably little damage is done if the specimen is obtained from near the center of the lesion, with a minimum of trauma. The advantages of having made an absolutely positive diagnosis before instituting treatment of any kind are obvious.

The surgical treatment of carcinoma of the tongue has been the accepted form of therapy. As in surgical treatment of cancer elsewhere, it is necessary to remove the lesion with a very wide margin. Even in the earliest cases, the most conservative operation finding favor with the surgeons is hemisection. In the more extensive cases, complete amputation of the tongue is done, often with the removal of the floor of the mouth. These operations are not only terribly mutilating, but also carry with them a high mortality, even in the most skilled hands, and are productive of but few cures.

During the past few years, a number of physicians have treated cancer of the tongue by electric coagulation, usually in conjunction with radiotherapy. In capable hands, the results are frequently satisfactory.

The treatment of carcinoma of the tongue with radium has many advantages. In the first place, there is no primary mortality. In contrast to this, we see a primary mortality in the surgical treatment varying from 10 per cent. to 30 per cent., depending on the extent of the lesion. Secondary death, due to hemorrhage or infection, is far less common after radium than after surgery.   A palliative result can be obtained in a majority of the cases with radium treatment; while, even if the patient survives the operative procedure, he is left with greatly impeded speech and is able to eat only with great difficulty and there is frequently increased rapidity of growth.   It is not possible at this time to estimate the percentage of cures by radium, because the method has not been in use long enough and because the majority of the cases which we are now seeing are the ones that the surgeons consider hopeless.   The percentage of cures for surgery is less than 20 per cent., even in picked cases.   The great disadvantage of radium in these cases is the painful reaction.   It is impossible to estimate the severity of this in advance. In some of our cases, the period of reaction was not long and the healing of the ulcer and softening of the lesion were prompt.   In others, the amount of suffering was out of all proportion to the extent of the lesion and the clinical appearance of the reaction.   We have not as yet been able to devise a satisfactory way of combating the reaction.

The ideal method of treating these cases is by the insertion of the tiny unscreened tubes of radium emanation.   This method has been described and was first used by Janeway and Quick of the Memorial Hospital of New York City.   At present, we feel that it is best to give the entire dose at one sitting and attempt to seed the entire indurated area with the tiny emanation tubes, each containing about 1 millicurie, inserting from five to ten or more tubes depending on the size of the lesion.   This gives an even, intense radiation throughout the tumor mass.   In inserting the tubes, we attempt to keep them within the carcinomatous tissue and do not intentionally place any of them in the surrounding normal tissues.   In addition, we sometimes crossfire from the surface by using a radium plaque or an applicator of a number of tubes.

The reaction occurs a little earlier following the use of buried bare tubes of emanation than following the surface application of radium.   It starts as a rule in about seven days, is usually at its height in from two to three weeks, and then gradually diminishes.   This reaction consists of an increase in the swelling, with burning pain, and often an increase in the size of the lesion due to ulceration following the separation of the slough.   A reaction on portions of the mouth adjacent to the area treated is a constant and often painful and unpleasant feature.   In favorable cases, after the height of the reaction has been reached, the lesion softens rapidly and then heals slowly.   Most of the patients complain of pain radiating to the ear.   This is sometimes of long duration, frequently outlasting the period of visible reaction.   Probably the next best method to that of burying bare tubes of emanation is the insertion of steel needles, containing radium element, into the tumor mass.   The number of these and the time of exposure depend on the strength of the needles and the size of the lesion. This method probably causes more tissue destruction than does the bare tube method and does not give as intensive a local radiation. The use of surface applications of tubes or plaques alone is certainly the least satisfactory form of therapy and can be expected to give no more than palliative results, except in the most superficial cases.

At the same time that the tongue lesion is treated, the cervical glands should receive a massive dose of roentgen ray, covering three areas, the front and the two sides. If there are palpable glands that are clinically malignant, these should be removed about two weeks after radiation, if they are operable. If they do not appear to be operable, bare tubes may be buried in them at the time of a partial operation, or inserted through the skin under a local anesthetic. If no glands are palpable, the patient should receive two or three courses of roentgen-ray therapy and be kept under close observation for as long as possible. Should glands develop under treatment, they should be operated on at once, and the roentgen-ray treatment continued after operation. During operation, bare tubes can be buried in any suspicious place. The technic of the roentgen-ray treatment is constantly being changed. During the last year, we have increased the distance and the screening considerably, and we are apparently getting better results. We have practically entirely given up the use of the radium pack to the neck in these cases as uneconomical and no more effective than the roentgen ray. It is probable that the newer deep therapy machines will still further improve our results.

During the last two and a half years, we have treated fourteen patients with carcinoma of the tongue, including two that were first treated just prior to the installation of the emanation plant at the University of California Hospital. Two of the patients were women. The ages varied from 36 to 93 years. Four had syphilis in addition to carcinoma. Four are clinically free of the disease, two at two years after treatment, one at one and a half years and one at six months. Five showed cervical metastases at the time treatment was instituted and five of the others developed an involvement of the glands during treatment. None of these patients survived. Ten are dead, or when last seen were in such condition that the end was only a matter of time. Several other patients received their first treatment but did not again report for observation or further treatment, and were not traced. It is possible that all our patients clinically cured will not remain well, but we have the satisfaction of having prolonged life without mutilation. It is reasonable to expect that with improved technic it will be possible to cure 25 per cent. of unselected cases of carcinoma of the tongue by radiation.

CANCER OF THE LIP TREATED BY ELECTRO-COAGULATION AND RADIATION *

GEORGE E. PFAHLER, M.D.
PHILADELPHIA

In the latest stages of cancer of the lip, neither radiation, electro-coagulation, nor any other form of treatment can be expected to cure the patient. Therefore, to cure cancer of the lip, as in any other form of cancer, it should be treated early and thoroughly. Thorough treatment of cancer of the lip means radiation, no matter what other form of treatment may be used in combination. I believe that a patient suffering with cancer of the lip does not get all possible chances of recovery unless radiation is given. Whether radiation should be used alone or combined with other treatment is a matter of careful judgment in the individual case. As a prophylactic measure, every point of irritation affecting the lip should be removed, such as irritation from a pipe, cigaret paper, excessive cigar smoking, traumatism, irritation from a jagged tooth, or excessive exposure to heat, cold and wind. Any fissure or crust formation on the lip that lasts for four weeks without complete healing should be looked on with suspicion. Practically every one of these lesions, especially if there is associated any induration at the base, is potentially malignant, if not actually so, unless due to syphilis. If patients are thoroughly treated in these early stages, practically all should get well.

RESULTS OF TREATMENT

I will review only the cases treated in my private clinic, because of the difficulties in tracing the patients in the hospital clinics. Many patients have been treated in the roentgen-ray departments of the hospitals. Most of these were postoperative or recurrent cases, and, in many instances, the patients did not consider themselves our patients, or looked on the postoperative treatment as an unnecessary annoyance, and often prematurely discontinued treatment. The recurrent cases were generally far advanced, and were referred to the department because there was nothing else to do. They were usually hopeless cases.

The early cases will, of course, give the best results, and, if treated thoroughly, all patients should get well. My records do not show that all do get well, but in the cases in which we failed the patients were difficult to manage. One had an associated syphilitic infection. He developed an extension in the cheek and jaw after seven years, and

* Read before the Section on Dermatology and Syphilology at the Seventy-Third Annual Session of the American Medical Association, St. Louis, May, 1922.

died during this stage, from pneumonia. It was always doubtful whether this induration about the angle of the jaw, but above the lower edge of the bone, was syphilitic or malignant, and he would not permit a section to be removed for microscopic examination. In another case in which we failed, the patient did not return after the first treatment. The third failure, I believe was due to insufficient treatment at the very beginning. While there was no local recurrence, an indurated ridge developed at the inner border of the original lesion and extended downward and outward toward the right submaxillary gland. The side of the cheek from the angle of the mouth to the submaxillary gland became indurated and undoubtedly malignant. The patient became discouraged; but at the time of the last visit the submaxillary gland was not palpable. It seems that the treatment given to the submaxillary region was efficacious.

In another case, eighteen months after the primary lesion had disappeared a metastatic lymph node developed in the submaxillary region. In looking about for the cause of this surprising fact, we found that. through some mistake in the office, he had not received treatment over these areas. While it is unfortunate for the man, it illustrates beautifully the importance of thorough treatment of the lymphatic areas by radiation, either with the roentgen rays or radium, at the time of beginning treatment of the primary lesion, and subsequently sufficient to insure thorough destruction of the cancer cells. This recurrent lymphnode has since been treated, apparently with success, by the insertion of radium needles.

In my private clinic, we have treated 105 cases of cancer of the lip: primary eighty, recurrent twenty, postoperative five. In eighty primary cases from my private records, seventy-four patients recovered. and have remained well from several months to eighteen years. Two died of a continuation of the disease, two have had a recurrence and in two the result is unknown.

I realize that such a record is not beyond criticism. because the duration of the results is variable, and other failures may have to be recorded. However, since the results obtained by my colleagues. Henry K. Pancoast and William L. Clark, correspond so closely to my own. and were obtained by similar technic, and since the results in the older cases are most satisfactory, I am led to believe that our enthusiasm is justified and that this method of treatment can be recommended.

The recurrent conditions are always more difficult to cure. In the twenty recurrent cases treated, only eight patients recovered. Much will depend on the promptness and thoroughness with which these patients are treated; but, in part at least, the results will depend on the nature of the cancer or the degree of malignancy. One must obtain prompt results from radiation or failure is likely to result. Thorough radiation by the roentgen rays, and by radium when it can be combined to advantage, from the very beginning is most important. I never like to have a patient referred to me after some one has used insufficient radiation over a considerable period of time, and then, having recognized failure, has concluded that perhaps more thorough radiation may produce good results. In such cases, unless the lesion is so situated that it can be destroyed by electrocoagulation, failure will be the rule.

The five patients given postoperative treatment have remained well, though in none was there a block dissection.

TECHNIC

In the treatment of malignant disease, probably more than in any other field, skill and keen judgment are required. One must understand the nature of the disease and its lines of distribution. One must then use enough radiation to destroy the cancer cells and at the same time do as little damage to healthy tissues as is possible. Boggs [1] says. "Too many failures have been accredited to radium, when, as a matter of fact, through inexperience and lack of proper study, only partial doses were given."

Electrocoagulation.—Electrocoagulation consists in the coagulation of the diseased areas by means of the heat produced by the high frequency current as it passes through the body from a point attached either to the Oudin current or to one pole of the d'Arsonval current. The Oudin current (unipolar) is used for small lesions, and the d'Arsonval current is used for the larger lesions. If the d'Arsonval current is used, one pole is attached to a pad or smooth metal electrode placed under the buttocks of the patient, while the active electrode is a point. This current is not selective in its action, but will destroy the tissues radiating outward from the point. One cannot use this current, therefore, in locations in which essential structures, such as important blood vessels or nerves, are located in the line of destruction. There will be a zone beyond the actual coagulation which will be superheated and will be sufficient to destroy cancer cells, but will not destroy the healthy tissue. In this way, one conserves tissue; and, as is shown by my own cases and by those shown by Clark,[2] the defect after the patient is well does not nearly equal the amount of diseased tissue removed. There is, apparently, a regeneration of a part of the tissue removed. The heat is generated in the tissues. It is the penetrative value of this form of heat that makes it more desirable than that obtained

---

1. Boggs, R. H.: Radium Treatment of Mouth and Throat. Pennsylvania M. J. **25**:22 (Oct.) 1921.

2. Clark, W. L.: Cancer of the Oral Cavity, Jaws and Throat. J. A. M. A. **26**:1365-1369 (Oct. 26) 1918.

by the thermocautery, which destroys only by transmitted heat and, therefore, is essentially more superficial. The destructive value of the current used can be learned only by experience, but experience can be obtained by practice with a piece of liver, or other meat. Such experience from practice with a piece of liver cannot be directly transferred, for the current value will vary with the shape of the lesion to be destroyed, whether small and prominent, such as a wart or mole, or flat and indefinitely outlined, as in carcinoma. The current value will also vary with the size of the mass or body to which the tissue to be destroyed is attached. The milliamperemeter is not of great value in judging the effects.

The tissue as it is destroyed by the high frequency current turns white, if it is coagulated; or is dried up, if small, and sparked through the air. (Desiccation.)

Selection of cases suitable for electrocoagulation is necessary. If the lesion is small, and its removal will not cause too serious a defect in the lip, I believe that such destruction will be followed by more prompt and more satisfactory results than by radiation alone. By such destruction, we macroscopically remove the diseased tissue just as the surgeon does with the knife, but we do it without opening any blood vessels or lymph channels. If the lesion is fairly large, I trim the destroyed tissue away with curved scissors, always carefully cutting within the destroyed area. In this way, one eliminates part of the disagreeable odor which accompanies the sloughing process.

If the cancer involves the entire lip, or even half of the lip, such preliminary destruction by electrocoagulation is impractical, unless one can foresee some means of closing the mouth by a subsequent plastic operation. If such a subsequent plastic operation is planned, the surgeon who is to perform the operation should see the patient and be consulted in advance, before the radiologist attempts the destruction. We have no more right to assume in advance what the surgeon's judgment and procedure will be than the surgeon has a right to assume what the judgment and procedure of the radiologist will be. Both specialties are developing too rapidly for either to take up the other as a side issue, and more will be accomplished by cooperation.

Generally speaking, I believe that, in these advanced primary cases, a thorough trial should be made first with applications of radium, and if it is skilfully applied, good results may be expected. In some cases, marked temporary improvement only may occur, and a stage is then reached in which the disease is at a standstill or may begin to progress in spite of radiation. At this stage, complete and thorough local destruction or complete surgical excision is probably the only procedure left. With the cooperation of skilful surgeons, I have had success in some such advanced cases.

RADIATION

Radiation is indicated in all cancers of the lip, no matter what other treatment is used, and sufficient radiation must be used actually to destroy the cancer cells. If a patient is to be operated on surgically, a preliminary radiation with a full erythema dose should be given over the lip and chin, and in the submental and submaxillary regions; and, after the operation, and two to three weeks after the preliminary treatment, similar radiation should be given. The patient should then be kept under observation for several years, and more radiation should be applied if there is the slightest sign of recurrence. This same sort of radiation should be added to electrocoagulation, and can be applied most practically by means of the roentgen rays. For this purpose, I use a 9-inch spark gap, with five milliamperes of current, through 6 mm. of aluminum filter, at a distance of 30 cm. for twenty-five minutes. The time must be governed by the radiation value of the individual instrument used.

If one possesses sufficient radium and sufficient skill in its use, most and perhaps all local cancers of the lip can be cured by this means. It will require more time, more skill, more patience than by the combination of electrocoagulation and radiation, but there will be more preservation of tissue and a better cosmetic result than can be obtained by any combination with surgery or electrocoagulation. Therefore, I can lay down no rule for the treatment of all cases. The circumstances surrounding the individual case should govern our procedure.

If radium is to be used for the local destruction of the cancer with preservation of the tissue, the local tissues must be kept saturated to the limit of toleration of the normal structures until the cancer entirely disappears.

If one has sufficient radium, the submaxillary regions can be treated by surface applications, properly screened.

If metastatic nodules are palpable, they should have preliminary radiation as described, and should then be dissected out surgically, or treated by the insertion of radium needles sufficient to destroy the disease.

Radium needles of 10 mg. each may be inserted, 1 cm. apart, throughout the diseased area, and left in place for eight hours. Following the insertion of radium needles into tissues, there is the production of fibrous nodules, especially when the needles are placed farther apart, and left in place sixteen hours. These nodules are composed of fibrous tissue and result from the necroses produced by the radium. They will lead the untrained to suspect malignant nodules or redevelopment of the disease. With our meager knowledge on this point, it will require considerable skill to be able to distinguish between the disease and the fibrous tissue. Therefore, I urge close observation, lest a false security lead to neglect of true malignant disease.

CONCLUSIONS

1. Any fissure or crust on the lip which lasts over a month should lead to suspicion of malignancy.

2. Local destruction by electrocoagulation, followed by thorough radiation, should effect a cure in practically all cases if patients are treated early.

3. Thorough radiation by radium or the roentgen rays should be given over the lymphatics draining the diseased area.

4. Recurrent carcinoma gives much less satisfactory results.

5. Metastatic lymph nodes should be treated by surface radiation and then by radium implantation or by excision.

TREATMENT OF CANCER OF THE LIP BY RADIATION *

EVERETT S. LAIN, M.D.

Professor of Dermatology and Radiotherapy, Oklahoma
University School of Medicine

OKLAHOMA CITY

At the meeting of this Association in New Orleans, 1920, I presented a paper before this Section,[1] "A Clinical Study of Epithelioma of the Lower Lip," in which I considered more especially the pathologic anatomy and clinical classification of epithelioma of the lower lip, as observed and recorded in the private practice of my associate, Dr. M. M. Roland, and myself. In this paper, I mentioned only briefly the technic of treatment and results. Today, I am presenting to you briefly our technic of treatment by roentgen ray and radium of 248 consecutive cases of cancer of the lip which have occurred in our private practice from Jan. 1, 1909, to Dec. 31, 1921.

Tracing by letter of inquiry to family physician or patient, or by other methods, the present condition of each patient or the cause of death, and correlating the facts from such a number of patients with cancer of the lips who have been treated is no small undertaking, as those who have had experience will testify.

Also, I shall repeat these diagnoses have been made largely from a clinical rather than a biopsy examination. Judging from statistics from the Mayo Clinic, as given by Broders,[2] and from the laboratories of Bloodgood, as quoted by Hazen,[3] not less than 96 per cent. of our cases were of the prickle or of the squamous cell variety.

This total does not include a smaller number of cases in which the patients have been treated by interns or nurses in the Oklahoma State University, and in other hospitals of our city in which our services were only of a supervisory nature. This review of patients treated includes a goodly number who were treated several years prior to that enduring work toward arithmetical computation of roentgen-ray

* Read before the Section on Dermatology and Syphilology at the Seventy-Third Annual Session of the American Medical Association, St. Louis, May, 1922.

1. Lain, E. S.: A Clinical Study of Epithelioma of the Lower Lip, J. A. M. A. **75**:1052-1055 (Oct. 16) 1920.

2. Broders, A. C.: Basal Cell Epithelioma, 1912 Mayo Clinic Reprint, read before Southern Minnesota Medical Association, Mankato, Jan. 20, 1919.

3. Hazen, H. H.: Prickle Cell and Basal Cell Skin Cancers, J. A. M. A. **64**: 958 (March 20) 1915.

technic which was done by MacKee,[4] Shearer and their co-workers. Also, much of our radium treatment covers a period antedating the more accurate methods of screening or filtering in order to get the effects of the more penetrating gamma rays.

Since about 1915, we have classified our patients into three groups, according to the location of the lesion upon the lip, and the degree of development, which to us also largely indicates the prognosis. This classification was presented in full in my former paper, and I shall repeat only briefly:

Group 1: Those lesions which are situated wholly on the cutaneous border of the lip, are not deeply indurated and are without palpable or other evidence of metastasis in adjacent glands.

Group 2: Those in which the lesion most commonly also overlaps the mucosa of the lip and are deeply indurated, and in which the adjacent submental or submaxillary glands are palpable. This group also includes a few cases of recurrences from former attempts at a cure by caustic applications or unsuccessful surgery.

Group 3: Those of obvious metastasis in more than immediately adjacent glands. Approximately, this entire group is composed of patients who have previously tried repeatedly some other methods of treatment and whose conditions are now hopeless so far as a final cure is concerned.

Medical literature on radiotherapy of cancer is becoming so voluminous and laboratory examination of radiated tissue has so frequently verified the following statements that they have become axioms to the experienced radiotherapist and are no longer debatable.

1. Immature and rapidly growing cells are more sensitive to radiations than those which have acquired their adult physiologic character. This is known as the law of Bergonie and Tribondeau. This change is more noticeable after radiations from the hard beta or the gamma rays of radium than after hard roentgen rays.

2. The most susceptible period in the life of this cell is the time of its division, when its nuclear life appears more amenable and accessible to this energy.

3. All types or characters of cells are not equally affected by the same degree or length of radiation, squamous or prickle cells and certain types of connective tissue cells requiring the greatest, basal lymphoidal and endothelic the least.

4. The lethal dose for a certain type of cell, such as the basal, may be only sufficient to stimulate to a more rapid growth a squamous or a connective tissue cell.

---

4. MacKee, G. M.: X-Ray and Radium in the Treatment of Diseases of the Skin, Philadelphia, Lea & Febiger, 1921, p. 134.

5. The shorter the waves of energy given off from radium or a roentgen-ray tube, the more penetrating and therefore the more effective are they in the disintegration of the cancer cell.

The more recent conjoined study of the physicist and radiotherapist has given to us a more accurate and scientific method of screening the rays so that roentgen rays and radium are now achieving cures in many cases of cancer formerly classified as inoperable or hopeless.

In the treatment of our cases, we have followed no invariable routine, except as regards certain proved or unquestioned procedures. One of the latter is the radiation of the submental and submaxillary glands by hard or gamma rays in all our cases of cancer of the lower lip.

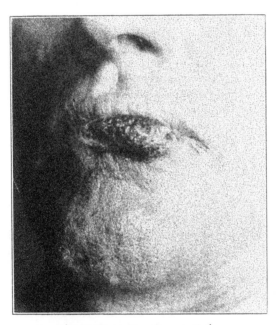

Fig. 1 (Class 1).—Cancer of lip.

The treatment of metastasizing areas has, in most cases, been given by roentgen ray, using M. A. of from 3 to 5, spark gap of from 6 to 10 inches (15 to 25 cm.), anode distance of from 8 to 18 inches (20 to 45 cm.) with filters from 1 to 4 mm. of aluminum. Later, we added from 0.25 to 0.5 mm. of copper, giving a time of twenty minutes to one hour each position. During the past two or three years, we have been giving a dosage to glands, expressed in modern terms, a K.V. 100, M.A. 5, focal distance from 16 to 18 inches (40 to 45 cm.), time from twenty-five to forty-five minutes, repeated as indicated in six weeks.

This variation in technic does not appear so inconsistent when I explain that our evolution in treatment has consisted of an increasing potentiality over a period of fourteen years. Considering the cycle-like development of the pathologic cells, and reviewing our total treatments as well as the opinions and statistics of others, we are fully convinced that two or three properly timed and filtered doses of radium applied within intervals of a few days are more destructive to any type of cancer cell than the total given at a single exposure. The so-called fractional dosage, with either roentgen ray or radium, is much to be feared, although it is more successful if a nearly lethal instead of a stimulating dose for the pathologic cell has each time been given.

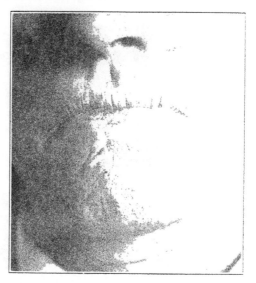

Fig. 2 (Class 1).—Patient shown in Figure 1, three years later.

Perhaps all radium specialists may not agree with our conclusions: still we have by experience been fully convinced that the destruction of a certain class of early and externally located basal cell cancers on the lips or elsewhere on the body may be more rapidly accomplished, and without an objectionable scar, by the use of the combined hard beta and gamma rays than by the gamma rays alone.

In a certain type of case under Group 1, in which there is a proliferating keratotic elevation with only a mild degree of infiltration, it has been our custom, first, to apply a 10 or 20 mg. plaque, screened with 0.10 mm. of aluminum for a period of two or three hours. This will cause, after ten or fifteen days, a reaction, which is followed, after twenty or thirty days, by degeneration and perhaps an exfoliation of

Before this reaction has begun or immediately after the first application, we apply a plaque of from 10 to 20 mg., with screening of 0.3 mm. of brass, for eight to twelve hours. This filter permits only about 5 per cent. of the hardest beta rays and yet utilizes all the gamma rays for deeper effects. Thus we produce, in from four to six weeks, a perceptible softening and perhaps a complete disintegration of deeper cellular structures of cancerous nature.

In the treatment of Class 2, lesions of deeper and more extensive development, or of the squamous or the prickle cell variety, we first apply a 10 or 20 mg. plaque of radium over the lesion, screened with 0.3 mm. of brass for from ten to fourteen hours, reinforced within a few days by a pack of from 100 to 160 mg. of radium screened with

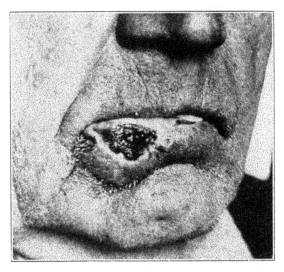

Fig. 3 (Class 2).—Cancer of lip, deeply infiltrated, involving submental glands.

2 mm. of brass and placed on a pad of gauze of from 1 to 3 cm. in thickness. This pack is located over regions of possible metastasis for a total of from fifteen to twenty hours and this application may be repeated within a few days until a total of from 2,000 to 3,000 mg. hours have been given.

In a certain class of indurated or deeply nodular cancers of the lips, we follow the applications of the plaques with as many radium needles inserted from 1 to 4 cm. apart as are necessary thoroughly to radiate the entire area of the cancerous growth. These are left for from three to five hours. Inserting the needles causes no severe pain if the entire growth is first injected with a 1 per cent. solution of procain.

We are indebted to Drs. Boggs, Clark, Pfahler and others for calling our attention to this valuable advancement in the application of radium to this class of cancers.

In tabulating our total number of cases of cancer of the lips, I wish to call attention to the following interesting findings:

Twenty-seven patients were examined and, after having the method of treatment explained and prognosis given, refused treatment.

In eight cases, or about 3.2 per cent., the lesions were located on the upper lip. Two of these patients were females.

In nine of the total number of cases of cancer of the lip the patients were females, and five of these were users of tobacco. Of Class 3, only three are now living and each still shows evidence of progressive cancer.

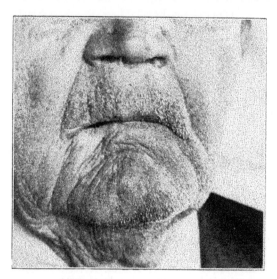

Fig. 4 (Class 2).—Patient shown in Figure 3; no evidence of recurrence three years later.

Each of the eight cases of Class 3 and ten cases under Class 2 were recurrences following caustics or surgery. Of eight deaths under Class 2, five followed the employment of caustics and three were postoperative cases.

If we eliminate from Class 1 one patient who died from a cancer on the hand, one who died from a sarcoma at the point of the shoulder and one who died from generalized lymphosarcoma, conditions which could scarcely be classed as metastases from the lips, our percentage of cures in Class 1 is 98 plus.

Under Class 2, we note that, since the beginning of the more recent and much improved methods of radiation with a heavy kilovoltage and radium packs, or, better still, when radium needles are inserted into the glandular metastasis, our percentage of cures promises to fall not far short of that of Class 1.

CONCLUSIONS

The cellular morphology of a cancer of the lip has less importance in the prognosis than the location or degree of development, or the age of the patient. We have repeatedly observed that, on account of a beginning atrophy of the lymph system, after a certain age the prognosis is better. Especially is this true in cancer of the lower lip.

TWO HUNDRED AND FORTY-EIGHT CONSECUTIVE CASES OF CANCER OF THE LIPS

Treatment and Results	Number	Percentage
Refused treatment	27	
Total taking one treatment only for palliative purposes or taking up some other form of treatment	13	
Total number of cases of upper lip involvement: Class 3, two patients, both now dead; Class 2, one living; Class 1, six, all living	8	
Class 3 (all postoperative or postcaustic treatment), total number of cases—each traced	8	
Total number of patients living more than one year, one; two years, much improved, though not well	3	
Class 2: Total number of patients treated (seven cases were postoperative or postcaustic)	35	
Unable to trace	3	
Patients living and well after one year	32	
Well after three years, 18 patients treated	13	72.2
Living and well more than five years, 14 treated; two died from other causes	12	
Class 1: Total number of patients treated to January, 1922	156	
Died of accident, two: committed suicide, one, each during first year	3	
Died of cancer during first three years, one of liver, one of deep cervicals, one of generalized lymphosarcoma and one of cancer on back of hand	4	
Total living after one year	101	
Total number of patients treated more than three years	89	
Total living, no recurrence	87	97.7

We believe that a prickle or a squamous cell cancer, in the early stage of its growth, will undergo degenerative changes under radiations from either radium or roentgen ray just as the basal cell variety does. They differ only in the amount of radiation necessary and the technic of its application.

Finally, we believe that sufficient statistics verified both by clinical and by laboratory findings have now accumulated to justify the conclusion that cancer of the lip is equally and perhaps more amenable to treatment by roentgen ray or radium than by surgery, and in most cases radiotherapy is to be preferred.

ABSTRACT OF DISCUSSION

ON PAPERS OF DRS. PARKHURST, HIGHMAN, TAUSSIG, PFAHLER AND LAIN

DR. GORDON B. NEW, Rochester, Minn.: I do not believe any one is more enthusiastic about the use of radium in malignant disease of the head and neck than I am, but I believe that a great deal of harm has been done both to radium therapy and to patients when surgical conditions are treated with radium alone. I also believe that the good end-results of the treatment of epitheliomas·of the lower lip with radium alone have been much overshadowed by the bad results. One must appreciate the fact that the diagnosis of these conditions must often be made microscopically. Fifty per cent. of questionable lesions of the lip are not malignant and must be excised for a microscopic diagnosis, so that the question of diagnosis must be considered in the cases of patients who are treated and cured with radium alone. If all lesions of the lower lip were excised for diagnosis, the mortality of epithelioma of the lip would be reduced a great deal; and I believe the cosmetic results in the cases I have seen treated surgically compare favorably with the results following·radium. The glands of the neck should be removed in all cases of cancer of the lip. Radium should be given before and after operation, but not used alone in these conditions.

DR. JOSEPH C. BLOODGOOD, Baltimore: The view I desire to emphasize is that at the present time the chief hope of preventing cancer is to get early cases, and I have demonstrated that 50 per cent. of the cases from which I have excised a V-shaped piece from the lip are not cancer. Another thing we must bear in mind is this: some people with cancer, who, before the days of publicity, waited so that we never saw them until they had hopeless metastases, now come to the physician early. Publicity has done that. We must also know what condition we are treating. We cannot make progress if we do not. Fifty per cent. of my last 100 cases clinically called cancer were not cancer. We have reduced the cases of cancer from 85 to 70 per cent. by excluding conditions that are not cancer; you cannot exclude cancer by reading the pathologic report. I want the sections and want them studied and restudied. The medical schools of the country have not the money to give us to make these investigations.

DR. F. J. EICHENLAUB, Washington, D. C.: Apparently dermatoses seen in the Middle West differ from those we see in Washington. I learn that ringworm of the scalp is cured by the application of a simple ointment. and now I learn that probably 98 per cent. of the cases of prickle cell cancer can be cured with radiotherapy. Our number of cases is small because we believe that prickle cell cancer of the lip is best treated with surgery. and so we send the patients to the surgeon. Of the fifteen patients we have treated. eight are dead or have recurrences; of the remaining seven. four have been well for only a year or two, so it is too early to call them cured. We have had one case treated just as a wart, then as a basal cell cancer. to the point of a third degree radiodermatitis. Before this reaction healed. the cancer recurred in the middle of the burn. When excised it proved to be a prickle cell cancer. This one case is enough to show that all prickle cell cancers cannot be destroyed by radiation. even when superficial and treated early. I cannot help but feel that surgery offers the best hope in prickle cell cancer of the lower lip.

Dr. William H. Guy, Pittsburgh: There seems to be a complete agreement in regard to prevention of malignancy about the tongue and lip by propaganda and publicity, and certainly we are all indebted to Dr. Bloodgood, if to any one, for what he has done to encourage this work. Further, there can be no divergence of opinion regarding the necessity for removal of points of irritation, and, in general, the application of oral hygiene, thus preventing malignancy in early cases that are definitely benign. There is a wide divergence of opinion, however, as to what is to be done after it is eventually determined that we are dealing with malignancy. Dr. Bloodgood's results are excellent, but I am not convinced that they are better than those obtained by other methods. We cannot attack every case in the same way and obtain the best results. Each and every case must be treated according to its own individual requirements. It would appear that in the early type of case classified as "local, likely malignant," without gland involvement, that either with surgery, electrocoagulation, or radium practically 100 per cent. are cured. In cases with gland involvement we find an increasing discrepancy of opinion. We have been told that nothing but excision of the mass with wide excision of the glands in the area will do. The difficulties of such a procedure are seen when we review the gland drainage of the area. All metastatic glands are not palpable, as we know, and many palpable glands are not carcinomatous, but inflammatory. A combination of methods, surgery, electrocoagulation and radiotherapy may be required in such a case. If absolute diagnoses are necessary, I favor biopsy, and this should always be preceded by the application of a heavy dosage of roentgen rays or radium. If these elements devitalize pathologic cells, radiation preliminary to either radical removal or biopsy is definitely indicated. There is still room for an honest difference of opinion in these cases. I am convinced that by a combination of methods and especially by the hypodermic method of using radium in both the primary growth and palpable glands, followed by intensive raying of the entire gland-bearing area, results at least equivalent to those obtained by advance surgery may be attained.

Dr. Richard L. Sutton, Kansas City, Mo.: I was much interested in Dr. Bloodgood's suggestion regarding tobacco as a causative agent in cancer of the mouth. In the Middle West, sunburn probably plays a more important part than tobacco. We see many cases of lip involvement. Seborrheic keratosis of the keratoid type not infrequently is followed by the development of carcinoma, usually of the prickle cell type. The fact that primary lesions are much easier to cure than secondary ones was first pointed out, I believe, by the late Dr. Heidingsfeld of Cincinnati. In those cases in which carcinoma recurs in scar tissue, one gets into all sorts of trouble. This is especially true in those cases in which caustics (such as arsenic paste, and similar agents) have been used. A cancer quack can take a simple, uncomplicated case of basal cell cancer of the skin, a case that could be cleaned up in a short time with radium, or even with a curet and acid nitrate of mercury, and by the use of some "simple, farm remedy," convert it into a lesion which involves not only the underlying periosteum, but the bone as well; and the patient is promptly placed beyond the possibility of a permanent cure. Dr. Elmer Twyman of Kansas City has called attention to the fact that as a rule in carcinoma of the lip the lesion exhibits a tendency to travel laterally downward, instead of directly downward. In my work with him, we have found best a combination of methods, radium and cautery for the mouth and tongue lesions, with erythema doses of roentgen ray in the submaxillary and submental localities. Carcinoma of the lower lip so often develops from keratoses. Only an eagle-eyed genius can know when all of the keratosis has been included in the excised area, and if it has not been, recurrence is prompt, and extension rapid, along the line of the scar.

Dr. G. A. Wyeth, New York: Dr. Taussig said that he has prolonged life in cases of carcinoma of the tongue without mutilation, and he consoles himself with this although he says he has had only a fair number of recovered patients. I think if he had mutilated a little more at the start he would have prolonged more lives and prolonged life longer. As Dr. Taussig said, many men have reported excellent results with electrocoagulation in the treatment of carcinoma of the tongue. It is not hard to understand how these excellent results have been obtained. The use of heat in the tissues from within, or endothermy, as I like to call it, greatly reduces the danger of metastasis and the likelihood of recurrence. How? Before a malignant area is touched it is completely surrounded by a wall of coagulation necrosis which destroys or seals off the blood vessels and lymphatics to and from the part. A specimen for microscopic section can now be taken with impunity, after which the whole malignant area is coagulated in situ and then cut out with scissors as an inert, necrotic mass rather than as a group of viable cells. Endothermy comprises two different technics, as developed by Dr. Clark of Philadelphia—desiccation for lighter work, coagulation for heavier work—and through them the operator has a wide range of destruction at his command. This is my reason for thinking we have fewer recurrences than surgery unattended has.

Dr. C. H. Ball, Tulsa, Okla.: If 50 per cent. of cases are not cancer, why perform a mutilating operation? If the condition can be eradicated by radium or roentgen ray, why not try that first instead of mutilating the patient? In my experience with the roentgen ray, results have been the same as Dr. Lain's. The roentgen ray removes the cancer and effects a cure in 98 per cent. of the cases. Why, if you obtain 98 per cent. cures, should you resort to any other method? Traumatic interference breaks down the natural resistance of the body, and metastases occur much sooner.

Dr. T. C. Kennedy, Indianapolis: I cannot agree with Dr. Bloodgood about his cures by surgery. If that is true, we have poor surgeons in the West. During the last year I have had nine patients come to me for radiation who had been operated within a year or a year and a half. He is certainly doing better work than our surgeons in Indiana. I have had many cases of carcinoma of the lip in the last few years and our results have been uniformly good. I do not mean that we cure all cases, for no method will do that; but in the treatment of cancer of the lip our results are so successful that I believe every patient should be treated with radium before operation is resorted to. If you treat the patient for a few weeks and the condition does not yield, it is not too late for operation. I think in every case the roentgen ray should be used before operation is advised. I do not know whether I understood Dr. New correctly, but I think he said he preferred operation. The cosmetic results from radium are far superior to any surgical results, and if we can cure these patients in this way, why operate? If there are any cancer cells, we are far more likely to spread them by operating than we are to cure them. I am satisfied that in cancer of the lip radium is more successful than surgical treatment.

Dr. F. W. Cregor, Indianapolis: I think we have no right to call these cases cancer until they have been proved to be cancer. Fifty per cent. of Dr. Bloodgood's cases called clinically cancer were proved not to be cancer. I do not think we should attack his position. I can subscribe to the position of Dr. Guy and of Dr. New, and I can also visualize an injury to normal tissue cells about these growths as the result of intensive roentgen ray or radium therapy. It seems to me like sending an army of cripples out to perform the functions of able-bodied men. According to Kinlock, the roentgen-ray burns that do not heal within a year become carcinomatous because of the traumatism of the normal tissue cells by the roentgen ray; so that if we are attempting to destroy these cancer cells which possess a very high radiosensibility, we must realize that we are injuring tissue cells that possess a lesser degree of sensibility, even though we are not destroying the cancer cells as we hope to do.

Therefore, I believe that the agent that destroys the macroscopically pathologic tissue, and the employment of radium, or especially roentgen rays, in the surrounding tissues afterward, in a dosage of not sufficient strength to impair normal tissue, but which we may hope will destroy pathologic tissue, is the method of choice.

Dr. John H. King, Nashville, Tenn.: Every case is a law unto itself, and we cannot use the same treatment in all. If we are treating a lesion on the lip, we should know the type of cancer and determine whether we are going to treat it with the roentgen ray, radium or electrocoagulation. If a case is treated by radium, the glands of the neck, submaxillary and submental, should receive deep roentgen-ray treatment or blunt dissection. I do not think we have a right to dismiss a patient without giving him the advantage of those two procedures. We know that many cases will recur, and we cannot say which they will be; if it is in our power to prevent these recurrences I think we should do so. Therefore, we should have a blunt dissection, a careful one, and a thorough radiologic treatment. A few weeks ago I had a case of recurrence in the submaxillary gland, that was quite large. I used the needle and heavy roentgen ray. The tumor-like formation disappeared remarkably quickly after three weeks. As the submaxillary and submental glands are the ones we first see affected, why can we not insert our radium needles in the areas we cannot strike with the rays? We cannot strike these glands because we cannot see them, but why cannot we do this as a prophylactic measure? It causes little discomfort, and we can leave them in for three, four or six hours as a prophylactic measure before any enlargement is observed.

Dr. Moses Scholtz, Los Angeles: One of the essayists has discussed roentgen-ray therapeutics in chronic nonmalignant inflammatory dermatoses, such as acne, lichens, psoriasis, eczemas, etc. There seem to be two points of view. The roentgen-ray experts and advocates of massive doses are looking for the largest dose that will not produce unpleasant after-effects. Another thing is to look for a minimum dose that will give the desired results. I think dermatologists should adopt the second point of view. There are essentially two dermatologic conditions calling for massive doses: malignancy and tinea of the scalp. In chronic inflammatory dermatoses we will get along much better with small fractional doses. I believe that in this group of dermatoses it is not only permissible, but distinctly helpful, to combine small fractional roentgen-ray treatments with exposures to ultraviolet light. By this means of additional sensitization we are able not only to reduce the number of roentgen-ray treatments to a minimum, but also the size of individual doses. I seldom use more than one-eighth or one-seventh of a skin unit with a spark gap of from 4 to 6 inches in chronic eczemas, lichens, acnes, etc. I cannot see the advisability of using one-fourth of a skin unit for many weeks in acne, a condition so benign and yielding so readily to therapeutics. Only very few, truly exceptional, cases would justify such heroic treatment. An overwhelming majority of acne cases will yield to ultraviolet light alternating with casual roentgen-ray treatments of much smaller aggregate dosage.

DR. I. L. McGLASSON, San Antonio, Texas: I take it from Dr. Bloodgood's and Dr. New's remarks that they meant the best type of surgery and perhaps compare it with ordinary radiotherapy. Then the results are not 100 per cent. perfect. All surgeons are not the best surgeons, nor are all radiotherapists the best in their line. All these things should be taken into consideration in discussing this subject in an effort to arrive at a conclusion. Dr. Bloodgood's statement is broad even for so eminent an authority. I am satisfied with my present treatment of cancer of the lip. I think I have overlooked something good in not following Dr. Pfahler's method of electrocoagulation, and I think that his plan is well worth while. Many patients with recurrence of cancer of the lip are sent to us by surgeons, and in these cases we get the worst results. If we have a failure, they say that radium is no good. I am curious to know whether the friends who talk against radium actually use it and have a sufficient amount. I think we should report our end-results, good or bad, until we can show something definite.

DR. DAVIS W. GOLDSTEIN, Fort Smith, Ark.: I do not believe that in cases of cancer of the lip there can be any routine treatment. If we see a patient who has received no previous treatment, we believe that patient should receive radiotherapy. It does not make any difference whether you use radium, the roentgen ray or electrocoagulation to destroy the tumor. We formerly used carbon dioxid snow for the local lesion, with good results. Whatever method is used, the glands should be irradiated. If the patient has received previous treatment, I believe it is a surgical case. The cell is weakened by previous treatment, and it will not regenerate. I have had numbers of failures after the lesions were treated with caustics. The mucous membrane of the oral cavity is the most resistant of all tissues of the body to radium, and whether you use surgery, caustics or what-not, it is essential to take care of the lymphatics either by radium, roentgen-ray or complete block dissection.

DR. EARL D. CRUTCHFIELD, Galveston, Texas: Some years ago I made a study similar to Dr. Parkhurst's. It seems to me that the reaction in these cases is more a reaction of the cell to particular environment under which the attack occurs than a definite specific reaction to the basal cell or the prickle cell epithelioma. Drs. Highman and Rulison spoke of the stimulating roentgen-ray dosage. In an incomplete study during the last eighteen months I have not been able to see any evidence of stimulation in any form of roentgen-ray dosage. I am not sure that the roentgen ray ever stimulates. The stimulation or reaction which may occur can be explained as a biologic reaction of the normal cells rather than as a stimulating reaction to the roentgen ray. In no case have I been able to see that mitoses were produced by the roentgen ray. One point in regard to surgery of the lip: Two or three years ago I studied serially sections of tumors of the lip which had been excised. Apparently on first examination many of these tumors seem to be small, localized lesions, but if serial sections are made, very often one is able to find small scattered cell nests in the edges of the lesions. The question then arises. When may we completely remove a lesion? If we knew that, then, perhaps, surgery would be the method of choice, for a great plastic surgeon; but if a piece of the lip is excised no man has the judgment to say whether or not the excision has been sufficiently extensive. We know that if ever a malignant growth is cut through, the possibility of metastases becomes very great. Therefore, since irradiation by the roentgen ray shows such a large percentage of cures radiation is certainly the method of cure; and electrocoagulation, which seals off everything, should be used as the method of removal.

Dr. Ben R. Kirkendall, Columbus, Ohio: I am glad that Dr. Pfahler has told us what to do for cancers of the lip that have been treated with roentgen rays but not cured. If we can cure these cases with electrocoagulation and not make them worse, it is a new method that can help us out. I think a great many nonmalignant growths of the lip would become cancers eventually. They are probably precancerous lesions, and the results we obtain with radium and the roentgen ray seem to be almost perfect in these cases. Dr. Lain's paper, with its statistics, shows almost perfect results with radiation, so why perform a mutilating operation first. That should not be resorted to until it is necessary. I believe that these patients, whether treated by radiation or surgery, should all be irradiated under the jaw where glandular involvement may occur. I wish to caution about the application of radium after roentgen-ray treatment in cases of cancer of the lip. I have had several cases of cancer of the lip in which the patients have first been treated, I suppose, with massive doses of roentgen ray. When they came to me there was probably more radiation in the growth than could be determined. We have been told not to treat with radium or roentgen ray until from four to six weeks have elapsed since the previous treatment. I have waited as long as four months to apply radium following roentgen ray and have had the whole lip slough off in two cases. Dr. Pfahler's electrocoagulation might have taken care of these patients and prevented this mutilation.

Dr. H. J. Parkhurst, Toledo, Ohio: There is at least one difficulty attending the use of arsphenamin as a therapeutic test in differentiating between epithelioma and syphilis: the arsenical preparations often seem to accelerate the development of a malignant process when it is present. Therefore, great caution is necessary. Concerning the subject of the tissue reaction in malignant epitheliomas, the literature contains few references; and this work has been offered with the hope of stimulating investigation along this line.

Dr. R. H. Rulison, New York: Dr. Scholtz says he combines the roentgen ray with the ultraviolet light. I have had no experience with this. In general, perhaps, we are too conservative, but if we have an erythema, due, possibly, to a simple sunburn, we are likely to postpone treatment and wait for it to subside, and on that basis I think we would not care to combine the two methods. Dr. Crutchfield makes the criticism that in one place we speak of the stimulating effect of the roentgen ray. Whether there is such an effect, I do not know. I have no defense to offer for using it, except that there are certain authorities who think this may happen. It seems to me we are not accomplishing much in the discussion because of the difference in terms.

Dr. Laurence Taussig, San Francisco: As I have tried to point out, the diagnosis of carcinoma of the tongue is difficult to make in many instances. Dr. Parkhurst pointed out the possibility of stimulating the growth by arsphenamin but, having made up our minds as to the probable diagnosis, we must treat it with that diagnosis in mind, being ready to change our method of attack whenever indicated. I think the main thing in carcinoma of the tongue is to make a correct diagnosis as early as possible in order to institute proper treatment.

Dr. George E. Pfahler, Philadelphia: We should treat each patient as an individual, and adopt the best treatment for each individual case. I have seen recurrences follow operations by the best surgeons in the country, whose names if mentioned would produce no doubt of their ability or good judgment. It must not be forgotten that the purchase of an amount of radium, either large or small, is no more a certainty of efficiency in its use than the purchase of a set of surgical instruments will guarantee a good operation. In my treatment with electrocoagulation, I always outline the surrounding edge in each case so that I know just how much is going to be taken away. That also seals off the lymphatics and blood vessels. I then trim it off with a pair of scissors, and at times the upper portion of that lesion can be sent to the pathologist for examination. There is no bleeding, which proves that I have actually sealed off the blood vessels and lymphatics. I give radiation over the lip and chin and the submaxillary and submental areas. This should be added to any other form of treatment. When there are palpable lymphatic glands, I am not sure whether these had better be treated first by general radiation and then excised, or whether we had better treat with general radiation and then introduce radium needles into the lymph nodes. I think we must let time tell us which is best.

Dr. E. S. Lain, Oklahoma City: Dr. King has asked me what I think of the treatment with radium needles introduced into all metastasizing glands or where metastasis might occur. I think this is good procedure though not as a routine treatment. This was done in one of our cases. As regards the standardization of roentgen-ray and radium treatments. I do not think such treatment can be standardized. Surgical or medical treatments are not standardized for any disease. If we should reach such a period, progress in therapy will cease. One thing that Dr. McGlasson mentioned I have also found true. Namely, in my Group 3, the advanced cases, all patients had previously been treated by plasters or by incomplete surgery. The radiotherapist has too long been made a "dumping ground" for hopeless cases, as has been said. You recall that twenty-seven of my patients did not take treatment, and that was largely due to our resolve not to be made a dumping ground for all cases in which other forms of treatment had failed. As regards the claim of a cure in 98 per cent. of squamous or prickle cell malignancies, Dr. Pfahler misunderstood me. I said that Hazen, quoting from the Bloodgood laboratory, reported that most cancers of the lips were of the squamous or prickle cell variety. I said that we have been able to effect a cure in 97.7 per cent. in Class 1. In Class 2. in which the glands were freely palpable and in which we had other evidence of metastasis, we have a percentage of 72.2 per cent. of apparent cures after three years. Our methods have improved during recent years, though had we combined other methods, such as Dr. Pfahler's electrocoagulation method. other patients might have been cured. Let me repeat that I do not believe we should entirely exclude surgery in the treatment of cancer of the lips. I do. however. insist that when we consider all phases of the patient's welfare and compare statistics on the various methods of treatment, we shall find in the use of radium and roentgen ray the most acceptable method.

CUTIS VERTICIS GYRATA *

REPORT OF CASES

HARRY E. ALDERSON, M.D.

Clinical Professor of Medicine (Skin Diseases), Stanford University
Medical School

SAN FRANCISCO

Cutis verticis gyrata has been well described by various authors since the first report by Jadassohn at the Ninth German Dermatological Congress in Berne. A recent interesting report and review of the literature by Wise and Levin [1] describes the first example of the anomaly observed in America. As far as I know, the cases that I am presenting constitute the second and third reported in this country.

The condition is characterized by the appearance of deep furrows and convolutions in the upper posterior portions of the scalp more or less resembling cerebral convolutions. By many it is regarded as a congenital tendency to furrowing which becomes pronounced later in life. My first patient comes in this category. Some believe that the process is usually intensified by local inflammation. My second patient comes under this classification.

Through the courtesy of Professor Lesser, I had the privilege of seeing a case in Berlin in 1912, so the scalp that I am presenting here constitutes the second well developed example of the condition that I have seen.

My first patient's scalp, preserved in Kaiserling solution No. 4, is here presented for your inspection. My second patient, presenting the deformity in its early stages, refused to part with his scalp. A photograph will be published later.

As will be noted on studying the gross specimen and photograph, the appearances suggest neurofibroma. We thought (and hoped) that it was that condition but microscopic study failed to disclose the presence of nerve tissue, and there were no lesions elsewhere. ,

REPORT OF CASES

History.—An apparently healthy Jewish girl, 15 years old, had had an oval well circumscribed sessile tumor with numerous convolutions covering most of the back of the head since birth. It had slowly grown larger, with deepening of the sulci. The growth had progressed more rapidly during the last few years. It had never been painful.

---

* Read at the Forty-Fifth Annual Meeting of the American Dermatological Association, Washington, D. C., May 2-4, 1922.

1. Cutis Verticis Gyrata—Report of a Case. Wise, Fred. and Levin, Oscar L.: Interstate M. J. **25**: No. 5, 1918.

She had always been in good health with the exception of occasional head-ache and nausea in the morning. She also had had measles. pertussis and parotiditis in early childhood, with no sequelae. There had been no accidents, operations or local infections, and the scalp had never been inflamed. For several years she had had occasional general headache and nausea in the morning.

Her eyes, ears, nose and throat had always been normal, and there never had been marked glandular swelling. She did not have goiter. There was no evidence of past or present disease of the respiratory systems. Her mentality was quite good.

Examination.—The skull was dolichocephalic in form. In the occiput and extending almost to the top of the head was an oval, sessile tumor with a

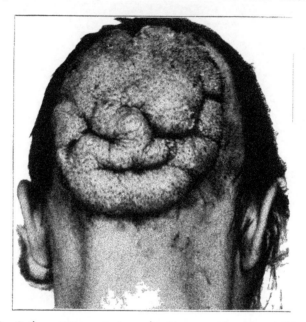

Fig. 1.—Cutis verticis gyrata in a girl. 14 years old, with a dolichocephalic type of skull. The hair was shaved for operation.

sharply defined, slightly constricted base. It was about 15 cm. in its broadest diameter and was elevated about 1.5 cm. at its highest point. It presented three main horizontal furrows and five secondary ones with convolutions like those of the cerebrum. These furrows were narrow and deep. The skin was loose and soft, and through it many firm round nodules 0.5 to 1 cm. in diameter, resembling sebaceous cysts, were plainly felt. When the scalp was shaved for the operation, the skin was seen to be normal in appearance. The hair was long, thick and black. It grew evenly over the entire tumor mass. The rest of the scalp was normal.

Eyes: The pupils were equal, regular and reacted to light and accommodation. The conjunctivae, eyelids and lashes were normal.

Nose: There was no obstruction or discharge.

Ears: The hearing was good. There was no discharge.

Mouth: The teeth were good and well kept. The tongue protruded normally. The tonsils were fairly large but apparently not diseased,

Neck: There were a few small palpable glands in the posterior cervical triangles. There was no goiter. There were no abnormal pulsations.

Chest: The cardiovascular and respiratory systems were normal.

Abdomen: The abdomen was flat. There were no masses or areas of tenderness. The liver and spleen were not palpable. The reflexes were normal.

Unfortunately, complement-fixation tests were not made. However, there was no personal or family history suggesting syphilis, and there were no stigmas.

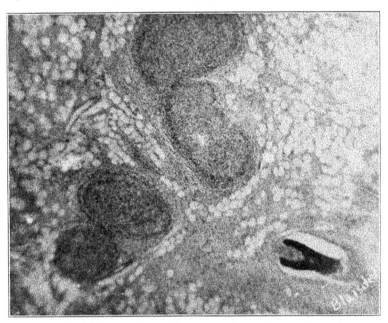

Fig. 2.—Four fibrous cords in corium. Note adipose tissue and hair follicle. Van Gieson stain.

Treatment.—Dr. Phillip K. Gilman, associate clinical professor of surgery, Stanford University Medical School, to whom I am indebted for the privilege of reporting the first case, removed the growth in its entirety and applied Thiersch grafts from the thigh. There were no particular difficulties connected with the procedure. The patient, after having been observed regularly for six weeks, was dismissed in "excellent condition." Since then our social service department has been unable to locate her.

Histologic Findings.—A piece of the growth from the summit of a convolution, including the skin, was fixed and hardened in formaldehyde solution. Sections were stained with hematoxylin and eosin, Mallory's connective tissue stain, van Gieson's stain and silver nitrate.

The tumor, preserved by the Kaiserling method No. 4, is presented for inspection. This work was done by Dr. F. E. Blaisdell, associate professor of surgery (surgical pathologist) of Stanford University.

The epidermis showed pronounced acanthosis with slight hyperkeratosis. In the upper corium the collagen showed lessened affinity for the acid stain. There were numerous young connective tissue nuclei and dense collections of pigment here and there. The blood vessels were quite numerous, dilated and their walls were not thickened. There were occasional plasma cells. Fat cells were rather numerous even in the upper regions.

The lower corium showed the chief changes. Here there were large cords or whorls of connective tissue, the bundles running in every direction. In between them were many fat cells. These structures extended down into

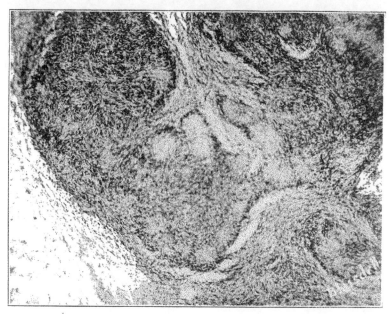

Fig. 3.—Fibrous cords under higher magnification. Hematoxylin and eosin stain.

the subcutaneous tissue where they were numerous. Many of these bundles were packed closely together.

The collagen in places took the acid dye intensely. The numerous sebaceous glands were quite large. The hair follicles were normal. Occasionally there was seen dense perifollicular infiltration of small round cells which extended the full length of the hair. Some apparently independent collections of these cells in serial sections belonged to the perifollicular deposit. No polymorpho-nuclear leukocytes were seen. The sweat glands were normal. No nerve tissue was seen.

Comment.—The general appearances and certain special features suggested a congenital connective tissue growth involving the skin. The signs of inflammation here and there were apparently incidental results

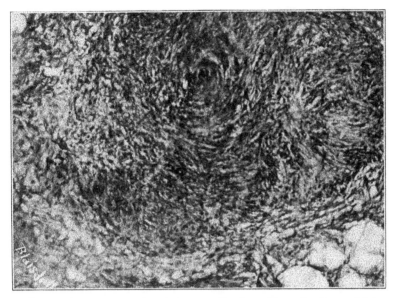

Fig. 4.—Fibrous cord under higher magnification. Note whorling and interlacing of fibers. Van Gieson stain.

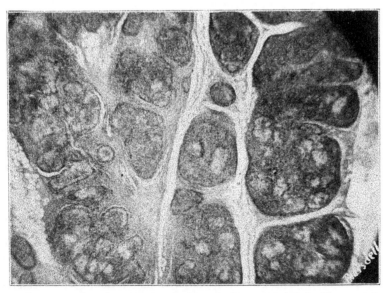

Fig. 5.—Portion of growth in subcutaneous tissue, showing the fibrous cords. Hematoxylin and eosin stain. Low magnification.

of slight traumatism. The nodules feeling like sebaceous cysts probably owed their characteristics to the arrangement of the numerous thick fibrous bundles and the uneven distribution of the fat.

Summary.—We have a case of cutis verticis gyrata in an otherwise normal girl, 15 years old, in good health (barring occasional headache and nausea). The condition had existed since birth and had increased in size during the development of puberty with the natural increase in activity of the pilosebaceous system. There was no history of past inflammation, as observed by various authors. The patient had a dolichocephalic type of skull, thus differing from the patients in most cases reported, in whom the brachycephalic type prevailed.

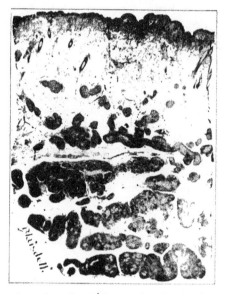

Fig. 6.—Section through entire thickness of scalp, showing growth in corium and subcutaneous tissue.

CASE 2.—I have another case under observation at the present time, in its earlier stages. The patient, a prosperous Jew, 54 years of age, obese, has a brachycephalic type of skull, a short thick neck and rather tightly drawn scalp. In the occipital region there is a deep narrow horizontal, tensely drawn, permanent furrow with a smaller curved offshoot from the same just above its right outer third. The condition has existed four or five years only. It is gradually becoming more accentuated. The hair is black, thick and normal. The patient has a seborrheal skin with typical seborrheic dermatitis in the occiput, umbilicus, groins and internatal region. The obstinate seborrheic eczema seems to be a factor in the process. I believe that the chronic inflammation there is resulting in connective tissue proliferation with consequent accentuation of the cutis verticis gyrata.

I have seen several similar but less marked cases in which the scalp was not diseased. One can see conditions approaching this in almost any crowd. A brachycephalic head with a short fat neck seems prone to develop horizontal and secondary furrows in the occiput. It is only cases showing increasing persistence of these furrows in the occiput and higher, of course, that can be regarded as early examples of cutis verticis gyrata. When chronic local folliculitis or eczema develops, naturally connective tissue proliferation occurs, and eventually the thickening of the corium and subcutaneous tissue results in the formation of this deformity.

DISCUSSION

DR. FRED WISE, New York: I reported with Dr. Levin what we thought was a typical case, but we were unable to perform a biopsy, which detracted from the value of the report. The second case in New York was presented by Dr. Fox two years ago.

The interesting point in Dr. Alderson's paper lies in the fact that the lesion is different from those described in the literature, the difference being that this is a decidedly circumscribed elevated growth and does not run into the scalp as all the other cases do, and I am inclined to believe that it should be interpreted as a nevus. It is a form of cutis verticis gyrata, but of nevus origin. The other cases described in the textbooks as nevus cerebelliformis are probably examples of this. The microscope reveals the facts, and the histology in those cases must be different from that described by Dr. Alderson.

Another statement occurring in the literature is that there are probably two very different types of cutis verticis gyrata, one in which there is a marked inflammatory process and the other in which no inflammatory reaction has ever been present.

DR. HARRY E. ALDERSON (closing): This summer more material from the specimen will be worked up thoroughly; sections from every part of the growth will be studied, and a complete report will be sent in later for publication.

PHYSICAL PRINCIPLES UNDERLYING THE DEVELOPMENT OF HIGH VOLTAGE ROENTGEN-RAY APPARATUS *

C. N. MOORE, M.D.

SCHENECTADY, N. Y.

Until recently, most roentgenotherapy was practiced with voltages up to approximately 100,000 applied to the roentgen-ray tube. The roentgen rays generated at these voltages produced definite biologic reactions at or near the surface of the body. Because of their comparatively low penetrating power, however, these rays were rapidly absorbed by the tissues, and it was difficult to deliver any effective amount to a point much below the surface without injury to the overlying tissue.

Figure 1 gives a visual picture of absorption of roentgen rays as they pass through matter. It shows a cube of lead glass which was placed beneath a half inch opening in a lead diaphragm and exposed for several hours to the rays from a tube operating with four milliamperes at 200,000 volts (peak). This glass becomes brown under the influence of roentgen rays, and the intensity of the coloration indicates the intensity of the roentgen-ray beam at different depths below the surface of the glass. It will be noticed that the color is very dark at the surface and gradually becomes lighter as the depth increases. This illustrates the physical problem involved in deep roentgenotherapy, which, as I have said before, is one of getting sufficient roentgen-ray intensity at a point much beneath the surface of the body.

In the past, the use of multiple ports of entry and of cross-firing was resorted to in an endeavor to increase the intensity beneath the surface. Results obtained by this method are illustrated by Figure 2. In this case, a similar glass cube was exposed from four sides in succession and an area will be seen in the center of the cube where the combined roentgen-ray beams have produced an effect nearly equal to that produced by any one beam at the surface.

During the last few years, the tendency has been toward the use of higher voltages, in an attempt to increase the ratio of depth to surface dose. It is the physical principles underlying this method of attack that I am to review in this paper. Tubes to operate at the higher voltage and apparatus to produce this voltage had to be developed, and the

---

* Read before the Section on Dermatology and Syphilology at the Seventy-Third Annual Session of the American Medical Association, St. Louis, May, 1922.

experimental work involved in this development was undertaken only after careful physical measurements had shown that a greater intensity at a depth could be produced by the use of higher voltage.

That the results of these measurements may be understood more clearly, let us first consider the beam of roentgen rays coming from any roentgen-ray tube. By means of a Bragg spectrometer and ionization

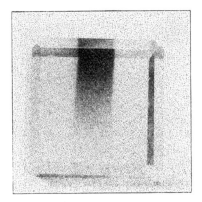

Fig. 1.—Absorption of roentgen rays in matter shown by color produced in cube of lead glass.

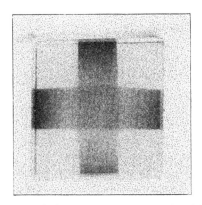

Fig. 2.—Cross-fire technic illustrated by color produced by roentgen rays in lead glass cube.

chamber, we may analyze this beam, and plot the spectrum, just as we would analyze the beam of light from an incandescent lamp. In doing so, we find that it is a composite beam made up of waves of varying lengths. Figure 3 presents a spectrum of the roentgen-ray beam operating at 40,000 volts,[1] and we find that the wave lengths vary from

---

1. Hull: Am. J. Roentgenol., 1915.

0.3 Å to 0.8 Å,[2] with a maximum of intensity at about 0.4 Å. We know that the shorter the wave length, the more penetrating power the roentgen-ray wave has, so that we are interested in anything that will give us a shorter wave length and a greater intensity of this shorter wave length.

Figure 4 shows the effect on the wave length and intensity of increasing the potential applied to the roentgen-ray tube. At 40,000 volts, the shortest wave length is about 0.3 Å, and this decreases to about 0.1 Å at 90,000 volts. At the same time, the intensity of the waves of shorter length has tremendously increased. There are still a lot of long wave lengths present, however. The same thing holds true as we go to still higher voltages, as is shown in Figure 5,[3] which gives the spectrum at 165,000 volts. Here the shortest wave length is 0.075 Å. The wave length of the gamma rays from Ra-C is approximately 0.004 Å. According to the work of Ellis in England, it would require a voltage of 3,000,000 on the tube to produce roentgen rays of this short

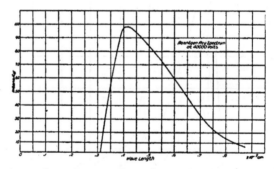

Fig. 3.—Spectrum of roentgen-ray beam from tube operating at 40,000 volts.

wave length. It is evident from these measurements that increasing the potential applied to the tube results in the production of a greater quantity of more penetrating rays.

For the purpose of cutting off the longer or less penetrating rays, it is customary to pass the roentgen-ray beam through some filter, a sheet of aluminum or copper, before it reaches the body. The effect of such a filter is shown in Figure 6,[4] in which the upper curve shows the spectrum at 70,000 volts without any filter and the lower curve the spectrum with a 3 mm. aluminum filter. It can be seen that the aluminum has reduced the intensity of the soft radiation (long wave

2. The Angström unit, 10^{-8} or $\frac{1}{100,000,000}$ cm. is the standard unit for expressing wave length.

3. Duane: Am. J. Roentgenol., March, 1922, p. 169.

4. Hull: Am. J. Roentgenol., 1915.

lengths) much more than that of the penetrating rays, but there is still a considerable amount of soft radiation left. This could, of course, be considerably reduced by the use of a great thickness of aluminum or a sufficient thickness of some denser material, such as copper, but not without cutting down the intensity of the useful penetrating rays to a small fraction of its original value. But we have already noted the effect of increasing the potential applied to the tube. Therefore, we are able to combine the two, higher voltage and greater filtration, to obtain a sufficient intensity of the more penetrating rays. This is

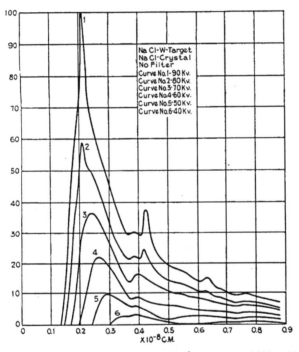

Fig. 4.—Roentgen-ray spectra from tubes operating at from 40,000 to 90,000 volts.

shown in Figure 7,[5] where we have plotted the intensities through different thicknesses of copper filters at various voltages of from 175,000 to 298,000. It will be noticed that for any voltage the intensity falls off rapidly with increasing thickness of filter, and that for any one filter thickness, for example 1 mm., the intensity increases rapidly with the voltage. When high intensity of penetrating radiation is desired, there is a strong argument in favor of the use of high voltage with sufficient filtration.

5. Coolidge and Kearsley, Jr.: Am. J. Roentgenol., February, 1922, p. 98.

So far we have been considering the roentgen-ray beam before it reaches the body of the patient. In deep roentgenotherapy, what we are interested in is the nature of the beam after it has passed through a certain amount of tissue on its way to the diseased area. To determine the physical characteristics of the beam within the body, we are accus_ tomed to choose some material, such as water, which has about the same abso:bing power as the body, and measure at some desired depth in the water, by means of the ionization chamber, the roentgen-ray intensity

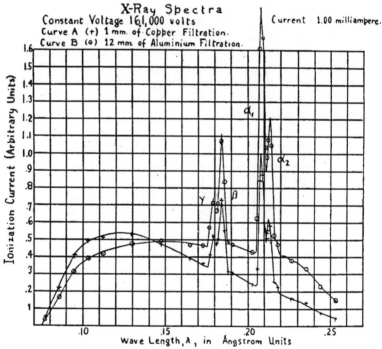

Fig. 5.—Roentgen-ray spectrum from tube operating at 165,000 volts.

with tubes operated at various voltages and with filters of various thicknesses. The results of such measurements are given in Figure 8.[6] Here we have plotted the percentage intensity beneath 10 cm. of water with the roentgen-ray tube operated at voltages of from 200,000 to 250,000, and with the roentgen rays filtered through 0.5 and 1.0 mm. of copper. With one-half millimeter of copper as a filter, the roentgen_ ray intensity beneath 10 cm. of water is 14.75 per cent. of what it is at the surface of the water when 200,000 volts are applied to the tube.

6. Coolidge and Kearsley, Jr.: Am. J. Roentgenol., February, 1922. p. 88.

while it is 17.25 per cent. if 250,000 volts are employed. A similar increase is shown with 1 mm. of copper filter. The curves indicate clearly that, up to 250,000 volts at least, the percentage depth intensity increases with increased voltage and that it is greater the thicker the filter.

A third factor enters into the question of percentage depth dose; namely, that of distance from the focal spot to the surface of the body. In any particular case, the distance from the surface to a point beneath at which the roentgen rays are to be delivered is a constant, and the ratio of this distance to the total distance from the focal spot becomes less as the latter distance is increased. At low voltages, it was impossible to greatly increase the focal spot skin distance because the roengen-ray intensity decreases inversely in proportion to the square of the distance; that is, the greater the distance, the less the intensity. We have seen, however, that this decrease in intensity may be compensated for by increased potential applied to the tube, and increased filtration of the roentgen-ray beam.

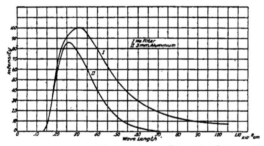

Fig. 6.—Roentgen-ray spectra at 70,000 volts with and without aluminum filter.

As a fourth factor, we have to consider the size of port of entry in regard to its effect on the percentage depth dose. The results of measurements made to determine the effect of varying this factor are given in Figure 9.[7] These curves show the percentage depth dose beneath 10 cm. of water for rays filtered through 3 mm. of aluminum, 10 mm. of aluminum, and 1 mm. of copper for three ports of entry, 5 by 5 cm., 10 by 10 cm., and 15 by 15 cm. It is evident from these curves that, within these limits, the percentage depth dose increases as the size of port of entry is increased. The explanation of this lies in the fact that roentgen rays in passing through matter generate secondary roentgen rays, and the effect of these secondary roentgen rays is added to that of the original beam. The greater the amount of

---

7. Krönig and Friedrich: Physikalische und biologische Grundlagen der Strahlen-therapie, 1918, p. 122.

matter subjected to the action of the original beam, the greater the amount of secondary rays generated, and, therefore, the greater the percentage depth dose. As has already been pointed out, the shorter the wave length of the roentgen ray, the greater the amount of rays which will pass through a certain amount of tissue. The combination of

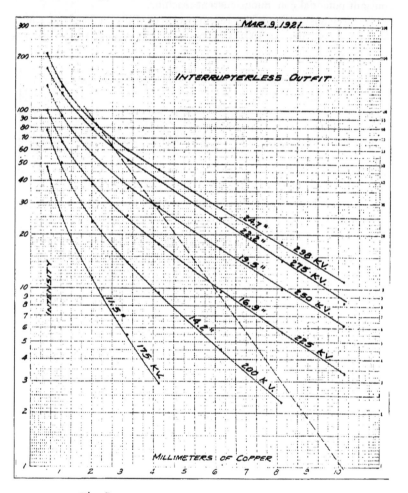

Fig. 7.—Absorption curves through copper filters.

higher voltage and larger port of entry is, therefore, effective in increasing the percentage depth dose.

Roentgen-ray tubes and generating apparatus are now available for operation at voltages of 200,000 and some experimental work has been done at voltages of 300,000. The tube developed for this work is of the hot cathode type with solid tungsten target, similar to that used at lower voltages except that the bulb is slightly larger and the arms somewhat longer, to prevent arcing along the surface of the glass. Experience has shown that these tubes operate most satisfactorily when excited from a high tension transformer with mechanical rectifier, or from a constant potential continuous current machine.

As previously stated, the recent work of Ellis in England shows that we should get, at 400,000 volts, radiation similar to the gamma

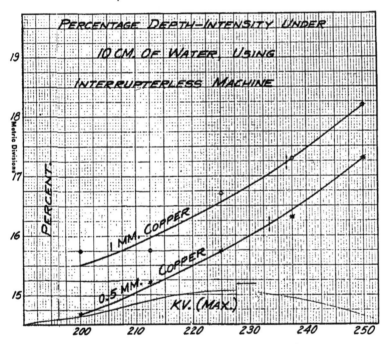

Fig. 8.—Percentage depth dose beneath 10 cm. of water.

rays of Ra-B, and at 3,000,000, radiation similar to the gamma rays of Ra-C. Though we may not be able to go to 3,000,000 volts, we may well be able to go high enough to increase materially the amount of roentgen-ray energy which can be transmitted through different mediums.

CONCLUSIONS

1. Increasing the voltage applied to the roentgen-ray tube increases the intensity of the roentgen rays produced. The intensity of the more penetrating rays increases much more rapidly than that of the less penetrating rays.

2. At any definite voltage applied to the roentgen-ray tube, increasing the thickness of filter decreases the roentgen-ray intensity but increases the proportion of the more penetrating rays in the roentgen-ray beam beneath the filter.

3. With a definite thickness of any filter, increasing the voltage increases the ratio of depth to surface dose.

4. With a definite voltage and filter, increasing the target skin distance increases the ratio of depth to surface dose.

5. Increasing the size of the port of entry increases the ratio of depth to surface dose.

6. Roentgen-ray tubes and generating apparatus are available for operation at 200,000 volts.

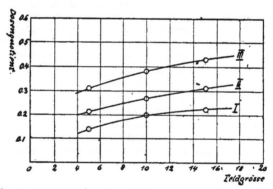

Fig. 9.—Effect of size of port of entry on percentage depth dose.

ABSTRACT OF DISCUSSION

Dr. William Allen Pusey, Chicago: We are under obligations to the physicists for introducing waves of higher voltage and shorter wave length but deeper penetration. Anyone who said such things are not useful would be stupid, but I would call attention to the fact that for the present these are technical, physical problems rather than problems in therapeutics. There is undoubtedly a propaganda for the use of roentgen-ray apparatus to produce enormous voltage. Many factors are involved in that problem about which we are uncertain. It is undoubtedly true that when we get more familiar with the use of roentgen-rays produced by such high voltage we will be able to attack deep lesions with more intelligence than we can now. I would, however, point out that in undertaking to treat these lesions with this new method we are not working with more intelligence than we have had. I know in the old days, when we treated with the old gas tubes, we were able to produce appreciable effects in deep lesions. I am sure no one who has seen a myoma of the uterus treated by this method will doubt that we could produce deep effects then. With the new apparatus, we have to know how much effect we are producing and how much effect we are getting. There is considerable difference in the opinion regarding this—one that the effect is produced by the direct voltage and the other that it is produced by the square of the voltage. We should keep an open mind and I think we are not yet in a position to be convinced that these enormous voltages are what we need. Recently I had the opportunity to see the work of Barlow with enormous doses of radium in animals. The deep effects produced in animals were exactly analogous with the effect produced on the skin by roentgen rays. They were so strikingly similar that you could almost use the one set of photomicrographs to illustrate the work. The chief thing that came to me in seeing this work of Barlow was the seriousness of an attempt to bombard a man's internals with this enormous penetration. I would not like to be regarded as undertaking to minimize the usefulness of the experiments presented today by Mr. Moore, but I would exercise the caution of a, perhaps, congenitally conservative man by saying that these questions before us are largely academic.

Dr. Harold N. Cole, Cleveland: I was much impressed with the fact that with a certain voltage, after you have used a certain amount of filter, no matter how much filter you use you get the same straight line of intensity. I should like to know about the amount of filter indicated with a machine with 60,000, one with 80,000 and one with 120,000 volts, respectively. This is a very important point and if you reach a certain amount of filter and no more will make any difference in the line, that is something we should know about.

Dr. F. J. Eichenlaub, Washington, D. C.: As dermatologists, I am sure that we have learned a great deal from this paper. I think the facts brought out by Mr. Moore demonstrate that the dermatologist will never need the 200,000 volt machine. Furthermore, the statement that filtration decreases the intensity is very interesting, because it strengthens the plea of Dr. MacKee that the rays we want in dermatology are the unfiltered rays. In dealing with basal cell cancer, acne, and other diseases of the skin for which we use the roentgen rays, we want the unfiltered rays which give the greatest intensity in the superficial tissues.

Dr. William H. Guy, Pittsburgh: As dermatologists, we are, of course, vitally interested in the physical properties of roentgen rays, and are in sympathy with all attempts to improve apparatus and technical details. However, the bulk of our pathology is very superficial and we use by preference unfiltered rays with moderate powers of penetration, using the minimum amount that will prove effective. Heavy dosage of highly penetrating rays may produce deep seated vascular changes that are not only unnecessary but are also likely to be productive of late undesirable results. By increasing the distance between the anode and the skin, one may reduce the enormous disproportion between surface and depth dosage due to divergence of rays. When additional penetration is desired, filters are indicated. I am rather skeptical as to the highly touted value of these very high voltage machines; certainly in dermatologic practice they are not needed.

Dr. C. N. Moore, Schenectady, N. Y.: Any discussion of the particular results obtained by the use of low or high voltage is, of course, entirely out of my province. The answer to the question as to what type of rays produce the best results should be left to the physicians who apply the rays. One point I would like to correct in Dr. Pusey's discussion, and that is the impression that you may have roentgen rays so penetrating that they are not absorbed at all in going through matter. It is a physical fact that roentgen rays of any kind are absorbed to a certain extent. A definite thickness of matter will absorb a certain percentage of the rays and the next equal thickness will absorb the same percentage of those rays which were not absorbed in the first layer. In regard to Dr. Cole's question as to the proper thickness of filter to use at the various voltages employed in roentgen-ray work, it would depend on what intensity was desired beneath the filter. As you remember, the curves showing the relation between intensity and filter thickness for any definite voltage indicated that the intensity always decreased as the filter thickness was increased. The fact that the curves became straight lines beyond a certain filter thickness simply showed that further filtration did not change the quality of the roentgen-ray beam.

LUPUS ERYTHEMATOSUS ACUTUS DISSEMINATUS HEMORRHAGICUS *

REPORT OF A CASE

MOSES SCHOLTZ, M.D.

Dermatologist, Graduate School of Medicine, Los Angeles Medical Department,
University of California, Los Angeles County and
Kaspare Cohn Hospitals

LOS ANGELES

The following case is reported, both because of the extreme rarity of the condition, and because of the several interesting clinical features of the case. The case was referred to me by Dr. D. Edelman of this city.

REPORT OF CASE

Aug. 5, 1920, Mrs. C. M., aged 31, mother of two children, consulted her family physician about two red patches on the forehead and on the chest. She had noticed the patches for the first time two weeks before. They caused burning and itching and grew steadily bigger. She had also been complaining of weakness, severe headaches and of general ill feeling for the last six months. The family physician had found a large amount of albumin in the urine and had prescribed a general and dietetic regimen. He referred the patient for a dermatologic diagnosis.

Skin Findings.—The examination revealed a very sharply defined, acutely inflamed area, occupying the nasal bridge, descending symmetrically on both cheeks and presenting a typical bat-wing shape. The patches were not bright, angry red, but rather deep red and livid. They showed a very slight infiltration, with a greater turgescence at the border and a perceptible flattening of the central parts, which were paler and gave a suggestion of mild sclerosis or atrophy. The surface of the patches was rather greasy and smooth, showing fine dirty white tightly adherent branlike scales. An irregularly shaped square patch, about 2 by 3 inches (5 by 7.5 cm.), of the same clinical characteristics was found on the upper third of the sternum.

Physical Examination.—Examination revealed: head and neck: no exophthalmos, thyroid palpable but not enlarged, oral cavity presenting no abnormalities. Chest: heart of normal size, shape and position, heart tones clear and distinct. Lungs: definite right apical retraction and fibrosis, dulness to flatness, supraclavicular to fourth interspace; breath sounds exaggerated, bronchial blow with harsh inspiration; left base lung excursion restricted with a reduction of vesicular breathing; inspiration productive of cloudburst of crackling. Impression of the chest condition: chronic fibroid tuberculosis (quiescent), and left basal adhesive pleuritis. The abdomen was rotund; there was no distention, and fat was retained; no masses were palpable, and there were no tender areas on deep palpation; liver, kidneys, spleen were not palpable. Superficial and deep reflexes were present, but there was no Argyll Robertson pupil, nor ataxia.

---

* Read before the Section on Dermatology and Syphilology at the Seventy-Third Annual Session of the American Medical Association, St. Louis, May, 1922.

Laboratory Findings.—Examination of the blood revealed that bleeding time was normal and coagulating time greatly prolonged (Howell's method). Hemoglobin was 63 per cent., the red blood cells numbered 3,200,000, the color index was 0.95; the leukocytes numbered 5,200. Differential leukocyte count revealed: polymorphonuclears, 136 (68 per cent.); lymphocytes, 50 (25 per cent.); large mononuclears, 11 (5.5 per cent.); transitionals, 3 (1.5 per cent.); total, 200 (100 per cent.). The red blood cells were normal in size, regular in shape and took the stain evenly. No nucleated red blood cells or blood parasites were seen, and no abnormal leukocytes. Platelets diminished in numbers. The blood culture was sterile; the Wassermann reaction, one plus. Examination of the urine revealed a trace of albumin. Microscopic examination of centrifugalized sediment revealed numerous red blood cells, pus cells and numerous bacteria. No casts were found.

Diagnosis.—The morphology and localization of the lesions on the face were so typical of lupus erythematosus that no other diagnosis was seriously considered. There were three unusual features: (1) an acute development; (2) the presence of constitutional symptoms, and (3) the presence of a clinically identical patch in the region of manubrium sterni—a distinctly seborrheic location. For this reason the possibility of an atypical seborrheic dermatitis was entertained temporarily in spite of the absence of seborrhea on the scalp, except a slight dandruff. Two per cent. salicylic acid in Lassar's paste was given.

Clinical Course.—Two weeks later, I was again called to see the patient at her home. She was confined to bed, complaining of weakness and feverish spells at night. There was a considerable extension of the lesions of the face, forming large symmetrical butterfly-shaped areas of the classic type of lupus erythematosus, extending down on the cheeks and also on the forehead. Beyond the sharply defined borders of the main areas appeared numerous small, discrete, though not nearly so sharply marginated, maculopapular lesions, ranging in size from that of a hemp seed to that of a coffee bean. These lesions were dusky red and perfectly smooth, suggesting papular lesions of erythema multiforme type. A few days later, multiple lesions of the same type appeared on the right arm and on the following days successively on both elbows, gluteal regions, legs and other parts of the body. A few similar maculopapular lesions could be seen on the hard palate. The patient complained persistently of a burning sensation in the large patches on the face and sternum, but the disseminated lesions on the limbs and trunk did not cause any discomfort.

At this time, the large patches on the forehead, cheeks and sternum had undergone a most peculiar change. They had suddenly developed a diffuse oozing of a hemorrhagic character, not merely a blood serum, but what seemed to be pure blood. In fact, it was, clinically, a striking picture of a cutaneous hemorrhage spontaneously developed. Blood was oozing slowly, forming heavy hemorrhagic crusts. Bleeding could not be stopped by pressure, but it was easily controlled by 1 : 1,000 epinephrin ointment. Gradually, the patches on the face lost their originally sharply marginated borders, fused with disseminated maculopapular lesions and formed rather diffuse areas of erysipeloid hue, covering practically the whole face. Similar changes took place in the sternal patch.

The rash, as a whole, had attained its maximum; it remained stationary for a week, and gradually began to recede. During this time, the patient had irregular and intermittent elevations of temperature up to 102 F., which also gradually went down to normal.

The treatment consisted in the administration of quinin hydrochlorid, 5 grain capsules, four times a day, and 5 grain capsules of calcium lactate, four times a day, given at alternate hours.

By September 30, about two months after the appearance of the first patches, all skin lesions had cleared up completely. The patient improved sufficiently to be up and about, and I withdrew from the case, leaving the patient in charge of the family physician.

Subsequent History.—The attending physician reported that the subsequent course was unexpectedly rapid and dramatic. In spite of the apparent improvement, the patient did not recover completely. There were, as before, indefinite complaints with no other clinical findings but persistent albuminuria, red blood cells, pus cells and hyaline, granular and blood casts in the urine. At one time, small purpuric spots appeared scattered over the body. December 17, the patient became unconscious and died, with a typical picture of uremia. At the partial necropsy examination made by Dr. A. Zeiler, no active tuberculous lesions were found, but a well expressed pyonephrosis.

REVIEW OF THE LITERATURE

As the foregoing clinical report shows, this was a case of acute hemorrhagic disseminated type of lupus erythematosus with a fatal termination—a case in which no active tuberculous lesions were found and in which the only source of focal infection responsible for the whole symptomatology proved to be pyonephrosis.

Cases of this type are extremely rare. One of the earliest cases of lupus erythematosus disseminatus was reported by Hardaway,[1] in 1889. The patient, aged 26, having discoid patches of lupus erythematosus on the face for several months, developed bullae, after some irritating local medication fever, with hemorrhagic crusts, enlarged lymphatic glands, coma and acute tuberculous pneumonia, resulting in death. Fordyce,[2] in 1896, reported a case of a woman, aged 25, who, after having discoid patches on the face for many months, developed multiple similar patches, disseminated on arms and hands, at the beginning of pregnancy. At the end of pregnancy, the eruption cleared up, leaving behind atrophic marks.

Pernet,[3] in 1908, quoted a series of ten cases of lupus erythematosus acutus disseminatus reported up to date: among these were one case of his own, three reported by Kaposi, one by Boeck, one by Koch, two by Jadassohn, one by Short and one by Heath. Strangely, he does not mention the cases of Hardaway and Fordyce. Gray,[4] in 1914, reported a case of a young woman suffering with pneumonia who developed

1. Hardaway: J. Cutan. Dis. **7**:447, 1889.
2. Fordyce: J. Cutan. Dis. **14**:89, 1896.
3. Pernet: Etude Clinique, Paris, 1908, p. 135.
4. Gray: Brit. J. Dermat. **26**:356, 1914.

patches of lupus erythematosus with hemorrhagic bullae on the face and hands. After the resolution of pneumonia, the rash cleared up also, but reappeared later as ordinary discoid patches.

Ravogli,[5] in 1915, reported a case of lupus erythematosus of discoid type in which, after injections of 0.01 mg. of tuberculin, a disseminated form of lupus erythematosus developed with fever and early death from miliary general tuberculosis.

Barber,[6] in 1915, reported a case in which, after recurrent attacks of discoid patches for several years, the lesions spread acutely on the face, body and limbs, associated with elevations of temperature, up to 104 F. A pure culture of *Streptococcus longus* was obtained from the intestines. After the improvement brought about by sour milk treatment, no streptococci were found in the feces, only *Bacillus coli* and allied bacilli being present. Ijiri,[7] in Japan, reported, in 1915, three cases of acute lupus erythematosus disseminatus. Ehrman,[8] in 1917, reported the case of a soldier who, after an injection of infected tuberculin, developed disseminated acute erysipelas-like lesions on the face, trunk and limbs. The lesions developed later into chronic discoid patches.

Brown,[9] in 1917, reported the case of a boy, aged 11, in whom patches of lupus erythematosus appeared on the ears. Four weeks later, he developed fever and vomiting; the patches disseminated on the nose, cheeks, fingers and toes, and the gums bled. As the rash faded, the patient developed pneumonia, and died four days later. There was no tuberculosis in the family, and the tonsils had been removed three years before.

Several cases were reported in 1920. Highman[10] reported the case of a woman, aged 51, who had discoid patches of five weeks' duration. She developed erysipeloid areas on the face and hands, with elevation of temperature and prostration. The lesions were proved histologically to be lupus erythematosus.

An interesting case was reported by Low and Rutherford.[11] The patient had discoid patches on the face for years; she also had pyorrhea and subacute nephritis. The skin lesions cleared up after the extraction of teeth and vaccine treatment, but recurred after each of four attacks of bronchitis which the patient had in four and a half years, with complete disappearance of the eruption between the attacks. In the sputum

5. Ravogli: J. Cutan. Dis. **33**:266, 1915.

6. Barber: Brit. J. Dermat. **27**:365, 1915.

7. Ijiri: Ztschr. f. Dermat. **15**: (July) 1915.

8. Ehrman: Wien. klin. Wchnschr. **30**:669, 1917.

9. Brown: New York M. J. **106**:931 (Nov. 17) 1917.

10. Highman, W. G.: Lupus Erythematosus Disseminatus, Tr. New York Dermat. Soc., Arch. Dermat. & Syph. **1**:227, (Feb.) 1920.

11. Low and Rutherford: Brit. J. Dermat. **32**:326 (Nov.) 1920.

were found streptococcus and staphylococcus. The patient died from intercurrent diphtheria. At necropsy, no active tuberculosis was found, but there were extensive chronic lesions in the lungs. Streptococcus was cultured from the blood.

Graham Little [12] reported a case in which discoid patches of seven months' duration on the nose spread all over the body, with elevation of temperature. Tuberculous glands were present. Whitfield [13] reported a case of acute lupus erythematosus with a fatal termination. The necropsy findings were negative. Sequeira [14] reported the case of a woman, aged 37, in which discoid patches appeared on the nose, covered its whole surface and then spread to other parts of the body, fingers and toes. On the hands were purpuric and hemorrhagic lesions; on the right calf appeared bullous lesions. The temperature was normal. There was no albuminuria. He cited another acute case, with a temperature of 103 to 105 F. Ormsby [15] cited two fatal cases of lupus erythematosus acutus (unpublished) with the lesions of erythema multiforme type scattered on the body. McLeod [16] recorded a fatal case of acute lupus erythematosus with nephritis. The eruption cleared up as the nephritis grew worse.

The analysis of the literature on the subject leaves an impression that many writers did not sufficiently differentiate between the acute and disseminated types of lupus erythematosus. A case may be disseminated but not necessarily acute. Many cases of disseminated lupus erythematosus run a chronic course throughout. They may develop from a discoid type or be disseminated from the start. They may also start as an acute disseminated type and run into a chronic discoid type. Such cases should not be termed acute disseminated lupus erythematosus. Only cases which start acutely, assume a disseminated form and run acutely throughout can be regarded as a pure type of acute disseminated lupus erythematosus.

From this point of view, the cases reported by Hardaway, Fordyce, Ravogli, Barber, Ehrman, Low and Rutherford, and Graham Little can hardly be considered as pure types of acute disseminated lupus erythematosus, but rather as a chronic disseminated type with an acute exacerbation. On the other hand, cases reported by Highman, Gray, Brown, Whitfield and Sequeira answer all qualifications of acute disseminated lupus erythematosus. The present case is the sixth of this class. In the remainder of the series of sixteen cases reported, the available data are not sufficiently detailed to determine their type.

12. Graham Little: Brit. J. Dermat. **32**:272, 1920.
13. Whitfield: Brit. J. Dermat. **32**:272, 1920.
14. Sequeira: Proc. Roy. Soc. Med. **13**:27 (Feb.) 1920.
15. Ormsby: Diseases of the Skin, Philadelphia, Lea & Febiger, 1921, p.698.
16. McLeod: Brit. J. Dermat. **20**:236, 1908.

As to the other salient features, out of twenty-seven reported cases of lupus disseminatus, seven terminated fatally, those reported by Hardaway, Short, Brown, Low and Rutherford, Whitfield, Ravogli and McLeod. The present case is the eighth fatal case.

As to the hemorrhagic lesions, they were present only in four cases of the series, those reported by Kaposi, Hardaway, Gray and Sequeira. The present case is the fifth.

PATHOGENESIS

The pathogenesis of lupus erythematosus is notoriously a controversial issue. It seems that the study of acute forms of lupus erythematosus would hold out a better promise to establish a definite pathogenesis. This has not been the case. The analysis of twenty-seven case reports cited in the foregoing shows a diversified pathogenesis.

One point has been settled; namely, that tuberculosis, regarded for a long time the sole or the main cause of lupus erythematosus, can be definitely excluded in many cases. It was present in the cases of Hardaway, Ehrman, Ravogli and Graham Little. On the other hand, in two fatal cases of acute lupus erythematosus cited by Torok, no tuberculosis was found at necropsy. In the cases of Cranston Low, Whitfield and Brown also, the necropsy findings were negative. Of twelve cases of disseminated lupus erythematosus reported by Jadassohn, only two showed active tuberculosis, and in two others it was inactive. Barber, in two of his cases, found focal streptococcic infection in the intestines in one and in the tonsils in the other. In Fordyce's cases, the outbreak was caused by pregnancy. Pneumonia was a factor in the cases of Shamberg, Gray and Brown.

The present case shows one pathogenic factor only—a pyogenic nephritis. It is of interest to note that nephritis in this case is not secondary to some local or general infection or toxemia, but is a primary lesion, responsible both for the skin lesions and for the fatal termination, and present in the clinical picture from the very start to the finish.

The theory of a multiple and diverse pathogenesis of lupus erythematosus has been advanced and accepted by several observers, among them Brooks, Jadassohn, Hartzell and Pusey. The study of the reported cases and of the present case strongly substantiates this view.

MORPHOLOGY

The morphology of the present case was extremely interesting. The initial patches on the forehead and the sternum were of the classic type of lupus erythematosus. The subsequent lesions which developed, when dissemination took place, were of maculopapular type, strongly suggesting generalized erythema multiforme.

For a while, the eruptive areas on the face strongly suggested an erysipeloid appearance in the color of the general configuration, the only difference being that the involved area did not show one solid uninterrupted surface, but a confluent one, of many small ill defined patches separated by small interspaces of normal skin. The papular lesions on the trunk and limbs were characteristic of the fugaceous small papular type of toxic exudative erythema multiforme.

It is of interest to note that the skin lesions cleared up completely with the subsidence of the acute attack and that no other skin lesions, with the exception of small scattered purpuric macules, developed later when the case entered its grave and ultimate stage. Apparently, the skin lesions of lupus erythematosus in the present case were merely a temporary and incidental feature of the whole clinical picture of pyogenic toxemia.

The most striking morphologic feature of the case was a hemorrhagic exudate that developed on the initial patches on the face and the sternum at the acme of the acute stage. The exudate was diffuse, capillary, purely hemorrhagic, of bright arterial character. It was, apparently, due to intense vascular engorgement and was associated with a marked subjective feeling of burning. It did not yield to pressure but was easily controlled by epinephrin ointment. It presented a perfect picture of diffuse cutaneous hemorrhage. Hemorrhagic lesions in the form of vesicles, bullae and purpuric macules were recorded by Kaposi, Hardaway and Gray and, as purpuric and discrete hemorrhagic lesions, by Sequeira, but I did not find any references to diffuse hemorrhagic lesions, as in the present case.

LUPUS ERYTHEMATOSUS VERSUS ERYTHEMA MULTIFORME

In correlating and interpreting the fact that the initial patches are of typical discoid type of lupus erythematosus, and that subsequent disseminated lesions strongly suggest papular erythema multiforme type, two modes of explanation present themselves as the most plausible. The first is that, in certain cases reported as lupus erythematosus acutus disseminatus, the two conditions of lupus erythematosus and of erythema multiforme, induced by different pathogenic factors, were two independent clinical entities, merely coexisting in one person, without any pathogenetic relationship and only apparently merging into one clinical picture. In other words, we may assume that erythema multiforme has been superimposed by an intercurrent infection or toxemia on lupus erythematosus, and that in such cases erythema multiforme may overshadow, disguise and even modify the original discoid patches of lupus erythematosus. This assumption is particularly plausible in cases in which, after the termination of intercurrent infection or toxemia, the lesions return to the original discoid type.

The other explanation of the morphologic transformation observed in these cases raises an important issue as to whether lupus erythematosus is a definite clinical entity or merely a certain clinical type of skin reaction potential of multiple etiology. This interpretation would closely link lupus erythematosus with erythema multiforme. As mentioned before, this point of view has already been voiced by Fordyce, Hartzell, Pusey and other writers, who point out the existence of borderline types between lupus erythematosus and erythema multiforme. The present case admits only the second interpretation. We cannot assume in this case an intercurrent infection or toxemia that has superimposed erythema multiforme on lupus erythematosus, since we have here only one pathogenic factor—pyonephritis responsible for all the symptoms and skin manifestations in the case.

What factor determines this morphologic transformation, and why disseminated lesions do not have the slightest clinical resemblance to the discoid patches, can be suggested only in a conjectural form. Possibly, the very intensity and rapidity of the pathologic process prevents lesions from developing into ordinary discoid type.

SUMMARY

1. The female sex is preponderant in cases of lupus erythematosus acutus.

2. Lupus erythematosus acutus may be due to focal infection from the kidneys.

3. Lupus erythematosus acutus may present lesions of diffuse cutaneous hemorrhages.

4. Skin lesions in lupus erythematosus acutus may clear up in spite of the unfavorable continuation of the systemic condition.

5. Acute lupus erythematosus is a herald of focal infection and calls for a thorough search for it.

6. Lupus erythematosus acutus is in close pathogenetic relationship with erythema multiforme.

7. A stricter differentiation should be exercised in reporting cases as lupus erythematosus acutus disseminatus. A case may be disseminated without being acute. Only cases which start acutely and run as such throughout should be termed lupus erythematosus acutus disseminatus.

DISCUSSION

DR. W. H. GOECKERMAN, Rochester, Minn: This case strikes at fundamental pathology responsible for dermatoses. Within the last few years I have seen two cases of acute disseminated lupus erythematosus come to necropsy. Both had been under the observation of a dermatologist and clinician for several months, and it was impossible to find any evidence of tuberculosis. An exploratory abdominal section was made because of the indefinite abdominal symptoms present, and even then we were unable to find any evidence of abdominal tuberculosis; but at the postmortem examination both cases showed involved abdominal glands, and the organism was demonstrated definitely in smears. I was impressed with the fact that we could not clinically determine the presence of tuberculosis when only the abdominal glands were involved. Gennerich, within the last year, reported a case in which he found definite gland pathology, but he was not willing to say that it was tuberculosis. I kept these observations in mind and determined that on the first occasion I would attempt to treat a case along the line we were treating Hodgkin's disease, with deep roentgen-ray therapy. About six or eight months ago a case was presented that somewhat resembled that of Dr. Scholtz'. The patient had marked lesions in the mouth; his hair had practically all dropped out. A week after the first treatment he had decidedly improved. A few weeks later the symptoms had all disappeared, the hair had grown in and he had gained in weight. I heard from him last week, and he said that he was doing the chores on his brother's farm, and none of the cutaneous lesions had reappeared. As to whether we learned anything about the etiology of lupus erythematosus in this case, I would not venture to say; but I wish to call attention to the desirability of repeating this form of treatment in other appropriate cases.

Dr. Everett S. Lain, Oklahoma City: I am especially pleased to hear another confirmation of an opinion I have held since the work of Rosenow on focal infections, namely, that lupus erythematosus is also a result of focal infection. My attention was first directed to this relation by seeing a patient with both herpes zoster and lupus erythematosus. I have many times seen clinical evidence of this apparent relationship. I am trusting that some one may prove or disprove this theory. It is my opinion that lupus erythematosus is merely a skin reaction to a toxin, probably having various foci of pathogenesis.

Dr. William T. Corlett, Cleveland: The etiology of lupus erythematosus has been for many years the subject of controversy, and the prevailing opinion as to its causation has shifted from time to time, the latest being that it is due to the presence of one or more foci of tuberculosis. Before Dr. Stokes published his interesting and complete article on his findings in a number of cases I was inclined to the opinion, my clinical experience at least had led me to so believe, that lupus erythematosus was not associated with tuberculosis, because in the cases I had seen there had been no evidence, so far as I was able to determine, of an infection of tuberculosis—that is, generalized or marked tuberculosis. Dr. Stokes, however, led me to believe that there might be insignificant foci in various parts of the body that had been overlooked by the ordinary means of examination, and since reading his article I have sought more carefully for evidence of tuberculosis whenever lupus erythematosus presented itself. I have never been convinced, however, that it was the only cause of the disease, and I am glad to hear another view, a little broader it may be, set forth in regard to its etiology. I still feel, however, that the last word has not yet been said as to the etiology of lupus erythematosus.

Dr. Marcus Haase, Memphis, Tenn.: I recall the case of an elderly woman who had three attacks of acute disseminate lupus erythematosus. I saw her in the last attack and she had none of the fixed type of lesions. From the information I received from her physician, a general practitioner, I learned that the attacks had disappeared within from three to five weeks of their onset, and that they came on suddenly. When I saw her, she had lesions on the face, over the upper arms and on the chest. The family physician said that the lesions she had during this third attack could not be differentiated from those he had seen in the two previous attacks. This woman was suffering from pyelonephrosis at that time and was under the care of an internist. What I wish to bring out is that if her two previous attacks were similar to the one she had at that time, then this case could not have been mistaken for a case of erythema multiforme, and while I am not positive of my diagnosis of acute lupus erythematosus, at the time I saw her it was my opinion that she had that disease.

Dr. WILLIAM FRICK, Kansas City, Mo.: With all our studies of lupus erythematosus we have not been able to find any direct connection between that disease and tuberculosis. It seems to me that the preponderance of opinion would be that it is a toxic condition, and I do not see why we should not have a toxic condition producing lupus erythematosus in a tuberculous case, whether of the lungs or elsewhere. This paper seems to confirm the belief that lupus erythematosus is due to a toxic condition and may be due to conditions other than tuberculosis, and at the same time it may develop in a patient with tuberculosis. In other words, it may be due to various causes.

Dr. RICHARD L. SUTTON, Kansas City, Mo.: At present, we can divide these cases into two distinct types, the acute and the chronic. The acute is almost always, if not invariably, due to tuberculosis, and the chronic is a symptomatic manifestation of any one of a number of factors. For many years, I have shared the opinion of Drs. Chipman, Lain, Stokes, Highman and others, that focal infection plays an important part in the causation of many of the chronic cases, and I do not believe that any patients with chronic lupus erythematosus should undergo a course of treatment until this possibility has been thoroughly investigated. Hartzell has recently reported a case in which the removal of an infected tooth was followed by a spectacular disappearance of the cutaneous lesions, and many English observers likewise have called attention to focal infection as a probable etiologic factor in the chronic type of the disease.

Dr. MOSES SCHOLTZ: To me the point of interest was the morphologic relationship between lupus erythematosus and erythema multiforme. Here we had the typical lesions of lupus erythematosus superseded and modified by lesions of erythema multiforme. The question is, Were these both due to the same etiologic factor? In my opinion cases like this suggest that lupus erythematosus is not an independent clinical entity but merely a certain type of skin reaction; and I was glad to hear at least one opinion to substantiate this view.

NEW FINDINGS IN PEMPHIGUS VULGARIS

PRELIMINARY COMMUNICATION

KAREL GAWALOWSKI, M.D.

Assistant in Dermatology, Bohemian Skin Clinic, Charles University

PRAGUE, CZECHOSLOVAKIA

Pemphigus vulgaris and the other clinical forms of the pemphigus group have so far had an obscure etiology. Neither the nervous and infectious nor the French toxic theories have been proved. Samberger's[1] new work on the lymphatic reaction brought a new light on this problem. It shows that the bullae in pemphigus being on a non-inflammatory basis are caused by hyperproduction of lymph which becomes accumulated in the epidermis (active lymphatic edema). Prof. Samberger says in his textbook:[2] "This active edema is brought on sometimes by the contraction of the blood vessels from a vasomotor irritation. The edema, however, cannot be produced by irritation of vasomotors; it results from the hypersecretion of the lymph. The hypersecretion of the lymph did not even in these cases result from a vasomotor irritation; it was incited by the oxygen starved tissues." And further: "In some cases, not in all by any means, the irritation of the vasomotors can become the indirect cause of them (urticaria, pemphigus)."

The serious condition of patients suffering from pemphigus suggests a serious internal disturbance, probably a disturbance of internal secretions.

What endocrine glands would first attract our attention? If we take for our starting point those cases caused indirectly by a vasoconstriction we logically come first to the suprarenals, as it is epinephrin that causes an energetic vasoconstriction.

In view of the fact that Samberger's theory presumes the correctness of Heidenhain's theory that the lymph is secreted by the blood capillaries, and the correctness of Mareš's hypothesis, which asserts that by hyperproduction of the lymph an organism provides a sufficient flow of blood and thus of oxygen, the possibility presents itself that epinephrin may cause a hypersecretion of the lymph not only indirectly through the vasomotors, but also directly by increasing the secretory capacity of the blood vessels.

1. Samberger: Das Menschliche Oedem, Arch. f. Dermat. u. Syph., 1921, No. 132, p. 42. Die lymphatishe Hautreaktion, Wien. klin. Wchnschr., 1918.

2. Samberger: Vseobecna dermatologie. II vyd. Praha. Unie, 1920.

A hyperadrenalinemia would be the cause of the trouble, and naturally there would be other evidences of its existence. Experimentally, little is known about the effect of repeated small doses of epinephrin. Other experimental facts show a series of effects of epinephrin from which it is possible to construct a theoretical picture of the disease caused by hyperadrenalinemia, little known clinically, and observed at most in the course of pluriglandular syndromes.

The main changes can be expected in functional disturbance of other endocrine glands. For the basis of our consideration can be taken the Eppinger-Falta-Rudinger scheme, modified by Aschner, and well founded experimentally and clinically, in spite of the fact that some have lately doubted its correctness (Weil).

Blum, in 1901, after an injection of epinephrin noticed glycosuria. Hyperglycemia is also known. We can, therefore, expect glycosuria or hyperglycemia as a result of a functional disturbance of the pancreas. Judging from the scheme, we can further expect hypovarism, loss of menses, thinning of regional hair, and finally hyperthyroidism, clinically manifested by thick hair, nervousness and tremor. Perhaps even premature grayness would occur.

Thyroid Hypophysis

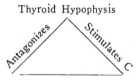

Ovary Pancreas Parathyroid antagonizes intensely (Chromaffin system).

Of the other experimental facts, the most interesting is the effect on the thermal regulation; on blood and blood circulation. It is known that after an injection of epinephrin the temperature of hibernating animals rises rapidly. Following repeated small doses we could expect an at least subjective internal sensation of warmth, accompanied by thirst; externally, however, there would be rather a sensation of cold. due to vasoconstriction.

The blood picture changes (Port-Brenow [3])—the number of white corpuscles increases with a relative increase in the number of polymorphonuclear leukocytes and a decrease of lymphocytes. So far as the blood circulation is concerned, no definite conclusions can be made. Any effect on the blood pressure under physiologic conditions has been denied (Gley [4]); nevertheless, a rise rather than a fall can be expected. Also, the effect on the kidneys is yet under discussion, and the relation between renal sclerosis and hyperadrenalinemia is doubtful (Volhard).

3. Port-Brenow in Weil: Innere Sekretion, Berlin, Springer, 1921.
4. Gley in Langlois, I. P., and Binet, L.: Presse méd., 1922, No. 18, p. 195

From this brief sketch of an assumed, clinically unknown disease, it appears that it is a chronic and serious condition, and also that many of the expected symptoms—deduced from the cited points of view—have not been observed as yet in pemphigus.

AUTHOR'S CASES

After a careful clinical examination of two patients, Mrs. H., 52 years old, and Mrs. I., 51 years old, we discovered many of the expected symptoms: the sensation of thirst, thick hair, thin regional hair and sensation of cold on the skin. Menses ceased at the age of 42 in the first and at the age of 48 in the second patient.

In the case of Mrs. H. the disease started in July, 1921, but she had felt weak since Christmas, 1920, and although she had never before perspired, a striking perspiration began. At present her skin is dry, fairly oily, with bullae all over the body. The skin is pale except in places of healed bullae which are pigmented.

Mrs. I. had a sudden onset at Christmas time, 1921, with blisters in the mouth. She had few but large bullae, especially over the abdomen and lumbosacral region. Her skin was dry, pale and fairly oily. Bullae healed with pigmentation. Both patients had ischuria and urinated twice daily from 500 to 600 c.c. in twenty-four hours. Metabolic investigation by Bang-Frejka's method revealed sugar in the blood (Mrs. H., 0.139 per cent., Mrs. I., 0.131 per cent.). A test for sugar in the urine was negative.

Judging from that fact, I presumed that the function of the pancreas was impaired, and expected a positive Loewi eye reaction. It was positive. Mrs. H. had a strong mydriasis, Mrs. I. a slightly less marked but definite mydriasis. Carried on with the patients' own serum, the reaction proved that the serum contained epinephrin, and at the same time it demonstrated the hypofunction of the pancreas. The Meltzer-Ehrmann test showed analogous results. Mrs. H.'s serum caused a definite mydriasis in the frog's eye; in the other case mydriasis was only slight if not doubtful. It is impossible to draw any quantitative deductions from this inexact reaction, but the difference in the degree of mydriasis, parallel in the two cases, proves that it was caused by the same substance—undoubtedly epinephrin.

The Leaven-Trendelenburg test was impracticable, owing to the fact that the venules of hibernating frogs were too narrow to allow the introduction of a cannula without thrombosis, so that the presence of hyperadrenalinemia was not directly proved.

The fact that patients with pemphigus showed a marked clinical improvement under the influence of diacetylamidoazotoluene (dimazon) ointment, and that new bullae did not appear enabled us to carry on a test for epinephrin glycosuria and glycemia and to ascertain whether a theoretically expected clinical aggravation would take place. To start with, we injected intradermally 0.2 mg. of 1 per cent. epinephrin solution to prevent an eventual severe reaction. Resulting urticaria was quickly absorbed; the surrounding skin became anemic; wheals did not form either at the point of injection or around it. A hypersecretion of the lymph from the contraction of the capillaires, from the starvation of the organism for oxygen, could be ruled out. Is there a possibility of direct influence on the secretion of the capillaries?

The injection of 1 mg. of 1 per cent. epinephrin solution caused in Mrs. H. a rise in blood pressure from 115 to 120, and in pulse rate from 108 to 120, with a maximum the tenth minute; moderate palpitation, mydriasis; sugar in the blood, before, 0.188 per cent., after one-half hour and four hours the same (!), sugar in the urine negative. The patient felt weak, even on the second day. Toward evening the first vesicles appeared and on the third day there was an abundant new crop all over the body in spite of constant applications of diacetylamidoazotoluene ointment. The clinical aggravation lasted over fourteen days.

Mrs. I.'s blood pressure rose from 105 to 125, her pulse from 98 to 110, with a maximum in twenty-five minutes; after ten minutes there were palpitation, tremor and mydriasis; sugar in the blood, before, 0.132 per cent., after two and one-half hours 0.377 per cent. (!); sugar in the urine was 0.2 per cent.; she urinated seven hours after the injection. The patient felt very weak for three days. Beginning with the second day, the erosions wept profusely for sixteen days, although dimazon ointment was applied. No new bullae and no edema of the ankles occurred.

Theoretical reasoning caused me to expect an early rise of sugar content and a slow decline. That explains the error made in the first case, in which the blood was taken after one-half hour and then after four hours only, so that the rise of sugar was missed altogether. In the second case one test only was made in the usual time—after two and one-half hours. In the first case, with a greater hyperadrenalinemia (Mrs. H.), there was a lesser reaction; in the second case, with lesser hyperadrenalinemia, there was greater reaction; in both there was a striking increase of lymphatic reaction and an aggravation of the general condition.

The patients were put on a milk diet and fourteen days after the epinephrin injection, a glucose test was made. One hundred and fifty gm. in 500 c.c. of water were administered after breakfast without sugar. Mrs. H. vomited 160 c.c. and retained only about 100 gm. of glucose. Results by the Maclean method were:

Mrs. H., before the test: 0.118 per cent., urine negative; after one hour 0.143 per cent., after two and one-half hours 0.1 per cent. (technical error), after four hours 0.134 per cent.; first urination after nine hours, sugar negative. The maximal rise was missed; a slow decline is evident.

Mrs. I., before the test: 0.131 per cent., urine negative; after one hour 0.187 per cent., after two hours 0.208 per cent., after four hours 0.134 per cent.; sugar after nine hours, 0.15 per cent.

The slow decline of sugar is striking and analogous to diabetic curves; the rise, however, is lower and resembles the curves observed in exophthalmic goiter by Rosenberg. It shows a lowered assimilation limit for carbohydrates, as in hyperthyroidism.

On milk diet, the nitrogen content in twenty-four hours was found to be: Mrs. H., 3.82 gm., 600 c.c. of urine, specific gravity 1.015; Mrs. I., 7.20 gm., 551 c.c. of urine, specific gravity 1.016—a considerably reduced nitrogen elimination in the first, and a moderate one in the second case. In the blood serum: Mrs. H., 42 mg. per 100 c.c.; Mrs. I., 40 mg. per 100 c.c., also a reduction. It is impossible to draw any conclusions. An attempt at nitrogen balance (in the food and in the urine) would be more enlightening. Both patients tolerated meat rather poorly, and mastication was difficult on account of mouth lesions.

A water test (one and one-half liters of tea being used) showed a normal renal permeability for water. The stools showed partially digested muscle fibers and a few fat globules. Urine diastase tested by the MacKenzie-Wallis method was normal (20-26 units). The results would point, then, toward a hypofunction of the internal secretion of the pancreas and a lowered trypsin secretion, while lipase and diastase were normal.

Blood Picture: Few eosinophils—Mrs. H. 0.33 per cent., Mrs. I. 0.5 per cent.; Mrs. H.: red cells 4,200,000, white cells 9,200, polymorphonuclears 69.33 per cent., lymphocytes 22.67 per cent. Mrs. I.: red cells 2,060,000, white cells 10,200, polymorphonuclears 82 per cent., lymphocytes 10.5 per cent. These findings would also agree with those of a hyperadrenalinemia. According to the findings both cases present a disturbance of internal secretions, characterized by hypopancreatism and hyperthyroidism, with a great probability of hyperadrenalinemia and hypovarism.

The disturbance is a mild one in every respect, and its functional character is well in accord with the usual negative necropsy findings. The facts bear out the theoretically deduced correlations. We had further to ascertain whether some known experimental facts are not at variance with the hypothesis that epinephrin increases the secretory capacity of the blood capillaries.

Camus, in 1904,[5] demonstrated that epinephrin increases the lymph flow in his experiment on the thoracic duct, from which a larger amount of lymph was escaping after an injection of epinephrin. The presence of hyperglycemia might cause an objection, as the sugar in the blood might be considered the real cause of the increased amount of lymph. The sugar should be classified as one of Heidenhain's lymphagogues of the second degree, which increase the amount of lymph by abstracting the water from the tissues. How could we, however, explain the fact that after the administration of epinephrin, edema develops, as it did in the case of Mrs. I., if not by the presumption that lymph is produced in a large amount by the capillaries and that its outflow is hindered?

That epinephrin is not a lymphagogue of the first degree was proved by Biedl, who in his series of experiments with injections of extracts of crawfish muscle and other lymphagogues never obtained a glycosuria when epinephrin was injected. Judging from this experiment, the authors conclude that lymphagogues of the first degree are antagonists of epinephrin in their effect on the pancreas (Ev. the liver).

Equally well founded seems the explanation that not the lymphagogue but the secreted lymph is the real antagonist, as was demonstrated by another experiment of Biedl. Epinephrin did not cause glycosuria (in dogs) if from 80 to 100 c.c. of lymph were previously injected. Biedl says that internal secretion of the pancreas, contained in the lymph, counteracts epinephrin, a fact that cannot be disapproved experimentally, except probably by injecting the lymph of a depancreatized animal (dies soon) into another one of the same species.

If the hypothesis that lymph itself counteracts the effect of epinephrin on the liver is correct, we can judge from it, as well as from the assumed effects of epinephrin on lymph secretion that epinephrin regulates the production of the lymph, and the lymph regulates the effect of epinephrin on the liver (and possibly other organs). In other words, epinephrin thus automatically prevents an increase of its own amount over the degree necessary to life.

Viewed from this standpoint, the formation of bullae in pemphigus vulgaris appears to be a disturbance of internal secretion, an expression of a defensive reaction on the part of the organism against epinephrin autointoxication (toxemia). Increased lymphatic reaction following the injection of epinephrin in our patients makes this presumption probable.

Therapy that would prevent the formation of epinephrin or counteract this action would furnish a clinical proof. Epinephrin production

---

5. Camus in Lucien. N.. and Parisot. I.: Glandes surrénales. Paris. 1913. p. 214.

can be limited (only temporarily, as compensation soon takes place) by operative removal of a suprarenal or by impairment of the medullary portion by the roentgen ray. The condition of the patients rules out the first procedure. The second should be used only when there is no other possibility, as Stephan [6] showed recently that doses controlling the action of the medulla destroyed completely the cortex, which is very sensitive. A damage to the cortex would result in a still greater production of sugar from glycogen. The splendid work of Ioshitomi Tokumitsu [7] demonstrated that the cortex and the pancreas are synergists. There is another possible procedure. H. H. Dale [8] proved that an alkaloid isolated from Secale cornutum, ergotoxin, counteracts the effect of epinephrin on the organs innervated by the sympathetics and also on the blood vessels. The question remains, however, whether the minute doses permissible in men, 0.05-0.13 mg., would be therapeutically efficient. In animals, poisoning with ergotoxin prevented the action of epinephrin. Dixon [9] obtained similar results with apocodein in doses of 0.02 gm. It has the disadvantage of acting as a purgative, thus abstracting water from the organism. Further findings and results will be announced later.

SUPPLEMENT

The glucose test was repeated in the case of Mrs. H. and 50 gm. were given. Sugar in the blood before the test was 0.105 per cent., after one-half hour 0.157 per cent., after one hour 0.131 per cent., and after two hours 0.108 per cent. Sugar in the urine after three-quarters of an hour was weakly positive, after one and one-half hours, strongly positive.

Clinically, there were at the same time many bullae. In former tests the sugar had not been found in the urine, probably because a catheterized specimen was not obtained (on account of the lesions on the genitals), and after several hours sugar concentration in the urine was slight.

The epinephrin test was repeated in the case of Mrs. I. (0.6 mg.). Sugar in the blood before the test was 0.131 per cent., after one-half hour 0.174 per cent., after one hour 0.170 per cent., after two hours 0.134 per cent., and after three hours 0.131 per cent. Sugar in the urine was positive after one hour. Blood examination showed at the

6. Stephan: München. med. Wchnschr., 1922, No. 10, p. 339.

7. Tokumitsu, Ioshitomi: Mitteil. aus. d. pathol. Institut der Kais. Univer. zu Sendai, Japan 1:161, 1921.

8. H. H. Dale in Schafer, E. Sharpey: Les glandes à secretion interne, Ed. 2, Paris, O Doin, 1921, p. 95. For other references see Beidl: Innere Sekretion, III. Aufl. Wien., 1916, Urban 1 and Schwarzenberg.

9. Dixon in Schafer: Les glandes à secretion interne.

same time before and after injection 1 per cent. eosinophils, although the white cells, especially the lymphocytes, increased considerably.

Mrs. H. showed a striking change in her general condition and many bullae; she had 22 per cent. eosinophils with a decrease in neutrophils; sugar diastase increased to 50 units.

In general, these tests corroborate our former results. In regard to Bauer's work, we intend to test the uric acid of the blood and urine by the bromhydrate method.

The latest literature brings three interesting communications: Trendelenburg has proved that epinephrin disappeared in the arterial capillaries and thought it was under the effect of some ferment.[10]

Pulay has found hyperglycemia in urticaria.[11]

Vallisnieri and Coli[12] have found that the serum of patients with pemphigus has a weak effect on the suprarenals and none on other organs.

The whole conception remains a hypothesis; either the success of suggestive treatment or the results of pathologic and histologic examinations of necropsy specimens will bring the solution. This hypothesis helped us to discover the new facts and if it does not accomplish any more, it will have done its duty.

---

10. Zentralbl. f. Herzkrankheiten, 1921, p. 7.
11. Klin. Wchnschr., 1922, No. 9.
12. Biochem. e. terap. speriment., 1921, No. 7.

Abstracts from Current Literature

THE EARLY MANIFESTATIONS AND RATIONAL TREATMENT OF TABES DORSALIS. H. F. STOLL, Am. J. M. Sc. **163**:723 (May) 1922.

Particular stress is laid on the points of physical examination, especially emphasizing the Argyll Robertson pupils, diminished or absent knee reflexes, areas of anesthesia and tabetic pains. Blood and spinal fluid examinations should also be considered carefully in arriving at a diagnosis. The usual mercury and arsphenamin courses of treatment are recommended with intraspinal treatment if improvement does not follow, using the original Swift-Ellis method.

ALASTRIM OR KAFFIR MILK POX. L. M. MOODY, Ann. Trop. M. & Parasitol. **16**:21 (March) 1922.

A description is given of an eruptive fever called alastrim which occurred in Jamaica as an epidemic from May, 1920, to March, 1921. After an incubation of from ten to fourteen days the disease developed abruptly with pyrexia, headache and backache, followed in three or four days by an eruption of papules which soon changed to vesicles and pustules.

The areas involved, the temperature curve and the general symptomatology closely resemble variola.

Patients previously vaccinated had cases of a milder type, and the opinion is given that alastrim and vaccinia belong to the same group but are slightly different as one disease almost completely immunizes against the other.

CLINICAL CALORIMETRY XXX. METABOLISM IN ERYSIPELAS. W. COLEMAN, D. P. BARR, E. F. DUBOIS and G. F. SODERSTROM, Arch. Int. Med. **29**:567 (May) 1922.

Ten experiments showed an increase in metabolism of from 19 to 42 per cent. above the average normal, this increase being roughly proportional to the degree of fever. The regulation of body temperature is similar to that observed in malaria during high continuous fever, and no specific differences were found between the metabolism in erysipelas and in typhoid fever, the protein metabolism being greatly increased in both.

JAMIESON, Detroit.

SKIN IRRITANTS: EXTERNAL AND INTERNAL. C. G. LANE, Boston M. & S. J. **187**:108 (July 20) 1922.

Six hundred records of the Massachusetts General Hospital Out-Patient Skin Department in which there was a diagnosis of dermatitis or dermatitis venenata were studied. Ten per cent. were due to exposure to woods and plants, 20 per cent. to the applications of medicinal agents and 11 per cent. to industrial factors. This group includes cases from accidental contact with irritating substances, also cases in which substances are applied with intent to deceive. Skin eruptions from ingestion of food and drugs are referred to. Case reports of various groups are cited.

PUSEY, Chicago.

A NOTE ON GENERAL PARESIS AT THE DANVERS STATE HOS-
PITAL. H. M. WATKINS, Boston M. & S. J. **187**:137*(July 27) 1922.

From 12 to 17 per cent. of all admissions to this state hospital for the
insane show evidence of syphilis in some form. Sixty-seven cases have been
studied and routine treatment outlined. Twenty per cent. are able to "carry
on" outside the hospital by the aid of the social service department, and 77 per
cent. of those in the hospital are able to do some form of useful work.

LANE, Boston.

CASE OF ERYTHROEDEMA (THE "PINK DISEASE"): AND THE
QUESTION OF ACRODYNIA ("EPIDEMIC ERYTHEMA").
F. PARKES WEBER, Brit. J. Child. Dis. **19**:17 (Jan.-Mar.) 1922.

The author refers to a case which he has lately reported (abstract, ARCHIVES
DERMATOLOGY AND SYPHILOLOGY **4**:708 [Nov.] 1921) as "A Condition Resembling
Lupus Pernio in a Child." That title well describes the appearance of the
child's extremities, but other features have suggested that the condition might
better be classified as "erythroedema," ninety-one cases of which have been
reported in Australia. Subsequently, Weston (*Arch. of Pediat.* **37**:513, 1920)
reported eight cases; Byfield (*Am. J. Dis. Child.* **20**:347, 1920, abstr., ARCHIVES
DERMATOLOGY AND SYPHILOLOGY **3**:659 [May] 1921) has described a series of
seventeen; Emerson (*J. A. M. A.* **77**:285, 1921, abstr., ARCHIVES DERMATOLOGY
AND SYPHILOLOGY **4**:546 [Oct.] 1921), Cartin and Zahorsky have also reported
cases. In America, this affection has been called "acrodynia." A really fitting
name is yet to be found; the author is of the opinion that "acrodynia" is a
poor one, for it alludes to only a single symptom of the complex.

The patients are usually under 4 years, and the symptoms, which usually
last about two months. include irritability, muscular asthenia, mental changes
and an erythroderma of the extremities and often of the face as well, desquamating frequently and with an ill-defined border (differing thus from the eruption in pellagra, as well as by its predilection for the palms and soles). It
is not known whether the cause is a fault in nutrition or whether the condition is an infectious neuritis, possibly postinfluenzal.

DERMATOPOLYNEURITIS (ACRODYNIA: ERYTHROEDEMA).
H. THURSFIELD and D. H. PATERSON. Brit. J. Child. Dis. **19**:27 (Jan.-
March) 1922.

In a female child, aged 1 year, a typical picture of the syndrome described
in the foregoing abstract appeared, of six weeks' duration. Acute intussuscep-
tion brought the case to necropsy, where no gross abnormality could be found.
In a second case, that of a child, aged 18 months. the temperature varied
between 98 and 104 F.

PARKHURST. Toledo. Ohio.

A CONDITION SOMEWHAT RESEMBLING LUPUS PERNIO IN A
CHILD. SEQUEL: QUESTION OF ERYTHRO-EDEMA (THE
"PINK DISEASE") AND ACRODYNIA ("EPIDEMIC ERYTHEMA").
F. PARKES WEBER, Brit. J. Dermat. & Syph. **34**:111 (April) 1922.

Describing a case demonstrated before the Dermatological Section of the
Royal Society of Medicine on April 21. 1921. in which the patient exhibited
circulatory deficiency of the extremities and ulcerations of feet. hands and

nasal septum, Weber states that the condition at that time might have been termed "acrodermatitis chronica mutilans." Acting on the suggestion of Sequeira that the case might be a severe form of erythro-edema, Weber investigated the subject, and he concludes that that diagnosis was correct. He then reviews the literature of erythro-edema by Australian authors and of acrodynia by American authors, and concludes that the two diseases are in all probability identical. Weber's case resembled closely Byfield's cases in his paper on "A Polyneuritic Syndrome Resembling Pellagra-Acrodynia Seen in Very Young Children."

BRIEF NOTES ON EPIDERMOPHYTON RUBRUM, CASTELLANI, 1909 (TRICHOPHYTON PURPUREUM, BANG, 1910) AND TRICHOPYTON VIOLACEUM VAR. DECALVANS, CASTELLANI, 1913. WITH REMARKS ON "ECZEMA MARGINATUM" ("TINEA CRURIS SEU INGUINALIS") IN JAPAN AND "LA LI TOU" OR "PARASITIC FOLLICULITIS" ("TINEA DECALVANS" PRO PARTE) OF SOUTHERN CHINA. M. Ota, Brit. J. Dermat. & Syph. **34**:120 (April) 1922.

Following investigation of cases seen in Japan and Manchuria, Ota concludes that the commonest type of tinea cruris seen in those countries is due to *Epidermophyton rubrum*, Castellani, 1909. In his examination of three cases of Chinese "la li tou" *Achorion schoenleini* was isolated twice and *Trichophyton violaceum* var. decalvans once, and the writer concludes that the Chinese term covers at least two diseases, favus and "tinea decalvans" of Castellani.

CASE OF SCLERODERMA (SCLERODACTYLY TYPE) WITH ADRENAL INSUFFICIENCY. J. H. Sequeira, Brit. J. Dermat. & Syph. **34**:124 (April) 1922.

Sequeira reports the findings in a case of extensive scleroderma in which exhaustive investigations were made. The blood pressure showed a great increase following injection of epinephrin, and Sequeira says that this is incontestable evidence of suprarenal inadequacy. He proposes grafting suprarenal tissue into the patient, and expects to report his results at an early date.

PRIMARY EPITHELIOMAS OF THE SKIN. J. Darier, Brit. J. Dermat. & Syph. **34**:145, 1922.

In this paper Darier discusses the question of the relative malignancy and the sensitiveness to radiotherapy of the different types of skin cancer. He confines himself to three types, the prickle cell and basal cell epitheliomas and a third type, which he styles the metatypical. After reviewing briefly the clinical and histologic findings of the first two types, he discusses the third type in detail, saying that it has not been described previously.

He says that this third type constitutes from 10 to 15% of the cases of epithelioma. It is usually seen on the face, and notably on the nose, but it also occurs on the scalp, neck and in other locations. Clinically it is difficult to distinguish from the basal cell epithelioma, and its nature is often suggested because of its resistance to radiotherapy. It usually begins as a grayish red, rather soft and translucent appearing projecting tumor; but sometimes it appears as an erosion or as a destructive and mutilating ulcer. Its development is more rapid than that of the basal cell type, but it may remain stationary for some months or years and then extend rapidly and produce deep ulceration. The lymph glands may become involved, and general metastases may occur.

Histologic examination is usually necessary to make an absolute diagnosis, and two types are seen microscopically. In both of these types, which are described fully, there are some features of both the basal and prickle cell epithelioma. Differentiation of this type is important because of the more serious prognosis in this form as compared to the basal cell epithelioma.

In a general way the author outlines the treatment of epithelioma as follows:

1. By complete and radical surgical excision: operable prickle cell and circumscribed metatypical epithelioma.

2. By radiotherapy: basal cell epitheliomas without deep invasion.

3. By intensive radiotherapy or radiopuncture: prickle cell epitheliomas which are not operable but completely accessible, also the deeply destructive basal cell or metatypical varieties.

HAEMATOGENOUS INFECTION IN TRICHOPHYTIA. E. Bruusgaard, Brit. J. Dermat. & Syph. **34**:150, 1922.

After reviewing briefly but comprehensively the clinical types and some experimental considerations of trichophytids, Bruusgaard discusses the possible sources of these eruptions. He feels that in most cases these exanthems must be considered of hematogenous origin, because of the acute form, the general symptoms, the symmetry of the eruption, etc.

He states that if we take the view that the exanthems are of hematogenous origin and due to trichophyton, we have to prove that the fungus can spread through the blood vessels to the skin. Hitherto efforts to cultivate the fungus from the blood or to discover it in sections of extirpated nodes or spots have been unsuccessful.

He then reports the case of a man, 68 years of age, suffering with kerion Celsi of the chin and submaxillary region, who developed an eruption of an erythema nodosum type on the forearm. They were able to demonstrate spores in a lesion excised from the arm, the organisms being found both in the tissue and in the blood vessels. *Trichophyton gypseum* from the lesions on the arm was identical with that grown from the lesions on the chin. This is, then, the first instance recorded in which hematogenous spread of trichophyton has been demonstrated.

PSEUDO-ALOPECIA AREATA. Haldin Davis, Brit. J. Dermat. & Syph. **34**: 162, 1922.

Davis described a condition in which children have exhibited patches on the scalp, to superficial examination resembling ringworm patches, but which fail to yield any stumps containing fungus. The affected patches are of small size, as a rule, and are covered with stumps, which characteristically are broken off very close to the scalp. Even when effectually seized they do not come out easily like the stumps in alopecia areata. On microscopic examination the chief point of interest is that the distal end of the stump is frayed out, and the hair is apparently split up into a number of bundles. In no case has there been more than one such patch on the head, and the patch has always been situated on the anterior part of the crown, or at the side, above and in front of the ear.

Davis believes that it is the scratching or rubbing of the spot by the patient which causes the breakage of the hair close to the scalp. They are thus in reality artefacts, not intentionally or even consciously produced. In support of this view he cites the nature of the stumps, the invariably single lesion, and the easily accesible site of the eruption. For this condition he suggests the name pseudo-alopecia areata, if it is advisable to give it any name at all.

With this idea in mind, Davis has reconsidered the outbreak of "epidemic alopecia areata" described by him as it occurred in an orphan asylum for girls, in 1914, and he thinks that the large number of cases seen at that time were cases of the factitious type described in the foregoing resulting from the effect of mass suggestion.

A NOTE ON THE USE OF FLAVINE-STARCH POULTICES IN ECZEMA. J. Ferguson Smith, Brit. J. Dermat. & Syph. **34**:166, 1922.

Smith recalls the common use (in Scotland particularly) of cold starch poultices for the treatment of acute dermatitis, but states that previously no antiseptics, except boric acid, have been used with it, because the older antiseptics will not be tolerated when used in a strength sufficient to make them effective. The flavines are, however, comparatively non-irritating in efficient strength, and their activity is enhanced rather than diminished in the presence of a serous discharge.

He has recently treated patients with severely infected "seborrheic" eczema of the head and groin with encouraging results, using the following preparation:

Four tablespoonfuls of rice starch and 10 grains (0.65 gm.) of acriflavine are mixed with a little cold water, one pint of boiling water is added, and the mixture is boiled with constant stirring until it thickens. When nearly cold it is poured on a dressing cloth so as to form a layer half an inch (12.7 mm.) thick. When quite cold and set it is covered with a single layer of gauze or butter muslin, and applied to the part. It is changed three or four times a day, and at each change the part is bathed with acriflavine 1:1,000 in 0 85 per cent. sodium chlorid. These applications should be continued until it is considered that more stimulating remedies may be safely applied.

CLINICAL AND HISTOLOGICAL STUDIES ON THE PATHOLOGICAL CHANGES IN THE ELASTIC TISSUES OF THE SKIN. A. Kissmeyer and Carl With, Brit. J. Dermat. & Syph. **34**:175 and 221, 1922.

Kissmeyer and With have studied the subject of pathologic changes in the elastic tissues of the skin from both the clinical and the microscopic aspects.

Detailed findings of changes occurring in various conditions are grouped under the following headings:

(1) Degeneration of newly-formed elastic tissue in scars.
(2) Elastic tissue degeneration in transplantation patches.
(3) Elastic degeneration in granulation tissue.
(4) Pseudoxanthoma elasticum.
(5) Yellowish color of skin from various causes.

As a result of their observations they conclude that the different clinical forms are not characterized by histologically different aspects, as stated by Arzt and Bosselini.

Different forms of elastic degeneration show themselves partly by a quantitative increase in elastin; as an irregularity in thickness, the fibers most often becoming thicker; frequently there appears a peculiar curling up of the elastic fibers into balls. Simultaneously with this the elastin seems to show a greater inclination to break. With this is seen rarely a formation of amorphous masses of elastin. It is characteristic of all changes that they leave a narrow belt uninvolved under the epidermis. Only under this do the changes commence which occupy the papillary body and the upper part of the cutis, but they do not go deeper into this (except in pseudoxanthoma elasticum).

. In senile degeneration the degenerative changes are often diffuse. In scars, either traumatic or inflammatory, the degenerative changes are most frequently localized. In pseudoxanthoma elasticum the changes are more strongly pronounced; the collagen bundles, in connection with the elastin, have formed small, sharply defined tumor-like formations, of which the main histologic characteristic is a strong curling up and granular necrosis of the elastic fibers and "elastorrhexis." The more deeply seated changes in pseudoxanthoma elasticum were possibly due to its development at an early age.

The elastic degeneration, produced by the continued influence of the weather over long periods on the parts which are exposed thereto and are especially susceptible on account of special structure, is found first and foremost in senile degeneration, but also in "presenility" in traumatic scars and in scars from transplantation and burns, just as after granulation processes, because the newly formed elastic tissue is less capable of resisting the factors mentioned.

The small elastomas and the elastic degeneration seen now and then in tuberculous and syphilitic lupoids must presumably be regarded as a further development of the degeneration process of the normal elastic tissue dependent on the inflammation and different from the slow degeneration of regenerated and therefore less resistant elastic tissue.

It has been tried before to discriminate between histologic types of elastic degeneration, but it is impossible because the histologic aspect may be identical in the different conditions and only contingent on the process.

To attempt a morphologic classification discriminating between diffuse and circumscribed forms is impossible, because the senile elastic degeneration is not always diffuse, and because pseudoxanthoma elasticum is sometimes circumscribed and sometimes diffuse.

The writers suggest the following classification on an etiologic basis:

1. Diffuse senile degeneration.

2. Presenile degeneration, no doubt of newly formed elastic tissue in scar from traumas, burns, transplantation, and after granulation processes, which is less capable of resisting the weather. Approximate to this group must be counted colloid-milium.

3. Pseudoxanthoma elasticum.

4. The small elastomas seen now and then in tuberculous and syphilitic lupoids, which presumably arise on a basis of an acute degeneration by inflammation, and as a further development of the degeneration of the normal elastic tissue which is found more or less pronounced in chronic granulation processes.

SYPHILIS OF THE TESTICLE CONFINED TO THE EPIDIDYMIS. A. REITH FRASER. Brit. J. Dermat. & Syph. **34**:195, 1922.

Fraser reviews the subject of syphilitic involvement of the epididymis independent of testicular involvement, and cites numerous authorities to show that such involvement can occur. The time of involvement of the epididymis varies in wide limits—from two months to 18 years after infection—according to the literature, but the majority of cases occur during the early secondary period. An acute interstitial epididymitis and gummatous formation are the two types recognized. The acute type has to be differentiated from gonorrheal epididymitis, while the chronic form has to be distinguished from chronic gonorrheal epididymitis, tuberculous disease or new growth.

Fraser then reports a case of syphilitic interstitial epididymitis occurring eighteen years after infection. The condition was bilateral, being acute on one side and chronic on the other. There was unilateral implication of the vas, but the testes, prostate and seminal vesicles were uninvolved. There was no other evidence of syphilis.

CLINICAL NOTE—LEUCONYCHIA STRIATA. KNOWSLEY SIBLEY, Brit. J. Dermat. & Syph. **34**:238, 1922.

A case of familial leukonychia is reported.

A CASE ILLUSTRATING THE ASSOCIATION OF VON RECKLING-HAUSEN'S DISEASE WITH DERANGEMENT OF INTERNAL SECRETION. ERNEST MALLAM, Brit. J. Dermat. & Syph. **34**:239, 1922.

This article contains the report of a case of von Recklinghausen's disease which the author feels is associated with a destructive tumor of the pineal gland. Many of the tumors disappeared following an attack of mumps associated with orchitis.

. SENEAR, Chicago.

SYPHILIS OF THE LUNG. A. FRIEDLANDER and R. J. ERICKSON, J. A. M. A. **79**:291 (July 22) 1922.

This article deals only with the acquired type. The necropsy incidence is from 0.14 to 0.3 per cent. Pathologically, the commonest forms are fibroid induration and gumma. There are no distinguishing diagnostic features. Roentgenologic evidence is of some value but is not conclusive. In the presence of symptoms of pulmonary tuberculosis, with negative sputum and a positive Wassermann reaction, syphilis of the lungs may be suspected, and the patient may be subjected to intensive antisyphilitic therapy.

This report records the pertinent facts of six cases.

MICHAEL, Houston, Texas.

OBSERVATIONS ON THE POISONOUS NATURE OF THE WHITE-MARKED TUSSOCK-MOTH. H. H. KNIGHT, J. Parasitol. **8**:133 (March) 1922.

In cocoon hunters and also experimentally lesions resembling urticaria were developed with swelling, pain and sometimes fever, these symptoms lasting two or three days. It was found that barbed hairs located in prominent tufts on the dorsal surface of the caterpillar apparently became hooked in the pores of the skin and could be removed only with difficulty. The poison glands may not be fully developed until the larva is nearly full grown.

A mucilaginous pulp of purslane leaves was found to be an excellent palliative.

RADIUM THERAPY OF CANCER OF THE MOUTH AND THROAT. C. E. FIELD, N. Y. State J. M. **22**:121, 1922.

This is an interesting article containing valuable details of technic.

SOME STUDIES IN THE EARLY TREATMENT OF CONGENITAL SYPHILIS. T. G. GIVAN, N. Y. State J. M. **22**:127, 1922.

This is a valuable report of a series of infants and children treated at the Long Island .College Hospital. It is demonstrated that the most important factor in the treatment of congenital syphilis is to begin treatment long before birth. Of twenty-seven cases in which the mother received energetic treatment during pregnancy, the infant gave a negative Wassermann test in twenty; in the remaining seven the Wassermann test was not taken. Of fifteen cases in which the mother received no treatment during pregnancy, the Wassermann test was positive in eleven; in only four of these was the Wassermann test changed to negative by postnatal treatment. The treatment recommended for the children is mercury by the mouth and by intramuscular injections, and also neo-arsphenamin intravenously or intramuscularly.

A CLASSIFICATION OF NEUROSYPHILIS WITH SOME REMARKS CONCERNING THERAPY. LEON H. CORNWALL, N. Y. State J. M. **22**: 316 (July) 1922.

The author makes a classification of varieties of neurosyphilis on the basis of the tissue involved—meningeal, vascular, parenchymatous, etc.—with illustrative cases. Good results were obtained with intraspinal therapy in certain cases in which intravenous therapy had failed. The author insists on the necessity of spinal fluid examination in all cases of syphilis.

WILLIAMS, New York.

CONCERNING THE NATURE OF BENIGN LYMPHOGRANULOMA. J. SCHAUMANN, Acta dermat.-ven. **2**:409 (April) 1922.

In the sputum of his Case 1 (described in the *Annales*, 1917, p. 375), the author has found the bacilli of bovine tuberculosis, as proved both morphologically and culturally, as well as by animal inoculation. He concludes that the syndrome of benign lymphogranuloma, including lupus pernio, Boeck's sarcoid and the erythrodermic form of benign lymphogranuloma (*Annales*, 1920, p. 561) is probably always the result of infection during childhood with the bovine tubercle bacillus, by way of the tonsils and respiratory tract rather than by way of the gastro-intestinal tract.

THE NEWER PRECIPITATION REACTIONS IN SYPHILIS. H. BOAS and B. PONTOPPIDAN, Acta dermat.-ven. **2**:419 (April) 1922.

The authors have done the third modification of Meinicke's reaction in 463 serums and sixty-three spinal fluids; they have tried the Sachs-Georgi reaction in 880 serums and seventy-two spinal fluids, using the second modification of the original technic. Serums from cases of tabes and paresis, with both methods, especially that of Meinicke, gave disappointing results. Occasionally a nonspecific reaction is obtained with the Sachs-Georgi technic; but not in any special pathologic conditions, as in the case of the Wassermann reaction, which has been found positive in malaria, scarlatina, and so on. In conclusion, it is stated that the two reactions are valuable only as supplements to the Wassermann reaction. Although easy to perform, the reading is very difficult and requires a trained serologist.

RECURRENT MIGRATING LYMPHANGITIS. O. Michaelis, Acta dermat.-ven. **2**:440 (April) 1922.

Two rather ill-nourished women presented this affection, the symptoms consisting in the appearance, for a few days at a time, of one or two nodules, in various locations about the thighs. These nodules were not sharply circumscribed, were not especially sensitive, and were sometimes erythematous. In both cases, they had first appeared after an attack of epidemic influenza, during which the patient had received injections of camphorated oil in the thighs. In the absence of a biopsy examination, the author rules out erythema induratum and ordinary foreign body tumors, concluding that the symptoms are a result of the oil injections in a soil of latent tuberculosis.

COMPARATIVE STUDIES OF TWO DIFFERENT EXTRACTS IN THE WASSERMANN REACTION. K. Heden, Acta dermat.-ven. **2**:451 (April) 1922.

The author describes in detail his method of preparing an ethereal extract of human heart muscle for use as antigen in the Wassermann reaction, his purpose having been to obtain a sharper reaction by having the colloid in a state of very fine dispersion. Lesser's technic for the preparation of ethereal heart extract is also given, and the results of Wassermann tests made during a period of six years, in 23,891 cases, both Lesser's and the author's antigen having been used in each case. All stages and conditions of syphilis, congenital and acquired, were included in the series, as well as cases for diagnosis, and the author's extract seemed to give distinctly better results throughout.

A CASE OF LEUKODERMA FOLLOWING PARAPSORIASIS. J. Almkvist. Acta dermat.-ven. **2**:468 (April) 1922.

A man, aged 26, presented an eruption of lichenoid parapsoriasis of three months' duration when first seen by the author in April, 1920. After fruitless treatment, he disappeared. Later he returned, and it was then found that the old lesions had disappeared after repeated exposure to the sun at an island resort. In their place were leukodermic spots, set in a deeply tanned background, and there was a sparse scattering of new papules.

A SECONDARY ERUPTION RECURRING IN SYPHILIS FOURTEEN YEARS AFTER INFECTION. N. Rhodin, Acta dermat.-ven. **2**:521 (April) 1922.

In 1908 and 1909, the patient had had a macular and later a papular eruption, with a Wassermann reaction which was positive, and became negative under mercurial treatment. In January, 1922, he returned with eroded papules in his mouth. *Spirochaeta pallida* was found in smears from the lesions, and the Wassermann reaction was strongly positive.

THE TREATMENT OF PSORIASIS BY NONSPECIFIC SEROTHERAPY. B. Cederquist, Acta dermat.-ven. **2**:522 (April) 1922.

In nine cases, the author has lately injected an immunizing vaccine prepared from gonococci cultures at three-day intervals, in doses from 25,000,000 to 2,000,000,000, each injection, barring severe reactions, consisting of twice the previous amount. Those who showed no general reaction to the injection did not yield to the treatment; but, in those who reacted more or less violently, the psoriatic lesions often disappeared quickly. In three of the latter, new psoriatic lesions appeared.

SUBCUTANEOUS INJECTIONS OF NEO-ARSPHENAMIN IN THE INTERSTITIAL KERATITIS OF CONGENITAL SYPHILIS. C. Cabannes and J. Chavannaz, J. de méd. de Bordeaux **94**:10 (Jan. 10) 1922.

These injections were given three times a week in the gluteal region, in such a way that the same spot was not injected more often than once a month. A 1 per cent. solution of procain was also employed. There were no untoward results and no discomfort was felt. In the four cases reported, twenty injections seemed to bring about a great improvement.

BIOLOGIC RESEARCHES ON THE FLOCCULATION REACTION OF THE SACHS-GEORGI TEST IN SYPHILIS. S. Nicolau and A. Banciu, Ann. de dermat. et syph. **6**:97 (March) 1922.

The authors have separated the end-substance into its several parts and have found that the patient's serum used in the reaction retains its power of flocculation, as demonstrated by placing it in contact with more of the antigen. This property is destroyed by heat. It is thought to be due to the presence of a catalytic agent of the nature of a diastase. The addition of complement to the serum-antigen mixture temporarily inhibits the flocculation; this protective combination is not stable, however, being destroyed by heat or by the lapse of time.

THE INFLUENCE OF TYPHOID INFECTIONS ON THE BORDET-WASSERMANN REACTION. Mestchersky, Ann. de dermat. et syph. **6**:116 (March) 1922.

The author cites two cases of typhus and one of typhoid, recently seen by him, in which persistently positive Wassermann reactions became persistently negative after the febrile infection. The hyperpyrexia is considerd to be the probable cause of this apparently favorable action.

MACROGLOSSIA WITH LESIONS OF THE CHEEKS AND BUCCAL MUCOSA. L. Chatellier, Ann. de dermat. et syph. **6**:121 (March) 1922.

A firm, nodular thickening, furrowed in places and covered by a pale, apparently scarred mucosa, had lead several times to an erroneous diagnosis of syphilis, with futile antisyphilitic treatment. The condition had probably always been present, and the author classifies it as a nevus (not hemangioma or lymphangioma).

CARDIAC SYPHILIS FORTY-FOUR YEARS AFTER THE CHANCRE. A. Nanta and Cadenat, Ann. de dermat. et syph. **6**:124 (March) 1922.

In a man, aged 74 years, with gummas of the scrotum and a sclerogummatous infiltration of the tongue, there was a partial heart block, illustrated by a polygraphic tracing; all these lesions soon disappeared under antisyphilitic treatment.

SYPHILIS RESISTING ARSENIC AND MERCURY, YIELDING WITH BISMUTH. Guibert, Ann. de dermat. et syph. **6**:126 (March) 1922.

A penile chancre in which the spirochetes were found grew larger under treatment with a fair amount of mercury and neo-arsphenamin. This therapy was then discontinued and the intravenous injection of bismuth salts begun, a local application being used on the lesion; improvement was immediate.

THE TREATMENT OF SYPHILIS WITH ARSPHENAMIN EXCLU-SIVELY (TEN YEARS' EXPERIENCE). R. Krefting, Ann. de dermat. et syph. **6**:193 (May) 1922.

In serologically negative cases with initial lesions, the author considers five injections usually sufficient, one given every fifteen days, the average adult male receiving from 0.5 to 0.6 gm. at a dose, the adult female from 0.3 to 0.4 gm. In cases of primary syphilis, with a positive Wassermann reaction, he recommends continued treatment, an interval of three or four weeks elapsing after the first course of five injections. In the secondary and later stages, he has had good results. He considers reinfection a not infrequent occurrence. Spinal puncture for diagnostic and therapeutic purposes is decried, and also the idea of the so-called "provocative Wassermann."

CANCER OF THE NECK OF THE UTERUS AND SYPHILIS. C Audry and P. Suquet, Ann. de dermat. et syph. **6**:206 (May) 1922.

Just as syphilis is considered to be the most frequent underlying cause of carcinoma of the tongue, the authors agree with Bertrand (*Bruxelles medical,* Jan. 15, 1922, p. 144), whose statistics showed it to be present in an over-whelming majority of cases of uterine cancer. Their own series of ninety-one cases shows a positive Wassermann reaction in 66 per cent., which is surely far above the normal.

ETIOLOGIC AND HISTOLOGIC CONSIDERATIONS APROPOS OF AN EPIDEMIC OF FOLLICULAR KERATOSIS. Rocamora, Ann. de dermat. et syph. **6**:209 (May) 1922.

Fourteen cases appeared simultaneously in an institution, the ages of the patients ranging between 7 and 13 years. All had been previously healthy, and there was no sign of tuberculosis or tinea. The lesions were grouped in some cases on the extensor surfaces, in others on the flexor, and there was also a sparsely scattered eruption elsewhere; the hands and feet were free. The element was a pinpoint follicular protrusion with an adherent horny plug, there being scarcely any sign of acute inflammation. Microscopic study verified this. A small coccus was found, not unlike that which Sabouraud has described.

These cases are classified separately under the heading of "follicular keratoses."

A CONTRIBUTION TO THE STUDY OF LUPUS PERNIO. R. Rabut, Ann. de dermat. et syph. **6**:227 (May) 1922.

The literature is reviewed, with special emphasis on the work of Schaumann (*Annales,* 1917, p. 537, and 1919, p. 385), who considers lupus pernio a part of the syndrome of benign lymphogranulomatosis, associated with sarcoid. The author describes a case of his own, showing Boeck's sarcoid and lupus pernio, with possible gradations between the two, partially demonstrated histologically. In concluding, he takes a middle course and subdivides the many cases which are given this diagnosis, classifying some as chilblains, some as lupus erythematosus, others as lupus vulgaris and perhaps the remainder in Schaumann's group, possibly including the sarcoids, the angiokeratoma of Mibelli, granuloma annulare and the angiodermites, which Gougerot calls "lupus pernio en plaques."

PARKHURST, Toledo, Ohio.

A CASE OF TRICHOPHYTOSIS IN AN ADULT. E. RIVALIER (Milian), Bull. Soc. franç. de dermat. et syph. **29**:128, 1922.

A woman, aged 30, had probably had the infection since childhood. The involvement was extensive, the scalp being its only site; the organisms seemed to be of the microsporon endothrix variety, but they had not yet been identified by cultures.

CONGENITAL KERATOSIS FOLLICULARIS (DARIER'S DISEASE). LOUSTE and BARBIER, Bull. Soc. franç. de dermat. et syph. **29**:130, 1922.

The patient, a woman, aged 36, was underdeveloped both physically and mentally. Some of the lesions were said to have been present since birth, and the final involvement was general, with certain sites of predilection. The lesions were of all possible types, according to their age and location. The oral mucosa was free. A biopsy examination confirmed the diagnosis. In addition, scabies was present, and also a vesiculopustular eruption, which was said to appear for a few days at each menstrual period.

A CASE OF PARTIAL SCLERODERMA. M. HUGEL, Bull. Soc. franç de dermat. et syph. **2**:15, 1922.

The patient spent four years in the war, during which time he suffered severe trauma to his leg on several occasions. Following this, his leg became swollen and movement of the joints was restricted. Soon after this subsided the skin of the leg became hard and sclerodermic.

The author used thiosinamin and sodium salicylate with good results. He believes the condition might have been due to trauma.

VERRUCOUS ERYTHRO-KERATODERMA EN NAPPES. SYMMETRICAL, PROGRESSIVE AND CONGENITAL. HUDELO et al. Bull. Soc. franç. de dermat. et syph. **2**:45, 1922.

The author presented a boy, aged 16 years, with circumscribed areas of keratoderma, on an erythematous base. The parts affected were the scalp, face, ears, neck, arms, forearms and hands. The eruption, which began at the age of 4 years, was symmetrical and congenital except on the scalp. There was no familial history, no history of syphilis, and the Wassermann reaction was negative.

The histologic section showed marked hyperkeratosis, and atrophic or absent sebaceous glands.

ATYPICAL PRECOCIOUS MALIGNANT SYPHILIS CURED BY BISMUTH. LINGUAL LESION OF UNDETERMINABLE NATURE. LERI, TZANCK and WEISMANN-NETTER. Bull. Soc. franç. de dermat. et syph. **29**:56, 1922.

This was a case of pustular, crusted and deeply ulcerated generalized lesions which appeared fifteen days after the chancre. The patient had no lesions of the mucous membrane nor any general adenopathy. The Wassermann reaction was strongly positive.

The patient received six injections biweekly of 0.2 gm. of a bismuth preparation. The fever disappeared, and the lesions cleared quickly. On the posterior third of the tongue appeared a cream colored lesion which was painless, noninfiltrated and persistent. The question arose whether this lesion was due to bismuth or syphilis or whether it was independent of both.

McCafferty, New York.

GENERALIZED EPIDERMOMYCOSIS. Louste and M. Laurent, Bull. Soc. franç. de dermat. et syph. **29**:134, 1922.

In a young man, aged 17, an erythematosquamous plaque appeared at one corner of the mouth, with tiny vesicles about its periphery. Within fifteen days, the trunk, arms and thighs were also involved, the patches being numerous and resembling those of pityriasis rosea. The microscopic examination of the scales showed the presence of segmented mycelia, but the organism had not yet been identified.

PITYRIASIS RUBRA PILARIS AND PSORIASIS ASSOCIATED. Hudelo, Boulanger-Pilet and Cailliau, Bull. Soc. franç. de dermat. et syph. **29**: 136, 1922.

In a boy of 10 years, an attack of measles was followed by a generalized eruption with the clinical and histologic characteristics of pityriasis rubra pilaris. There being signs of endocrine disturbance, thyroid extract was prescribed. One month later, among the lesions of pityriasis rubra pilaris typical psoriatic patches appeared. Their nature was shown histologically.

ERYTHROPLASIFORM DYSKERATOSIS OF THE VULVAR MUCOSA. Hudelo, Oury and Cailliau, Bull. Soc. franç. de dermat. et syph. **29**:139, 1922.

The lesions, in a woman, aged 55, had first been noticed in 1907, and in 1916 were removed by the curet, only to recur two years later. As the name tells us, they were smooth red plaques, histologically the site of dyskeratosis. The authors are struck by their resemblance to the lesions of Bowen's precancerous dermatosis, with which they may be identical.

A PEMPHIGOID ERUPTION OCCURRING IN THE COURSE OF A SPASMODIC SYRINGOMYELIA. G. Milian and Lelong, Bull. Soc. franç. de dermat. et syph. **29**:142, 1922.

The eruption was of twenty-eight days' duration in a patient of 66 years, being especially located on the forearms, which were the chief sites of the syringomyelic involvement. There was a 16 per cent. eosinophilia.

A NOTE REGARDING THE ETIOLOGY OF RECURRENT HERPES. Milian and Perin, Bull. Soc. franç. de dermat. et syph. **29**:147, 1922.

The vesicular contents in two cases of recurrent herpes facialis produced a nonphlyctenular keratitis in rabbits, and a similar result was obtained after inoculation from an apparently sterile and negative culture which had been made from the original lesions.

A CASE OF ERYTHROKERATODERMA EXTENDING IN GEOGRAPHIC PLAQUES. E. JEANSELME, P. CHEVALLIER, BURNIER and PERIN, Bull. Soc. franç. de dermat. et syph. **29**:150, 1922.

In an otherwise apparently healthy girl, aged 18 years, erythematous plaques had begun to appear ten years previously, and the eruption had gradually spread, involving the upper and lower extremities, especially on their extensor aspect, the face and neck, and the trunk, slightly. The palms and soles were affected. The lesions answered the description, clinically and histologically, of congenital ichthyosiform erythroderma. A sister, aged 16 years, had been similarly afflicted since the age of 8. The flexures were remarkably free from the eruption.

A LINEAR NEVUS CORRESPONDING TO DISTRIBUTION OF EIGHTH CERVICAL AND FIRST DORSAL NERVES WITH CERVICAL RIB. A. LERI and A. TZANCK, Bull. Soc. franç. de dermat. et syph. **29**:156, 1922.

A pigmented verrucous unilateral linear nevus was associated with cervical rib on the same side, suggesting that the two may have arisen from the same structural defect.

A DIRECT-LOADING FREEZING CAUTERY. LORTAT-JACOB, Bull. Soc. franç. de dermat. et syph. **29**:158, 1922.

An apparatus is described which was designed to supplant the carbon dioxid snow pencil. It has given better results than the older method in the clinic. A cylindrical container is filled with the desired amount of solid carbon dioxid and acetone is added. To one end of the small cylinder, copper applicators of various sizes may be attached, and at the other end is a gauge similar in appearance to the sliding tire-air-pressure gauge, by which the pressure of application is measured.

THE SYMPATHETIC SYSTEM AND THE ENDOCRINE GLANDS IN LINGUA GEOGRAPHICA. A LEVY-FRANCKEL and E. JUSTER. Bull. Soc. franç. de dermat. et syph. **29**:163, 1922.

Four cases are cited to show a possible relationship between disturbances in the thymus, thyroid and gonads and the occurrence of the lingual eruption. In two, the administration of a thyroid compound was followed by fading of the lesions.

THE SYMPATHETIC FACTOR IN THE NITRITOID CRISIS OR VAGO-TONIC CRISIS. E. JUSTER, Bull. Soc. franç. de dermat. et syph. **29**:168. 1922.

In twelve patients, including nine females, the author found an oculocardiac reflex which indicated the presence of a vagotonic state; all of these had been subject to nitritoid crises. The phenomena of this crisis are said to result from a simultaneous parasympathetic stimulation and sympathetic paralysis. Therefore, it seems that vagotonic persons would be more susceptible. Acidity of the arsenical drug, or a lowered alkaline reserve in the blood, serve to precipitate the crisis; therefore, great care must be used in the preparation of the solution. Furthermore, vagotonic patients should receive a preceding prophylactic injection of epinephrin. The administration of belladonna, three times a day, is also advised, with a view toward combating the vagotonic state.

PRESENTATION OF A SEROLOGIC SCALE. Lacapere and Gerbay, Bull. Soc. franç. de dermat. et syph. **29**:175, 1922.

By accurate quantitative measurement, employing decreasing amounts of the patient's serum for the Wassermann and Hecht reactions, the authors have found what they consider to be a useful gage to follow in treatment. With a fixed "positive" standard, the reaction may be hyperpositive or hypopositive, the symbols Ho(x3), Ho(x5), Ho(x30), etc., representing degrees of hyperpositivity, while Ho represents the normal positive and H2, H4, H6, etc., indicate the degree of hypopositivity. A curve may be plotted in each case as treatment is checked up.

In the authors' opinion, many cases in which the Wassermann reaction seems irreducible have really been strongly hyperpositive and are becoming less and less so under treatment.

GENERAL THERAPEUTIC RESULTS OBTAINED BY THE USE OF AMINO-ARSENOPHENOL (132) INTRAMUSCULARLY IN THE TREATMENT OF SYPHILIS. E. Jeanselme, Pomaret and M. Bloch, Bull. Soc. franç. de dermat. et syph. **29**:182, 1922.

This product contains 40 per cent. of arsenic, and is said to be much more stable than neo-arsphenamin. Its injection intramuscularly is said to be less painful than that of the soluble salts of mercury. The authors usually inject 0.12 gm. every other day, 0.24 gm. every fourth day, or 0.36 gm. every seven days, giving a minimum total dose of 2.36 gm. within forty-one days in primary syphilis and 2.80 gm. within fifty-three days in the secondary stage. The clinical and serologic results are similar to those obtained by the arsphenamins, and the authors have found that it can usually be given safely to patients who do not tolerate the intravenous medication.

A CASE OF CANINE ITCH IN MAN. W. Dubreuilh, Bull. Soc. franç. de dermat. et syph. **29**:185, 1922.

The owner of a dog suffering from itch had contracted the affliction from his pet. The sites usually involved in scabies were unaffected. By careful search, the canine itch mite, an organism slightly longer than *Acarus scabei,* was found in a miliary vesicle on the man's arm. No itch mites could be recovered from the dog, which had been treated by a veterinary.

LICHEN PLANUS SUPERVENING IN THE COURSE OF NEO-ARSPHENAMIN TREATMENT. J. Montpellier, A. Lacroix and P. Boutin, Bull. Soc. franç. de dermat. et syph. **29**:186, 1922.

Briefly alluding to cases reported by others in 1921, the authors describe one in which a typical eruption of lichen planus appeared after the second injection of neo-arsphenamin, in a man, aged 36. Continued administration of the drug was followed only by extension of the eruption. However, after a rest of two and a half months, the patient returned; and the lesions disappeared after the fourth injection of a new series of neo-arsphenamin.

SCLERODERMA IN PLAQUES AND BANDS. Vedei, G. Giraud and P. Boulet, Bull. Soc. franç. de dermat. et syph. **29**:188, 1922.

The lesions, in a woman, aged 22, had first appeared in her sixteenth year, two years after puberty. Plaques occupied the right breast and left shoulder, while bands traversed the length of the left upper extremity, including the thumb and forefinger, and also the right leg and foot. There was diffuse infiltration of both thighs.

There was nothing to support theories of nervous or infectious etiology, and there seemed to be no endocrinopathy.

A PRELIMINARY NOTE ON THE USE OF TARTROBISMUTHATE IN THE TREATMENT OF SYPHILIS. J. Nicolas, G. Massia and J. Gate, Bull. Soc. franç. de dermat. et syph. **29:** R. S. 29, 1922.

For several months, the authors have been using this medication. They consider it superior to mercury and only slightly inferior to the arsphenamins, so far as its immediate clinical effect is concerned. It has rather serious inconveniences: the injections are painful, stomatitis is frequent and albuminuria often occurs. Therefore, the drug is to be used cautiously, the oily suspension seeming preferable, in doses of 0.2 gm. every six or seven days for five, six or seven injections. The intramuscular route is always employed.

A CASE OF TERTIARY CONGENITAL SYPHILIS OF THE MEDIAL PREMAXILLA. J. Nicolas, J. Gate and D. Dupasquier, Bull. Soc. franç. de dermat. et syph. **29:** R. S. 34, 1922.

In a boy, aged 13 years, with the stigmas of congenital syphilis, there was a loosening of the upper medial incisors of several weeks' duration; and examination of the palate revealed ulceration and a fistula, the medial premaxilla being involved. Under treatment with neo-arsphenamin, the lesions healed, after sequestrums had been removed; the two teeth remained loose. The authors are about to publish an article dealing with the manifestations of syphilis in the medial premaxilla.

PEMPHIGUS FOLIACEUS. Pautrier and J. Roederer, Bull. Soc. franç. de dermat. et syph. **29:** R. S. 37, 1922.

In a man, aged 44 years, otherwise in fairly good health, there was a generalized eruption of pemphigus foliaceus of nine years' duration, only the palms and soles being spared. The hair was rather sparse and the nails were slightly involved. The Wassermann reaction had been twice positive, in the absence of any history of syphilis. Various forms of treatment, including mild antisyphilitic therapy, were tried, without result.

PAINFUL DERMATITIS HERPETIFORMIS WITH A MENINGEAL REACTION. Pautrier, Bull. Soc. franç. de dermat. et syph. **29:** R. S. 41, 1922.

In August, 1921, a man, aged 74, first noticed extremely pruritic erythematous patches on the scrotum, which soon spread and were set with vesicles. The usual sites of predilection were soon involved, and there was an eosinophilia of 19 per cent. in the circulating blood, and of 45 per cent. in the contents of the vesicles. Painful sensations accompanied the usual pruritus. The spinal fluid contained six lymphocytes per cubic millimeter and an increased amount of albumin, which may have had something to do with the sensory disturbances.

A CASE OF PITYRIASIS RUBRA PILARIS. O. ELIASCHEFF and ZIMMERLIN, Bull. Soc. franç. de dermat. et syph. **29**: R. S. 43, 1922.

A typical eruption of general distribution is described in a boy, aged 16 years; it had started on the palms and soles in May, 1920. The patient was underdeveloped, and there may have been an endocrine factor.

A CASE OF ELEPHANTIASIS NOSTRAS. HUGEL, Bull. Soc. franç. de dermat. et syph. **29**: R. S. 46, 1922.

In a man, aged 38, there had been a swelling of the right lower extremity for twelve years, constantly increasing. About the ankle, the skin was folded and hyperkeratotic. The patient had always lived in one locality.

The histologic features were: hyperplasia of all the elements excepting the elastic tissue, thick-walled vessels surrounded by an infiltration including plasma and mast cells, and dilatation of the lymphatic vessels.

A CASE OF ACANTHOSIS NIGRICANS ACCOMPANYING GASTRIC CARCINOMA. PAUTRIER, Bull. Soc. franç. de dermat .et syph. **29**: R. S. 50, 1922.

A man, aged 35, had had abdominal distress for six years. A laparotomy, in August, 1921, revealed the presence of gastric malignancy and a gastro-enterostomy was performed. One month later, following an intense pruritus, the lesions of acanthosis nigricans appeared, located especially in the great flexures.

A NEW MEANS OF LOCAL ANESTHESIA. S. CHAUVET, L'Hopital **10**: 193 (April) 1922.

The "gazotherme," a portable apparatus for anesthetizing prior to dental and minor surgical operations, is said to be efficient and without drawbacks. A stream of oxygen is directed accurately against the part to be anesthetized, its temperature being gradually reduced by means of a controllable cooling coil containing carbon dioxid, until the field has been frozen.

THE PATHOGENESIS AND TREATMENT OF EDEMAS. MAURIAC, J. de méd. de Bordeaux **94**:103 (Feb. 25) 1922.

The theories of causation of the various acute and chronic edemas are reviewed, but especial consideration is given to nephritic edema, which can be removed, the author believes, by the administration of potassium and calcium salts, these ions replacing the undesirable majority of sodium ions.

PARKHURST, Toledo, Ohio.

RECURRING URTICARIAL CRISES DUE TO WOOL. R. DAMADE, J. de méd. de Bordeaux **94**:111 (Feb. 25) 1922.

A woman experienced these attacks every time she slept on a certain wool mattress, but the symptoms were gradually becoming less marked. The wool itself is blamed, rather than agents employed in its bleaching.

FRENCH SOCIETY OF DERMATOLOGY AND SYPHILOGRAPHY. Presse. méd. **30**:228 (March) 1922.

Dermatitis from "Kabyline": Hudelo presented a patient who had a dermatitis of the thorax which began in the axillae as a result of wearing a corsage containing a ruby red dye of kabyline. The eruption became generalized after using a weak sulphur ointment.

Alopecia Areata, Syndrome of Irritation from the Large Sympathetic Nerve: Lévy-Frankel presented a patient who had a war wound involving the nerves at the elbow. The involvement of these nerves caused atrophy of the scapular muscles, vasomotor and thermic changes, tachycardia with emotivity and finally alopecia areata of the beard and scalp. From this idea and the coexistence of alopecia areata with exophthalmic goiter, zona and scleroderma, the author concludes that irritation of the large sympathetic nerve plays a rôle in the genesis of alopecia areata.

Origin of Dyshidrosis: Sabouraud observed a typical case of dyshidrosis and made cultures. The cultures were sterile. It is his opinion that in true dyshidrosis one never finds fungi. Brocq shared this opinion. Darier has seen some mycelial filaments in certain cases of dyshidrosis. The search is often long and difficult.

Hemodiagnosis of Hereditary Syphilis: Leredde thought hereditary syphilis is unrecognized in 95 per cent. of the cases. He studied the presence of alterations in the blood of presumptive hereditosyphilitic patients. If one used a recognized treatment, namely, arsphenamin, one found quite often an elevation of hemoglobin, more often an increased number of red cells and frequently a diminution of mononuclears.

Syphilitic Reinfection: Lepinay reported a case of reinfection. The first chancre was excised and the patient received a prolonged treatment of arsphenamin and mercury. The second chancre appeared not far from the scar of the first chancre, and contained some spirochetes. The new chancre appeared in due time after suspicious coitus. The partner was examined and mucous patches of the vulva were found.

Apropos of a Case of Reinfection: Lacapere gave the history of a patient who had a chancre on the balanopreputial fold and after three years developed a second chancre on the internal aspect of the prepuce. The Wassermann test was negative the first time and the second time positive, in spite of treatment.

Jeanselme made some reservations here because a search for the spirochete was not made in the first chancre, and the patient did not seem to have been treated in a particularly intense manner.

Researches on Acidosis in the Course of Post-Arsenical Erythroderma: Pomaret and Blamoutier showed in the course of postarsenical erythroderma that the subjects attacked are in a state of acidosis. They found the acidosis coefficient high in both the blood and urine. The authors have not been able to ascertain whether the acidosis precedes or results from the arsenical medication.

Brocq displayed much interest at this statement and thought it quite important in order to determine when to discontinue the administration of arsphenamin in susceptible patients.

THE SYNDROME OF THE CORPORA STRIATUM OF SYPHILITIC ORIGIN IN THE AGED. Lhermitti and Comil. Presse méd. **30**:280 (April) 1922.

The authors believe that the symptoms so frequently associated with paralysis agitans are due to a latent syphilis involving the corpora striatum and the pyramidal system.

They cite two cases in which the clinical picture was that of Parkinson's disease, but which at necropsy revealed lesions characteristic of syphilis. It is their opinion that many of these parkinsonian cases are truly syphilitic in origin, even if the analogy is negative. They strongly advocate antisyphilitic treatment in these cases and assure good results if persisted in.

RADICULAR DISTRIBUTION OF THE NEVUS AND OF VITILIGO.
KLIPPEL and MATHIEU—Pierre Weil, Presse méd. **30**:388 (May) 1922.

The authors believe nevus and vitiligo are closely associated in their etiology. Many authors support the nervous theory in nevus, while others favor the vascular theory. In the former theory it may be due to a primitive alteration of the neurax, and occurs late in fetal life; in the latter or vascular theory it is due to an alteration of the vascular walls and occurs early in fetal life. The radicular topography is more frequently observed.

Vitiligo appears in a similar manner and is due to local conditions (trauma, syphilitic scars, etc.), as well as to nervous alterations, which are perhaps the more common. Its symmetrical appearance is clearly radicular and must be associated with nervous alterations. Infectious diseases, such as leprosy, tuberculosis, etc., may also cause vitiligo.

THE ETIOLOGY OF LEISHMANIOSIS. JOYEUX, Presse méd. **30**:643 (April) 1922.

There are two types of leishmaniosis, the visceral and cutaneous. The visceral type is characterized by a splenic hypertrophy associated with fever and subdivides itself into two categories: one type existing in India and called kala-azar, the other observed in the Mediterranean valley and affecting only children.

One also recognized two kinds of cutaneous leishmaniosis. The first, the more serious, invades sometimes the mucous membrane and is seen in Brazil. It is the ulcer of Bauru. The second variety is the Oriental button, boil of Biskra or Aleppo button.

The etiology of the Oriental button has been studied for fifteen years. In 1904, the Sergents of Algeria stated that they believed the phlibotome, which is similar to the mosquito but smaller, transmitted the disease. In 1921, the Algerian authors verified their hypothesis by experimental work. They ground up some *Phlibotomi papatasi* sent from Biskra and used the product for inoculation into the forearm of a person. At the end of three months they obtained a typical Oriental button and in its serum they found some *Leishmaniae*. The authors, however, have not proved how the phlibotome conserves the virus, as the Oriental button exists only during the winter, and at this time the insect or phlibotome is hibernating in the larvae stage.

McCAFFERTY, New York.

THE DEVELOPMENT OF SKIN AND HAIR PIGMENT IN THE HUMAN EMBRYO AND THE CESSATION OF PIGMENT FORMATION IN GRAY HAIR (CAUSE OF CANITIES). BLOCH, Arch. f. Dermat. u. Syph. **135**:77-108, 1921.

While hair pigment is developed in the fifth embryonal month, the skin pigment is postembryonal and probably due to the influence of light. The specific Dopa reaction in the epidermis can be positive before pigment is traceable. The function of the pigment-forming Dopa oxydasis in the hair matrix cells accounts for the color of normal hair.

A CASE OF ULCERATIVE SKIN DISORDER OF THE ECTHYMA GANGRAENOSUM TYPE (WITH PYOCYANEUS BACILLUS). FREI and WIENER, Arch. f. Dermat. u. Syph. **134**:106-118, 1921.

Pustular and ulcerative infiltrations occurred with peripheral spreading probably due to *Bacilli pyocyaneus*. The effect of a pyocyaneus vaccine which was administered also pointed to this etiology.

THE PARTIAL ANTIGENS ACCORDING TO DEYCKE-MUCH IN TUBERCULOSIS CUTIS. FRIED, Arch. f. Dermat. u. Syph. **136**:386-400, 1921.

Sixty-three patients were treated with "partigenes." This therapy did not prove superior to tuberculin treatment.

THE PIGMENTATION OF THE SKIN OF GRAMPUS GRISEL'S CUV. KRUEGER, Arch. f. Dermat. u. Syph. **136**:408-415, 1921.

The belief that all epidermis cells are able to form pigment under the influence of light is incorrect. The author believes that the germ plasm takes part in the pigment formation, as the embryo in utero shows the same differences in the distribution of the chromatophores and the quantity of pigment as the skin in later life.

A CONTRIBUTION TO THE PHOTOMETRY OF THE ULTRAVIOLET LIGHT. PASSOW, Arch. f. Augenheilk. **90**:123-126, 1921.

Time and distance of exposure to quartz light is indicated by the various colors of photometer paper which had been exposed in various sessions. This is used for judging the relative intensity of a quartz lamp.

SPECIFIC INFLAMMATIONS IN ANUS AND RECTUM. GOTTSTEIN. Berl. klin. Wchnschr. **58**:36, 1921.

The author reports the following cases:
(1) Periproctic abscess with gonococci in a virgin; (2) extensive rectal and anal tuberculosis with involvement of skin, and (3) extensive destruction of anus due to lupus.

EXPERIMENTAL PROPHYLAXIS OF SYPHILIS. WORMS. Berl. klin. Wchnschr. **58**:39, 1921.

Prophylactics should be applied after coitus and not before coitus.

BROMODERMA TUBEROSUM. HOFFMANN. Berl. klin. Wchnschr. **58**:51. 1921.

The administration of 400 gm. of potassium bromid caused the development of pain size, partly eroded papillomatous proliferations on the legs of a boy of 11 years. The urine test was bromid positive.

METHOD FOR PREPARING SOLUTIONS AT ANY TIME. Sagi, Berl. klin. Wchnschr. **58**:52, 1921.

The substance in question, e. g., neo-arsphenamin, is placed in a special ampule, and covered with a layer of sterile paraffin (for thermolabile substances use paraffin whose melting point is from 28 to 32 C.). The solvent is then poured on this layer and the ampule sealed. When the solution is required for use the ampule is placed in warm water. The paraffin then melts and sinks to the other end.

ROENTGEN RAY IN TREATMENT OF CARCINOMA. Fraenkel, Berl. klin. Wchnschr. **58**:298, 1922.

The author says that treatment of carcinoma depends, chiefly, on the condition of the collagenous tissue, as the latter, in his opinion, is connected with the endocrine system, and is influenced by the thymus and thyroid glands. The aim of irradiation treatment should be to stimulate the function of the collagenous tissue in the sense of nonspecific stimulation treatment. The direct irradiation of a carcinoma cell is, therefore, probably a wrong idea in carcinoma therapy.

CONTRIBUTION TO THE KNOWLEDGE OF THE LEPTOTHRIX ANGINA. Fuerbringer, Berl. klin. Wchnschr. **58**:437, 1921.

This is the report of a case in which the leptothrix buccalis was cultivated from the inner surface of the tonsils. Therapeutically, gargles with menthol are advised.

TREATMENT OF ERYSIPELAS WITH TINCTURE OF IODIN. Lämmerhirt, Berl. klin. Wchnschr. **58**:1389, 1921.

A strip, two fingers broad, of tincture of iodin is painted on and along the edge of the lesion. A second strip should be painted on the healthy surrounding tissue within 3 c.c. from the lesion.

SUGILLATIONS IN TABES. Pineas, Berl. klin. Wchnschr. **58**:1530, 1921.

This is a report of three cases of tabes with the rare symptom of circumscribed subcutaneous hemorrhages, which developed spontaneously, chiefly on the lower limbs. All of these patients suffered from syphilitic heart and circulatory disturbances.

ARSPHENAMIN ERUPTIONS. Kusnitzky and Langner, Berl. klin. Wchnschr. **58**:1534, 1921.

The authors advise three exposures, under 0.5 mm. of aluminum, to the roentgen ray. This relieves itching and stimulates cornification.

THE LIPOLYTIC CAPACITY OF THE WHITE BLOOD CORPUSCLES. Nees, Biochem Ztschr. **124**:156-164, 1921.

Not only lymphocytes but also leukocytes have a lipolytic effect and cannot be distinguished in this respect. For tracing the lipolytic ferments both in the lymphocytes and leukocytes a soil is used containing three parts of hogs' lard, one part of wax and methyl red.

AHLSWEDE, Hamburg, Germany.

INVESTIGATION OF THE PATHOGENESIS OF IODID AND BROMID ACNE. H. HAXTHAUSEN, Dermat. Ztschr. **35**:54 (Nov. 1921.

It seems possible that the action of iodid and bromid on the diffusion of different substances causing inflammation plays a part in the production of iodid and bromid acne. The altered luetin reaction after iodid is quoted as one basis of this, in addition to some bacterial experiments. It is impossible to determine whether such an action of the iodids and bromids is either the proper or only explanation for the eruption. It would seem also that the iodid and bromid were themselves not directly responsible; but it was the action of these salts on substances called forth by them from the body which resulted in changes leading to the eruption. No solution to the problem is offered.

NEURODERMATITIS AND CARCINOMA OF THE CLITORIS IN A YOUNG GIRL. H. MILLER, Dermat. Ztschr. **35**:70, 1921.

A unique history is presented of a girl, 24 years of age, who had been under observation by dermatologists for some years, and who had been presented before dermatologic societies at one time or another, so that the sequence of events could be vouched for. She presented a neurodermatitis of the genital region, and then successively, papillomas and carcinomatous degenerations. According to Fohr, there were twelve carcinomas of the clitoris among twenty-two reported carcinomas of the genital region in young women.

DARIER'S DISEASE, WITH REPORT OF A CASE. H. LIPPERT, Dermat. Ztschr. **35**:76, 1921.

A characteristic case of Darier's disease in a man of 35 years is described. The author's conclusions are: Darier's disease is a congenital disease, which is also hereditary, and as a rule it manifests itself about puberty. The cause is related to an unknown disturbance of the internal secretory mechanism of the body, and may be related to the cause of tumors, especially to the group of malignant epithelial tumors. Organotherapy has been reported as giving favorable results, but in no case has cure resulted. The reason is that Darier's disease is primarily a germplasm disturbance. Organotherapy therefore is only symptomatic therapeutics. Of all other methods of treatment, the roentgen ray in repeated doses is the best for cosmetic and certain results. The bibliography includes articles as recent as 1920.

ACTIVATION OF PROTOPLASM AND OSMOTHERAPY, WITH ESPECIAL REFERENCE TO INTRAVENOUS GRAPE SUGAR INJECTIONS. W. SCHOLTZ, Dermat. Ztschr. **35**:127, 1921.

Egg white, terpentine, milk fats, sulphur, hypertonic and hypotonic solutions of salt and sugar have been used in this type of treatment. The diseased or altered cell is more deeply influenced by these substances than the healthy cell. Little is known definitely concerning the mechanism of the action of this form of treatment. Among the diseases of the skin treated with injections of grape sugar intravenously, exudative eruptions were quickly and favorably influenced. Several patients with grave cases of pemphigus were treated, and the large bullae disappeared after only a few injections. Dry eczemas and psoriasis were treated; likewise bacterial affections. The spirochetes of syphilis diminished in active syphilis. Injections of grape sugar are recommended for severe exanthems following arsphenamin and mercury.

SO-CALLED "FIXED" AND ORDINARY URTICARIAL RECURRENT EXANTHEMS FOLLOWING ARSPHENAMIN AND MERCURY. C. GUTMANN, Dermat. Ztschr. **35**:135, 1921.

Three patients are described. The first presented a typical example of the so-called fixed exanthem following administration of neo-arsphenamin; the second presented an acute, urticarial eruption of short duration and symptoms of angioneurotic edema after a single intravenous injection of novasurol; and the third presented a universal urticaria accompanied by high temperature after an injection of neo-arsphenamin and novasurol (in combination in the same syringe) and the same picture recurred after injection of neo-arsphenamin and silver arsphenamin. Singularly, similar eruptions appeared after intraspinal injections of 1.5 or 1.6 mg. of sodium arsphenamin. No essential differences could be detected in these three cases. No other complications were noted in these patients.

GOODMAN, New York.

XANTHOCHROMIA IN THE CEREBROSPINAL FLUID. LESCHKE, Deutsch. med. Wchnschr. **47**:376 (April 7) 1921.

Xanthochromia of the spinal fluid is due to the formation of bilirubin from red blood corpuscles. It is traced with the diazo-reaction. Xanthochromia is frequent in hemorrhagic inflammations and hemorrhages of the central nervous system.

A NOTE ON REVACCINATION. SOBERNHEIM, Deutsch. med. Wchnschr. **47**:672 (June 16) 1921.

Experiments with rabbits concerning vaccine immunity proved that a reactionless revaccination effects a strong antibody formation, and thereby an increased immunization. Whether this also refers to the human body must still be proved.

SYPHILIS OF THE EYE. IGERSHEIMER, Deutsch. med. Wchnschr. **47**:738 (June 30) 1921.

The author found that *Spirochaeta pallida* is nearly always located in that layer of the cornea which borders the eye chamber. He therefore injected arsphenamin into the front eye chamber of rabbits with satisfactory results.

EARLY NEUROSYPHILIS. WEIGELDT, Deutsch. med. Wchnschr. **47**:1018 (Sept. 1) 1921.

Neurorecurrences are explained as previously existing foci, which are provoked by arsphenamin. Prognostically, there does not exist a predisposition in nerve syphilis for metasyphilis. Tabes is considered a genuine late syphilis. Intraspinal medication is not advised, except as an ultima ratio. Arsphenamin therapy cannot prevent late syphilitic involvement of the nervous system.

ROENTGEN-RAY DOSAGE IN RELATION TO ROENTGEN-RAY BURNS. KURTZAHN, Deutsch. med. Wchnschr. **47**:1326 (Nov. 3) 1921.

After inunctions with mercury, the radiosensitiveness of the skin is frequently increased. The author mentions a case of trichinosis in a patient who developed roentgen-ray ulcer (there was no overdosage). He ascribes the ulcer to the increased radiosensitiveness of the skin caused by the trichinosis.

SOFT CHANCRE VACCINES. Stümpke, Deutsch. med. Wchnschr. **47**:1331 (Nov. 31) 1921.

This is a short report on active immunization of soft chancre. The difficulties lay in the preparation of suitable cultures of streptobacilli. Ordinary agar was used with the addition of 1, 5 or 10 per cent. human or rabbit blood. Treatment, exclusively with vaccines prepared from these cultures with sodium chlorid solution, plus phenol, distinctly hastened healing of chancrous lesions.

RADIOTHERAPY OF CARCINOMA WITH STIMULATING RAYS. Fraenkel, Deutsch. med. Wchnschr. **47**:1396 (Nov. 17) 1921.

The author advises small doses which suffice to destroy fully developed carcinoma cells, while incompletely developed carcinoma cells may resist even the most heavy exposures. It is, therefore, not possible to destroy the carcinoma cells. The author advises the stimulation of all endocrine glands. This is more important than to influence the carcinoma directly.

A NEW METHOD OF PREPARING SOILS FOR CULTIVATING BACTERIA. Brunhübrer and Geiger, Deutsch. med. Wchnschr. **47**:1397 (Nov. 17) 1921.

This is a preliminary report of a new soil prepared from higher fungi for the cultivation of bacteria.

THUMB CARCINOMA IN COBBLERS. Stahr, Deutsch. med. Wchnschr. **47**:1452 (Dec. 11) 1921.

Stahr reports the development of a deep cancroid down to the bone on the thumb of a cobbler's apprentice aged 17. The author holds that repeated pricking and mechanical irritation through handling certain pointed tools accounts for the disorder. The "oat-epithelioma on the tongue of rats which are fed exclusively with oats is probably caused in a similar way. The author compares the cobbler's carcinoma with xeroderma pigmentosum. While in the former the external irritation predominates and the internal disposition plays no rôle, in the latter, the internal disposition alone is the important factor.

NEUTRALIZATION OF REACTIVITY OF SYPHILITIC SERUMS BY FORMALDEHYD. Dold, Deutsch. med. Wchnschr. **47**:1485, 1921.

The addition of formaldehyd inhibits or neutralizes the precipitation which normally occurs in Dold's turbidity reaction. As formaldehyd has a strong dehydrating effect and thereby impedes swelling processes, it is assumed that swelling or dehydrating processes must have some relation to the precipitations in the Wassermann, Sachs-Georgi, Meinicke and Dold reactions. Formaldehyd should not be used for preserving serums.

THE BIOLOGY OF THE SKIN. Gans, Deutsch. med. Wchnschr. **47**:1495 (Dec. 8) 1921.

Intracutaneous injection of endocrine gland extracts causes reddening and infiltration of the vaccinated skin part in healthy persons. In men, the reaction is weaker but more lasting than in women. In pregnant women the addition of pregnant plasm or pregnant serum considerably increased the reaction.

THE EFFECT OF INTRAVENOUS GRAPE SUGAR INJECTIONS ON THE SKIN. Scholtz and Richter, Deutsch. med. Wchnschr. **47**:1522, 1921.

This method of treatment was particularly effective in eczema, erythemas and pemphigus. Pruritus was also well influenced. In gonorrhea and syphilis local reactions were observed. From 16 to 30 c.c. of a 50 per cent. solution were administered from four to eight times in the course of eight to fourteen days.

INCREASED EFFECT OF ARSPHENAMIN IN COMBINATION WITH GRAPE SUGAR. Steinberg, Deutsch. med. Wchnschr. **47**:1523, 1921.

The author found almost double the therapeutic effect of neo-arsphenamin when combined with grape sugar injections. Experiments were made with 0.2 gm. neo-arsphenamin and 3 c.c. of a 30 per cent. grape sugar solution. This combination also proved more effective than Ringer's mixed injection of 0.2 gm. neo-arsphenamin and 0.015 gm. mercuric chlorid. The spirochete disappeared from lesions in forty-two hours.

ACTIVATION OF ARSPHENAMIN PREPARATIONS BY METALS. Kolle, Deutsch. med. Wchnschr. **48**:17 (Jan. 5) 1922.

Neo-arsphenamin plus silver arsphenamin forms neo-silver arsphenamin, a new compound, the toxicity of which is not increased even after twenty-four hours' exposure to air, nor is this product precipitated by carbon dioxid snow contrary to the silver arsphenamin. Neo-silver arsphenamin combines the therapeutic advantages of silver arsphenamin with the solubility of neo-arsphenamin.

TREATMENT OF BURNS. Tunger, Deutsch. med. Wchnschr. **48**: No. 3, 1922.

The author recommends the following ointment for noninfected wounds caused by burns: beta-naphthol resublimed, 0.25 gm.; eucalyptus oil, 2 gm.; olive oil, 5 gm.; soft paraffin, 25 gm.; hard paraffin, 67.75 gm. This should be warmed and then painted on with a hair brush.

CIRCUMCISION TUBERCULOSIS. Wolff, Deutsch. med. Wchnschr. **48**: No. 3, 1922.

The author reports fifty-eight cases of tuberculosis following ritual circumcision. He prefers irradiation and iodoform-glycerin injections to surgical treatment.

DAMAGE TO THE RETINA BY ULTRAVIOLET LIGHT. Schanz. Deutsch. optische Wchnschr. **7**:438, 1921.

Degeneration of the center of the retina which is generally noticed in advanced life, in all cases years after the exposure, should be avoided by wearing euphos glass spectacles, which weaken the effect of the ultraviolet rays.

INFLAMMATION AND THE NERVOUS SYSTEM. Kauffmann, Klin. Wchnschr. **1**:12 (Jan. 1) 1922.

The author reports the development of a serious dermatitis on the leg, after oral administration in two days of 8 gm. of potassium iodid. Local application to the lesions of a diluted tincture of iodin caused the development of a vesicular eruption. As the vesicle formation was sharply defined, and strictly limited to the area treated with iodin, a direct peripheral irritation of the vessel system is assumed.

MAMMARY SECRETION AND BREAST CRISES IN TABES. BIBERSTEIN, Klin. Wchnschr. **1**:68 (Jan. 8) 1922.

This is the report of the fifth known case of this curious disease. Sudden painful attacks in the breasts are followed by uninterrupted secretion of a fatty sero-sanguineous fluid. In one case there was colostrum, in three others a secretion of pure milk.

PIGMENT GENESIS IN THE EYE AND THE NATURE OF THE PIGMENT GRAIN. MIESCHER, Klin. Wchnschr. **1**:173, 1922.

This is the report of an examination of the eyes of chickens, rabbits and guinea-pigs with the Dopa reaction. The pigment forming process in the eye is the same as in the skin though a positive Dopa reaction of the pigment of the retina was found only in a certain stage of embryonal life. As to the pigment mother substance, it is not yet proved that this takes its origin from the cell nucleus.

LASTING EFFECT OF SILVER ARSPHENAMIN. BRÜNING, Med. Klin. **17**:1293 (Oct. 23) 1921.

Several years' experience has proved that ten injections of neo-arsphenamin administered in three weeks cause clinical symptoms to disappear within five months. With silver arsphenamin administered under similar conditions and in the same dosage, the results attained were distinctly better.

WHICH CHEMICAL PROCESSES CAN TURN CALOMEL WHEN ADMINISTERED PER OS INTO A DANGEROUS POISON? SCHUMACHER, Med. Klin. **17**:1485 (Dec. 4) 1921.

Weak sodium chlorid and hydrochloric acid solutions do not, while alkaline carbonate solutions do immediately, turn a large part of the calomel into soluble mercury compounds. This reaction can therefore not take place in the stomach but exclusively in the intestines. Intestinal paresis, ileus and hernia can cause calomel to be turned into a dangerous poison.

VAGOTONIC MANIFESTATIONS OF THE SKIN AN EXPRESSION OF URATIC DIATHESIS. PULAY, Med. Klin. **18**:79 (Jan. 15) 1922.

The author distinguishes five groups of pruritus: (1) as a vagotonic symptom, (2) as an uratic symptom, (3) in diabetes, (4) in hypertonia, (5) in chronic uremia. In all groups, the blood shows an increased percentage of uric acid. Therapeutically, cinchophen combats the cause, and atrophin the vasomotor symptoms.

NEO-SILVER ARSPHENAMIN TREATMENT OF SYPHILIS. FABRY and WOLFF, Med. Klin. **18**:106 (Jan. 22) 1922.

This is the report of 100 cases of syphilis in all stages treated with from ten to seventeen injections, averaging from 0.2 to 0.5 gm. of neo-silver arsphenamin twice weekly. In a few cases only, edema of the face and eyelids was seen, otherwise there were no disturbances, no fever, headaches, eruptions and no angioneurotic syndrome. In general, authors do not advise its combination with mercury.

EFFECT OF SILVER SALTS ON THE CELL. SCHUMACHER, Med. Klin. 18:159 (Jan. 29) 1922.

If metal salts are made to act on cell smears or sections, a silver nucleus picture is obtained. Protoplasm absorbs little silver and stains a light brown, while the nucleus takes up more silver and becomes dark brown.

THE ECZEMATOID FORM OF SKIN DIPHTHERIA. BIBERSTEIN, Med. Klin. 18:168 (Feb. 51) 1922.

The author saw a large number of cases of eczematoid diphtheria in children suffering from so-called "ear eczemas." Laudé has already described this form of skin diphtheria.

EFFECT OF TRYPAFLAVIN (ACRIFLAVINE) IN DISEASES OF THE BUCCAL AND PHARYNGEAL CAVITY, WITH SPECIAL REFERENCE TO THRUSH. MAIER, München. med. Wchnschr. 68:49, 1921.

Stomatitis and thrush were well influenced with sprays of a 1 per cent. aqueous trypaflavine solution. Rinsing of the mouth with acriflavine solution and dissolving of sugared tabloids containing 0.5 per cent. of acriflavine proved effective.

ARTIFICIAL CULTIVATION OF BACTERIA IN BUCCAL AND PHARYNGEAL CAVITY. REIS, München. med. Wchnschr. 68:325, 1921.

All attempts to cultivate foreign bacteria in the buccal cavity have hitherto failed. The author put *B. coli* on the tonsils and succeeded in nine cases in proving its presence after fifty-four days. As *B. coli* are strong antagonists of the ordinary buccal flora, and particularly of diphtheria bacilli, it should prove practical to attempt a "displacing-therapy," in the sense that diphtheria bacilli on tonsils are destroyed or pushed aside by *B. coli,* cultures of which should be painted on the tonsils for this purpose.

NEURORELAPSE AFTER COMBINED SERONEGATIVE PRIMARY SYPHILIS. NATHAN, München. med. Wchnschr. 68:487 (April 22) 1921.

Energetic arsphenamin treatment (3.1 gm. silver arsphenamin and 0.95 gm. mercuric salicylate in a period of two months) of a case of primary syphilis with a negative Wassermann reaction was followed by a serious neurorelapse. During the course of the latter the serum Wassermann reaction was negative while the spinal fluid was positive in all reactions. The author therefore advises that all patients with primary seronegative cases should submit to at least two, possibly three, "courses" of combined arsphenamin and mercury treatment.

GAS POISONING IN THE ROENTGEN-RAY ROOM. LOENNE, München. med. Wchnschr. 68:1519 (Nov. 25) 1921.

A surplus of ozone, the quantity of which is difficult to determine, is certainly the damaging factor. The author found 0.2 mg. of ozone, some nitrous acid and hydrogen dioxid, in 1 cubic meter of air in a room, after intense use of the roentgen-ray apparatus.

LOCAL REACTIONS OF INTRACUTANEOUS AOLAN INJECTIONS. GAUNÜTZ, München. med. Wchnschr. 68:1585 (Dec. 9) 1921.

Aolan is a sterile and toxin-free milk albumin solution for nonsyphilitic protein body treatment. In the treatment of gonorrhea the reaction which occurs is not specific but is seen also in patients without gonorrhea.

COMBINATION OF VARIOLOID AND LATENT SYPHILIS. HILLENBERG, München. med. Wchnschr. 68:1624 (Dec. 16) 1921.

The syphilitic infection was proved by a maculopapular eruption and positive Wassermann test. The varioloid ran its usual course.

MEINICKE'S THIRD MODIFICATION. RUETE, München. med. Wchnschr. 69:83 (Jan. 29) 1922.

The author found the Wassermann reaction superior to Meinicke's test for examining spinal fluids.

ROENTGEN-RAY TREATMENT OF PERNIO. LENK, München. med. Wchnschr. 69:87 (Jan. 20) 1922.

The author recommends irradiation in all stages of pernio. The dose should be from one-third to one-half pastille under 0.5 mm. of aluminum and should be repeated in a fortnight if necessary.

INCREASING THE EFFECT OF ARSPHENAMIN ON THE NERVOUS SYSTEM. KALBERLAH, München. med. Wchnschr. 69:114 (Jan. 27) 1922.

This is the report of experiments with rabbits which were given 0.1 gm. neo-arsphenamin, either alone or in combination with methylene blue or Bismarck brown. The ashes of the brain of the rabbits that were given the combined treatment contained from two to three times the quantity of arsenic. The author then discusses the possibilities of bringing the arsphenamin nearer to the diseased nervous tissue. He calls attention to the experiments of Embden, who showed that activity, also inflammatory processes and fever render the cell membranes more permeable.

A METHOD OF DEMONSTRATING SPIROCHETES IN FROZEN SECTIONS. STEINER, München. med. Wchnschr. 69:121 (Jan. 27) 1922.

The section is first treated with a 10 per cent. alcoholic solution of mastic. then it is put into a 0.1 per cent. silver nitrate solution at 37 C. for twenty-four hours, then into a milky mastic solution, and finally into a fresh solution of 5 per cent. hydrochinon.

COMPLEMENT PRESERVATION. HAMMERSCHMIDT, München. med. Wchnschr. 69:121 (Jan. 27) 1922.

The author recommends an addition of 10 per cent. sodium acetate to complement for preserving it.

PATHOGENESIS OF SYPHILIS MALIGNA. UMANSKY. Schweiz. med. Wchnschr. 51:48, 1921.

The author bases his explanation of the development of syphilis maligna chiefly on the following points: (1) concomitant disorders such as tuberculosis, malaria, alcoholism, pregnancy, etc., which encourage this development, also (2) differences in the quantity and quality of the virus, and (3) the lack of inherited resisting power. The general opinion, endorsed chiefly by Hecht, is that the system is in such weakened state that the antibody production practically ceases. The author proposes to replace the name syphilis maligna by "lues allergica."

EXPERIMENTAL TAR CANCER. Bloch and Dreifuss, Schweiz. med. Wchnschr. 51:1033 (Nov. 10) 1921.

The authors tried to discover which particular substance in crude tar has the special carcinoma provoking capacity. They found a constituent which boils at 300 C., is soluble in benzene, and which, when freed of phenols, bases and the lower carbohydrates, provoked carcinoma in 100 per cent. of the cases (white mice).

THE EFFICIENCY-INCREASING EFFECT OF ROENTGEN RAYS AND THEIR IMPORTANCE FOR A THEORY OF EFFECT OF DRUGS. Cattani, Schweiz. Rundschau f. Med. 21:44, 1921.

Small doses generally stimulate the growth of plants, bacteria, etc. Stimulation of growth of human hair has not yet been made use of therapeutically. Ray stimulation therapy (small doses) corresponds to protein body treatment. Many therapeutic agents (tuberculin, organotherapeutic preparations, collargol), also apparently specific agents, act as nonspecific protein bodies if injected parenterally (intramuscularly, intravenously). Small doses stimulate the defensive action of the body cells, large doses inhibit. A drug has only a specific effect because it is directed to one special kind of cell. All kinds of stimulation of a cell have the same effect, they only differ in intensity.

FURTHER THERAPEUTIC EXPERIENCES WITH ROENTGEN RAYS. Stark, Strahlentherapie 12:4, 1921.

The following dosages may interest the dermatologist as they are somewhat unusual and resemble the technic generally applied in gynecology:

1. Eczema: dose, 1 pastille under 0.5 mm. of zinc, or 0.5, 0.66 and 0.8 pastille, or, a few times, 1 pastille under 3 mm. of aluminum. Cure was effected after two exposures.

2. Lupus vulgaris and tuberculosis cutis: dose, 1 pastille under 0.5 mm. of zinc; repeated from three to four times.

3. Carcinoma: dose, 1 pastille under 0.5 mm. of zinc. Seven of ten cases of carcinoma of the face were healed with from one to three exposures.

THE LOOSE FILTER. Hirsch, Strahlentherapie 12:260, 1921.

Loose's metal salt crystal filter did not differ in effect from a 5 to 6 mm. aluminum filter. The biologic effects also corresponded to those of the aluminum filters.

INVESTIGATIONS OF INDENTITY OF NEO-ARSPHENAMIN OF IMPORTANCE TO THE PRACTITIONER. L. Kolfer and A. Perutz, Wien. klin. Wchnschr. 34:594, 1921.

The possibility of substitution of false neo-arsphenamin of German origin for the original gives especial importance to the tests detailed. Before opening the ampule, the identifying signature, serial number, packing of the container and labels should be examined. The color of the salt should be of the characteristic yellow, and the quality of the division should be that of known neo-arsphenamin. The physician requires a simple test to be used with each injection solution prior to use. The test should be one which while not absolute could distinguish most of the known false products. Reduction of silver nitrate solution is a feasible test. This may be made either with the solution by adding a few drops of the neo-arsphenamin solution to a 10 per cent. solution of silver nitrate, or by using a piece of filter paper previously impregnated with silver nitrate solution. If the test is used with the two solutions, a black precipitate is formed. The few drops of neo-arsphenamin dropped upon the filter paper from the syringe will cause a brown discoloration at the borders of the drop which will turn black in a few minutes. Nessler's reagent gives a black precipitate. Millon's reagent gives a dirty brown precipitate. Alcoholic solution of bichlorid gives a light yellow precipitate. There is a canary yellow precipitate formed with tincture of iodin. If Lugol's solution is used, yellow results, which becomes red. Bromin water gives a yellow to reddish brown precipitate. Ferric chlorid gives a violet shade to the solution. This reaction may also be performed with filter paper. There is a pretty reaction with hydrogen peroxid. If one mixes a 10 per cent. neo-arsphenamin solution with a 3 per cent. hydrogen peroxid solution, the neo-arsphenamin is decolorized, and in a few seconds red results. If the hydrogen peroxid is used in stronger solution, the decolorization lasts only part of a second, and the red appears. If one mixes the 3 per cent. hydrogen peroxid with a few drops of neo-arsphenamin a yellow precipitate is formed, which does not dissolve on further addition of neo-arsphenamin solution.

Some of the substitutes for neo-arsphenamin in falsified ampules have been: (1) barium sulphate and lead chromate; (2) silica, ocher, rye flour and lead chromate; (3) barium and calcium sulphate, lead chromate and napthol yellow; and (4) sand, sodium bicarbonate and ocher.

These are sometimes detected by not going into solution, and this would be the first step indicating falsification. Any suspicion of substitution would be absolutely confirmed by chemical analysis. The tests used by the chemists differ of course from those set forth for the physician.

INTRAVENOUS TREATMENT OF OBSTINATE ITCHING DERMA-TOSES. STRASSBERG, Wien. klin. Wchnschr. **34**:595, 1921.

Autoserum and grape sugar treatment, after bleeding. was particularly effective. No benefit was derived from physiologic sodium chlorid solution injections.

ACTIVE IMMUNIZATION WITH EXTRACTS OF FETAL SYPHI-LITIC LIVER. JACOBI, Ztschr. f. d. ges Neurol. u. Psychiat. **73**: No. 4, 1921.

The author prepared extracts from fetal syphilitic liver and applied these for stimulating the defensive action of the body in the sense of a nonspecific protein therapy. Regular injections of the extracts caused a rise in temperature and anaphylactic symptoms, while the therapeutic effect was doubtful. The author believes that his extracts act as nonspecific proteins. and besides. that they effect a certain specific active immunization.

SEBORRHEA FACIEI IN LETHARGIC ENCEPHALITIS. Stiefler, Ztschr. f. d. ges. Neurol. u. Psychiat. **73**:455, 1921.

In two cases of epidemic lethargic encephalitis which ran a typical course, there was the curious symptom of a swollen, extremely greasy skin of the face. The secretion of grease was so abnormal that a central origin, i. e., functional disturbance, was assumed in the corresponding cerebral center.

GUMMA OF OVARY WITH POSITIVE SPIROCHETE FINDINGS. Kubinyi and Johan, Zentralbl. f. Gynäk. **46**: No. 2, 1922.

The right ovary of a woman of 20 was completely destroyed by nodular gummas. The Wassermann reaction was two plus. Levaditi staining revealed *Spirochaeta pallida*. This is the first case reported of a gumma of the ovary with *Spirochaeta pallida* in acquired syphilis.

IMPORTANCE OF DOMESTIC ANIMALS IN THE SPREADING OF TUBERCULOSIS. Kempner, Ztschr. f. Tuberkul. **34**:570-574, 1921.

Of nineteen strains of tubercle bacilli in the dog, sixteen were of the typus humanus and three only of the typus bovinus. Of five strains in cats, three were typus humanus. Domestic animals are therefore a permanent source of infection and require attention in this respect.

PRIMARY MELANOSARCOMA OF THE PENIS. Peters, Ztschr. f. Urol. **16**:1, 1922.

This is the fifth case reported in the literature. Contrary to the others, the tumor in this case developed in advanced life. The development was rapid with ulceration. Metastases caused the death of the patient.

SPONTANEOUS OCCURRENCE IN THE RABBIT OF A SPIROCHETE RESEMBLING THE PARASITE OF SYPHILIS. Klarenbeek, Zentralbl. f. Bakteriol., Parasit. u. Inf. **87**:203, 1921.

The author could not find either morphologic or tinctorial peculiarities for *Spirochaeta pallida hominis*. He believes the rabbit spirochete is only a variety of *Spirochaeta pallida hominis* and therefore calls it a *"Treponema pallidum varietas cuniculi."* The disorder itself he calls a "spirochetosis" or "lues cuniculi."

Ahlswede, Hamburg, Germany.

Society Transactions

PARAPSORIASIS GUTTATA. Presented by DR. EISENSTAEDT.

A Russian, aged 28 years, presented a skin disorder which was said to have developed at the age of 19 after the patient had been swimming. He was ill at that time with cough and fever. The lesions began on the flexor surfaces of both arms and gradually spread over the body, except on the face. There had been occasional remissions. His general health was good. He was drafted in 1917 and served overseas. The lesions consisted of an eruption over the trunk and limbs of faintly pink, lenticular spots, slightly infiltrated and covered with dry, adherent scales.

DISCUSSION

DR. PUSEY said that he thought it was always well to show these cases, if for no other reason, in order to get them grouped in the mind. Dr. Pollitzer objected to the term parapsoriasis, but Dr. Pusey thought it was fortunate that a generalization had been made showing the relation of the various types of cases, and the name parapsoriasis had obtained such wide usage to denominate the group that it was a useless effort to try to replace it, even by a more suitable name.

DR. EISENSTAEDT asked Dr. Mitchell whether there was any unanimity of opinion in regard to these cases being grouped as a tuberculid, as Civatte had maintained.

DR. MITCHELL said that he knew nothing about tuberculosis in this connection.

A CASE FOR DIAGNOSIS. Presented by DR. EISENSTAEDT.

A man, aged 30 years, who presented lesions on the left hand, four months previously had noticed a slight redness on the dorsum of the left hand. About one month previously papules appeared around the eye, which discharged a diffuse watery fluid. Lesions later appeared about the back of the neck, and still later on the toes of the left foot. A mucoid substance exuded from lesions on the toe. The lesions had later become verrucous in character. The Wassermann reaction was negative. He was admitted to Cook County Hospital with the examining room diagnosis of infected ringworm. Treatment had consisted of application of Whitfield's ointment.

DISCUSSION

DR. SENEAR thought the lesion about the left eye, if taken alone, would pass as a nodular, serpiginous syphilid. Those on the hand and back of the neck were unquestionably of the same character, but they did not look at all like the one about the eye. He did not think it was a fungus infection for the lesions were all too deeply infiltrated. There seemed to be no follicular involvement, such as one would expect to give rise to a deep fungus infection. The lesions on the back of the neck seemed to be clearing at the center and if examined closely some nodules could be seen. At the right side of the neck there were some outstanding follicular pustules which looked as if they might be the primary lesions which had ruptured and discharged. He considered the whole picture puzzling, but thought the lesion on the face was morphologically late syphilis.

Dr. WAUGH said that if the lesions appeared at the time the patient stated syphilis was the logical diagnosis. At first glance the case suggested lupus, but it was hard to conceive of lupus becoming so extensive in that length of time.

Dr. STILLIANS said that he thought the diagnosis lay between lupus and blastomycosis.

Dr. EISENSTAEDT said that he thought the lesions on the hand suggested either a verrucous tuberculosis or blastomycosis. The later lesions that Dr. Senear had called attention to on the back of the neck he called miliary abscesses. They had searched for blastomycetes but had found none. Dr. Zeisler had seen the patient and diagnosed lupus, and a section examined microscopically showed only distinct giant cells. Dr. Eisenstaedt thought the case could be regarded as lupus. The verrucous character of the lesions on the hand and also on the neck had been changed considerably by the use of Whitfield's ointment. The Wassermann reaction was negative. The sections would be examined more carefully and stained for blastomycetes.

TUBERCULOUS GUMMATOUS LYMPHANGITIS.   Presented by Dr. EISENSTAEDT.

The patient was a Mexican, aged 21 years. He complained of painless, multiple swellings of the left foot and thigh and of the neck. Those of the foot and thigh had been present for three years and those of the neck for one week.

He had stubbed his toes some weeks before the lesions had appeared. The trauma was followed by diffuse swelling of the middle toe and of the ankle. The toe had subsequently been amputated, and a discharging sinus still was present. Two weeks later swellings appeared in the left groin. Pain was a prominent symptom at first, but the lesions later became painless. The swelling in the neck was painless but was increasing in size, and there was some difficulty in swallowing.

He had taken a considerable amount of medicine during the last year, chiefly iodids. The Wassermann reaction was negative, as was also roentgenray examination for osteitis and osteomyelitis. Tubercle bacilli had been found in direct smear from the skin lesions in the groin after puncture.

Dr. Eisenstaedt wished to know whether to classify the case as a tuberculous gummatous lymphangitis, and considered it interesting because at first glance there was a great resemblance to sporotrichosis.

The histopathology revealed a chronic infective granuloma but was not typical for the usual type of tuberculous lesion. Guinea-pig inoculation was positive to the extent that an acid-fast bacillus answering the morphologic and staining requirements of *B. tuberculosis* was regained from the spleen of the guinea-pig.

DR. MITCHELL said that he thought the case was interesting. The picture of the foot taken alone looked like a Madura foot, but the lesions in the groin were not hard and showed no resemblance to that.

DR. SENEAR asked whether this case resembled the tuberculous type of sporotrichosis that Dr. Eisenstaedt described, or was it rather a tuberculosis resembling sporotrichosis?

DR. EISENSTAEDT was impressed with the resemblance to sporotrichosis at first glance. The lesions were definitely along the course of the lymphatics. Cultures for blastomycosis were negative. They had found tubercle bacilli, and the smears were examined carefully by Dr. D. J. Davis, who said that the organisms were definitely tubercle bacilli. Their reason for making the stain was that the case might be a nocardiosis, as reported by Dr. Guy. Finding the tubercle bacillus on direct smear in association with osteomyelitis, for which amputation was done, he thought made the diagnosis clear. The involvement of the foot was more extensive than is usual in sporotrichosis, but they had three cases at the Cook County Hospital in all of which there had been amputation of the fingers for lesions of sporotrichosis.

Dr. Eisenstaedt considered the case one of tuberculosis resembling sporotrichosis.

A CASE FOR DIAGNOSIS. Presented by DR. STILLIANS.

A Jewess, aged 45 years, a piano teacher, for two years had had paroxysms of pain in the small of the back, groin and vagina, followed by severe itching in the groins and about the vulva, less severe on the abdomen, the back of the thighs, arms, palms and backs of the hands. The skin lesions had appeared after the attacks of itching had slowly progressed.

At the time of presentation the patient had patches of lichenification on the inner, upper surface of both thighs. The patches were sharply defined. slightly elevated and pinkish. There were similar small patches on the arms. backs of hands, about the knuckles and the bend of the elbows, and on the back of the neck. The palms were hyperkeratotic in patches.

The white blood count was 12,200. Differential count: polymorphonuclears. 65 per cent.; small mononuclears, 28 per cent.; large mononuclears. 5 per cent.: eosinophils, 2 per cent. The blood sugar was 100 mg. to 100 c.c.

DR. PARDEE said that he could see no connection between the disorder and the menopause. The pain in the back and the lesions in the groin he thought indicated a parasitic trouble. He did not see the hands. but if there were lesions on them it suggested the analogy of a case he had had a long time ago, which was quite similar and in which no etiologic factor was ever developed; but the woman recovered under treatment with intestinal anti-septics with colonic lavage, which cleared up her long standing toxemia. Whether it was in spite of this treatment or because of it he did not know.

DR. HURLBURT said that he was impressed with the similarity to a surface infection. He did not see any connection between the constitutional symptoms and the cutaneous manifestations.

DR. SENEAR said that he thought it was a fungus infection. The sharp definition of the lesions in the groin and those of the palms if seen alone would suggest a probable fungus infection, and the same thing was true in the axilla. In spite of the fact that no fungus had been found, he thought this was the diagnosis, and that there was no connection with the constitutional symptoms described.

Dr. EISENSTAEDT said that he thought it was a fungus infection.

Dr. MITCHELL said that he thought the lichenification might have been induced by a fungus infection which was certainly not active at present. It had probably been started by a fungus, but he did not think any would be found now.

Dr. STILLIANS said that he was especially interested in the case on account of the beautiful lichenification, and said it was the finest and most artistic marking he had ever seen.

Book Reviews

RADIUM THERAPY. By Frank Edward Simpson, A.B., M.D., Professor of Dermatology, Chicago Policlinic. Cloth. Price, $7. Pp. 391, with 166 illustrations. St. Louis: C. V. Mosby Company, 1922.

In a moderate size volume the author has attempted to cover the entire subject of radium therapy from both theoretical and practical standpoints. The result is a creditable and interesting book. It is the second work on radiotherapy to have recently come from the pen of a dermatologist. While MacKee's book on "X-Ray and Radium in the Treatment of Diseases of the Skin" confines itself to dermatologic therapeutics, the work of Simpson covers in a more cursory way the entire field of radium therapy in medicine. The present book is the work of a man of large experience in general radium therapy and is written in a clear, scholarly and conservative manner.

The book contains 383 pages, fifty-nine of which are devoted to a rather cumbersome general bibliography. The number of the authors referred to in this text is naturally rather small. About half of the book deals with the physics and biologic action of radium and the general principles of dosage and technic, while the remaining half deals with the treatment of individual diseases. Of the six chapters dealing with different branches of medicine, the one on dermatology covers a little more than fifty pages. Barely a dozen pages, however, of this chapter are devoted to text, the remainder being utilized for illustrations.

In the chapter on dermatology the author mentions the following main groups of diseases in which he states that "radium offers a possibility of use:" malignant and benign tumors, chronic infections, inflammatory and granulomatous infiltrations of uncertain nature, hypertrophies, neuroses and disorders of the appendages of the skin. In the treatment of keloid the writer considers radium to be the method of choice. Special attention is paid to the treatment of various types of nevus, including the use of flexible cloth applicators in the treatment of port wine marks. Contrary to the opinion of some other authorities, the writer advocates the use of radium in pigmented nevus, stating, however, that great care should be used in "order not to give excessive doses." In lupus vulgaris he considers radium of only limited use "being distinctly inferior to the Finsen light." Among inflammatory diseases amenable to radium treatment he mentions with special favor psoriasis of the nails and lichen simplex. In lupus erythematosus he considers that radium is "one of our most valuable agents." Warts and papillomas are discussed briefly, and excellent photographs are given showing results of treatment in sycosis. The subject of epithelioma and sarcoma is dealt with at some length in the chapter on general surgery and is illustrated by some rather striking photographs.

The numerous and excellent photographs showing results of treatment form a feature of the book. In addition there are many tables, charts and illustrations of apparatus. Glazed paper has been used throughout the book. Typographical errors are conspicuous by their absence, and the clearness of type and general appearance of the volume reflect credit on the publishers.

SURGICAL AND MECHANICAL TREATMENT OF PERIPHERAL
NERVES. By Byron Stookey, A.M., M.D., Assistant Surgeon, New York
Neurological Institute. With a Chapter on Nerve Degeneration and Regen-
eration by G. Carl Huber, M.D., Professor of Anatomy and Director of
Anatomical Laboratories, University of Michigan. Cloth. Price, $10 net.
Pp. 273, with 225 illustrations. Philadelphia: W. B. Saunders Company, 1922.

The treatment of peripheral nerve injuries has had a varied history, not
always happy, and one of the most valuable heritages that has come to us
from the great war is the advance that has been made in this field. The
abundant material from the war gave opportunity for the testing of different
methods in large numbers of cases and for the application of newer theories,
up to then experimental, to the human nervous system. The results have been
most interesting and valuable, and have proved that the nearer nerve surgery
approaches nerve histology the better are the results obtained. To the neurologist, this seems axiomatic, but unfortunately it has not seemed to be so
to many surgeons in the past, or they could not have devised joining operations
based on tendon surgery without considering nerve fibers as individuals. The
modern neurosurgeon is a neurologist, well grounded in the anatomy, histology
and physiology of the nervous system. When peripheral nerves are to be
treated, the neurosurgeon should be somewhat of an orthopedist as well, for
much of the preliminary and after-treatment is orthopedic.

In this book, the author quite satisfies the foregoing requirements. His
approach is primarily anatomic and histologic. To a neurologist, the book
contains much of interest. Each nerve and plexus is considered first from
the point of view of its embryonic development, with many clarifying references to the phylogenetic, and these points are then collected to form the basis
for surgical principals. Operations are described in detail, and considerable
space is given to the expectation of results. In places, one could wish that the
author's material had been larger, but this is in good measure offset by an
extended review of the literature and a compilation of the experience of others.
The numerous illustrations add a great deal to the book both in enhancing
the appearance and in supplementing the text.

The book opens with a chapter on the anatomy of the spinal nerve, in
which is reviewed much of the newer work on development. Dr. Huber's chapter on nerve degeneration and regeneration contains a wealth of material in
surprisingly compact form. The reviewer does not know where in English one
may find a better exposition of the subject, for the knowledge of which we
owe so much to Dr. Huber's original work. The following chapters on surgical
methods would interest the surgeon more than the neurologist.

Following these chapters, the author considers in detail the various nerves
and nerve plexuses in which injury is likely to occur, and methods of their
repair. Never does the author wander away from the anatomic and histologic
features of his problem, and one is impressed that he approaches his surgery
with the histologic eye. His plan of presentation is consistent throughout. A
point of interest to neurologists and neuro-anatomists is the description of
anomalous nerve distribution and supply as explaining atypical paralyses and
failures of operative results. The author describes and pictures in diagram
many of these anomalies which have been described by others. The chapter
on nerve tumors seems somewhat sketchy. Causalgia and amputation neuromas
form the subjects of the last two chapters.

From the point of view of the neurologist, this book contains much that is of interest and of value, which lies in good measure in the author's clear presentation of the anatomy and development of nerves. It should serve as an easy reference book both for the anatomy of peripheral nerves and for the indications in and prognosis for nerve injuries. It is likely that the general surgeon may glean from it more than would the neurosurgeon, and one may feel glad that it will carry to the general surgeon the neurologist's point of view, which considers the peripheral nerve as a histologic structure. The general makeup of the book is pleasing, and the diction is clear and makes for easy reading.

Index to Current Literature

DERMATOLOGY

Acne. Methods of Cultivating and Identifying Bacillus Acne. H. L. Begley, Philippine Islands Med. A. J. **1**:229 (Nov.-Dec.) 1921.

Acrodynia in Infants: Report of Cases. J. Zahorsky, Missouri State M. A. J. **19**:296 (July) 1922.

Actinomycosis. B. Galli-Valerio, Schweizer. med. Wchnschr. **52**:607 (June 15) 1922.

Actinomycosis, Copper Sulphate in. R. von Baracz, Zentralbl. f. Chir. **49**:634 (May 6) 1922.

Actinomycosis, Primary Pulmonary. Deutsch. med. Wchnschr. **48**:801 (June 16) 1922.

Addison's Disease, Subsequent Course of a Case of. L. G. Rowntree, J. A. M. A. **79**:556 (Aug. 12) 1922.

Anthrax Hazard in Pennsylvania Tanneries. H. F. Smyth, Am. J. Hygiene **2**:346 (July) 1922.

Anthrax, Treatment of. T. Biancheri, Policlinico **29**:718 (May 29) 1922.

Anthrax, Treatment of. L. Conti, Policlinico **29**:720 (May 29) 1922.

Arsenical Poisoning, Acute. W. H. Willcox, Brit. M. J. **2**:118 (July 22) 1922.

Blastomycosis, Local: Report of Case. M. Haase, E. R. Hall and C. H. Marshall, J. A. M. A. **79**:820 (Sept. 2) 1922.

Blue Spot, Mongolian, in Bordeaux. Boisserie-Lacroix, J. de méd. de Bordeaux **94**:355 (June 10) 1922.

Burns, Cause of Death from. R. A. Vaccarezza, Rev. asoc. méd. arg. **35**:48 (Jan. to April) 1922.

Burns, Modern Treatment of. A. de Moraes, Brazil-med. **1**:242 (May 13) 1922.

Cancer, Roentgen-Ray Treatment of. E. H. Molesworth, M. J. Australia **2**:1 (July 1) 1922.

Corpus Cavernosum, Plastic Induration of. Montpellier et al., Ann. d. mal. vén. **17**:523 (July) 1922.

Dermatitis, Exfoliative, Following Silver Arsphenamin. Loyd Thompson, J. A. M. A. **79**:628 (Aug. 19) 1922.

Dermatology, Ultraviolet Rays in. D. Carvalho, Brazil-med. **1**:255 (May 20) 1922.

Dermography, White. A. Sézary, Ann. de méd. **11**:403 (May) 1922.

Eczema. H. B. Mills, New York M. J. & Med. Rec. **116**:125 (Aug. 2) 1922.

Eczema, Infantile. H. Spohn, Canad. M. A. J. **12**:461 (July) 1922.

Eczema Parasiticum. J. W. Jones, Georgia M. A. J. **11**:253 (July) 1922.

Epidermophytosis. A. M. Greenwood, Boston M. & S. J. **187**:176 (Aug. 3) 1922.

Epithelioma on Hand, Surgical Treatment of. A. Manna, Policlinico **29**:753 (June 5) 1922.

Erysipelas Associated with Streptococcal Septicemia, Two Fatal Cases of. J. H. Pollock, Irish J. M. Sc. **5**:172 (June) 1922.

Erysipelas, Treatment of, by Vaccines. J. R. Russell, Brit. M. J. **2**:15 (July 1) 1922.

Exanthem Subitum. Report of Five Cases. A. Goldbloom, Canad. M. A. J. **12**:467 (July) 1922.

Face and Lips, Fatal Outcome of Certain Cases of Staphylococcus Infections of. W. Martin, Ann. Surg. **76**:13 (July) 1922.

Furuncles of Ear Canal. J. A. Glassburg, New York M. J. & Med. Rec. **116**:135 (Aug. 2) 1922.

Furunculosis, Iodid of Potassium Ionization in. Lacquerrière, J. de radiol. **6**:284 (June) 1922.

Gangosa in Hainan; Report of Case. N. Bercovitz, China M. J. **36**:203 (May) 1922.

Gangosa. Should Gangosa Be Removed from Nomenclature of Tropical Medicine? W. M. Kerr, Am. J. Trop. M. **2**:353 (July) 1922.

Glanders in Man; Two Cases. Said Djémil, Bull. Soc. méd. d. hôp. de Par. **46**:820 (May 26) 1922.

Granuloma, Telangiectatic Pedunculated. G. Anzilotti, Policlinico **29**:301 (June 15) 1922.

Granuloma, Ulcerating (Granuloma Inguinale). H. Goodman, J. A. M. A. **79**:815 (Sept. 2) 1922.

Herpes Zoster, Bilateral. E. Hillenberg, Klin. Wchnschr. **1**:737 (April 8) 1922.

Leprosy, Bacteriology of; Diphtheroid in Leprosy. E. L. Walker, Am. J. Trop. M. **2**:293 (July) 1922.

Leprosy, Treatment and Prognosis of. P. Harper, Brit. M. J. **2**:39 (July 8) 1922.

Leprosy, Treatment of. Gac. méd. de Caracas **29**:79 (April 15) 1922.

Lips and Face, Fatal Outcome of Certain Cases of Staphylococcus Infections of. W. Martin, Ann. Surg. **76**:13 (July) 1922.

Lip, Precancer Lesion of. G. Anzilotto, Riforma med. **38**:411 (May 1) 1922.

Manson. Patrick Manson as a Dermatologist, Appreciation of. J. M. H. Macleod, J. Trop. M. **25**:163 (June 15) 1922.

Measles, Prophylaxis of. P. Nobécourt and J. Paraf, Presse méd. **30**:497 (June 10) 1922.

Mongolian Blue Spot in Bordeaux. Boisserie-Lacroix, J. de méd. de Bordeaux **94**:355 (June 10) 1922.

Psoriasis, Etiology of. Bettmann, Deutsch. med. Wchnschr. **48**:762 (June 9) 1922.

Psoriasis, Treatment of. L. Hudelo, Paris méd. **12**:525 (June 24) 1922.

Psoriasis, Treatment of, by Manganese. J. Moore, Brit. M. J. **2**:41 (July 8) 1922.

Quartz Light Therapy in Skin Diseases. E. L. Oliver, J. A. M. A. **79**:625 (Aug. 19) 1922.

Recklinghausen's Disease. Mamerto Acuña and F. Bazán. Prensa méd. Argentina **9**:12 (June 10) 1922.

Roentgen Rays. Use of, in Diseases of Skin. G. E. Richards. Canad. M. A. J. **12**:478 (July) 1922.

Roseola, Transient, in Recurrent Fever. Oettinger and Halbreich. München. med. Wchnschr. **69**:778 (May 26) 1922.

Scarlet Fever, Epidemiologic Study of, and Its Control in Army Camps. E. B. Maynard, Mil. Surgeon **51**:25 (July) 1922.

Scarlet Fever, Etiology of. IV. Variation or Types of Alkali-Producing Organism in Scarlet Fever. R. W. Pryer, J. Lab. & Clin. M. **7**:592 (July) 1922.

Scarlet Fever, Some Diagnostic Points in. H. R. Mixsell **116**:159 (Aug. 2) 1922.

Scleroderma. G. A. M. van Balen, Nederlandsch. Tijdschr. v. Geneesk. **1**:1078 (May 20) 1922.

Scleroderma, Treatment of. G. Tognini, Riv. crit. de clin. med. **23**:133 (April 25) 1922.

Skin Diseases, Quartz Light Therapy in. E. L. Oliver, J. A. M. A. **79**:625 (Aug. 19) 1922.

Skin Irritants: External and Internal. C. G. Lane, Boston M. & S. J. **187**:108 (July 20) 1922.

Skin, Peculiar Discoloration of, Probably Resulting from Mercurial Compounds (Calomel) in Proprietary Face Creams. W. H. Goeckermann, J. A. M. A. **79**:605 (Aug. 19) 1922.

Skin. Suggestions in Treatment of Certain Diseases of Skin. J. M. King, New Orleans M. &. S. J. **75**:17 (July) 1922.

Skin, Use of Roentgen Rays in Diseases of. G. E. Richards, Canad. M. A. J. **12**:478 (July) 1922.

Sporotrichosis. F. W. Cregor, J. A. M. A. **79**:812 (Sept. 2) 1922.

Sporotrichosis, Case of Disseminated Gummatous Sporotrichosis, with Lung Metastasis. L. M. Warfield, Am. J. M. Sc. **164**:72 (July) 1922.

Ultraviolet Rays in Dermatology. D. Carvalho, Brazil-med. **1**:255 (May 20) 1922.

Variola in Bagdad. H. C. Sinderson, Edinburgh M. J. **29**:18 (July) 1922.

Variola, Violet Ray in Treatment of. P. Romeo, Boston M. & S. J. **187**:215 (Aug. 10) 1922.

Verrucae Plantares, Extensive Case of. G. P. Lingenfelter, Colorado Med. **19**:147 (July) 1922.

SYPHILOLOGY

Abortions and Syphilis. R. E. Seibels, South Carolina M. A. J. **18**:175 (June) 1922.

Abortion, Stillbirths and Infant Mortality, Syphilis in Relation to. W. G. Cosbie, Am. J. Obst. & Gynec. **4**:40 (July) 1922.

Arsenic, Elimination of, in Urine of Syphilitic Patients After Intravenous Injection of Arsphenamin. C. Weiss and G. W. Raiziss, Arch. Int. Med. **30**:85 (July) 1922.

Arsenicals, Action of, Adaptation of the Organism Thereto and Poisoning Therefrom. K. Ullmann, Wien. klin. Wchnschr. **35**:502 (June 1) 1922.

Arsphenamins and Hemoclastic Crisis. J. Golay and Benveniste, Ann. d. mal. vén. **17**:481 (July.) 1922.

Arsphenamin and Mercury Intravenous Injection. H. Boas and B. Pontoppidan, Ugesk. f. Læger **84**:645 (June 8) 1922.

Arsphenamin, Biologic Reactions of. III. Immediate Toxicity as Contrasted with Late Ill Effects, and Rôle of Agglutination in Production of Former. J. Oliver and S. S. Yamada, J. Pharmacol. & Exper. Therap. **19**:393 (July) 1922.

Arsphenamin, Bleeding Time Under. A. Sézary, Bull. et mém. Soc. méd. d. hôp. de Par. **46**:862 (June 2) 1922.

Arsphenamin by Subcutaneous Injection. J. Minet and R. Legrand, Rev. de méd. **39**:230 (April) 1922.

Arsphenamin Dermatitis. W. Heyn, Deutsch. med. Wchnschr. **48**:767 (June 9) 1922.

Arsphenamin, Elimination of Arsenic in Urine of Syphilitic Patients After Intravenous Injections of. C. Weiss and G. W. Raiziss, Arch. Int. Med. **30**:85 (July) 1922.

Arsphenamin, Fatal Cerebral Disturbances from. C. Hart, Med. Klin. **18**:444 (April 2) 1922.

Arsphenamin, Silver, Exfoliative Dermatitis Following. Loyd Thompson, J. A. M. A. **79**:628 (Aug. 19) 1922.

Arsphenamin Treatment of Syphilis, Prophylactic. W. Schänfeld, München. med. Wchnschr. **69**:811 (June 2) 1922.

Backache, Syphilitic. W. Thompson, Am. J. M. Sc. **164**:109 (July) 1922.

Bismuth in Treatment of Neurosyphilis. J. M. Agramunt, Siglo méd. **69**:397 (April 15) 1922.

Bismuth in Treatment of Syphilis A. Machado and A. E. Area Leite, Brazil-med. **1**:195 (April 22) 1922.

Bismuth in Treatment of Syphilis. U. Paranhos, Brazil-med. **1**:311 (June 10) 1922.

Bismuth Treatment of Syphilis, Present Status of. H. Haxthausen, Hospitalstidende **65**:342 (June 10) 1922.

Bismuth, Treatment of Syphilis with. H. Müller, München. med. Wchnschr. **69**:547 (April 14) 1922.

Bleeding Time Under Arsphenamin. A. Sézary, Bull. et mém. Soc. méd. d. hôp. de Par. **46**:862 (June 2) 1922.

Cerebrospinal Fluid and Syphilis. Nonne, Prensa méd. Argentina **9**:33 (June 10) 1922.

Chancre, Syphilitic, in Ear. E. Conde Flores, Gac. méd. de Caracas **29**:11 (Jan. 15) 1922.

Chancres, Syphilitic, Unusual Locations for. Müller, Deutsch. med. Wchnschr. **48**:803 (June 16) 1922.

Chancre, Tuberculous. J. A. Nixon and A. R. Short, Brit. J. Surg. **10**:44 (July) 1922.

Ear, Syphilitic Chancre in. E. Conde Flores, Gac. méd. de Caracas **29**:11 (Jan. 15) 1922.

Epinephrin. By-Effects of Neo-Arsphenamin and How to Prevent Them; with Special Reference to Epinephrin. H. Reinhard-Eichelbaum, Deutsch. med. Wchnschr. **48**:804 (June 16) 1922.

Flumerin—A New Mercurial for Intravenous Treatment of Syphilis: First Report of Chemical, Animal and Clinical Experiments and Results. E. C. White, J. H. Hill, J. E. Moore and H. H. Young, J. A. M. A. **79**:877 (Sept. 9) 1922.

Formalin Test for Syphilis: Some Conditions Controlling Gel Formation. A. G. Holborow, Lancet **2**:274 (Aug. 5) 1922.

Formol-Gel Reaction in Blood Serum of Syphilitics. C. A. Watson, Canad. M. A. J. **12**:469 (July) 1922.

Formol-Gel Test for Syphilis, Value of. S. Ramakrishnan, Indian M. Gaz. **57**:254 (July) 1922.

Gangrene of Fingers Associated with Secondary Syphilitic Lesions. G. Guillain and C. Kudelski, Bull. et mém. Soc. méd. d. hôp. de Par. **46**:917 (June 9) 1922.

Gangrene of Penis, Syphilitic. E. Orphanidès, Ann. d. mal. vén. **17**:516 (July) 1922.

Genital Lesions, A Study of Four Hundred and Eighty-Five Cases with. J. R. Driver, J. A. M. A. **79**:867 (Sept. 9) 1922.

Heart Disease, Syphilitic. S. A. Meza and J. Paulis, Rev. españ. de med. y cirug. **5**:199 (April) 1922.

Hecht's Modification of Wassermann Test. W. Loele, München. med. Wchnschr. **69**:885 (June 16) 1922.

Hemoclastic Crisis and Arsphenamins. J. Golay and Benveniste, Ann. d. mal. vén. **17**:481 (July) 1922.

Infant Mortality, Abortion and Stillbirths, Syphilis in Relation to. W. G. Cosbie, Am. J. Obst. & Gynec. **4**:40 (July) 1922.

Intestine, Small, Acquired Syphilis of. R. Schmidt, Beitr. z. klin. Chir. **126**: 61, 1922

Kahn Precipitation Test in the Diagnosis of Syphilis: A Preliminary Study. H. L. Keim and U. J. Wile, J. A. M. A. **79**:870 (Sept. 9) 1922.

Lung, Syphilis of. J. Lecaplain, Bull. et mém. Soc. méd. d. hôp. de Par. **46**:930 (June 16) 1922.

Mental Disease, Syphilis in. H. Hoven, Arch. méd. belges **75**:393 (May) 1922.

Mercurial Compounds (Calomel) in Proprietary Face Creams. Peculiar Discoloration of Skin Probably Resulting from. W. H. Goeckermann, J. A. M. A. **79**:605 (Aug. 19) 1922.

Mercurosal, Intravenous Injection of, in Treatment of Syphilis. W. T. Williams, Canad. M. A. J. **12**:401 (June) 1922.

Mercury, Anaphylaxis to. Gougerot and Blamoutier, Bull. et mém. Soc. méd. d. hôp. de Par. **46**:868 and 873 (June 2) 1922.

Mercury. Simultaneous Arsphenamin and Mercury Intravenous Injection. H. Boas and B. Pontoppidan, Ugesk. f. Læger **84**:645 (June 8) 1922.

Myopathy with Inherited Syphilis. G. Milian and Lelong. Bull. et mém. Soc. méd. d. hôp. de Par. **46**:893 (June 2) 1922.

Neo-Arsphenamin, By-Effects of, and How to Prevent Them; with Special Reference to Epinephrin. H. Reinhard-Eichelbaum, Deutsch. med. Wchnschr. **48**:804 (June 16) 1922.

Nervous System. Results of Treatment in Syphilis of Nervous System. R. Hearn, Brit. M. J. **2**:37 (July 8) 1922.

Neurosyphilis, Asymptomatic, Studies in. J. E. Moore, Bull. Johns Hopkins Hosp. **33**:231 (July) 1922.

Neurosyphilis, Asymptomatic, Studies in. IV. The Apparent Rôle of Immunity in the Genesis of Neurosyphilis. A. Keidel, J. A. M. A. **79**:874 (Sept. 9) 1922.

Neurosyphilis, Bismuth in Treatment of. J. M. Agramunt, Siglo méd. **69**: 397 (April 15) 1922.

Neurosyphilis, Bismuth in Treatment of. Evrard, Ann. d. mal. vén. **17**:525 (July) 1922.

Neurosyphilis, Classification of: Concerning Therapy. L. H. Cornwall, New York State J. M. **22**:316 (July) 1922.

Neurosyphilis, Early. Nonne, Prensa med. Argentina **9**:68 (June 20) 1922.

Paralysis, Amyotrophic, Early in Tabes. W. Schmitt, Med. Klin. **18**:436 (April 2) 1922.

Penis, Syphilitic Gangrene of. E. Orphanidès, Ann. d. mal. vén. **17**:516 (July) 1922.

Reticular Fibers in Syphilis and Other Cutaneous Diseases, Occurrence and Significance of. E. Zurhelle, Deutsch. med. Wchnschr. **48**:724 (June 2) 1922.

Rheumatism, Deforming Articular, of Syphilitic Origin. H. Dufour and Geismar, Bull. et mém. Soc. méd. d. hôp. de Par. **46**:970 (June 23) 1922.

Serum, Opacity of Mixture of, and Wassermann "Antigen" in Progressively Increasing Concentrations of Sodium Chlorid. J. Holker, J. Path. & Bacteriol. **25**:291 (July) 1922.

Sigma and Wassermann Tests. W. T. Collier, Lancet **2**:274 (Aug. 5) 1922.

Silver Arsphenamin, Exfoliative Dermatitis Following. Loyd Thompson, J. A. M. A. **79**:628 (Aug. 19) 1922.

Spirochaeta Pallida in Sperm. R. Lakaye, Arch. méd. belges **75**:385 (May) 1922.

Stillbirths, Abortion and Infant Mortality, Syphilis in Relation to. W. G. Cosbie, Am. J. Obst. & Gynec. **4**:40 (July) 1922.

Syphilis, Abortive Treatment of. P. Pediconi, Policlinico **29**:937 (July 17) 1922.

Syphilis, Acquired, of the Small Intestine. R. Schmidt, Beitr. z. klin. Chir. **126**:61, 1922.

Syphilis, African, Tabes in Two Europeans from. A. Sézary and J. Alibert, Bull. et mém. Soc. méd. d. hôp. de Par. **46**:816 (May 19) 1922.

Syphilis and Abortions. R. E. Seibels, South Carolina M. A. J. **18**:175 (June) 1922.

Syphilis and the Cerebrospinal Fluid. Nonne, Prensa méd Argentina **9**:33 (June 10) 1922.

Syphilis and Other Cutaneous Diseases, Reticular Fibers in, Occurrence and Significance of. E. Zurhelle, Deutsch. med. Wchnschr. **48**:724 (June 2) 1922.

Syphilis and Yaws, Relation Between, as Observed in American Samoa. J. C. Parham, Am. J. Trop. M. **2**:341 (July) 1922.

Syphilis, Bismuth in Treatment of, II. Parreiras Horta and P. Gans, Brazil-méd. **1**:183 (April 15) 1922.

Syphilis, Bismuth in Treatment of. A. Machado and A. E. Area Leite, Brazil-med. **1**:195 (April 22) 1922.

Syphilis, Bismuth in Treatment of. U. Paranhos, Brazil-med. **1**:311 (June 10) 1922.

Syphilis, Bismuth in Treatment of. H. Grenet et al., Bull. de l'Acad. de méd. **87**:658 (June 13) 1922.

Syphilis, Bismuth Treatment of. P. Wolfer, Schweizer. med. Wchnschr. **52** 703 (July 13) 1922.

Syphilis, Cerebrospinal, Types of, in China. A. H. Woods, China M. J. **36** 206 (May) 1922.

Syphilis, Clinical Diagnosis of. H. A. Dixon, Canad. M. A. J. **12**:470 (July) 1922.

Syphilis, Congenital. G. Stümpke, München. med. Wchnschr. **69**:551 (April 14) 1922.

Syphilis, Congenital, and Eruption of First Teeth. E. Moody, Missouri State M. A. J. **19**:295 (July) 1922.

Syphilis, Developments in Diagnosis and Treatment of. L. W. Shaffer, U. S. Naval M. Bull. **16**:1011 (June) 1922.

Syphilis, Diagnosis and Treatment of. G. W. Payne, Kentucky M. J. **20**:393 (June) 1922.

Syphilis, Early Clinical Diagnosis of. H. Colman, Med. Klin. **18**:437 (April 2) 1922.

Syphilis, Expression of Eyes as Sign of. A. Chelmonski, Rev. de méd. **39**: 172 (March) 1922.

Syphilis, Family; Its Relation to Public Health. E. Hess, Penn. M. J. **25**:693 (July) 1922.

Syphilis in Mental Disease. H. Hoven, Arch. méd. belges **75**:393 (May) 1922.

Syphilis in Northern Africa. G. Lacapère, Ann. d. mal. vén. **17**:493 (July) 1922.

Syphilis in Relation to Abortion, Stillbirths and Infant Mortality. W. G. Cosbie, Am. J. Obst. & Gynec. **4**:40 (July) 1922.

Syphilis, Intracutaneous Gelatin Reaction in. A. Busacca, Wien. klin. Wchnschr. **35**:523 (June 8) 1922.

Syphilis. Intravenous Injection of Mercurosal in Treatment of Syphilis. W. T. Williams, Canad. M. A. J. **12**:401 (June) 1922.

Syphilis. The Kahn Precipitation Test in the Diagnosis of Syphilis: A Preliminary Study. H. L. Keim and U. J. Wile, J. A. M. A. **79**:870 (Sept. 9) 1922.

Syphilis, Modern Treatment of. L. W. Harrison, Brit. M. J. **2**:1 (July 1) 1922.

Syphilis. Myopathy with Inherited Syphilis. G. Milian and Lelong. Bull. et mém. Soc. méd. d. hôp. de Par. **46**:893 (June 2) 1922.

Syphilis of Central Nervous System, Results of Treatment in. R. Hearn. Brit. M. J. **2**:37 (July 8) 1922.

Syphilis of the Lung. J. Lecaplain, Bull. et mém. Soc. méd. d. hôp. de Par. **46**:930 (June 16) 1922.

Syphilis of the Tonsil. J. May, Rev. méd. d. Uruguay **25**:485 (June) 1922.

Syphilis, Present Status of Bismuth Treatment of. H. Haxthausen. Hospitalstidende **65**:342 (June 10) 1922.

Syphilis, Prophylactic Arsphenamin Treatment of. W. Schönfeld. München. med. Wchnschr. **69**:811 (June 2) 1922.

Syphilis, Reinfection with. Carle, Ann. d. mal. vén. **17**:497 (July) 1922.

Syphilis, Serodiagnosis of, by Flocculation. C. Bruck, Deutsch. med. Wchnschr. **48**:825 (June 23) 1922.

Syphilis, Spontaneous Cure of. F. Lesser, Med. Klin. **18**:824 (June 25) 1922.

Syphilis. Ten Cases of Delayed Congenital Syphilis. E. D. Spackman. Lancet **2**:65 (July 8) 1922.

Syphilis—Three Years' Observation. E. J. Trow, Canad. M. A. J. **12**:455 (July) 1922.

Syphilis, Treatment of, with Bismuth. H. Müller, München. med. Wchnschr. **69**:547 (April 14) 1922.

Syphilis, Treatment of, with a French Arsenical. J. A. Ortiz. Semana med. **1**:798 (May 18) 1922.

Syphilis, Value of Formol-Gel Test for. S. Ramakrishnan. Indian M. Ga⁻ **57**:254 (July) 1922.

Syphilitic Backache. W. Thompson, Am. J. M. Sc. **164**:109 (July) 1922.

Syphilitic Lesions. Gangrene of Fingers Associated with Secondary Syphilitic Lesions. G. Guillain and C. Kudelski, Bull. et mém. Soc. méd. d. hôp. de Par. **46**:917 (June 9) 1922.

Syphilitic Serums in Relation to Specificity of Immunity Reactions, Properties of. J. Holker, J. Path. & Bacteriol. **25**:281 (July) 1922 .

Tabes, Amyotrophic Paralysis Early in. W. Schmitt, Med. Klin. **18**:436 (April 2) 1922.

Tabes in Two Europeans from African Syphilis. A. Sézary and J. Alibert, Bull. et mém. Soc. méd. d. hôp. de Par. **46**:816 (May 19) 1922.

Teeth. Eruption of First Teeth and Congenital Syphilis. E. Moody, Missouri State M. A. J. **19**:295 (July) 1922.

Tonsil, Syphilis of. J. May, Rev. méd. d. Uruguay **25**:485 (June) 1922.

Urine of Syphilitic Patients After Intravenous Injections of Arsphenamin, Elimination of Arsenic in. C. Weiss and G. W. Raiziss, Arch. Int. Med. **30**:85 (July) 1922.

Venereal Battalion, Development of. C. M. Williams, Mil. Surgeon **50**:177 (Aug.) 1922.

Venereal Disease in Nürnberg, Spread of. L. Voigt, München. med. Wchnschr. **69**:861 (June 9) 1922.

Venereal Disease, Prophylaxis of. V. Hernández Usera, Bull. Porto Rico M. A. **16**:114 (June 30) .1922.

Via Veneris. H. H. Rutherford, Mil. Surgeon **50**:173 (Aug.) 1922.

Wassermann and Sigma Tests. W. T. Collier, Lancet **2**:274 (Aug. 5) 1922.

Wassermann "Antigen" and Opacity of Mixture of Serum in Progressively Increasing Concentrations of Sodium Chlorid. J. Holker, J. Path. & Bacteriol. **25**:291 (July) 1922.

Wassermann Reaction. A. Dulière, Arch. méd. belges **75**:510 (June) 1922.

Wassermann Reaction as Index of Cure, with Special Reference to Value of Cold Fixation in Technic of Test. C. H. Shearman, M. J. Australia **1**: 656 (June 17) 1922.

Wassermann Reaction, Relative Value of Human and Guinea-Pig Complement in. A. F. Hayden, Brit. J. Exper. Path. **3**:151 (June) 1922.

Wassermann Test, Hecht's Modification of. W. Loele, München. med. Wchnschr. **69**:885 (June 16) 1922.

Wassermann Test in Spinal Fluid. Cestan and Riser, Ann. d. mal. vén. **11**:365 (May) 1922.

Wassermann Test, Standardization and Preservation of Complement Serum for. E. H. Ruediger, J. A. M. A. **79**:551 (Aug. 12) 1922.

Wassermann Variations: A Study of the Serums of Seventy-Five Patients by Eight Laboratories. L. J. Palmer, J. A. M. A. **79**:724 (Aug. 26) 1922.

Yaws and Syphilis, Relation Between, as Observed in American Samoa. J. C. Parham, Am. J. Trop. M. **2**:341 (July) 1922.

Archives of Dermatology and Syphilology

| Volume 6 | NOVEMBER, 1922 | Number 5 |

A PRELIMINARY STUDY OF THE EXPERIMENTAL ASPECTS OF IODID AND BROMID EXANTHEMS *

UDO J. WILE, M.D., CARROLL S. WRIGHT, M.D.

Professor and Instructor, Respectively, of Dermatology and Syphilology,
University of Michigan Medical School

AND

NED R. SMITH, M.D.

Intern in Internal Medicine, University Hospital

ANN ARBOR, MICH.

The experimental aspects of the various dermatoses associated with and following the ingestion of various medicaments have received little attention from dermatologists. This is quite readily understandable when one realizes that such investigation involves the most intricate problems of biochemical and physicochemical research. For this reason, therefore, most of the articles dealing with the question of drug eruptions from their experimental side have been written by physiologic chemists.

Notwithstanding the fact that most of our experimental evidence comes from those not primarily interested in dermatology, valuable contributions from the side of cutaneous medicine have been made, in calling attention to the appearance of such rashes and in properly ascribing the cause to the offending drug. We are, therefore, indebted to dermatologic literature for the first descriptions and the etiologic factors involved; and, moreover, in not a few cases, to productive research attempting to explain the ultimate cause.

With the introduction into the practice of medicine, notably in the last three decades, of an enormous number of synthetic drugs, there has been a correspondingly increasing number of cases of so-called idiosyncrasy or susceptibility to such medicaments, such being mani-

* Read before the Forty-Fifth Annual Meeting of the American Dermatological Association, Washington, D. C., May 2-4, 1922.

* Studies and contributions of the department of dermatology and syphilology of the University of Michigan, service of Dr. Udo J. Wile.

fested by reactions on the part of the digestive, the nervous and the arterial systems, and, most important, the cutaneous covering. It is safe to state that probably no synthetic drug has ever yet been introduced which, in isolated cases, has not given rise to symptoms of intolerance, with their associated cutaneous manifestations. These, as is well known, vary from the most evanescent type of erythema to lesions actually so destructive as to impair function and to endanger life. The greatest diversity of lesion and the greatest variability of intensity can occur with each and any drug; the process is the same, the difference only in the intensity of the reaction.

Lacking accurate experimental evidence, the occurrence of exanthems following the ingestion of drugs has been ascribed by various writers to such vague terms as idiosyncrasy, susceptibility, chemotaxis, toxicity, and, of late years, allergy and anaphylaxis.

Granting that, in enormous doses, practically all drugs of therapeutic value are distinctly toxic to the human organism, it is evident from the outset that, in a given case of intolerant reaction to such drug on the part of the skin, two factors surely come into consideration: (1) the poisonous quality of the drug itself, and (2) the human organism in its relation to the drug. All synthetics, and most drugs, are prepared with extreme care with regard to their actual toxicity, long before their introduction into medical practice. Their therapeutic application, moreover, is always fixed at a point much below the minimum lethal dose. The natural source for investigation as to the effect of the minimum lethal dose on the person who nevertheless reacts is in the person himself.

Some drugs in common use are so frequently associated with mild manifestations on the skin that the occurrence of these manifestations is regarded as almost physiologic. Thus, for example, as is well known, pustulation occurs so frequently in the administration of iodid of potash that it is stated by some that iodid only reaches its physiologic effect when the skin reacts in the form of pustules. We believe this conception to be quite as erroneous as the former acceptance of the physiologic reaction of mercury when the stage of salivation had been reached.

Exanthems following the ingestion of synthetics, although common enough, occur usually in isolated instances, and the manifestations are, as a rule, of such a fleeting nature that the investigation of these eruptions from the biochemical side is extremely difficult, owing to the lack, over a sufficient period of time, of the proper material. Laboratory animals, furthermore, do not lend themselves readily to experimentation for this purpose.

The universal use, notably in group cases, of iodids in the infectious granulomas, and of bromids in neurologic disorders, such as epilepsy, has for obvious reasons, therefore, led to a greater degree of experimentation with these two drugs than with any others. It is highly probable, also, that a suitable explanation, based on proper experimentation, for the occurrence of iododermas and bromodermas in their various forms would suffice as an adequate explanation for the occurrence of exanthems and rashes due to the ingestion of other drugs. The bromids have been more extensively investigated than have the iodids.

Notable contributions in foreign literature bearing on the subject have been made by Adamkiewicz,[1] Szadek,[2] Laudenheimer,[3] Von Wyss,[4] Ulrich,[5] Ellinger and Kotake;[6] and in this country by Sollman and Pilcher,[7] Kolmer and his associates,[8] Engman and Mook,[9] and by Osborne.[10] The earliest investigators on the subjects of both bromid and iodid were led to believe that the reaction in the skin was due to the liberation of the free halogen in the blood, and its irritant action directly on the skin or on the blood vessels of the skin. Color, perhaps, was lent to this view by the discovery that all of the secretions of the body contained the offending drug, after ingestion. All glandular

1. Adamkiewicz: Die Ausscheidungswege des Jodkaliums beim Menschen, Charité-Ann. **3**:381, 1878.

2. Szadek: Casuistik des Brom-exanthems, Arch. f. Derm. **20**:599, 1888.

3. Laudenheimer: Ueber das Verhalten der Bromsälze im Korper in des Epileptikers, Neurol. Centralbl. **16**:538, 1897.

4. Von Wyss: Ueber das Verhalten der Bromsältzer in menschlichem und tiereschen Organismus, Arch. f. exper. Path. u. Pharmakol. **55**:263, 1906: Ueber das Verhalten der Bromsaltzer in menschlichem und tiereschen Organismus. Arch. f. exper. Path. u. Pharmakol. **59**:186, 1908. Von Wyss and Ulrich: Die Bromtherapie der Epilepsie auf experimenteller Grundlage, Arch. f. Psychiat. **46**:197, 1909-1910.

5. Ulrich: Footnote 4, third reference.

6. Ellinger and Kotake: Die Verteilung des Broms im Organismus nach darreichung unorganischer und organischer Brompreparata. Arch. f. exper. Path. u. Pharmakol. **65**:87, 1911.

7. Sollmann and Pilcher: Endermic Reactions. J. Pharmacol. & Exper. Therap. **9**:309, 1916-1917; ibid. **10**:147, 1917. Sollmann: The Fate of Iodin. Iodids and Iodates in the Body, J. Pharmacol. & Exper. Therap. **9**:279, 1917.

8. Kolmer, J. A.; Matsunami, Toitsu, and Broadwell. Stuart. Jr.: The Effect of Potassium Iodid in the Luetin Reaction, J. A. M. A. **67**:718 (Sept. 2) 1916. Kolmer, Immerman, Matsunami and Montgomery: The Effect of Certain Drugs upon Skin Reactions, J. Lab. & Clin. Med. **2**:401, 1916-1917. Kolmer: Mechanism and Clinical Significance of Anaphylactic and Pseudo-Anaphylactic Skin Reactions, Proc. Pan-Am. Scien. Cong., Sec. 8, Pub. Health & Med. **10**:287, 1917.

9. Engman and Mook: A Contribution to the Histopathology and History of Drug Exanthems, J. Cutan. Dis. **24**:502, 1906.

10. Osborne, E. D.: Iodid in the Cerebrospinal Fluid. with Special Reference to Iodid Therapy, J. A. M. A. **76**:1384 (May 21) 1921.

structures, including the sebaceous glands and sweat coils, eliminated the drug, and, in the case of the latter, the elimination took place on the surface of the body. The acid reaction in secretions from the sweat and sebaceous glands was thought by earlier observers to liberate iodid and bromid in their free state, with the resultant irritation phenomena.

As early as 1878, Guttman [11] reported the occurrence of bromid in the contents of pustules in a patient taking 12 gm. of bromid a day. This observation, however, has not been confirmed by subsequent investigations. In the same year, Adamkiewicz,[1] investigating iodid, established its presence in all body fluids following ingestion, and stated that he had found it also in the pus of iodid acne, using as his reagent a starch paste for its detection. Both of these observers regarded the cutaneous reaction as due to the free halogen liberated by the acid with which it came in contact in and about the structures of the skin.

It is noteworthy that, in 1885, Tilbury Fox,[12] in reporting a case of bromoderma, stated that the histologic examination of the lesions did not bear out this theory, in that, in his case, neither sebaceous nor sudoriparous glands were found to be in the least involved in the process. In 1888, Szadek,[2] after studying bromodermas and establishing that these varied from simple erythema to urticaria, nodules, bullae and phlyctenulae, came to conclusions similar to those held by Guttman.[11] From his chemical studies and the histologic study of Neumann, he regarded the bromexanthem as starting in an irritation phenomenon from the sebaceous apparatus.

This belief, namely, that the native halogen was, by an actual irritation, responsible for the eruption, persisted until about 1897, and, in the face of experimental evidence to the contrary, is still held by some. At this time, Laudenheimer,[3] with much material for the study of epilepsy at his disposal, made a careful chemical observation of the behavior of bromid in the various tissues of the body in a large number of patients. He demonstrated a very definite phenomenon for bromid, which differs materially from the behavior of either chlorid or iodid in the body. His researches, subsequently substantiated in 1910 by Von Wyss,[13] and since that time by others, demonstrated that the ingestion of bromid led to a gradual piling up of the drug and a gradual replacement by it of the chlorid content of the tissues. That is to say, a patient taking bromid at once showed in the urine a marked increase

11. Guttman: Bromreaktion des Inhalts von Aknepustuln nachlangen Bromkaliumgebrauch in einem Falle von Agrophobie, Virchows Arch. f. path. Anat. **74**:541, 1878.

12. Fox, Tilbury: Brom Eruption, Brit. M. J. **2**:971, 1885.

13. Von Wyss: Footnote 4, third reference.

of a chlorid excretion. The bromid at the outset was excreted by the urine in far smaller quantities than it was ingested. Not only did this take place in the circulating blood, but it was demonstrated that the chlorin ion of the gastric juice was replaced by bromin (Nencki and Simanowski [14]). The various symptoms of brominism, apart from the cutaneous reactions, namely, stupor, pallor, emaciation and psychic disturbance, Laudenheimer attempted to explain as manifestations of chlorid hunger or chlorid deficiency. This is interesting in substantiation of his explanation that the reintroduction of large amounts of chlorid into the system gradually reestablished the normal chlorid content of the tissues, with a relief of the symptoms of bromism. It is also interesting, in this connection, that the introduction of chlorid in excess into the system has a marked beneficial effect upon the bromodermas.

Similar investigations conducted by Nencki and Simanowski,[14] Von Wyss,[4] and also Ulrich,[5] and by Büchner and Fessell,[13] substantiated the results of Laudenheimer. Fessell [15] showed that chlorid elimination markedly increased, as evidenced by its appearance in the urine after bromid intake, and that, further, after bromid and sodium chlorid were given together, the bromid was much more rapidly eliminated. Von Wyss,[16] and later Von Wyss and Ulrich,[17] in a careful study of the behavior of bromid in the animal and human organism, showed definitely that the elimination lagged far behind the intake, and that long after the withdrawal of the drug its presence could be detected in the urine. Von Wyss stated that if this were so, either bromin remained somewhere in the body in close union and bound up with protoplasm, or else it remained not fixed but, for some unknown reason, not as readily eliminated by the kidney, as iodid and chlorid; or that it is eliminated into the intestine and continually reabsorbed, being slowly eliminated by the kidney, establishing thus a more or less continuous digestive cycle for the drug. By intracutaneous injection, he determined that the chlorin ion could be displaced in the gastric juice of the stomach by the bromin ion. He concluded that bromid in the body is removed slowly, for some unknown reason, through the kidney, and that a constant reabsorption by the gastric and intestinal mucosae occurs; which accounted for its piling up in the system. He further determined, by careful tissue analysis, that the circulating blood, and notably the serum, contained the bulk of the bromid held back in the

---

14. Nencki and Simanowski: Studien über das Chlor und die Halogene im Thierkörper, Arch. f. exper. Path. u. Pharmakol. **34**:313, 1894.

15. Fessell: Ueber das Verhalten des Brom im Thierkörper. München. med. Wchnschr., Series 2 **46**:270, 1899.

16. Von Wyss: Footnote 4, first reference.

17. Von Wyss and Ulrich: Footnote 4, third reference.

system. The remarkable ability of bromid to replace chlorid was further established by the interesting findings of Ellinger and Kotake,[6] who, by careful chemical quantitative analysis, determined that those organs and tissues in which there were the largest amounts of chlorid contained the largest amount of bromid, in experimental animals to whom bromin had been fed.

Von Wyss and Ulrich [17] did not regard the cutaneous manifestations of bromid ingestion as symptomatic of bromid intoxication, nor in any way related to what they were pleased to call chlorid deficiency in the explanation of other forms of brominism. They regarded the cutaneous lesions as due to the liberation of free bromin on the skin, giving rise to exquisite irritation phenomena, thereby enabling the existing pus organisms on the skin to become pathogenic, with the resultant formation of the lesion. Laudenheimer,[3] however, was inclined to regard the cutaneous reaction as actually a symptom of brominism, that is, as due to chlorid deficiency.

In 1906, a noteworthy article appeared in the French literature by Pasini.[18] His contribution is valuable because he demonstrated that it was quite impossible for free bromin to exist in the pus, as was recorded by Guttman;[11] that if one added actual bromid in vitro to albumin solutions, it was impossible to detect the drug until the albumin was destroyed, or until such a high degree of oxidation occurred by the addition of concentracted acid that it could be liberated; and that this degree of acidity could never occur in the normal chemistry of the animal body. Following experiments involving the implantation of actual bromids subcutaneously into laboratory animals, he stated his belief that the salts of bromin exercised a chematactic action, and that resultant cutaneous reaction was one of chemical irritation.

These views were held tenable by Jacquet, Leloir and Vidal [19] only so far as such irritation prepared the soil for subsequent activity of the common pus organisms. About the same time, Auspitz, and also Crocker,[20] advanced the theory that the cutaneous reactions were due to a direct action of the drug on the vasomoter centers.

In 1906, Engman and Mook [9] presented a paper before the American Dermatological Association on the "Histopathology and the Theory of Drug Eruptions." Their contribution is noteworthy in that they stated that the pustular contents of iodid and bromid eruptions, not only in simple pustules but also in open ulcers, were sterile, and that the micro-organisms of the skin could, therefore, not be held

18. Pasini: Sur la pathogenie des eruption bromiques, Ann. de dermat. et syph., Series 4 **7**:1, 1906.

19. Jacquet, Leloir and Vidal: Etude d'un cas de bromisme cutané polymorphe, Ann. de dermat. et syph., 1889, p. 981.

20. Crocker: Eruptions from Bromid and Iodid, Brit. M. J. **2**:1208, 1893.

responsible for the appearance of the lesions. They likewise called attention to the tendency of iodid and bromid eruptions to localize themselves in the seborrhic and acne areas. Another interesting point in connection with their presentation was the demonstration of iodid in the pus from iodid lesions. Bromid was not satisfactorily investigated in their cases, on account of the difficulty of finding a specific bromid reaction. In their contribution, Engman and Mook express the opinion that the lesions resulting from the ingestion of both drugs are liable to occur at points of previous inflammation, that actual trauma may precipitate an eruption, and that the glands or follicles of the skin take no specific part in the production of the lesions. They suggest a disturbance of equilibrium induced by various factors producing a toxin, which in turn causes irritation and various local inflammatory symptoms. Herein is the first suggestion that, in the occurrence of bromid and iodid lesions, an altered disturbance of the blood might be held responsible.

Considerable impetus to the study of the mechanism of all drug exanthems, notably those caused by iodid and bromid, was given by the careful studies of Kolmer and his associates,[8] and of Sollmann.[21] Sollmann's and Pilcher's [7] studies were carried out with the idea of determining the local effect of various drugs on the production of cutaneous lesions. An enormous number of drugs were tried out, both by intracutaneous inoculation and by the ingenious use of the *Mucuna* method. This consists in the application of the dried stiff hairs of a leguminous seedpod, rubbing these on the skin, and following it by solutions of the drugs to be investigated. In a later study, Sollmann [21] investigated the fate of iodin, iodids and iodates in the body. His studies led him to the inevitable conclusion that iodin exists in the tissues of the body only as iodid, that it could never be liberated free in the body or from the body surface, because to liberate the free halogen would require a hydrogen-ion content, that is to say, an acidity far stronger than can possibly exist in the human organism. He also demonstrated that the iodin existed loosely bound with protein, in which it was readily dialyzable.

Kolmer [22] investigated the behavior of iodid and drug exanthems from the side of a possible allergy or anaphylaxis. In an extensive monograph published in 1917, Kolmer [23] concludes that skin reactions are either specific anaphylactic in nature; pseudospecific or nonspecific protein reactions; or traumatic reactions; that iodid and bromid increase the nonspecific action by facilitating the activity of nonspecific pro-

21. Sollmann, Torald: Footnote 7, third reference.
22. Kolmer: Footnote 8, first and second references.
23. Kolmer: Footnote 8, second reference.

teolytic ferments and the production of protein poison through the removal of antiferment. It will be noted here that this bears directly on the administration of iodid and bromid as they affect anaphylactic conditions caused by protein poison, and is in no way an attempt to explain the mechanism of iododermas and bromodermas. The suggestion, however, that the presence of iodid and bromid in the blood can and does materially affect true allergic reactions no doubt bears in a very distinct way on the nature of reactions caused by these drugs themselves. Kolmer's investigations in this field were inspired by the work of Sherrick,[24] who, in 1915, determined that nonsyphilitic patients could be made to react with a typical pustule with the luetin test, if before or after the test was made they were taking iodid of potash.

In summing up the total evidence at present in our hands, we are confronted with a mass of contradictory facts:

1. The theory that iododermas and bromodermas can be caused by the liberation and the presence of the free halogen in the tissues.

2. That the presence of the salts of these halogens increases the virulence of the normal cocci of the skin, with resulting infection.

3. That they are the phenomena of chemical irritation.

4. That they are vasomotor phenomena.

5. That they are due to an altered condition of the blood, and that the lesions themselves are sterile.

6. That they are closely allied to the phenomena of local sensitization or allergy.

It was in an attempt to shed at least some light on this problem that the studies herein noted were begun about a year and a half ago.

Our experiments covered the following problems:

1. The corroboration of previous results for the determination of iodid and bromid in body fluids.

2. The study of the elimination of bromid in the urine and the replacement of chlorid by it in the tissues.

3. Investigation as to the presence of iodin and bromin or their salts in the local lesions of bromoderma and ioderma.

4. Bacteriologic studies of the lesions to determine the absence or presence of pus organisms.

5. Percutaneous tests on patients taking salts of bromin and iodin, in the attempt to determine a skin sensitization.

6. An attempt to produce cutaneous bromid reaction in conditions of acidosis.

---

24. Sherrick, J. W.: The Effect of Potassium Iodid in the Luetin Reaction, J. A. M. A. **65**:404 (July 31) 1915.

7. The investigation as to the existence of specific precipitins in the blood for bromid and iodid.

With respect to the determination of bromid and iodid in the body fluids, it may be briefly stated that in the case of iodid this is a matter of extreme ease. In tissues containing organic material, such as the circulating blood, it is, however, necessary, before testing for either iodid and bromid, to destroy the organic material. We found the easiest way to do this was by digesting the organic material with sulphuric acid, distilling the material, and testing for the drug in the acidulated distillate. The final test employed was that of shaking out iodin with either chloroform or carbon disulphid in the presence of nitric acid and sodium nitrite. Under these conditions, iodin was found, even if only a small quantity had been ingested, in the circulating blood, the urine, the sweat and the saliva. So delicate was our test under these conditions that we could determine easily the presence of iodin in 10 c.c. of blood fifteen minutes after the ingestion of 5 grains (0.3 gm.) of potassium iodid. After distilling over and acidulating the distillate, even a few drops of the original 10 c.c. were found to contain iodin.

In the case of bromid, great difficulty was encountered in that the established chemical tests for bromid are markedly interfered with by the presence of chlorid. We finally determined on the best method for the detection of bromid as follows: The suspected material was oxidized with a solution of potassium permanganate in the excess of sulphuric acid. In organic material, this maneuver was carried out as in the case of testing for iodid by first digesting with sulphuric acid and distilling. Under these condition, we found bromin in patients ingesting the drug, in the blood, the urine, the sweat and the saliva. under the same circumstances that iodin was found.

In our investigations, we had an opportunity of making tests in a large number of cases, the patients in the iodid group being syphilitic and having taken the drug over a long period of time. and the patients in the bromid group, for the most part, being afflicted with and treated for various neurologic disturbances, including epilepsy. In no case were we able to determine the presence of the slightest trace of either drug in the local lesions, and it is our belief that this does not occur. except so far as there may be an admixture of the blood serum in the local lesion. We examined at one time an enormous amount of pus gathered from several patients. who were taking large amounts of iodid. The addition of the smallest quantity of iodid of soda (2 or 3 drops to a 1 : 1000 solution) to such a mixture. followed by dilution. enabled us to determine iodid very readily. In the sample. however. in which iodid existed as a possible unknown. that is to say. in the pure pus recovered from many pustules from several different patients. our most delicate test failed to reveal a trace of the drug. It should be noted here that our test is much more delicate than the test with starch paste.

In this connection, attention might well be called to the enormous nodular bromoderma which not so infrequently occurs in nursing infants whose mothers are taking bromid for epilepsy, or other cause. The largest amount of such bromid ingested by the mother is voided in the urine, and but a small amount exists in the milk. It is hardly conceivable, therefore, that in such cases an enormous lesion could be caused by the actual presence of the drug itself.

In the blister content in all cases in which iodid and bromid are ingested, both drugs were easily recoverable.

The belief that the typical iodid acne is a physiologic reaction we believe to be erroneous. We found that a large number of patients could take relatively enormous doses of iodid without the slightest sign of a pustule, and we were able to establish, moreover, that when a tendency to pustulation occurred, it apparently bore no relation to the amount of the drug given. Patients receiving such small amounts as 5 or 10 grains (0.3 to 0.6 gm.) developed a rash at times; others again, under like conditions, maintained over many weeks, developed no pustules. The same condition pertained to doses as high as 200 grains (13 gm.) per diem; some reacted with pustulation; others, under like conditions, did not.

We can corroborate the findings of Engman and Mook that patients who had a pre-existing acne or seborrhea seemed to develop the acne more readily than did others.

It is regrettable that we had no opportunity to examine the contents of a bullous iododerma. If the contents of such bullae are analogous to the fluid of an artificial blister, one might expect in such cases to find the salt present.

To determine the excretion of chlorids in patients taking bromid, twenty-four hour urine was examined from day to day with respect to the chlorid content. It is to be noted that the normal chlorid content of the urine varies so greatly that a normal had to be fixed for each case before the necessary examinations could be made. Having established the normal for the individual, it was noted, after the ingestion of bromid, that an increase in chlorid output began about the second or third day, this increasing markedly up to about twice the amount of normal for that individual; after which a gradual fall toward normal occurred, notwithstanding the fact that the drug was continued during this time. The normal, however, was not reached in these cases until a considerable time after the drug had been withdrawn.

A most interesting observation in this connection occurred in a case of pemphigus. The patient received potassium bromid, 20 grains

(1.3 gm.) three times daily. About the third day after this had been begun, he broke out with an enormous crop of new blisters. The contents of these blisters were found to contain bromin, more easily demonstrable than in any other material examined. The urine showed a slight increase in chlorid at the outset, and a decided fall after the appearance of the blisters. After this fall, the amount remained well below the patient's normal.

In the investigation of the behavior of iodid toward the normal chlorid in the urine, no change was found. This is entirely in accordance with the fact that iodid is readily and rapidly eliminated through the kidneys. A suggestion is here tenable that the ultimate mechanism of iododerma may differ materially from that of bromoderma.

In our bacteriologic studies, in cases of iododerma and bromoderma, we were unable to substantiate the result of Engman and Mook in finding such lesions sterile. Cultures from pustules were made with great care, the lesions being first cauterized and the cultures being made from the depth of the lesions. All cases examined revealed uniformly large colonies of staphylococci.

To determine whether or not there existed in normal patients not ingesting either drug, and in those partaking of the drug, a cutaneous sensitization, solutions of potassium bromid and potassium iodid were injected cutaneously and intracutaneously. For the normals, we ourselves were the controls. The remainder of the skin tests were carried out on patients ingesting either salt. From our studies thus conducted, it was found that no cutaneous sensitization could be determined, either in patients already ingesting iodid and bromid, or in those not ingesting it who subsequently might develop pustulation. All cases, both of controls and of individuals ingesting the drug, were negative to percutaneous tests, both injections and scarifications.

When a certain concentration of both salts had been reached (the saturated solution), minute abscesses, in no way to be regarded as specific reactions, occurred in all cases.

Investigation of the effect of bromids in patients suffering with acidosis was based on the possible assumption that the replacement of chlorid in the blood by bromid might lead to a change in the blood reaction. It is a well-known fact that patients in a state of cachexia and acidosis are extremely prone to auto-infection, with the development of furuncles and carbuncles. Such conditions are frequently seen in the acidosis of diabetes and starvation, and the acidosis of marasmus, in malnutrition, and in the cachexia following acute infectious fevers. The suggestion followed here was that the local lesions following ingestion of the bromid might possibly be infections in the skin due to an altered alkaline reaction in the blood. To determine this, bromid in small doses was given to diabetic persons and to patients who, for other reasons, were suffering from milder or severer grades of acidosis, it having been recognized that the administration of small amounts of the drug could in no way be harmful to these patients. In no case did the administration of bromid under these conditions result in a spontaneous bromoderma.

To determine under such conditions whether a protein injected into the skin could in this way influence the production of a lesion, tiny droplets of typhoid vaccine were injected intracutaneously at various sites. These injections were followed in a few days, in a patient receiving a small amount of bromid, by the appearance of pustules entirely analogous to those of the pustular bromoderma. They persisted but a short time, however, and disappeared even during the time that the patient was ingesting bromid.

In order to determine the possible existence of precipitins in the blood which might perhaps be held responsible, or in some way allied to the local phenomena, small amounts of varying solutions of iodid of potash and bromid of potash were added to the blood serums of patients ingesting both drugs, as well as to normal bloods. It is conceivable that our technic was at fault, but we must, for the present, report uniformly negative results in these experiments.

COMMENT

From our results, certain definite things appear to have been established:

1. The pustules of iodid, also of bromid, acne are not sterile. Bacteria, therefore, cannot be eliminated as a factor, possibly, and probably, secondary in the production of such lesions. That they cannot be primary is undoubtedly shown by the fact that certain forms, at least of the cutaneous manifestations following the ingestion of these drugs, do not occur as pustules. The erythematous, urticarial and pure bullous types cannot in any way be associated with a bacterial cause.

2. Iodid and bromid exist in the body fluids following their ingestion, but are not found in the purulent material from acneform lesions. Their easy demonstration in the sweat, and their presence in the highest concentration in the blood serum, no doubt accounts for their previously reported presence in the local lesions as a contamination.

3. Percutaneous sensitization tests for iodid and bromid are uniformly negative, and cannot, therefore, be used to indicate ingestion susceptibility.

4. The ready substitution in the body fluids of chlorid by bromid leads to the hypothesis that the ultimate cause of this reaction in the skin differs somewhat from that caused by iodid. This replacement

may well lead to a change in the reaction of the circulating blood, and such change, it is conceived, might readly play a part in the production of bromid lesions.

5. The percutaneous introduction of foreign protein in the presence of a circulating blood containing bromid resulted, in one case, in lesions simulating those caused by bromids spontaneously. This reaction is, no doubt, parallel to the experiment of Sherrick with luetin in the presence of circulating iodid.

6. Precipitins in the blood serum were not demonstrable, at least by the addition in vitro of solutions, in minute quantities, of bromid and iodid salts to the blood serums.

7. The local phenomena of iododerma and bromoderma do not find their explanation on simple bacterial nor simple chemical grounds. The ultimate explanation probably lies in a complex biochemical reaction. The classification of such cutaneous phenomena, however, as true sensitization or allergy is as yet unjustifiable in the light of present knowledge.

DRUG ERUPTIONS FROM THE CLINICAL ASPECT

WITH SPECIAL REFERENCE TO THE RECENT MEDICAMENTS *

FRED WISE, M.D.

NEW YORK

AND

H. J. PARKHURST, M.D.

TOLEDO, OHIO

Whoever has read Prince A. Morrow's [1] monograph on drug eruptions will surely sympathize with us in our effort to present the subject
of "Drug Eruptions from the Clinical Aspect" with the greatest possible
expedition; with Morrow's work before us, we feel that little more can
be said. The eruptions of his day are, with a few additional examples,
those of today. The best course to follow, it seems to us, is to forbear
from burdening you with a reiteration of the well-known cutaneous
manifestations resulting from the use and abuse of the older drugs, and
to devote what time and space is at our disposal to a consideration of
eruptions provoked by the recent medicaments. Among the latter are
included such widely used drugs as barbital, medinal, adalin, bromural,
phenobarbital (luminal), cinchophen, pyramidon, melubrin, acetylsalicylic acid, hexamethylenamin, phenolphthalein and the various
arsphenamins.

DEFINITION

As used today, the term "drug eruptions" is synonymous with
dermatitis medicamentosa; that is, eruptions resulting from the introduction into the body of drugs which undergo absorption and elimination. The older definition of the term "drug eruption" embraces a
much broader field and is interpreted by Morrow in this sentence: "In
the proper signification of the term, drug eruptions embrace all con-
gestive and inflammatory changes in the skin caused by the external and
internal use of drugs."[2] Today, the term dermatitis venenata is used
to designate eruptions resulting from contact of irritant materials with
the skin.

CLASSIFICATION

What Morrow said with regard to classification thirty-five years ago
still holds good at the present time; namely, that "a classification based

* Read at the Forty-Fifth Annual Meeting of the American Dermatological
Association, Washington, D.C., May 2-4, 1922.

1. Morrow, Prince A.: Drug Eruptions, in Selected Monographs on Dermatology, London, The New Sydenham Society, 1893. (The monograph was
first published in 1887.)

2. This signification would exclude argyria.—T.Colcott Fox.

upon the anatomical form of the lesions produced by drugs is impracticable. The very multiformity of the lesions forbids any such attempt, for while the irritant action of a particular drug may, in one individual, be manifested by a single elementary lesion, the same drug may produce, in another individual, eruptive elements of dissimilar forms."

CERTAIN PHASES OF THE SUBJECT OMITTED

References to certain phases of the subject are omitted in this paper. Among these are:

1. Combined eruptions of dermatitis medicamentosa and dermatitis venenata, such as occur after the application of a belladonna plaster, absorption through the skin resulting in a general toxic rash, together with a local reaction at the site of the plaster, or, a local and general mercurial eruption following the application of blue ointment to a limited area of the skin.

2. Eruptions resulting from the simultaneous employment of more than one remedy, as mercury and arsphenamin, or mercury and potassium iodid. The European literature deals with several recently published articles on this aspect of the subject.[3]

3. Various types of stomatitis, as those provoked by mercury and the arsphenamins.

4. The general constitutional symptoms associated with drug eruptions; for example, malaise or fever, and injury to the viscera.

5. Eruptions occurring at the site of and around the point of injections of certain drugs; for example, arsphenamin necrosis from faulty technic; or, zosteriform skin necrosis after intramuscular injection of mercury succinimid, recently described by Jadassohn[4] and by Saphier.[5]

---

3. Gutmann, C.: The Treatment of Syphilis with Neo-Arsphenamin-Novasurol (Bruck) and with Neo-Arsphenamin-Cyarsal (Oelze). Berl. klin. Wchnschr. **58**:1233 (Oct. 17) 1921. Menze, H.: Exanthems from Recurrence of Syphilis During Treatment with Arsphenamin and Arsphenamin-Mercury: Influence of Predominant Conditions on the Wassermann Reaction and Allergy. München. med. Wchnschr. **68**:1290 (Oct. 7) 1921. Levin, Ernest: Localized, Recurrent, So-Called Fixed Exanthems After Arsphenamin and Mercury. Dermat. Wchnschr. **72**:278 (April 9) 1921. Gutmann, C.: So-Called Fixed and Generalized Urticarial Recurrent Exanthems After Arsphenamin and Mercury. Dermat. Ztschr. **35**:135 (Dec.) 1921. Mergelsberg, Otto: A Case of Hypersusceptibility Toward Mercury and Silver Arsphenamin. Dermat. Ztschr **31**:12? (Sept.) 1920. Heller, Julius: Further Communications as to the Occurrence of Severe Arsenical Melanosis and Hyperkeratosis After Combined Neo-Arsphenamin and Mercuric Salicylate Treatment. Arch. f. Dermat. u. Syph. **130**:309 (March 31) 1921; Berl. klin. Wchnschr. No. 46, 1918.

4. Jadassohn, J.: Zosteriform Skin Necrosis After Intramuscular Injections of Mercuric Succinimid, München. med. Wchnschr. **68**:852 (July 8) 1921.

5. Saphier, J.: Zosteriform Skin Necrosis After Intramuscular Injections of Mercuric Succinate, München. med. Wchnschr. **68**:394 (April 1) 1921; Another Case of Zosteriform Skin Necrosis After Intramuscular Injections of

DRUG ERUPTIONS FROM THE NEW ARSENICAL PREPARATIONS (ARSPHEN-
AMIN, NEO-ARSPHENAMIN, SILVER ARSPHENAMIN, ETC.)

From the clinician's point of view, the different eruptive phenomena provoked by the arsphenamin compounds are of considerable interest. Certain phases of the subject may be arbitrarily itemized as follows:

1. Attempts to classify types of eruptions.

2. Occurrence of peculiar forms of eruption. Among these are the so-called "fixed" eruptions, analogous to those following antipyrin and phenolphthalein administration. Lichenoid and lichen planus-like dermatoses, and even true lichen planus, are included under this heading. In the literature are found articles describing posteruptive manifestations under the titles of pemphigus foliaceus, hemorrhagic purpura, leukomelanoderma, Raynaud's syndrome, stomatitis, aplastic anemia and so forth.

3. Occurrence of the ordinary arsenic eruptions from the use of arsphenamin. Among these are dermatitis exfoliativa, hyperkeratoses, palmar and plantar keratodermas, pigmentations, erythemas and so forth; herpes zoster.

4. Argyria from silver preparations.

5. The influence of arsphenamin eruptions on the course of syphilis; "esophylaxis," a term applied by E. Hoffman to a phenomenon involving the reversal of a positive to a negative Wassermann reaction, after a severe arsphenamin eruption.

ATTEMPTS AT CLASSIFYING TYPES OF ERUPTIONS

A classification of the different eruptions provoked by the arsphenamins presents the same difficulties that are encountered in trying to classify the eruptions from arsenic itself. The whole gamut of cutaneous lesions, from faint erythema to squamous-cell cancer, from mild freckling to deep-seated melanoderma, is included under the term arsenical dermatitis. Arsenical zoster also comes under this heading.

Stühmer [6] classifies arsphenamin dermatitis under three headings: (1) acute vasotoxic arsphenamin dermatitis; (2) subacute, anaphylactoid arsphenamin dermatitis, and (3) chronic arsphenamin dermatitis. The last is divided into early and late forms.

The acute vasotoxic dermatitis appears immediately, or within a few hours, or at most within one or two days after the injection. Included in this group are the eruptions appearing within this lapse of time, consisting of acute urticarial and erythematous rashes, as well as those limited to certain parts of the body and called "fixed" arsphenamin

6. Stühmer, A.: Arsphenamin Exanthems; Attempt at Classification; Practical Important Peculiarities of Chronic Arsphenamin Dermatitis, Dermat. Ztschr. **34**:304 (Oct.) 1921.

eruptions. In this type of eruption, Stühmer assumes that, for some unknown reason, there exists in certain areas of the skin a hypersusceptibility against arsphenamin oxids. He believes that these oxids are present to a greater or less extent even in the best preparations of arsphenamin. In this connection, he speaks of a so-called "oxidreaction." This may be primary, resulting from oxid formation in vivo, or secondary resulting from oxid formation in vitro. He believes that arsphenamin in the body may undergo oxidation and may be synthetized into an albuminous compound through a reaction produced by combination with normal serum. He believes that these various reactions result from a reaction toward the "oxid-protein-body" which is produced in this manner, and which he calls "oxid-toxin."

The subacute, anaphylactoid dermatitis appears from six to twelve days after the first injection of arsphenamin. The second and third injections have no bearing on the causation of the eruption, even though it becomes manifest at the time of the second or third treatment. It is characterized chiefly by the fact of its appearance after the first injection. The author believes this form of reaction to be analogous to serum sickness, which it resembles with respect to the localization of the rash, the temperature curve, the time interval after the first injection, and the fact that subsequent treatments may be administered without harm, after the subsidence of the reaction. Included in this group are the recurrent exanthems described by Nathan. In these, the rash appears from ten to fourteen days after the first injection, fades within a few days to a great extent, and then may partially recur. In this type, also, he found that it is safe to administer further treatment after the subsidence of the rash.

Chronic dermatitis is divided into early and late forms. The early form manifests itself at the termination of a course, after the fifth or sixth treatment; the late form, from several weeks to two or three months after the completion of a course of injections. These eruptions represent the severest types of dermatitis, often beginning as harmless looking follicular, urticarial or erythematous rashes on the extensor surfaces of the extremities. These soon may develop into a generalized dermatitis, going on to the characteristic erythroderma. With the continuation of the process, severe desquamation sets in, following which there may be the formation of hyperkeratoses, and marked changes in the hair and nails, together with pyodermic manifestations, the whole process presenting a severe and serious affection. Sometimes the eruption presents large plaques of weeping dermatitis with extensive areas of desquamation; there may be high fever, and the patient may die. This clinical course may obtain in both the early and the late forms; in the late form, however, the patient would seem to have withstood the ill effects of the drug, having no reaction whatever until several weeks have elapsed; then suddenly, and without apparent cause, the reaction sets in. Stühmer lays emphasis on a clinical feature of the chronic form of dermatitis which he considers of importance from the therapeutic standpoint; namely, the fact that after the partial subsidence of the acute eruption, the persistent erythroderma remains longest and is most severe in the areas of predilection to seborrheic dermatitis. He believes that patients with seborrheic skins are more susceptible to arsphenamin dermatitis.

Moore and Keidel [7] published a comprehensive paper on arsphenamin reactions, part of which goes into the subject of classification. They differentiate a mild and a severe group of reactions on the basis of their constitutional manifestations and their significance as regards the further treatment of syphilis. Urticaria, erythema and herpes comprise the mild group; mascular, maculopapular and exfoliative rashes, itching and stomatitis, the severe group.

Thirty-one reactions were observed in their series of twenty-three patients. Urticaria was seen six times, erythema once, herpes simplex twice, macular or maculopapular rashes five times, exfoliative dermatitis fourteen times, stomatitis twice, and itching once. The authors regard the macular and maculopapular rashes, the vesicular eruptions and exfoliative dermatitis as degrees of the same process. The rash "begins as a maculopapular or vesicular dermatitis, often limited to the extensor surfaces of the limbs, but rapidly spreading until the whole body is involved. In the milder cases, particularly of the macular or maculopapular type, the process may stop with this, and the eruption disappear in a few days. Frequently, there is a late fine branny exfoliation. In the more severe maculopapular, and especially the vesicular eruptions, marked scaling and exfoliation usually takes place, and the skin of the entire body is desquamated in large flakes. Often an entire palmar or plantar surface comes away intact. The rash is accompanied by the most intense and distressing itching. Usually, the exfoliation is complete in from three to four weeks, but in some cases healing may take much longer. Once or twice, it has been noted that several distinct exacerbations have occurred in the same patient, the skin continuing to exfoliate periodically for several months." Conjunctivitis, involvement of the buccal surfaces, with swelling and denudation of the tongue and buccal mucosae, may also occur.

Brauer [8] recognizes two groups of reactions, primary and secondary.

---

7. Moore, J. E., and Keidel, A.: Dermatitis and Allied Reactions Following the Arsenical Treatment of Syphilis, Arch. Int. Med. **27**:716 (June) 1921.

8. Brauer, A.: Contribution to the Subject of Arsphenamin Dermatoses, Dermat. Ztschr. **19**:800, 1912.

In the primary group, he includes the "genuine toxic exanthems," of which he saw sixteen instances in thirteen of 1,500 patients; nine were erythematous, scarlatiniform or morbilliform, with or without stomatitis; one was erythemato-urticarial, complicated by edema; two were exudative erythema multiforme; one was purpura rheumatica with erythema nodosum; and one was severe universal pemphigoid dermatitis. As secondary dermatoses, he classes herpes simplex and zoster, hyperhidrosis, alopecia, alterations in the nails, jaundice, melanoses following primary rashes and immediate macular and urticarial eruptions. He does not believe that these reactions are due to the actual toxic effect of the arsenic; the Herxheimer reaction is considered to be directly related to the urticarial eruptions, which are due to the destruction of foci of spirochetes in the skin.

THE SO-CALLED "FIXED" ARSPHENAMIN ERUPTIONS

On rare occasions, arsphenamin provokes so-called "fixed" eruptions. These are very much like those seen in persons susceptible to antipyrin and phenolphthalein. They consist of from one or more to several dozen sharply circumscribed, slightly elevated, smooth plaques. which may be pink, red, yellowish or brown; sometimes they leave no trace, at other times a moderate grade of pigmentation. They have a tendency to disappear in the intervals between the injections, only to reappear in situ after each administration of arsphenamin. Such cases were first described by German authors (Naegeli, Bitterling, Engwer and Josephson, Fuchs, Grütz, Hecht, Hofmann, Kraus, E. Levin. Nathan, Schoenfeld, Stern), and in one article by the French authors Thibierge and Mercier. More recent papers on the subject have been published by Leibkind, Süring and Gutmann.[9] Drs. Goldenberg and Chargin presented a patient with such a "fixed" arsphenamin eruption. before the New York Academy of Medicine, at one of last year's meetings of the section on dermatology. In this patient, a man. there were two or three well-defined, pink, elevated, round plaques on the thighs and trunk, from one-half to three-quarters inch (1.2 to 1.8 cm.) in diameter. They appeared shortly after an injection of arsphenamin. vanishing in the intervals between treatments. They closely resembled the plaques of an antipyrin rash. In a general way. this type of eruption simulates the fixed types of antipyrin and phenolphthalein dermatoses. As has been stated elsewhere.[10] those who have the

9. Gutmann, C.: Concerning So-Called "Fixed" and Generalized Urticarial Relapsing Exanthems After Arsphenamin and Mercury. Dermat. Ztschr. **35**:135 (Dec.) 1921. (This article furnishes references to the literature of "fixed" arsenical eruptions).

10. Wise, Fred, and Abramowitz, E. W.: Phenolphthalein Eruptions. Arch. Dermat. & Syph. **5**:297 (March) 1922.

opportunity to investigate this peculiar recurring and relapsing dermatosis must always bear in mind the possibility that the patient is taking either antipyrin or one of the numerous phenolphthalein preparations while undergoing his course of arsphenamin injections. The point of special interest in these "fixed" arsphenamin rashes lies in the fact that the lesions tend to relapse and to recur in situ, and to flare up quite markedly after each injection, to fade partly, with or without leaving pigmentation, in the intervals between injections, or to vanish entirely, without leaving a trace.

LICHENOID ERUPTIONS

Mention of lichenoid, lichen planus-like and apparently genuine lichen planus eruptions are found in the literature on arsenical dermatoses preceding the arsphenamin era. Brooke and Roberts,[11] in their paper on the British arsenical beer-poisoning epidemic, speak of rather frequent lichen planus-like rashes. Recently, several European publications have appeared dealing with lichenoid and lichen planus post-arsphenamin eruptions. Eruptions resembling lichen planus are reported by Kleeberg,[12] Buschke and Freymann,[13] Keller[14] and others.

Most of these accounts state that there is a "striking similarity," both clinically and microscopically, to lichen planus. Naturally, the pros and cons of the question as to whether the arsphenamin "lights up" a latent lichen planus in a patient subject to the disease, or whether the drug actually causes an eruption of lichen planus, are discussed by the various reporters. Buschke and Freymann content themselves by invoking the homeopathic dictum: Similia similibus curantur. Keller reports a case which in his estimation is an undoubted lichen planus, both clinically and histologically. Queyrat, Louis and Rabut[15] report a patient who suffered from recurring plaques of erythema of the body, associated with a lichen planus eruption of the tongue; Civatte pronounced a microscopic section from one of the tongue lesions true lichen

---

11. Brooke, H. G., and Roberts, Leslie: The Action of Arsenic on the Skin as Observed in the Recent Epidemic of Arsenical Beer Poisoning, Brit. J. Dermat. **13**:121 (April) 1901.

12. Kleeberg, L.: Clinical Aspects of Arsenical Exanthems, Therap. Halbmonatsh. **35**:370 (June 15) 1921.

13. Buschke, A., and Freymann, W.: Lichen Ruber-Like Arsphenamin Exanthems, Med. Klin. **17**:899 (July 24) 1921; Further Contribution to Lichen Ruber-Like Exanthem After Arsphenamin, Dermat. Wchnschr. **73**:945 (Sept. 10) 1921.

14. Keller, P.: Lichen Planus and Lichenoid Arsenical Dermatitis, Dermat. Wchnschr. **74**:9 (Jan. 7) 1922.

15. Queyrat, Louis and Rabut: Lichen Planus of the Tongue Appearing in a Syphilitic During the Course of an Arsenic Treatment, Together with Generalized Erythema Following Arsenical Injections, and Leaving Plaques of Pigmentation, Bull. Soc. franç. de dermat. et syph. 1921, No. 2, p. 39.

planus. In the discussion, Milian said that he believed that the arsenic injection provoked an exacerbation of a preexisting or latent lichen planus, while Thibierge contradicted him, saying he did not think that such an explanation was plausible.

Recently, one of our colleagues at the Vanderbilt Clinic, Dr. McCafferty, brought to us a patient from his service at the Presbyterian Hospital, in whom a lichen planus eruption, confirmed by microscopic examination, appeared after a course of arsphenamin and mercury injections. As Dr. McCafferty intends to report this case fully, a detailed account is omitted here. The patient was a negress, aged 40, with active syphilitic cutaneous lesions and atrophic scarring from preexisting eruptions. The Wassermann reaction was strongly positive. She received ten or twelve injections of arsphenamin and mercury, at weekly intervals. Toward the end of this course of treatment, a widespread lichen planus eruption appeared, being most pronounced on the trunk and extremities, while the lingual and buccal mucosae exhibited slightly elevated grayish plaques. The exanthem was associated with severe pruritus. She had never had an attack of lichen planus.

Among other unusual cutaneous reactions may be mentioned a case of hemorrhagic purpura, reported by Anwyl-Davies,[16] following injections of neo-arsphenamin. Deep melanosis and hyperkeratosis are reported by Nördlinger,[17] and by Heller [18] and others. Nicolas, Massia and Dupasquier [19] describe a patient with Raynaud's syndrome with gangrene, after neo-arsphenamin injections. A case of pemphigus foliaceus following the administration of the same preparation is reported by Nicolas and Massia.[20] Moore and Keidel [21] published a paper on stomatitis and aplastic anemia following arsphenamin treatment of syphilis. The literature on dermatitis exfoliativa and on icterus is abundant.

---

16. Anwyl-Davies, T.: Hemorrhagic Purpura Following the Therapeutic Administration of Neo-Arsphenamin, Brit. J. Dermat. & Syph. **33**:264 (July) 1921.

17. Nördlinger, A.: A Case of Deep Melanosis and Hyperkeratosis. Arch. f. Dermat. u. Syph. **131**:257 (April 30) 1921.

18. Heller, J.: Further Contribution on the Occurrence of Severe Arsenical Melanosis and Hyperkeratosis After Combined Neo-Arsphenamin and Mercuric Salicylate Treatment, Arch. f. Dermat. u. Syph. **130**:309 (March 31) 1921.

19. Nicolas, J., Massia, G., and Dupasquier, D.: Raynaud's Syndrome with Gangrene, of Neo-Arsphenamin Origin, Ann. de dermat. et syph. **2**:193 (May) 1921.

20. Nicolas, J., and Massia, G.: A Contribution to the Study of Arsenobenzolids; Pemphigus Foliaceus due to Arsenobenzol. Ann. de dermat. et syph **2**:145 (April 1921.

21. Moore, J. E., and Keidel, Albert: Stomatitis and Aplastic Anemia Due to Neoarsphenamin Treatment, Arch. Dermat. & Syph. **4**:169 (Aug.) 1921.

ORDINARY ARSENIC ERUPTIONS

In the early period of arsphenamin treatment, it was thought by many clinicians that the new arsenical preparations were not prone to give rise to the characteristic arsenical dermatoses which have always been associated with the prolonged use of the old arsenicals; namely, keratoses, palmar and plantar hyperkeratoses and melanoses. As time went on, case reports began to crop out here and there, so that the literature of the day contains a fairly large number of instances illustrating the hyperkeratotic and pigmentary by-effects in the skin of susceptible persons who had never taken arsenic, but who had received arsphenamin for syphilis. Among other writers, Heller [22] published two good articles on this phase of the subject. He reported three cases in which severe melanosis and hyperkeratosis occurred after combined neo-arsphenamin and mercuric salicylate treatment. After the publication of this report, he observed five similar cases in connection with the same combined treatment. Two of the patients had a cutaneous inflammation, without melanosis or hyperkeratosis. In two other patients, an intensive melanosis developed; in one, only hyperkeratosis. The last mentioned patient died so early that it was not possible to observe the melanosis. Six of the first described cases presented typical changes in the skin. None of the six showed any signs of idiosyncrasy in the beginning of the treatment, and in all the skin disease appeared toward the end of the treatment. None of them showed any signs of irritability toward mercury. Palmar and plantar hyperkeratoses were observed in all of the six patients. The anomaly of cornification was exhibited in Patients 3, 4, 5 and 6; the melanosis in Patients 1, 2, 4 and 6. Patient 5 died before the period in which the melanosis usually manifests itself. A striking example of palmar and plantar keratoderma is described and illustrated by Edmund Hofmann,[23] who also refers to the case reports of Heller,[22] Philip [24] and Pürckhauer.[25]

Herpes simplex and herpes zoster are comparatively frequent cutaneous manifestations following arsphenamin treatment. As to the

22. Heller, Julius: Further Communication as to the Occurrence of Severe Arsenical Melanosis and Hyperkeratosis After Combined Neo-Arsphenamin and Mercuric Salicylate Treatment, Arch. f. Dermat. u. Syph. **130**:309 (March 31) 1921; idem, Berl. klin. Wchnschr. **46**, 1918.

23. Hofmann, Edmund: Concerning Arsphenamin Exanthems, Dermat. Ztschr. **31**:1 (July) 1920.

24. Philip, Caesar: Arsenic Keratoses After Arsphenamin Injections, München. med. Wchnschr., 1915.

25. Pürckhauer: Arsphenamin Intoxication Running a Course with Fever and Dermatitis Exfoliativa, Developing into Arsenomelanosis and Arsenical Hyperkeratosis, München. med. Wchnschr. 30, 1917.

occurrence of malignant changes which are sometimes encountered in connection with arsenical keratoses, we have not as yet run across such a reference in the literature.

ARGYRIA FROM SILVER ARSPHENAMINS

No authentic case of postarsphenamin argyria has been recorded. Schlossberger's [26] report was based on hearsay evidence only.

THE INFLUENCE OF ARSPHENAMIN ERUPTIONS ON THE COURSE OF SYPHILIS: "ESOPHYLAXIS"

Erich Hoffmann [27] applied the term "esophylaxis" to a phenomenon observed in certain patients with severe arsphenamin reactions. In these patients, it was discovered that a strongly positive Wassermann reaction would become negative after an attack of arsphenamin dermatitis and would remain negative for a long time thereafter. Corroborative testimony to this effect has been offered by Buschke and Freymann,[28] Carl Bruck,[29] S. Levi [30] and F. Lesser.[31] The last named writer takes up the question in detail, stating that it could be proved only by the collection of statistics extending over at least two years.

Statistics as to the effect of mercury treatment and of insufficient treatment of tabes are not satisfactory, since they are not uniform. A comparison must be made between syphilitic patients who have had identical treatment and have been observed for the similar periods of time, to determine whether those with drug eruptions have had fewer clinical and serologic recurrences. Lesser discusses the theory that the skin has a defense reaction which protects the internal organs from the disease, which Hoffmann calls esophylaxis. This theory is supported by the fact that syphilitic persons who have had intense skin eruptions and frequent recurrences in the early stages have tabes and paresis more rarely than those who have had slight skin eruptions. Lesser's explanation of this is as follows: While the skin symptoms are visible.

---

26. Schlossberger, H.: Supposed Case of Argyria After Silver Arsphenamin. Therap. Halbmonatsh. **34**:608 (Nov.) 1920.

27. Hoffmann, Erich: Late Exanthems after Arsphenamin, Niederrh. Ges. f. Nat. u. Heilk., Med. Abt., Feb. 20, 1911; Abstr. Deutsch. med. Wchnschr., 1911, p. 2058.

28. Buschke, A., and Freymann, W.: Influence of Arsphenamin Exanthems on the Course of Syphilis, Berl. klin. Wchnschr., 1921, No. 15.

29. Bruck, Carl: Influence of Arsphenamin Exanthems on the Course of Syphilis, Berl. klin. Wchnschr. **58**:518, No. 20, 1921.

30. Levi, S.: Syphilis Following Toxic Exanthems. Berl. klin. Wchnschr. **58**:1137 (Sept. 19) 1921.

31. Lesser, Fritz: The Effect of Toxic Exanthems on the Course of Syphilis. Berl. klin. Wchnschr. **58**:1210 (Oct. 10) 1921.

those in the internal organs are latent, as is shown by the positive findings in the cerebrospinal fluid at the time of the eruption. As the cell infiltration in the early stage is a defense reaction against the spirochetes, it is to be assumed that such defense reactions are also taking place in the internal organs. This pronounced organic immunity will frequently bring about a cure of the syphilis, and if not, will protect the organs from late syphilis. Milder skin symptoms indicate weaker defense reactions, a lesser degree of immunity, more frequent recovery and more frequent late syphilis. Arguments against esophylaxis are furnished by the positive cerebrospinal fluid findings in the early period, the fact that the disease can be reproduced by inoculations with the cerebrospinal fluid with a negative blood Wassermann reaction, and the possibility of experimental inoculation with all the internal organs. Buschke and Freymann's assertions that slight erythemas have no effect, and only eczematoid eruptions with pronounced skin changes have any effect, are in contradiction to the usual findings that changes in the skin decrease the function of the organs. But the high fever which precedes or accompanies the exanthem may have a favorable effect on the course of the syphilis. The chronicity of syphilis may be due to its afebrile course.

A criticism of the opinion that syphilis is favorably influenced by arsphenamin eruptions is expressed by Benveniste.[32] Five examples are briefly reported which show that, although erythroderma coincides with the disappearance of the positive Wassermann reactions, this effect is only transitory, lasting but a few months; and usually a clinical relapse is observed when the Wassermann reaction becomes again positive. No beneficial influence is, therefore, to be attributed to the exanthems produced by arsphenamin. On the contrary, in view of the fact that arsenic cannot be used further, the prognosis becomes less favorable in these cases.

Another French author, Gougerot,[33] cites several examples favoring the theory of so-called "esophylaxis." He thinks that the explanation of the reversal of a positive to a negative Wassermann reaction, after the appearance of a toxic exanthem, may be referred to the assumption that the tissues have been more strongly impregnated with the drug than usual, that arsenic is retained in the body, or again that the fever which sometimes accompanies arsenical erythroderma has had a destructive effect on the spirochetes. It has also been suggested that

32. Benveniste, Elie: Exanthems Produced by Arsphenamin and the Evolution of Syphilis, Presse méd. **29**:904 (Nov. 12) 1921.

33. Gougerot, M.: Syphilitic Relapse with Visceral, Cutaneous, Mucous and Serologic Manifestations Soon After an Exfoliating Erythroderma, Consecutive to Treatment with Arsphenamin, Bull. et mém. Soc. méd. d. hôp. de Paris **37**: 1339 (Oct. 27) 1921.

the violent cutaneous reaction may cause "the production of defensive substances by the skin, which help the action of specific therapy." In his article, Gougerot mentions a series of cases in which the toxic eruptions produced a favorable reversal of the Wassermann reaction. But, in contrast to these, he also cites several examples in which no such reversal of the serologic findings took place. In one patient, there was a relapse within two months after the appearance of the toxic rash, with special localization in the nervous system and with the appearance of syphilitic cutaneous papules. In another patient, there was a relapse within two months after the toxic eruption, even before the latter was completely cured.

RECENT SYNTHETIC DRUGS

The large majority of the new synthetic remedies are capable of provoking eruptions in those who are susceptible. These are usually described as erythematous, urticarial, morbilliform, scarlatiniform, erysipelatous, bullous, erosive and so forth. It is probable that a great many of these eruptions, being ephemeral and causing no inconvenience to the patient, never come to the physician's notice. Simulating the acute exanthems, as many of them do, these eruptions are naturally of interest to both the dermatologist and the general practitioner. Scattered references are frequently encountered in the literature, and recently Lutz[34] has published a review of the subject. Among the remedies mentioned in his paper, some of the following are more or less freely prescribed in this country:

Barbital and Medinal (Sodium salts of Diethylbarbituric Acid and Diethylbarbituric Acid). Gregor encountered exanthematous rashes with fever after two or three small doses. The eruptions disappeared as soon as the drugs were withdrawn; renewed administration was followed by a rash more intense than the first. Weitz described a morbilliform, partly confluent itchy eruption and erythematous swelling of the face, with an increase in temperature in a girl, aged 22, who had been taking doses of medinal of unknown quantity. She died two days after the appearance of the rash. Pollitzer found, after barbital administration, a much darker morbilliform rash in a patient who had been taking 1 gm. of the drug every night. The rash was associated with red blotches on the cheeks and pharyngeal mucosa, and with erosions of the mouth and anus. Fernet and Mertens report the appearance of blebs within five minutes after the ingestion of barbital. In another case, the blebs appeared on the third day. They

34. Lutz, Wilhelm: Dermatoses from the Newer Remedies (Excepting Arsenic and Mercury), Therap. Halbmonatsch. **35**:480 (Aug) 1921, and **35**:52?, 1921. (This article furnishes references to the literature).

were localized on the external aspect of both forearms, their contents were cloudy, and they had no areolae. Localized, so-called "fixed" eruptions are described by Klausner, Zeisler, Glaser and Lichtenstein.

Codeonal (Codein-Barbital). Beyerhaus saw a patient develop bluish-red, severely itching plaques on the face and chest, later extending over the entire body, and associated with fever, within three hours after taking 0.18 gm. of the proprietary codeonal. It is not known whether these untoward effects were due to codein, as Beyerhaus seems to think, or to the barbital.

Adalin and Bromural (Bromidethylacetylcarbamid and Monobromisovalerylurea): In three cases, Fürbringer saw, on the day following the administration of adalin, an intense pruritus, and in a fourth patient, an attack of itching with urticaria which lasted twenty-four hours. Roeder saw similar cases. Walter met with a bromid acne as an untoward effect of adalin. Zetlin and Giorgio saw a pustular and tuberose bromid dermatitis after administration of bromural—a drug belonging to the same group as adalin. Loeb [35] reported six cases of adalin eruption. These appeared partly in the form of papular eczematoid eruptions of either the acute or the chronic variety, partly as erythematous, irregularly outlined, more or less edematous and infiltrated plaques, which showed some similarity to long standing forms of exudative erythema. Petechiae and telangiectases were noted in one case. Pigmentation may remain after the lesions subside. One patient had urticaria of the face. The eruption appeared in irregular, geographic outlines, with no tendency to coalescence. The sites were chiefly on areas subject to pressure from the clothing, or where the skin was irritated. The eruptions were symmetrical, and the mucosae were not involved. Pruritus was marked during the night; less troublesome during the day. The drug was given experimentally and produced the same eruption. In two patients, a long time intervened before the second administration of the drug. There was no rise of temperature. The eruption faded in about two weeks without leaving a trace, except mild pigmentation. Old people seem to be more susceptible.

Phenobarbital (Phenylethylbarbituric Acid): A universal erythema in two patients is mentioned by Gräfner; and a rubeolar rash on the chest, back, arms and thighs, with a red swelling of the face, disappearing at the end of a week with desquamation, by Fröderstrom. Several authors reported morbilliform eruptions. Juliusburger, Fürbinger, Haug and Emanuel describe a scarlatiniform exanthem. Several eruptions, some resembling measles and some scarlet fever, were seen by Strauss in five patients. In two of them, the rash appeared within a few days after taking doses of 0.05 gm. two or three times a day.

35. Loeb, H.: Concerning an Exanthem from Adalin, Arch. f. Derm. u. Syph. **131**:128 (April 30) 1921.

Luce and Feigel had a similar experience. In their cases, however, the rash was accompanied by a hyperemia of the conjunctivae, mouth and pharyngeal mucosae; in two instances, the fever was high, and, after four to seven days, disappeared, with desquamation. Konig and Meissner cite similar cases. Raecke saw one patient with an urticarial eruption. Curschmann saw three patients with eczematous eruptions and dermatitis. Exanthems which cannot be classified are described by Loewe, Zimmermann, Moerchen and Blickert. Fürer, König and Juliusburger, twelve hours after a subcutaneous injection of this drug saw a pea-size blister develop at the site of the injection. In one case, necrosis occurred. No such complications followed injections into the subcutaneous fatty tissue. Phenobarbital eruptions are frequently associated with lingual and oral erosions. At one of the recent meetings of the section on dermatology of the New York Academy of Medicine, Chargin presented a remarkable case of pemphigoid erosion of the entire tongue, in an epileptic girl who had been taking phenobarbital, and who had no cutaneous rash. These tongue and mouth eruptions closely simulate antipyrin and phenolphthalein erosions. Phillips [36] reports a case of severe poisoning from phenobarbital, accompanied by an extensive erythematous and morbilliform eruption, which itched severely, and swelling of the oral mucosae. This paper also describes a number of other cases previously reported.

Cinchophen (Phenylquinolincarboxylic Acid): After the use of this drug, Stiefler reports angioneurotic edema. Maranon saw an erysipelatous swelling of the face with chills, on two occasions, in one patient; thereafter, the drug was well borne. He also reports an intense pruritus in a patient who for months before had been taking the drug without any ill effects. Scarlatiniform, urticarial and mixed rashes are also reported. Oyarzabal saw a patient in whom an eczema on the back of the neck, previously induced by formaldehyd, was aggravated by the subsequent administration of atophan. Fricke saw herpes zoster make its appearance while the patient was under the influence of the same drug.

Pyramidon (Dimethylaminoantipyrin): Scherber and Weidenfeld report a case in which a single dose was followed by the appearance of two concentric, red, elevated circles on the left cheek. In a patient who had previously borne antifebrin well, Bechet observed the development of a large swelling of the lower lip and a severe pruritus of the face and neck, with an erythematopapular and partially urticarial exanthem with petechiae on the feet and legs. This rash appeared after the patient had taken pyramidon daily for four days. It disappeared entirely after three days.

36. Phillips, John: Phenobarbital (Luminal) Poisoning. J. A. M. A. **78**:1100
(A l 22 1922

Melubrin (Sodium salt of Antipyrinamidomethansulfonic Acid):
Krabbel reports an exanthem associated with this drug similar to that
following antipyrin. Mullers had a patient who, after taking 0.5 gm.
acetysalicylic acid daily, developed a few small papules on the arms.
After the acetysalicylic acid was replaced by melubrin (2 gm. daily)
there followed, two days later, an aggravation and extension of the
rash. It extended over the entire body, and became coarser and itchy.

Acetylsalicylic Acid: The eruptions described following acetylsalicylic acid ingestion are comparatively uniform. In some cases, within
an hour, swelling of the face, chiefly of the eyelids and lips appears,
generally accompanied by swelling of the nasal, buccal and pharyngeal
mucosae, frequently with intense general malaise. Some patients
develop urticaria, others a scarlatiniform rash, and still others conjunctivitis with edema of the eyelids. Kraus saw two cases of "dyshidrotic eczema" following the use of the drug.

Hexamethylenamin: Hilbert reports the case of a woman, who,
immediately after taking a tablespoonful of a 5 per cent. solution,
developed an intense itching and burning eruption over the body; half
an hour later, after a second dose, there appeared swelling of the
eyelids, redness of the conjunctivae, and urticarial wheals the size of
lentils, all over the trunk and scalp. Sachs reports a similar experience;
in his case, headache, tinnitus, a temperature of 40 C., and a light red
efflorescence on the trunk also developed.

Phenolphthalein: Eruptions from phenolphthalein were described
in detail at last year's meeting of this Association.[10] Since then, several
new examples of the eruption have been presented before various
medical societies, and three articles on the subject have been published;
one by Ayres,[37] dealing with the exanthem itself, another by Corson
and Sidlick,[38] who report urticaria from the habitual use of the drug,
and another by Rosenbloom,[39] who records a case of nasal herpes which
always recurred after the patient took a proprietary phenolphthalein
pill.

DISCUSSION

ON PAPERS OF DRS. WILE, WRIGHT AND SMITH, AND WISE AND PARKHURST

Dr. John H. Stokes, Rochester, Minn.: I am sure I voice the sentiment
of the Association when I say that to have heard these papers makes the trip
to Washington very much more than worth while. I believe that the essayists
deserve a unanimous vote of thanks for such a splendid presentation of such

37. Ayres, Samuel: Phenolphthalein Dermatitis, J. A. M. A. **77**:1722 (Nov.
26) 1921.

38. Corson, Edward F., and Sidlick, D. M.: Urticaria from Habitual Use
of Phenolphthalein: Report of a Case, J. A. M. A. **78**:882 (March 25) 1922.

39. Rosenbloom, Jacob: Report of a Case of Nasal Herpes Due to Ingestion
of Phenolphthalein, J. A. M. A. **78**:967 (April 1) 1922.

an intricate subject. It occurred to me that I might add something to the interest of the evening if I mentioned one or two of the observations made on our service by Dr. E. D. Osborne, who has been studying the chemical aspects of iodid administration.

Reactions to sodium iodid administered intravenously in doses ranging from 2.5 to 20 gm. a day are relatively rare. Patients who show pronounced reactions to potassium iodid by mouth tolerate sodium iodid intravenously without incident. Such reactions as occur are practically all of an anaphylactic type, including urticaria, erythema multiforme and local edemas of the eyelids and the larynx. Transient asthmatic symptoms may develop. If iodid acne develops, it is usually mild. We have seen no fungoid or bullous lesions. Dr. Wise mentioned the slow elimination of the bromids and the cumulative action. There is no cumulative action in the administration of iodid regardless of the method of administration or the dose. The drug has completely left the body within seventy-two hours after administration. Not over 5 per cent. of the iodid is eliminated in the stools. Practically all of it leaves the body through the kidneys.

In investigating the possible dissimilarities in action in the case of sodium and potassium iodids, Dr. Osborne made several interesting observations. Following the administration of sodium iodid by mouth there was a definite marked rise of the sodium content of the blood serum proportional to the size of the dose, with no change in the potassium content. In contrast to this finding, administration of potassium iodid by mouth did not produce a corresponding rise in the potassium content of the blood serum, but, on the contrary, a definite rise in the sodium content almost equal to that following the sodium iodid.

There is no special advantage in giving small doses intravenously. Administration by mouth creates a moderate sustained concentration. Intravenous administration of large doses creates peaks of high concentration followed by rapid decline. Only traces of iodin can be found in the serum proteins after the administration of sodium iodid by mouth. In direct contrast to this finding, from 7 to 26 per cent. of the iodin following the administration of potassium iodid by mouth was found in the serum proteins. Following intravenous administration of sodium iodid, from 6 to 9.9 per cent. of the iodin is found in the serum proteins.

Evidently an exchange of ions occurs in the process of absorption of potassium iodid. The potassium is replaced by sodium to a large extent. Whether in this exchange of ions the iodin from potassium iodid (I am now merely serving as a mouthpiece for Dr. Osborne) is absorbed in the same form as after sodium iodid, is open to question. Since the potassium is evidently absorbed to a very slight degree, the question naturally arises as to whether the iodin after potassium iodid unites with the protein, the fat or the inorganic constituents of the blood. Dr. Osborne's investigations suggest that the iodin in the form of potassium iodid by mouth forms a sodium protein combination while in the case of sodium iodid by mouth only traces of iodin enter into combination with the proteins. In a study not yet completed of two patients showing symptoms of iodism following the administration of sodium iodid by mouth, it was found that the iodin unites with the protein fraction to a greater extent than in normal persons. If iodin when administered in the form of potassium iodid unites with the serum proteins to a greater extent than when administered as sodium iodid the question at once arises as to whether this sodium protein iodin combination is the basis of the action of iodids, and an explanation of possible differences in the pharmacologic behavior of the two salts. These points must be made the subject of further study.

Dr. WILLIAM H. MOOK, St. Louis: Our work was done about seventeen years ago under very different circumstances than are possible in a modern hospital. It was done at the city poor-house where the laboratory facilities were crude; consequently, owing to faults of technic, the results of making cultures were negative In the histologic examination of this tissue we were struck by the marked changes in the capillaries surrounding these iodid lesions, and we concluded that there was a toxin in the blood that probably attacked the blood vessels instead of the glands of the skin themselves. Frequently they developed at sites of former traumas, especially of old healed acne lesions.

Dr. HERMAN GOLDENBERG, New York: Through my connection with a large general hospital and a close contact of the dermatologic department with the medical and surgical services, I have been able to see a great many drug eruptions, probably a much larger number than the average dermatologist. I do not wish to detain you with the enumeration of such ordinary eruptions as you see following the administration of bromids, acetyl salicylic acid, barbital, antipyrin and other coal-tar products, but I wish to report a few unusual drug manifestations which are not at all or only briefly described in textbooks.

I wish especially to call attention to scarlatiniform or morbilliform eruptions following the administration of digitalis or its derivatives, which I, not infrequently, observe, and similar universal eruptions from the use of hexamethylenamin. On the surgical side the same type of skin lesions is occasionally observed following the application of tincture of iodin over large patches for sterilization or the use of an iodoform gauze packing, not at the site of application, but through absorption from the skin. The type of bromid eruption resembling an erythema nodosum, of which Dr. Wise showed a photograph and stated that it was of rather frequent occurrence, is not universally known or described in textbooks. We see every year from three to six cases, generally located on the lower extremities, but also found elsewhere and anywhere on the body, and usually accompanied by a slight rise of temperature.

In addition, I wish to report briefly a number of cases of mouth lesions, either in connection with or independently of skin manifestations which I have seen in private and hospital practice. One of the cases is that of a phenobarbital eruption which was presented from my service by Dr. Chargin and referred to by Dr. Wise. The patient was a young girl who for a period of over two years had taken phenobarbital in doses of 4½ to 6 grains (0.3 to about 0.5 gm.) a day for epilepsy. The tongue was twice the natural size, raw, beefy and had a number of thin walled blisters, filled with blood. These blisters ruptured spontaneously or on the slightest trauma. The mucous membrane of the lips showed lesions resembling mucous patches and multiple hemorrhagic punctae. On admission to the hospital phenobarbital was withdrawn and at the end of the third week the mouth condition was almost normal. It was then given again, and the same eruption produced. A skin sensitization test for phenobarbital was negative. The urine still showed phenobarbital two and one-half weeks after its administration had been discontinued. The second case was that of a man of 40 years who consulted me for an eruption of the tongue consisting of swelling and numerous round and oval erosions without cutaneous manifestations. They resembled mucous patches so much that for the afternoon of the same day an appointment had been made by a colleague for an arsphenamin injection. In this case the lesions in the mouth were due to salipyrin. After being informed of the cause of his affection, the patient recollected that a year ago he had had a similar attack due to the same cause.

Another case was that of a woman who had suffered for two years with repeated attacks, beginning with itching of the hands and feet, sneezing and a watery discharge from the nose, and eruption of a bullous character in the groins, vagina, rectum, lips and mouth. The patient had made the rounds of dermatologists and had been put on a strict diet on the basis of skin sensitization tests, without any benefit. This eruption was due to cinchophen. When this drug was discontinued, the lesions promptly healed.

I have seen a similar case, following the administration of cinchophen, in a female patient with an erythematous and hemorrhagic eruption of the hands and fingers and a herpetic and bullous eruption on the roof of the mouth and the tip of the tongue.

A few weeks ago I saw a young girl with a generalized scarlatiniform eruption, after one dose of 1½ grains (0.097 gm.) phenobarbital. Three weeks later, this patient developed a peculiar erythema in the flush area of the face resembling a superficial lupus erythematosus and blebs in the mouth. suggesting a drug eruption. This patient had received two injections of phenolsulphonephthalein to test the renal efficiency. I mention this as a mere suggestion that the eruption may have been due to that drug.

Regarding the fixed arsphenamin eruptions which Dr. Wise mentioned in his paper and of which he said on account of their resemblance to antipyrin or phenolphthalein eruptions that one of these drugs might have been administered, I want to state that this was not the case in my patients. Furthermore, we were not able to produce an eruption in the patient with the arsphenamin eruption by the administration of phenolphthalein nor in the patient with the phenolphthalein eruption by the injection of arsphenamin.

You all remember the patient with the unusual eruption, resembling lichen planus, who was presented at our clinical meeting in Boston last year. The eruption followed the injection of arsphenamin. Drs. Wise, Highman and myself considered the condition lichen planus. Drs. Fordyce and Ormsby strongly contested this view, and proclaimed it an unusual arsphenamin eruption. This case resembled closely the one mentioned by the essavist and I now admit that in my opinion the view of my opponents was correct.

The facts mentioned by Dr. Wile, that bromids replace the chlorids in the body, has induced me for many years to give patients with bromid eruptions either a diet rich in salt or to administer calcium chlorid by mouth.

Dr. C. C. DENNIE, Kansas City: I would like to offer a suggestion regarding the chemical end of this proposition. I do not think consideration has been taken of what has been called the solution tension of metal. All metals have a solution tension, and iron has a greater one than copper: therefore, iron replaces copper in solution, and the copper is thrown out. The presence of sodium iodid in the blood when potassium iodid has been given can readily be explained on the basis that potassium has a greater tension than the sodium. and in that case the potassium would replace the sodium in the body cell and one would have the sodium eliminated and the potassium retained. When one gives sodium iodid the sodium will not replace the sodium there because it will have the same tension. It might be conceivable that it is the potassium in the cell combination thus retained that causes the trouble.

Dr. Jay Frank Schamberg, Philadelphia: It must have required a great deal of discriminating judgment on the part of Dr. Wise to give us his excellent digest of the literature on this subject. Dr. Wile's contribution acquires a permanent importance because he eliminates untenable hypotheses and his decisions are based on experimental evidence.

As I understood a reference by Dr. Wise, a writer quoted by him assumes that cases of arsphenamin dermatitis are due to the presence of "arsenoxid" in the drug. Ehrlich early stated that all lots of arsphenamin contained traces of arsenoxid, usually less than 1 per cent. I do not believe that we can incriminate arsenoxid as the cause. In the first place, from the use of 2,000 ampules of the same lot, one or two cases of dermatitis may develop. Second, compounds that have given rise to dermatitis were found by analysis not to contain an excessive amount of arsenoxid. Arsenoxid is both more toxic and more curative than arsphenamin, but there is no evidence that it is the cause of dermatitis.

We do not know the fate of arsphenamin, after it is introduced into the blood stream. We know that it produces rapidly a combination with the blood serum. We have produced in the test tube a combination with blood serum, a substance which we evaporated to solid form and after redissolving injected into animals, with results not differing greatly from those of arsphenamin.

In regard to phenobarbital, this drug has come into use extensively on account of its value in epilepsy; we must familiarize ourselves with the eruptions produced by it in order to be of aid to the practitioner.

I saw a man who had been taking 1½ grains of phenobarbital three times a day for three weeks. He presented an intense morbilliform eruption, with bloodshot eyes, with marked stomatitis and with hundreds of blebs over the trunk and studded profusely over the palms and soles. The case had been diagnosed by the practitioner as measles, but I said that I had never seen measles with such a slight rise in temperature and with numerous blebs. I regarded it as a phenobarbital eruption. I would be interested to know whether other members have seen a similar manifestation.

Barbital is apt to produce eruptions which simulate the exanthems. I am sure that many erroneous diagnoses of scarlet fever are made on account of confusion with drug eruptions. I recall a patient with a scarlatinoid rash and a temperature of 101 F. in whom the diagnosis of scarlet fever was made. We stopped the drug, and the symptoms all disappeared; we resumed the drug and the symptoms reappeared. I think we should determine in all drug eruptions whether a leukocytosis exists because its absence would operate against the diagnosis of scarlet fever. In the latter disease there is virtually always a leukocytosis.

Dr. Harold N. Cole, Cleveland: Some years ago some German research workers, who were studying drug eruptions to ascertain whether they were due to anaphylaxis, worked with potassium iodid. In 1910 I checked up this work. I withdrew some of the blood from patients with acute potassium iodid eruptions, injected the serum into guinea-pigs, and then gave some of the drug to the pigs. We could not confirm the work of the Germans. The same was also true in regard to copaiba eruptions.

Dr. Sigmund Pollitzer, New York: I am very much interested in this subject, but it is of such tremendous scope that it is impossible in the few minutes allowed for discussion to touch more than a few points.

It seems that we have at least two definite classes of effects in drug eruptions. First, it seems certain that the effect of arsenic on the epidermal struc--

ture is something entirely different from the effect produced by any other cutaneous irritant conveyed by the blood. Arsenic exercises a direct influence on the process of cornification. It is on the stimulation of this process that one of the therapeutic uses of arsenic is based. It needs only a slight over-stimulation of this cornification to produce the keratoses of arsenic.

With regard to the arsenic in certain organic compounds, it has effects of an entirely different class, presenting a group of symptoms of the erythema multiforme type of eruption. All of the new drugs, I think I am safe in saying all, produce eruptions of the erythema multiforme type—simple erythema, urticaria or scarlatiniform, morbilliform or purpuric eruptions; all of these are simply stages of the same process, which predicates an injury to the blood vessels.

As to the question of iodids and bromids, I remember the interest aroused by Adamkiewicz' announcement of the discovery of iodin in the pustules of iodid acne. It was soon pointed out, however, that the mere presence of iodin in these lesions proved nothing unless it could be proved that there was more in the lesions than elsewhere in the tissues, and of course such a quantitative demonstration was out of the question. Soon after that a number of observers —Duckworth, Thin, Ducrey, and others—showed that it was not true that the pathogenic process began in the sebaceous glands, but that it started in the epidermis over the papillae, and that the involvement of the sebaceous glands was secondary.

With all that has been said, we cannot get away from the fact that a drug eruption depends on something more than the drug. Most people may take these drugs without manifesting any cutaneous effects; there is always the drug plus the patient. That peculiarity in the patient we have been in the habit of speaking of as idiosyncrasy. I have no doubt the time will come when the meaning of idiosyncrasy will be understood, and we will know that it is, after all, a chemical process; but at the present time the nature of this is not understood, and notwithstanding the large amount of work accumulated and the excellent observations presented to us this evening, we do not yet understand it. The pathogenic process in these ills is still a mystery.

DR. CHARLES J. WHITE, Boston: In regard to the relation of bromids, I wish to relate this rather extraordinary experience. I was asked to treat an ulcer on the leg of a woman with a remarkably clear white skin. There was no hair and there were no varicose veins. The ulcer seemed remarkable. I asked many questions but received no answers of any value. I tried to heal this ulcer in various ways without success. I tried liquor ferri et potassii tartratis, scarlet red, a fuchsin paste solution, and finally applied surgical solution of chlorinated soda. The patient sent for me in the middle of the night, saying that something had happened. She was right. I have never seen such an explosion as had occurred in the skin of the patient's leg. I said, "You have not told me the whole truth," and she then said, "I will tell you something that I have never told anybody before. I am an epileptic; my attacks come on at night, and I have been taking bromids for years." This outburst seemed to me to be due to the combination of bromid and chlorin, and I would like to ask Dr. Wile to explain what he thinks of this episode. To my mind it does not seem to fit in well with his theory.

DR. SAMUEL E. SWEITZER, Minneapolis: In looking up the subject of drug eruptions I have been surprised to find recorded three deaths from the use of boric acid. I had previously considered boric acid as a mild and harmless preparation.

In April I saw an unusual procain eruption in a young woman who had been given a caudal anesthetic. The procain eruption came out within a few hours and presented itself as an acute eruption, which extended around the body in the region of the hip. It was, to me, a very unusual manifestation.

DR. CHARLES WALLIS EDMUNDS, Department of Pharmacology, Ann Arbor, Mich.: I wish I might add something to this discussion, but I came to learn. I have profited greatly by the papers I have heard, but have. been especially interested in the papers on drug eruptions and in knowing that the dermatologists, when it comes down to the fundamental causes, know no more than the pharmacologists, and they know very little.

Regarding the question of iodids and bromids: It has been known for a long time that there is a marked difference in the time of elimination. Iodid requires about forty-eight hours and bromid much longer. I think Fishman, in 1907, took 15 grain (0.97 gm.) doses of bromid, and found bromid in the urine fifty to fifty-five days afterward. This is very interesting when considered in relation to the chemical reactions of the two drugs. The fact is that the iodid is a foreign substance in the body, and the urine quickly gets rid of it, but as a matter of fact the kidney cannot differentiate between the bromid and chlorid ions. We are taking chlorid all the time, and it is therefore impossible to trace any definite dosage, but probably it is retained in the body just as the bromid is retained. The iodid is a foreign ion and we can trace it, but we cannot do this with the bromid. The kidney tubules apparently cannot differentiate between the bromid and the chlorid, and the bromid keeps circulating in the body for five or six weeks, which explains the difference in the rate of elimination of the two substances.

I was much interested in hearing of the giving of large doses of iodids intravenously. I think we are becoming more prone to give intravenous injections, and yet I wonder whether it is justified. For instance, the iodids and bromids taken by the stomach are absorbed in a few minutes, and large amounts will be absorbed within a very short time, making intravenous medication largely unnecessary. Sometimes the results from the administration of some drugs intravenously are rather unfortunate, and it is well to go a little more slowly. Some firms are putting out large numbers of drugs that can be given intravenously, but I think that pharmacologists are opposed to the administration of most of these drugs intravenously, thus subjecting the patient to a risk that attends the injection of these drugs directly into the blood stream, unless of course there is some definite indication for an extremely rapid administration of the drug.

DR. HARRY E. ALDERSON, San Francisco: I have a patient whose condition calls for the administration of iodids in the largest possible dosage, and yet she cannot take over 5 grains (0.32 gm.) at a time without having distressing symptoms. She develops a rapid heart, and she has coryza and all the other manifestations of iodism, without having acne. She also has symptoms of hyperthyroidism. At one time she was able to take as much as 30 grains (1.95 gm.) daily for a short period. Once when she had taken none at all for a month she insisted that the coppery taste persisted. As she is a very intelligent woman, I think her statement is worthy of consideration. I should like to ask what can be done with a patient showing this idiosyncrasy or hypersensitiveness.

DR. FRED WISE, New York: One of the points which Dr. Goldenberg brought up in his very interesting discussion was the use of phenolsulphonephthalein and the possibility of that drug producing an eruption. There is no question but that thousands of kidney tests are being made every day, and since we have not heard that any of these patients have had a rash, it seems obvious that there must be a vast difference in the chemical combination in the blood which results from the ingestion of phenolsulphonephthalein and phenolphthalein. I have too little knowledge of chemistry to say what the difference may be, but I think, in view of the fact that we do not get reports of eruptions following phenolsulphonephthalein, that it does not cause the eruption provoked by the phenolphthalein.

The well-known fact that iodids and bromids may provoke deep-seated subcutaneous nodules, bears out Dr. Wile's statement that the ordinary cutaneous bacteria do not play a leading rôle in the causation of iododermas and bromodermas.

In regard to Dr. Schamberg's saying that we should look for leukocytosis in skin eruptions, we have no experience except in bromid eruptions in which the leukocyte count was normal. Whether this holds good in phenobarbital eruptions, I do not know.

Among the points not touched on was the remarkable disappearance of antipyrin and phenolphthalein lesions in spite of the fact that the patient continues the use of the drug. That is a puzzle, and I do not know that any one has said anything that would explain this in any way. Stelwagon and some of the foreign writers say that the eruption will disappear while the patient is taking antipyrin, and may vanish permanently.

Another fact is that a patient may have a bromid eruption, and on stopping the bromids the eruption will persist for a year or longer. I have seen a case like this in a baby who had a bromid eruption from suckling the mother, and the eruption persisted for a year after the mother stopped taking the drug.

I would like to stress the point Dr. Pollitzer made, and that is the question of idiosyncrasy, which, of course, we can talk of in only a vague way. There are some drugs in which idiosyncrasy must play a much more important rôle than in others. Nearly every one may have an iodid eruption if he takes enough of the drug; people have arsphenamin eruptions.

I should like to have Dr. Wile make clear the point as to whether his patient with pemphigus received potassium iodid or bromid.

Dr. Udo J. Wile, Ann Arbor, Mich. (closing) : Dr. Goldenberg's discussion brings out a therapeutic suggestion of great value which we have had occasion to employ, and which is very instructive. He said he has been accustomed to give patients with a bromid rash sodium chlorid. The bromid dermatitis can be made to disappear quickly by the intravenous injection of physiologic sodium chlorid solution, which I am sure Dr. Edmonds would not disapprove. In one patient, a man, the bromid reaction was very severe, accompanied by stupor, pallor and palpitation; he was promptly relieved of the stupor and other symptoms after the administration of 100 c.c. of physiologic sodium chlorid solution. In another case the eruption disappeared very quickly after the intravenous injection of physiologic sodium chlorid solution.

I well remember the experiment of Bruch, which Dr. Cole alluded to, and it was one of the best examples of true allergy in the literature. Bruch was attempting to demonstrate iododerma on the basis of anaphylaxis. The patient he had as a control was in the hospital for gonorrhea and, according to his statement, had never taken any iodid of potassium. This blood was taken as a control, together with the serum of the guinea-pig and that of a patient who had iododerma; following this injection the guinea-pig immediately died with anaphylactic shock. Bruch then gave the patient a few doses of potassium iodid, and he immediately broke out with an inténse eruption. Bruch concluded that this man had a hereditary sensitization to iodids. This has never been substantiated.

Dr. Pollitzer's remarks regarding the type of dermatitis following intravenous administrations and that following ingestion are very interesting. I believe the two processes are distinctly different. That the effect when the drug passes through the digestive canal and when it passes through the blood is very different must be self evident. There is a great difference in the results after intravenous injection and after administration of the drugs by mouth.

I do not think Dr. White's case is difficult to explain if one accepts the fact that trauma is a local predisposing feature in drug exanthems. I think we have demonstrated this in the production of exanthems. I do not think it has anything to do with the replacement of the bromid in the blood with chlorin. I think the explanation in this case is based on the element of trauma.

Dr. Sweitzer's remarks regarding boric acid were interesting. I saw a patient this year who developed a marked erythematous rash each time he came in contact with the biborate solution with which his bladder was irrigated.

I wish to take issue with Dr. Wise's statement that any patient taking iodid of potassium will sooner or later develop an eruption. That is not so, and I am sure a large group can take amounts of this drug over many months without developing rash. Those who develop a rash do so after taking a few grains in some instances. This is perfectly manifest in the cases of nursing children who develop a nodular bromoderma from the breast milk of the mother who is taking a few grains of bromid. I believe our experiments have conclusively proved that there is no relation between the size of the dose, and the appearance of a rash in a given case.

INDUSTRIAL DERMATITIS AT THE MASSACHUSETTS GENERAL HOSPITAL *

C. GUY LANE, M.D.

Assistant Dermatologist, Massachusetts General Hospital

BOSTON

The papers of Fordyce,[1] Hazen,[2] Knowles,[3] White[4] and Pusey[5] have already pointed out the many occupations in which an irritation of the skin may be produced. They have described the types of eruption appearing as a result of employment in these various occupations, and have discussed the etiologic factors which have caused these irritated conditions. Of particular value is· the paper of Knowles, based on the study of more than 7,000 cases of eczema, which was presented in this city just ten years ago this month. A study of his paper, and of the other papers as well, emphasizes the importance of external causes in the etiology of these pathologic skin conditions. These authors have made a distinct contribution to our knowledge of such dermatoses, and rendered a real service to dermatology and to the afflicted patients.

But have we profited by this knowledge which they have given us? Have not their lessons been relegated to the background in the mass of dermatologic literature of the last ·few years? For instance, are we not likely to forget the frequency with which occupational cases are appearing in our clinics? Fordyce has stated that 2 per cent. of the total number of new cases at his skin clinic for 1911 constituted occupational dermatoses, and Knowles in 1913 and 1917 estimated that one sixth of all eczema was due to occupation. There is no doubt that at least the same percentage of our skin cases today will be found by careful study to be due to occupational factors.

---

* Read before the Section on Dermatology and Syphilology at the Seventy-Third Annual Session of the American Medical Association. St. Louis. May, 1922.

* From the Dermatological Clinic. Massachusetts General Hospital.

1. Fordyce, J. A.: Occupational Diseases of the Skin, M. Rec. **81**:207 (Feb. 3) 1912; Occupational Skin Diseases, J. A. M. A. **59**:2043 (Dec. 7) 1912.

2. Hazen, H. H.: Industrial Skin Diseases, J. Cutan. Dis. **32**:487 (July) 1914.

3. Knowles, F. K.: The External Origin of Eczema. Particularly the Occupational Eczemas, as Based on a Study of 4.142 Cases. J. Cutan. Dis. **31**:1i (Jan.) 1913; Eczema of External Origin. and Its Relationship to Dermatitis. J. A. M. A. **68**:79 (Jan. 13) 1917.

4. White, C. J.: Certain Occupations as Contributing Factors to Diseases of the Skin, Boston M. & S. J. **175**:35 (July 13) 1916.

5. Pusey, W. A.: Industrial Dermatoses. Their Sources. Types and Control, J. Indust. Hyg. **1**:385 (Dec.) 1919.

In this paper it is my purpose to act as the social service worker, that is, to attempt to do a little "follow-up work," and help "carry on" in this broad field in which these pioneers have shown the way. I shall discuss the occupational cases appearing at the Massachusetts General Hospital in the last few years, and emphasize the opportunity presented to us, as dermatologists, to contribute a still greater share to the work of preventive medicine.

FREQUENCY

In making this study of the cases of occupational dermatitis, it was found that no attempt had been made to group these cases in the diagnosis catalogue. Experience in the clinic had shown that the majority were given a diagnosis of dermatitis, dermatitis venenata or eczema. It has been necessary, therefore, to examine all records with the foregoing diagnoses in order to find the cases associated with the patient's occupation. For the three years 1919, 1920 and 1921, there were 921 cases of dermatitis or dermatitis venenata treated in the outpatient skin

NUMBER OF CASES AND NUMBER OF ADMISSIONS

	1919	1920	1921	Totals
Admissions to skin department.........	2,263	2,301	2,580	7,144
Cases of dermatitis	249	365	307	921
Cases of occupational dermatitis	22	47	37	106
Cases of eczema	....	522	564	1,086
Cases of occupational eczema	....	25	23	48
Total cases of dermatitis and eczema....	249	887	871	2,007
Total occupational cases...............	22	72	60	154

department. A critical examination of these records revealed 106 cases in which the occupation was a probable etiologic factor. In more of these cases the relation was not as clear cut and the evidence did not warrant including them in this group. In other words, there were 11.5 per cent. of the cases of dermatitis or dermatitis venenata which were probably industrial in origin.

In a similar manner, the 1,086 cases of eczema for the years 1920 and 1921 were examined. In this group there were forty-eight cases in which there was definite evidence on the record to show that the skin condition was probably derived from the patient's trade or occupation. There were, then, 4.4 per cent. of the cases of eczema from industrial causes.

The accompanying table shows the number of cases occurring in each year and the number of patients admitted to the skin department for each year.

For the year 1921 there were sixty occupational cases among 2,580 admissions to the skin department, so that the ratio of industrial cases to total admissions, so far as it is possible to ascertain, was 2.3 per cent. The ratio in 1920 was 3.1 per cent. The cases of eczema in 1919 have not been studied, but it is hoped to make still further investigation on this subject.

In the two years 1920 and 1921 there were 132 cases which were caused by occupational conditions. This is 7.1 per cent. of all cases of dermatitis, dermatitis venenata and eczema, or 2.7 per cent. of the total admissions to the skin department.

From a study of these records I feel that the actual percentage is larger than these figures show because of the number of cases, especially of eczema, in which the occupational factor was not mentioned. Furthermore, burns, infected conditions, keloids, etc., have not been examined from this point of view. I believe that it would be a conservative estimate to say that 4 or 5 + per cent. of the admissions to the skin clinic may be caused by occupational factors.

TYPES OF WORKERS

Examination of these 154 cases more closely shows that there were ninety-four, or 61 per cent., male, and sixty, or 39 per cent . female workers, all of them white. The ages varied from 16 to 82 years. There were thirty-one different occupations represented. Housework and allied work contributed forty-seven, the greatest number, to the group. Various washing powders, naphtha soap, soapine and brass polish are the agents most frequently mentioned as the exciting causes. Seven men are included in this group, their occupations providing opportunity for contact with washing powders and cleansing agents. The shoe workers, fourteen in all, formed the next largest class. There were twelve who handled dyes in some form or other. Paints, including furniture polish and varnish and various removers. accounted for ten. There were seven rubber workers. and seven who worked in candy factories, four of the latter among chocolate workers. There were six nurses in the group, and three men in whom cyanid was a probable factor. Among the others, the following types of workers were represented: machinist, photographer, silver polisher. packers (using hay, straw, etc.), baker, tanner, cement worker, nickel plater, tobacco worker, longshoreman, bleacher, upholsterer, waitress, gardener, necropsy room attendant, miller, acetylene worker, labeler, lumberman, farmer, wool worker and printer. A more detailed investigation of these cases is being undertaken, and a further report will be made in a later paper.

THE INDUSTRIAL CLINIC

The investigation of these cases has been greatly facilitated by the Industrial Clinic at the Massachusetts General Hospital. This is a separate clinic through which pass all cases of disease associated with industrial conditions, or any condition suspected of being associated with an industry. This clinic is one of the first, if not the first, industrial clinic established in a general hospital. The clinic has a very close association with the department of industrial hygiene in the Harvard School of Public Health, and, on the other hand, with the state department of labor and industries. It therefore offers an opportunity for the scientific study of occupational diseases, and also an opportunity for an accurate investigation of the conditions under which the disease or condition may have been acquired. It is possible, then, for a patient with an industrial skin condition, or one suspected of being such, to be referred to this clinic for investigation. This clinic will interview the patient, and report the case to the state department of labor and industries, which will send out an inspector to investigate the particular plant and the particular part of the work which this patient does. Furthermore, this clinic is in position to follow up the patient to make sure that he returns to the skin clinic at proper intervals for treatment; to attend to various details in connection with compensation, if time is lost, and to maintain close cooperation with the various industrial physicians in the vicinity.

PROPER METHOD OF DEALING WITH THESE DERMATOSES

The study of these cases has brought home to me very forcibly several facts which seem essential in the proper dealing with these dermatoses. In the first place, there is the wide variety of occupations in which a dermatitis may arise. The list which I have given discloses some of the types of work, but there are many others to which our attention has already been called. In the second place, there should be a more careful study of the patient. These occupational cases are likely to be lost in the rush of the clinic. They are likely to be considered as an ordinary type of skin disease, for they do not usually present unusual and therefore interesting manifestations. Some present the picture of an acute dermatitis of short duration. Others simulate an eczema of long standing. Others appear as burns, boils, etc., or as other common conditions. We are likely to write a few words of description on the record. We make a diagnosis of acute dermatitis, dermatitis venenata or eczema, or the like, and we prescribe some simple remedy for the relief of the present condition. Often, in the crush of the clinic, little thought is given to possible occupational factors, and still less attention is paid, I am afraid, if the patient is unable to understand or speak good English. The patient is dismissed to make way for the next one without an attempt to study the case or the working conditions. Let me use, as an example, certain cases of eczema in 1920, ninety-nine in all, in which the disease was practically limited to the hands and arms. In fifty-two of these the occupation was given as "housewife" or "at home." There was no indication on the record that the occupation of any of this group had been considered as a possible cause, and I have not included these among the occupational cases. But I believe that many of them were due to some element in their work. Such cases are lost, not only for the purpose of statistical study, but also for the purpose of investigating the industrial factors involved, and without the knowledge based on the study of such accumulated facts it is a difficult matter to take steps for the prevention of such skin conditions among susceptible persons.

In the third place, there should be a more exact analysis of the job, and a wider knowledge of trade processes and conditions. Pusey has already emphasized the necessity for "more knowledge of the factors which are important in the production of these diseases and in their prevention and control." It is not enough to know that a man is a painter or tanner or dyer or rubber worker. We should find out the active agent in producing his condition, or at least instigate an investigation of his working conditions, of the substances which he handles and of the effect of such factors on the skin. The fact that a man, aged 33, with an eruption on his arms, is a night pumper in a compressed gas factory means little till it is found that at intervals during the night he fills a generator with calcium carbid, wearing only cotton gloves. The same is true of the book packer who is found to handle new books and to have his hands become covered with stains from the covers, or the housewife who is working part of the time in a tobacco factory as a stripper, or the jeweler working with cyanid in the coloring room. The exact knowledge obtained in the study of the processes of vulcanizing and of printing has been of inestimable value in the proper handling of the dermatoses occurring in these occupations. A most valuable feature of the book on this subject by R. Prosser White [6] is the detail with which the trade processes are explained.

PREVENTION

In the fourth place is the fact that the prevention of these dermatoses should receive greater emphasis. There is, of course, the present skin condition to treat; but the real problem is the prevention of its recurrence and the prevention of a similar condition in other susceptible persons. The situation is analogous to the infectious skin conditions. We do not make a diagnosis of scabies or impetigo without taking steps for the prevention of its recurrence and for preventing the infection from appearing in others; but meanwhile we treat the existing condition. The same should be true in the case of the occupational dermatoses—the proper treatment should mean prevention.

---

6. White, R. P.: Occupational Affections of the Skin. Ed. 2. New York, Paul B. Hoeber, 1920.

We need, first, to realize the wide variety of substances responsible for these skin conditions; then to make a painstaking inquiry into the individual case, and to make a careful analysis of the work he is doing, and on this foundation attempt to build a rational procedure for his particular kind of work. There has been exact scientific work of this character in the last few years in the study of two occupations, and it seems reasonable to expect that further similar studies will eliminate the skin conditions resulting from other trades. I assume that most readers are familiar with the preventive work which has been done in the case of the vulcanizers and among the pressmen in the printing trade, but the importance of this research work warrants a brief review.

Among the vulcanizers it had been noted that eruptions appeared on the forearms and hands of men using hexamethylenamin as one of the accelerators in the vulcanizing process, especially in hot weather. Working on the theory that under the influence of the acid in the sweat the hexamethylenamin was broken down to formaldehyd, and later oxidized to formic acid, and thus causing an irritation, Shepard and Krall[7] used alkaline solutions for the immersion of the hands and arms of susceptible persons previous to going to work, and found that the condition did not appear.

Among the pressmen there were a number of workers with an eruption on the exposed surfaces. McConnell,[8] after a careful study of the working conditions, inks, cleansing processes, etc., found that by applying a mixture of hydrous wool fat or hydrous wool fat and oil before working, and by using a liquid soap and sawdust for cleansing purposes, the eruption could be prevented.

In both of these occupations the result was obtained by changing the working conditions without changing the man to another job. It is interesting to note that the first report issued by the committee which studied the eruptions among the vulcanizers recommended a change of work; but the later investigations made this unnecessary. This is the usual suggestion made in the treatment of these dermatoses. It is well to remember that there are the two possibilities, in this phrase, one to send the patient to another job, and the other to alter the process or the working conditions in some way. The former is the one usually employed, thus allowing the conditions to remain for the next susceptible person. It is not hard to imagine the difficulty with which a person acquainted with only one kind of work adapts himself to another kind, especially if he has worked at the first one all his life. The most

---

7. Shepard, N. A., and Krall, S.: Poisons in the Rubber Industry, India Rubber World **61**:75 (Nov. 1) 1919.

8. McConnell, W. J.: Industrial Dermatosis Among Printers, Pub. Health Rep. **36**:979 (May 6) 1921.

rational preventive measure, then, is the one directed toward rendering the working conditions as safe for the susceptible workers as possible.

SUSCEPTIBILITY

The study of these occupational cases emphasizes still further the fact that these persons with eruption caused by their work have undoubtedly become sensitized in some way to a particular substance, or that they are naturally susceptible. At any rate, to be still more indefinite, they are cases of idiosyncrasy or individual susceptibility. The fact so often used in arguing against these cases, that the condition cannot be due to the occupation because the one person affected is the only one in his room, or the only one affected among many who are using the same substances, or working under the same conditions, is no argument at all, of course. It is perfectly possible for only one person out of fifty or a hundred to have an eruption from handling dyes, or to be the only one out of a large gang of machinists who will be affected by oil, etc. I emphasize this fact because only recently before the industrial accident board an employer defended his case by bringing in man after man employed in the same process as the patient and exhibiting them to the board as examples of the fact that the process did not cause any irritation. The case was one of undoubted susceptibility, and yet the board, at last reports, had decided in favor of the employer. Moreover, the same fact is true in these cases that is true in cases of food sensitization, or of suspected food sensitization, because of positive cutaneous reactions; namely, that only a therapeutic test—the matter of omitting a certain food from the diet in one case, and the matter of omitting a certain process or a certain substance in the other case—is the only real test. It is also important to remember in this connection that there are cases of individual susceptibility to extremely minute quantities in the cases of foods and drugs, and that undoubtedly the same fact is true in connection with these occupational cases.

NOMENCLATURE

Finally, the very number of these fairly definite occupational skin conditions suggests the advisability of grouping these cases better for the purpose of statistical and preventive study. Can we not call attention to these dermatoses in a more forceful manner? Would it not help to emphasize them by giving them a more definite place in our official nomenclature? We have the term dermatitis medicamentosa applied to dermatoses from the absorption of medicinal agents. Why can we not adopt some term, such as "dermatitis industrialis" to be applied to this group of pathologic skin conditions resulting from the industry in which the patient is employed? The name "trade eczema" has the advantage of long usage, but it seems as if the time had come when we ought to cleave these cases of occupational skin conditions from the eczema group and segregate them in a group by themselves. One objection immediately raised is in regard to the multiform character of the lesions caused from various substances. The possible multiformity is apparent; but, as one thinks of dermatitis venenata with its erythematous, papular or. vesicular lesions, and of dermatitis medicamentosa with its macular, papular, pustular or verrucous lesions, such objections seem inconsistent. These are examples of a definite etiologic group, but with possible multiform appearance. The importance of this group in the economic and financial life of the employee who suffers such disability, and the loss in efficiency with the consequent financial loss to the employer, serve as an additional argument for the use of a definite name. If some term, such as "dermatitis industrialis," cannot be agreed on, let us at least adhere to the term occupational dermatitis, or agree to group these cases under one or the other of the diagnoses dermatitis venenata or eczema, and use the term occupational as a qualifying phrase, in order that they may be available for proper study.

CONCLUSIONS

1. Seven per cent. of dermatitis venenata and eczema, or almost 3 per cent. of all admissions to a skin clinic in a large hospital, were occupational in origin.

2. It is fair to estimate that 4 or 5 + per cent. of admissions to a skin clinic may be occupational.

3. A more careful study should be made of the individual patient.

4. A more exact study of trade processes should be instigated in case of questionable eruptions on exposed surfaces.

5. The consideration of preventive measures should be a greater factor as we see these cases in the clinic.

6. Some name, such as "dermatitis industrialis," or at least a more accurate place in our nomenclature, should be provided for this definite etiologic group of cases.

421 Marlborough Street.

ABSTRACT OF DISCUSSION

Dr. Richard L. Sutton, Kansas City, Mo.: I wish to thank Dr. Lane for his suggestion of the term, "dermatitis industrialis," for it fits these cases admirably. I also wish to recommend to my fellow dermatologists a splendid little book along this line, "Occupational Affections of the Skin," by R. Prosser White. It is one of the most useful volumes in my library. I found it almost encyclopedic in its scope.

Dr. Joseph Grindon, St. Louis: Attention has been particularly directed during the last several years to the importance of the subject of occupational diseases, and yet there remains a good deal to be learned in regard to occupational dermatoses. In the first place, what shall we call them? Certainly not "trade eczema." When the causative agent is determined we arbitrarily take the disease out of the "eczema" group and place it in the dermatitis group. The term "trade dermatoses" would be unobjectionable. There are several things to bear in mind in connection with these cases. First, we know only a small part of the subject, and we should all be on the lookout for new forms. Not only in our clinics but in our private practice we often forget to inquire into the occupation of the patient, whereas often the occupation would throw a light on the condition. These conditions sometimes lead to damage suits. There are some cases of malingering. Other cases are exemplified by that of a man with a congenital ichthyosis, which he attributed to his trade. Again, there are cases in which the patient honestly but erroneously believes that an eruption is due to something connected with his occupation. I recently saw a man who took a new job on Saturday. On Sunday he went out picnicking and Monday developed a toxicodendron dermatitis, which he honestly thought was due to his trade. At the same time we must be ready to do the patient full justice and not hastily determine that the condition is unconnected with his occupation when, perhaps, we are insufficiently informed. If we gave a little more thought to a matter spoken of by Dr. Lane, namely, special sensitization, we sometimes would feel that there was more in the contention of the employee. The responsibility of the physician is great. He should make it a matter of conscience and thoroughly consider the question before giving a decision.

DR. JEFFREY MICHAEL, Houston. Texas: I would like to add to the long list of industrial dermatoses another which occurs in the oil fields, due to crude petroleum. It has no clear-cut clinical features, except that the covered portions of the body are more affected than the uncovered. This is due to the fact, I think, that the clothing is saturated with the irritating oil.

DR. MOSES SCHOLTZ, Los Angeles: This subject interests the dermatologist as he is called on to determine whether the patient is entitled to compensation or not. The hardest thing I find is to tell whether the condition is ordinary eczema and whether it is systemic in origin or occupational. Whether we call it "eczema" or "dermatitis," the conditions are identical conceptions. It is simply a difference in nomenclature. I tried to differentiate morphologically. and my impression is that toxic eczema is likely to be less symmetrical than the occupational variety. Systemic eczemas are likely to affect any portion of the body while the occupational variety is most likely to affect the face. neck or hands. We often see the hands free, and we then have to assume dust or irritation through the air rather than direct contact as a cause. Another point is that the systemic eczemas are more likely to be fluctuating in their course, while those due to external irritation are likely to be more stable. If any one could give us a definite morphologic differentiation of systemic eczemas from those due to external irritants, it would be of great service.

DR. T. J. BURKE, Pittsburgh: I wish to call attention to a preparation in relation to these dermatoses, that known as "Lux." It is much used for washing shirt waists and other garments of that kind. There is nothing on the label or the instructions regarding its use to lead one to think that there is any danger in using it, but I have seen a number of cases in which it had caused a severe dermatitis.

DR. WILLIAM ALLEN PUSEY. Chicago: Dr. Lane touched on one point lightly—the necessity of a more intensive study of these occupational dermatoses. The great difficulty is that the industrial physician or surgeon is interested in other things and is not a trained dermatologist. What is needed, and what I believe is a possibility if it is gone after, is to get some of the foundations, or perhaps the U. S. Public Health Service, to make a real study of this condition. I know that young well trained dermatologists are in great demand, but I still think it is possible to have two or three of the young, well trained men devote their time to this question for two or three years. They could take with them some of the nestors of dermatology. We could be of help as consultants.

Dr. C. H. Ball, Tulsa, Okla.: My impression is that the main thing in a dermatitis is the peculiar idiosyncrasy of the individual. In a large establishment only a few men will have a dermatosis following an irritation of the skin. Possibly one of the worst cases I have ever seen was treated here in St. Louis by a well known dermatologist as dermatitis exfoliativa, and it was due entirely to a well known brand of hair dye.

Dr. S. Ayers, Jr., Los Angeles: I reported six cases of scleroderma with arsenic in the urine. Dr. Sutton had one of these cases. The history in several of the cases was very suggestive of an industrial dermatosis. One of these patients worked in a paper factory and examination of several samples of that paper showed a high content of arsenic. I think this is against the law now, but it is used nevertheless. Another one of the patients, a woman who kept a grocery store, used powdered arsenic in a dish under the counter for killing mice. The duration of her disorder was coincident with the use of the powder.

Dr. Lester Hollander, Pittsburgh: During the last year I treated four severe cases of vesicular dermatitis, affecting the hands and forearms, and in one instance spreading to the face, in workers in the photographic trade. After careful investigation I was able to determine that metol, which is used in the developing of photographs, was the offending agent. The chemical used was manufactured by the same concern in each instance. As I had a great deal of difficulty in clearing up these lesions, I communicated with the Eastman Kodak concern of Rochester, N. Y., regarding the necessity of medical investigation of industrial dermatoses. In this particular instance the industry itself had taken up the problem. Regarding the treatment, two things must be considered, especially when we are speaking of the acute type of trade dermatoses, the treatment of the condition itself and the prevention of its return.

Dr. Lane mentioned the fact that simply removing the patient from his work does not mean that the dermatologic condition is cured. I heartily endorse that view. Regarding the view of some writers that trade dermatoses depend on idiosyncrasy, in the four cases mentioned skin tests were utilized for the determination of the causative agent, but only two of the cases showed an erythema to metol applied in the form of a skin test. This makes one think guardedly how much of a factor idiosyncrasy really is in trade dermatoses.

Dr. A. J. Markley, Denver: It should always be borne in mind that the irritants with which one comes in contact in industrial occupations constitute only one of the factors in the production of these dermatoses. We know that each person has a certain amount of resistance, and when that resistance is broken down by internal conditions, improper diet or focal infection, it requires only a little external irritation to produce a dermatitis. It seems to me wholly unjust that a dermatitis involving the hands and face or considerable parts of the body should be attributed entirely to an external irritation when that irritation is simply the precipitating factor. It is not just to the patient that he should be dismissed with simply an amelioration of the condition from which he suffers. It is not fair to the patient and certainly not to the employer that the occupation be held wholly responsible for having induced an industrial dermatosis, and it is proper that we investigate the personal conditions of diet and of health of these patients.· It has been pointed out that only one of fifty employees may have such a reaction, and it has also been pointed out that removal from his work frequently fails to result in complete amelioration or disappearance of the symptoms. Unless we are prepared to inquire carefully into the entire condition, the internal cause as well as the external, we are not doing justice to the industry, to the patient, to the employer nor to ourselves.

Dr. David Lieberthal, Chicago: I want to stress the point that we should not say "occupational dermatitis" but "dermatoses."

Dr. C. Guy Lane, Boston: I did not talk about the occupations listed, but in my group there were thirty-one. I also wish to emphasize the careful scientific work done by the investigators of these two particular trades, among the vulcanizers and the pressmen. Dr. Sutton spoke of the book of Prosser White. I think it is particularly good in the way in which he explains the trade process. The malingerers have been spoken of and also the fact that all dermatoses appearing in workers are not industrial in origin. That must be taken into account every time. Dr. Pusey has brought up the necessity of studying, and I think we should certainly attempt to clear up these conditions. It was my intention to advocate the use of the the term "occupational dermatoses," in this group, but on talking it over with a member of the hospital nomenclature committee, there was some difficulty about including it among the other Latinized names and the term "dermatitis industrialis" seems very apropos. Someone mentioned the use of skin tests, but my experience with skin tests is that this is not a real test of susceptibility in these cases. The real test is the therapeutic test. Having the man stop his work for a period or changing the process proves the cause of the dermatitis better than any skin test can do.

Note.—The author agrees with the suggestions made in the discussion regarding "dermatosis" and believes that the better term to adopt in classifying this group is "dermatosis industrialis."

PROCAIN DERMATITIS AMONG DENTISTS *

HENRY KENNEDY GASKILL, M.D.

. PHILADELPHIA

One has only to turn back the pages of history to be reminded of the enthusiasm with which new inventions and remedies for the treatment of diseases have been hailed. Later, they have either been relegated to oblivion or have found their level in the treatment of a few conditions and often in a few selected cases. The roentgen ray is one of the best exemplifications of this, and the vaccines which were employed for every known ill from eczema to ingrowing toenails are a very close second.

It is equally true that, when an epidemic of disease sweeps the country, possibly becoming pandemic, there is always a certain amount of hysteria associated with it; as, for instance, there have been for the past several years epidemics of influenza; and every one who has a cold, no matter what the type, situation or degree, looks on it as a grip infection. At the present time, dentists have become more or less hysterical over procain or allied products; and if an eruption of any kind occurs on their hands, they promptly put the blame on these pain relieving remedies. The medical journals have published several articles on this subject, and unquestionably some of the cases have been directly referable to the irritation caused by the dribbling on the fingers or lack of care in preparation when giving hypodermic injections of procain and, in one instance at least, solutions containing cocain. But, after analyzing some of these published articles, and making careful investigations in my own cases, I am convinced that there are elements other than the direct action of these drugs to be considered. In speaking of the action of this class of drugs, I shall use the word procain, as that is apparently the most commonly employed, taking for granted that any one of them might have been responsible, unless otherwise noted.

True procain dermatitis is an extremely unfortunate type of disease in the case of the dentist, for it not only is a constant source of irritation and annoyance to him, but it also often deprives patients of a tremendous amount of relief that they cannot otherwise obtain; he is often loath to acknowledge the cause and may continue the use of the drug either from ignorance of its deleterious effects or because he does not want to believe and hopes it will soon get better. I believe that there are few persons so susceptible to the action of procain that it of itself will cause trouble; but it is an acknowledged fact that any one

---

* Read at the Forty-Fifth Annual Meeting of the American Dermatological Association, Washington, D. C., May 2-4, 1922.

working under the physical and mental strain to which men in this profession are subjected is liable to afflictions which would not occur in different surroundings. This disbelief as to the injurious effect of procain, has been substantiated by Dr. Herman Prinz, professor of materia medica and therapeutics in the Thomas W. Evans Museum and Dental Institute, School of Dentistry, University of Pennsylvania, who in a recent communication says:

We prepare in our Institute the solution as outlined below. We use about 25 or more quarts per year in our various clinics and we have never seen a single case of skin irritation or other disturbances of a local nature arising therefrom. Many dentists keep their syringes and needles immersed in various types of antiseptic solutions, which contain cresol, alcohol, formaldehyd, boric acid, benzoic acid, alkalies of various types and other compounds. When they use the syringe, they remove it with their hands, which possibly means more or less always contamination with these preserving solutions and I assume that some of the so-called anesthetic dermatitis may most likely find an explanation therein, although I do not deny that isolated cases of procain dermatitis may exist. Personally I have used procain since its introduction into dentistry in 1907 in many thousands of cases and I have not seen any single skin reaction therefrom. I have employed it to a very limited extent in powdered form directly upon wound surfaces in the oral cavity and have never seen from it any ill results.

I have had a number of cases of severe skin irritations observed on the fingers of dentists and in all of these cases I was able to trace the origin to the careless use of formaldehyd, which is so freely employed by dental practitioners in the treatment of infected root canals and also for sterilizing purposes.

Dentists have long hours of doing the most minute kind of work over nervous patients, and unless they are particularly phlegmatic, become more or less fagged before the expiration of the day, and in many cases deplorably so before the end of the year. Without this all important factor, the drug which has been of such enormous benefit to mankind might be relatively harmless. The powers of resistance are lower, and the largest organ of the body, the skin, does not have the same general tone that should normally exist. While physicians and surgeons are using these drugs frequently, they are not under the same continuous strain as are dentists; and while there may have been cases of procain poisoning among the former class, I have failed to find any recorded.

Procain is the hydrochloric salt of a synthetically prepared base, para-amino-benzoyldiethylamino-ethanol. Its solution is neutral in reaction. Caustic alkalis and alkaline carbonates precipitate the free base from the aqueous solution in the form of a colorless oil, which soon solidifies. It is incompatible with the alkalis and alkaline carbonates, with picric acid and with the iodids.

The solution is prepared by dissolving 1.5 per cent. of procain in physiologic sodium chlorid solution, by boiling. When this solution, which either should be freshly prepared or should not be older than about a week, is used, 1 drop of epinephrin to from 1 to 2 c.c., 2 drops to from 3 to 5 c.c. and 3 drops to 6 or more c.c. is needed. As stated, this addition of epinephrin is always made as needed. Solutions containing epinephrin must under no conditions be boiled, as that invariably decomposes the epinephrin. For this reason, so-called dental tablets containing epinephrin and epinephrin in combination should not be boiled in the solvent, but should be merely added to the boiled saline or the Ringer solution.

All glassware used in making this solution or in which the solution is kept should be alkaline free glass (so-called Jena or hard glass).

Ready-made solutions containing procain-epinephrin mixtures as obtained from supply houses in bulk, as well as those obtained in ampules, usually decompose within a reasonable time.

There are apparently two distinct types of eruption: (1) the papulo-vesicular on a markedly erythematous base, usually preceded by pomphlyx-like lesions, accompanied by intense itching, and with little tendency to spread to other parts of the body; (2) a thickened verrucous condition of the ends of the fingers with involvement of the nail bed and hypertrophy of the nail itself. Marked pain is experienced, due to fissuring. It is not unusual for these two types to coexist.

In a few of the following histories there is no doubt that the direct cause was procain, but it is also reasonably certain that it was planted on unusually susceptible tissue. The patients often say that they have been using the same chemical or dye for years without any harm to themselves, and it is difficult to understand why at this particular time they should suffer from its use. It is largely a question of resistance.

When we come to realize what this peculiar change is—what it is that takes place—perhaps on account of overwork, worry, improper eating, eating when tired or exhausted, eating food which is not adapted to the individual patient and, what is worse, not being content with three meals a day, or, probably the worst of all, constipation and its associated gastric symptoms, we will be in a position to treat more intelligently the conditions that arise. One other factor which is quite frequently overlooked is the relationship between the skin and the kidneys, as faulty elimination of the kidneys throws more work on the skin and changes to some degree the character of the sweat.

Lane [1] reports three cases, in each of which there was marked dermatitis following the use of procain—all in dentists of long standing;

---

1. Lane. C. G.: Novocain Dermatitis in Dentists, Dental Cosmos, 1921, p. 878.

the causative factor in one was particularly clearly defined, for when the patient used rubber gloves, he was entirely free from the eruption, but on the use of procain without the gloves, there was an immediate return. In all his cases, Lane verified his clinical observations by means of cutaneous sensitization tests.

If a clinical diagnosis has been made of procain dermatitis, a positive skin reaction is of the utmost importance, but a negative reaction does not necessarily mean that the clinical diagnosis must be eliminated, for too many factors enter into these cutaneous tests to make them absolutely reliable; but should the second and third tests prove negative, I should be strongly inclined to look for another cause.

Several dentists have told me that they are resorting to the cutaneous test, and others have asked me to do it for them. On finding it negative, they have continued using procain without fear, placing absolute reliance on the sensitiveness of this test. But they must bear in mind that the body resistance may be altered by so many different conditions that they may become susceptible to the irritation of that or any other drug at any time.

REPORT OF CASES

CASE 1.—Dr. H., first seen, April 4, 1921, presented an eruption on the hands which he said had been there for ten weeks, a typical papulovesicular eczema. The skin in several parts was exfoliating; at the joints were numerous fissures, and there was the usual intolerable itching. The patient was nervous and depressed, could not sleep and had frequent attacks of indigestion: in fact, he felt and looked sick. He attributed the eruption to the use of procain. It had been much better for a few days before my seeing him, but became much worse after the use of a new liquid soap. In the course of a few days this same type of eruption had extended to the face and to the feet and ankles. The patient was confined to his bed for several weeks, and on recovery was advised to take a sea trip. On his return, the last of July, the condition was almost entirely well; but, August 19, there was a slight breaking out on the face and fingers, and he told me that he had used procain with gloves but had unconsciously put his gloved hands to his face. From this time on, he steadily improved but was never entirely well. On October 29, there was a marked outbreak on the face, following the use of a medicated shaving soap. Under soothing lotions, this also promptly disappeared. I am willing to agree that at the outbreak of this eruption in February the cause of it was procain, but it might just as well have been any other irritant substance, as was proved by the later eruptions. This patient had been working hard, frequently at night, and was in an excessively nervous condition, with severe indigestion, largely the result of overwork and nervousness. The outbreak following the use of the medicated shaving soap was convincing, to me at least, that the prime cause was any irritating substance, though procain might just as well take the blame for it in the first instance.

As this patient regained his health, the eruption on the hands gradually improved, but there were frequent nerve racking exacerbations of the papulo-vesicular type, always yielding to treatment, consisting of total abstinence from work and the application of soothing lotions. We searched for every possible and impossible cause, realizing that it must be somewhere in his house or office. Finally, in discussing the kind of rubber gloves worn, I asked how long he boiled them, only to be told his attendant washed them in tincture of green soap and hung them up to dry. The cause was found and the condition cured.

CASE 2.—Dr. R. called me on the telephone, Oct. 10, 1921, saying that he had procain dermatitis. On examination, he had, on several fingers, pomphlyx lesions with occasional vesicles occurring in small groups, mildly inflammatory and accompanied by itching. They presented the characteristic linear formation, which made me feel that they were due to the action of some of the poisonous plants. The patient told me that he had been pulling weeds the previous week, and that while he felt the eruption on one hand was due to procain, he was equally sure it was due to the action of the weeds on the other. Personally, I am inclined to feel that procain played no part in this eruption, which disappeared promptly under mild, soothing remedies and roentgen-ray exposure. As he has since expressed it, his hands are constantly bathed in procain, as his practice is limited to extraction; and there has been no return.

CASE 3.—Dr. N. had been in practice only a short time when he came in with a ready-made diagnosis of procain dermatitis. He presented a thickened, fissured condition around the ends of the nails and around the matrix. There was little or no inflammation surrounding it, and no vesiculation. On microscopic examination, this was proved a typical case of ringworm, as unyielding to treatment as they usually are; but on account of the popular feeling regarding procain, this patient always felt he had had a more or less atypical form of that type of dermatitis.

CASE 4.—Dr. D. wrote me the following history: He had a severe case of procain dermatitis affecting both hands, particularly the finger nails, which became thickened and hornlike. He was treated several months for this condition before the cause was ascertained, and it disappeared only on discontinuance of the use of local anesthetics. To prove to his own satisfaction that one of this class of drugs was the cause, he conducted the following experiment: Taking Waite's solution, he shook the bottle and rubbed the cork on his arm every day for four days, at the expiration of which time red marks began to appear where he had rubbed in the solution, and the part began to itch. He continued to rub in this solution in the same way for several days; the spots were becoming larger and swelling until there were several blebs which ruptured with the resulting oozing and pus formation. He rubbed in the solution for ten days, and at that time was convinced that the cause of the inflammation or his hands was that which had produced the lesions artificially on his arm. As soon as he stopped these applications the arm began to heal, but the itching remained intense.

Undoubtedly, however, there are many other substances which would have caused his local irritation from friction. I can recall the case of a young boy who had six or eight peculiar looking lesions on his face, which did not seem to fit into any defined category. He was accused of producing them himself by some artificial means and finally confessed that he had been in the habit of pinching up the skin, wetting his finger with saliva and rubbing it vigorously until these spots appeared. In the case of Dr. D., a stronger irritant was used than saliva. After an interval of two weeks, he rubbed in a little more of the solution, with a violent reaction within five hours. He later tried a solution of pure procain, which produced exactly the same result as had been obtained from Waite's anesthetic. In this case, we have a suspected dermatitis confirmed by sensitization test of the skin carried out to a greater extent than the diagnosis warranted.

CASE 5.—Dr. S. A., aged 25, who consulted me, November 25, presented a severe dermatitis on both hands. On the dorsal aspect, it had been extended nearly half way to the elbow, and not quite so far on the inner surface. It was extremely inflammatory, and more or less covered with crusts and scales, with many points of exudation. There was considerable involvement of the nail bed, with a recession of the matrix and a slight thickening of the nails themselves. To use his own words: "About five weeks ago there appeared on the index finger of my right hand small lesions, like little grains of sand under the skin, gradually developing into red, scaly blotches with a liquid oozing out." Later, there appeared on the finger and thumb of the left hand the verrucous type of eruption, with a thickening around the nail. Three weeks later, the condition extended until there was presented the picture that has been described. Shortly after he noticed the first irritation on the fingers, he was in the woods picking autumn leaves. The severe eruption did not occur until two weeks after that time, but it is not probable that *Rhus* was a factor, especially as there was no history of susceptibility, he having handled the plants on other occasions with impunity. The cutaneous sensitization tests were negative; and, while the patient was absolutely convinced that procain was responsible for the eruption, there has been no recurrence, although he uses the drug freely, but with the greatest caution against its coming in contact with his fingers in any way.

CASE 6.—Dr. F. wrote me that he had been using a solution called Novol for a year, when the fourth finger of the right hand became affected. Thinking it was due to the soap he had been using, he discontinued that, but the condition gradually spread to the other fingers and the interdigital spaces. The eruption was of the same inflammatory character as described in the other cases. accompanied by intense itching, particularly at night. This continued for three months, when his attention was called to the fact that it might be due to the use of Novol and, on the discontinuance of the use of that drug. the lesions healed in about three weeks. This patient also rubbed into his arm a solution of pure procain every day for a week, with the resulting erythematopapular eruption, accompanied by intense itching. Dr. F. is now using Waite's cocain solution and is apparently having no trouble.

CASE 7.—Dr. S. first noticed a thickening around the nail bed of the left hand, with an accompanying inflammation and considerable irritation. A diagnosis of eczema was made by a local physician. and the patient was told to keep his hands out of water—about as sensible a thing to tell a dentist as to urge a neurasthenic inmate of the almshouse to take a trip to Europe. The condition healed promptly under complete abstinence from work. and the application of calamine liniment; but it returned as soon as he resumed practice. and after close questioning it was found that he had been using considerable quantities of formaldehyd. It was difficult to convince him that this was the probable cause as he had such a fear of its being procain dermatitis that he could see no other possibility. However, he discontinued using formaldehyd. is very careful with his injections. and there has been no recurrence in the last six months.

CASE 8.—Dr. K. had been using procain since 1912. with the exception of intervals during the war. when it was impossible to procure it. Later, its use was resumed, and early in October. 1920. the cuticle around the nails began to harden, and there was severe itching and cracking of the epidermis. At the same time, he also had a severe itching under the ring on the third finger of the left hand. (This, however, is not an unusual occurrence when men wash their hands frequently with soap, which collects under the ring and is very irritating). Within a short time, the inflammation extended over the back of the left hand; and later the right hand was also affected. There was considerable induration with fissuring at times, and superimposed staphylococcic infection. About the middle of November of the same year, he was away for two weeks and the hands greatly improved; but, on his return to the office, the itching and inflammatory symptoms returned, and he received active treatment, besides taking the precaution of always using rubber gloves while administering procain. Six months later, he gave the following report: "At the present time, the epidermis is healing under the finger nails of the left hand, but there is a slight dermatitis where the trouble originally started; and while using rubber gloves and exercising the greatest care, I believe that I am so sensitized that it takes only a minute quantity of procain to start the trouble again."

Case 9.—Dr. F., for several years, had a dermatitis on the hands during the summer. As soon as the late fall came on, he was entirely free from the eruption, which was practically the same as others herein described; but it returned again with absolute surety in the early summer. This man had his own truck garden and was accustomed to find pleasure and recreation in taking care of it himself. He not only weeded it, but picked his own vegetables. The occurrence of this eruption during a certain season made one suspicious; so he was induced to forego the pleasure of working in his garden the entire summer, and was absolutely free from any type of irritation. Later in the fall, he pulled up the dead tomato plants, and a severe dermatitis resulted within twenty-four hours, convincing him and me that it was a case of tomato plant poisoning and not caused by the use of procain.

In a recent letter from the H. A. Metz Laboratories, they offer no explanation. They are aware of the fact that frequent cases occur, but mention also that as far as they are aware no cases have been reported among surgeons, which they attribute to the fact that the latter class of professional men wear gloves when they operate. They suggest as a remedy that all dentists who are susceptible wear gloves. In this, as in many other dermatologic conditions, it is rarely difficult to effect a cure if complete rest can be secured; but how to prevent a recurrence is the serious question. Total abstinence from the use of the drug is one way; but this is undesirable, as patients are deprived of a wonderful anesthetic and the dentist of a part of his income, for someone else can handle the drug with impunity; the use of rubber gloves is another way, but that also has its disadvantages. I have several times advised the use of the following preparation for leather workers and those in kindred trades who are subject to irritation of the hand on account of certain chemicals, and it has proved of value; and I have suggested its use to several dentists and have had a few good reports: 25 per cent. of hydrous wool fat and 75 per cent. of petrolatum are heated in a water bath; 2 per cent of phenol is added, thoroughly mixed and allowed to cool in a jar. A small quantity of this is rubbed thoroughly all over the hands before an injection is made, and the excess is wiped off The taste is not especially unpleasant to the patient, though a small quantity of ointment of rose water can replace a part of the petrolatum.

While there is no doubt that procain and the allied products can produce a dermatitis, for any known drug will do this in a susceptible person under certain circumstances, yet I am inclined to agree with Dr. Prinz that the cases are rare, occurring only in those who possess a marked idiosyncrasy, and under particularly unfavorable conditions. It is not so common as is supposed by the dentists themselves, for they catalogue every eruption they may possess as due to that cause; and they are rather difficult to convince to the contrary in spite of their desire to use the drug. I have found few men who adhere strictly to the direction for the preparation and use of the anesthetic, and it may be that these personal deviations play a more or less important rôle in the production of certain dermatoses occurring on the hands.

Spruce and Sixteenth Streets.

INTRAMUSCULAR INJECTION OF TURPENTINE IN THE TREATMENT OF DISEASES OF THE SKIN *

OSCAR L. LEVIN, M.D.

Instructor and Chief of Clinic, Department of Dermatology and Syphilology
Cornell University Medical School and Clinic; Chief Dermatologist, United Israel-Zion Hospital

AND

EMIL ROSE, M.D.

Clinical Assistant, Cornell Medical Clinic; Adjunct Dermatologist,
United Israel-Zion Hospital

NEW YORK

Subsequent to the publication of Fochier's [1] paper concerning the beneficial effect of the fixation abscess in combating septic disease, many writers, chiefly German, reported good results in a multitude of general infectious conditions. It remained for Klingmüller [2] to introduce the injection of turpentine as a therapeutic agent in the treatment of diseases of the skin. A review of the literature on the subject reveals many enthusiastic reports. We have employed turpentine in the treatment of a large variety of skin conditions during the last year in order to test its therapeutic value.

REVIEW OF THE LITERATURE

Fochier advanced the "fixation abscess" theory in 1891. He believed that virulent septic infections form no pus foci. He sought to produce an artificial abscess by injecting subcutaneously turpentine oil that would "fix," exhaust and beneficially influence the general infection. He employed the fixation abscess in septic and pyemic processes, especially in puerperal fever, with excellent effect. He also believed that the fixation abscess has a great prognostic value, as no abscesses are formed by turpentine injections in severe infections. Among other enthusiastic sponsors of the fixation abscess theory are Senn,[3] Revilliod,[4]

* From the Department of Dermatology and Syphilology, Cornell University Medical School and Clinic.

1. Fochier, A.: Therapeutique des infections pyogenes generalisées, Lyons méd. **67**:555, 1891.

2. Klingmüller: Ueber Behandlung von Entzündungen und Eiterungen durch Terpentineinspritzungen, Deutsch. med. Wchnschr. **43**:1294, 1917.

3. Senn: L'Abscess de fixation, Dissertation, Geneva, 1898.

4. Revilliod, quoted by Senn: Dissertation, Geneva, 1898.

Gauthier,[5] Colladon[6] and Lépine.[7] They employed the artificial abscess with gratifying results in pneumonia, typhus and otitis media. Pic[8] used it with success in severe forms of erysipelas and other streptococcic infections. Sahli[9] and Hodel[10] administered turpentine with good results in influenza and pneumonia.

Klingmüller[11] deserves the credit for utilizing it and attempting to explain its action in a large number of skin diseases. Plato had used trichophytin successfully in 1901 for the treatment of deep tineas. In 1918, Klingmüller sought to find a substance, not containing bacteria or protein, that had the power to produce pus locally and that might be used in deep tineas instead of vaccines. First experimenting with croton oil, 0.01 c.c. in oil solution, he found that it caused severe local reactions. He then tried 0.001 c.c. solutions and found that the deep nodules of inveterate tinea barbae disappeared in a week. There was a local tissue reaction causing the patient considerable pain and some rise in temperature but no ill effect on the kidneys. He then tried croton oil in other pyodermias, such as furunculosis, with success. Pus decreased in the first twenty-four to forty-eight hours. On account of the severe local reactions, he substituted turpentine for croton oil, and he found that purified turpentine in 0.1 c.c. solutions in oil was less irritating. Leukocytosis was noted for two days following the injection. He ultimately found a strength of 20 per cent. of turpentine best suited for his purpose and recorded success in furunculosis, tinea barbae, impetigo and impetiginous eczema; especially gratifying were the results in tinea barbae of the most recalcitrant type after a single injection. Excellent results were also noted in acne, pityriasis rosea and lichen planus. In lupus vulgaris the effects compared favorably with those following tuberculin injections.

Becher[12] made an exhaustive study of turpentine therapy and made the following classification of his findings: 1. Excellent results are obtained in buboes, poorly healing wounds following operations for bubo.

5. Gauthier: Abscess de fixation chez les syphiques indication et modes d'action, Lyons méd. **117**:1021, 1911.

6. Colladon, quoted by Senn: Dissertation, Geneva, 1898.

7. Lépine: Sur une nouvelle methode de traitment de la pneumonie en imminence de suppuration, Semaine méd. **12**:72, 1892.

8. Pic: Abscess de fixation dans l'érysipele, Lyons méd. **117**:109, 1911.

9. Sahli, H.: Ueber die Influenza, Cor.-Bl. f. schweiz. Aerzte **99**:193, 1919.

10. Hodel, H.: Zur Behandlung der Grippen-pneumonie mit Colloidmetallen und Fixationsabscess, Cor.-Bl. f. schweiz. Aerzte, 1919, p. 610.

11. Klingmüller: Ueber die Wirkung von Terpentineinspritzungen auf Eiterungen und Entzündungen, München. med. Wchnschr., 1918, No. 33.

12. Becher: Ueber Terpentinölbehandlung mit besonderer Berücksichtigung ihrer anwendung in der Dermatologie, Dermat. Wchnschr. **71**:957, 1920.

chancroids, eczema, furunculosis, sweat gland abscesses and mastitis.
2. Good results are obtained in prurigo, pruritus, pyodermias, drug eruptions, posterior gonorrheal urethritis, epididymitis and acute prostatitis.
3. Turpentine therapy is helpful when employed in conjunction with
other remedies in ulcers of the leg, tineas, especially deep and indurated
ones, and in anterior gonorrheal urethritis.   4. Turpentine has no effect
in impetigo contagiosa, pyodermias in children and chronic gonorrheal
urethritis.   In 1919, Fischl [13] reported good results in tinea barbae.
Appel [14] reported good results with small doses of turpentine and stated
that he did not believe that the muscles have to be avoided in injecting
the drug, as first advised by Kingmüller.   In his experience the pain
was negligible.   Sellei,[15] in 1918, used an emulsion of turpentine oil,
camphor, anesthesin and liquid petrolatum with gratifying results in
acute and chronic eczema, prurigo and universal pruritus.   Fever and
severe pain were disadvantages.   Holzhauser [16] recommended turpentine in tinea barbae, when used in conjunction with trichophytin, and
in impetiginous skin conditions.

Müller [17] (1918) favored turpentine in tinea barbae, kerion and
pityriasis rosea.   In the same year Gravisch endorsed its beneficial
effect in tinea barbae and in all skin lesions with inflammatory exuda-
tions, such as acute eczema, dermatitis, drug eruptions, erythema multiforme, furunculosis and pyodermia.   Other reports indicate good
results with the use of the drug in tinea barbae.   Pöhlmann [18] (1919)
achieved success in the deep type of ringworm and in sycosis vulgaris.
Löwenfeld [19] (1919) and Michael [20] (1919) also obtained similar findings in the deep type.   Schubert [21] (1919) reported cures in tinea barbae,
sycosis vulgaris, furunculosis and swellings of the legs.

13. Fischl, F.: Ueber Therapie der Trichophytie mit besonderer Berücksichtigung ihrer tiefen Formen, Wien. klin. Wchnschr. **32**:94, 1914.

14. Appel, A.: Zur Technik der Terpentinbehandlung von Hautkrankheiten,
Dermat. Wchnschr. **71**:911, 1920.

15. Sellei, I.: Terpentinölinjection bei einigen Hautkrankheiten, Deutsch.
med. Wchnschr. **44**:1828, 1918.

16. Holzhauser and Werner: Trichophyia Vakzine mit Terpentin in der
Dermatologie, Deutsch. med. Wchnschr. **44**:1253, 1918.

17. Müller, F.: Die Behandlung der Trichophytie superficialis et profunda,
München. med. Wchnschr. **65**:697, 1918.

18. Pöhlmann: Diagnose, Verbreitung und Behandlung der Bartflechte,
Med. Klin. **15**: 1919, No. 6.

19. Löwenfeld, W.: Zur Frage der specifischen und unspecifischen Therapie
der Trichophytie, Wien. klin. Wchnschr. **32**:132, 1919.

20. Michael: Die Behandlung der Bartflechte, Therap. d. Gegenw., 1919,
No. 10.

21. Schubert: Erfahrungen mit Terpentininjection bei chirurgichen
Enkrankungen, Zentralbl. f. Gynäk. **43**:468, 1919.

Wederhake [22] (1917) approved of its use for streptococcus and staphylococcus infections in surgery. Rüte [23] (1919) recommended it in staphylococci infections such as furunculosis.

Meyer [24] (1918), and Schmidt [25] (1918) reported benefit from turpentine therapy in skin infections and ulcerating chilblains.

INJECTION OF RECTIFIED TURPENTINE IN DISEASES OF THE SKIN

During the last year we have treated, in private, clinic and hospital practice, more than two hundred patients with cutaneous diseases, with turpentine oil administered by deep intramuscular injection. Although a large variety of diseases were treated, those conditions which previously had been reported as benefited by this form of therapy constituted the great majority in our series. The diseases treated were mainly those in which an infectious agent is known to be the cause or in which, as in pityriasis rosea and pemphigus, some form of micro-organism may be the causative factor.

At first a 20 per cent. solution of turpentine in sterile olive oil was employed, but this produced too much pain. A 20 per cent. solution of rectified turpentine was then tried and found to give practically no pain. This also was given up for a solution of 15 per cent. rectified turpentine and 0.5 per cent. each of anesthesin and quinin hydrochlorid in olive oil, which solution corresponds to the proprietary preparation "terpichin." The technic employed for the injection was in all details similar to that followed for the intragluteal injection of insoluble mercury. The dose administered was 0.5 to 1 c.c. every four to seven days for adults, 1 to 2 minims (0.06 to 0.12 c.c.) once weekly for infants and children up to the age of 5, and 4 minims (0.24 c.c.) every four to seven days for older children.

Subsequent to the injection of the terpichin preparation no subjective complaints were reported except for the rare occurrence of pain in the kidney region. At times a trace of albumin was found in the urine. Injections were immediately discontinued when lumbar pain or albuminuria appeared. Following the injection of ordinary turpentine most of our patients complained of excruciating pain and infiltrations at the site of injection and fever. Some were so sick that they were compelled to remain in bed for several days. However, there were

22. Wederhake: Zur Behandlung des Puetpurfiebers mit Terpentin. Zentral'. f. Gynäk. **41**:843, 1917.

23. Rüte: Zur Frage der Terpentinbehandlung. Dermat. Ztschr. **28**:28. 1919.

24. Meyer, F. M.: Behandlung der Hautkrankheiten mit Terpentinöl. Berl. klin. Wchnschr. **55**:880, 1918.

25. Schmidt. E.: Ueber neuere Behandlungmethoden der Bartflechte. Berl. klin. Wchnschr. **58**:59, 1919.

several patients with severe furuncular and obstinate suppurative follicular lesions, who insisted on continuing treatment because of the almost immediate improvement in their skin condition.

No beneficial effect was observed in exudative nonvesicular dermatoseslike erythema, urticaria or purpura. In one case of severe bullous erythema multiforme, however, which had resisted all recognized methods of treatment, the injection of turpentine was followed by general improvement and the disappearance of the lesions.

Among the vesicular dermatoses no constant good results occurred except partial improvement, as manifested by a disappearance of the pustules in infected eczematoid conditions like eczematoid ringworm, infectious eczematoid dermatitis, impetiginous eczema and varicose eczema. In several varicose ulcers turpentine therapy produced cleaner lesions with a serous discharge and rapid formation of granulation and epidermal tissue. None of the patients with exanthems were treated for fear of causing renal complications. The lesions in three patients with pemphigus were not affected. In one of these the injections were administered in doses of 8 minims (0.5 c.c.) every four days for a period of three months, without effect.

The parakeratotic conditions treated were seborrheic eczema, psoriasis and pityriasis rosea. In the first two no change was noticed. Two cases of pityriasis rosea seem to have been aborted, new lesions did not develop and the old ones faded within ten days after the first injection. This deserves further observation.

No good results were obtained in the hyperkeratoses or in the erythrodermas with scaling. Acne simplex did not yield to turpentine therapy but in acne pustulosa and acne indurata the pustules and deep masses became less marked. It seemed that the turpentine produced improved cell metabolism with absorption of the pus and infiltration.

Although the attempt was made to test turpentine therapy in all dermatologic conditions, we felt that the main indication for its employment was in pyogenic infections of the skin, especially when associated with poor general tone. For this reason most of our cases belong in this group. In impetigo simplex, impetigo contagiosa and perléche the lesions did not disappear as quickly as when treated by local antisepsis. Improvement was the rule in impetigo of Bockhart. Excellent results were obtained in the deeper pyogenic infections accompanied by metabolic disorders and poor resistance. Ecthyma, furunculosis, sycosis vulgaris, lupoid sycosis, abscesses and erysipelas present a group of diseases in which turpentine should be employed as a valuable therapeutic adjunct.

Noteworthy among the cases of sycosis vulgaris were three which had previously resisted all methods of treatment, including roentgen therapy and vaccines, but which responded to turpentine injections as manifested by a disappearance of the follicular papules and pustules. It is suggested that these injections be employed in conjunction with roentgen therapy in conditions such as follicular infections, when antiseptic or irritating applications are contraindicated. The ravages of lupoid sycosis were stopped in two instances. In recurrent furunculosis cures were obtained by local cleanliness, applications of cool saline dressings, roentgen therapy, a diet low in carbohydrates and turpentine injections. In erysipelas the injection of turpentine was followed by a drop in temperature and local relief.

Lesions of the skin produced by the various fungi responded indifferently. Favus was not affected; tinea capitis of the superficial type did not react; kerion was only slightly affected; but in deep ringworm of the beard some good results were attained.

COMMENT AND DISCUSSION

No positive evidence exists to explain the mode of action of turpentine on the tissues of the body when administered by injection.

Klingmüller advanced the following theories: 1. Turpentine or its oxidation products circulating in the blood and lymph have a purely chemical action rendering the toxins inactive. 2. Turpentine or its oxidation products dispel from the lesion substances which attract the pathogenic fungi. The stronger power of the turpentine then renders the fungi inactive and enables the body to remove them. 3. The similarity between the action of turpentine and specific vaccines can be shown. The organism is stimulated to form substances which are toxic to pathogenic bacteria or have some sort of opsonic action. 4. Turpentine has a marked inflammatory action. If introduced into the circulation, the organism responds with the formation of antibodies and anti-inflammatory bodies. These may combat inflammation and pus formation and weaken or even destroy pathogenic bacteria. If these theories are true, a polyvalent antibody can be produced.

Becher concluded in his review on the opinions of investigators who studied the action of turpentine that there exists a wide difference in opinion. He believed that it is possible to influence favorably specific diseases with nonspecific vaccines and chemicals such as turpentine. He theorized that there may be an activation of the protoplasm or perhaps a group of actions: (1) leukocytosis; (2) irritation to formation of granulation, and (3) antitoxic action.

Rectified turpentine oil, which we employed in more than 90 per cent. of our cases, is formed from ordinary oil of turpentine by redistillation with lime water, in order to remove any acids and resin which may be contained in it. It is a volatile oil containing a large proportion of terpene, with comparatively little oxygen, and possesses a penetrating action. It has been shown that terpenes ($C_{10}H_{16}$) undergo a partial oxidation in the body and become terpenols $(C_{10}H_{15}OH)$. The odor of the original oil or of these derivatives may often be detected in the breath, showing that a small part is excreted by the lungs, and possibly traces may be eliminated by the skin. Some escapes by the kidneys.

It is our belief that just as the elimination of the terpenols or terpenes by way of the lungs and kidneys produces increased bronchial secretions and urinary output, excretion by the skin results in enhanced local cell metabolism. The effect is mainly that of irritation. The blood vessels dilate, a serous exudation with diapedesis of the erythrocytes and migration of the leukocytes follows, and the tissues of the skin are stimulated to new growth. This results in improved nutrition, improved absorption of waste products and tissue repair. The terpene products because of their chemotactic property also aid in phagocytic action against bacteria. It is also known that the terpenes in the body are slightly disinfectant.

The general effects produced by injections of turpentine may be similar to those of counterirritation. The local irritation causes reflex stimulation of the various centers in the medulla oblongata. The vasomotor change leads to an increase in blood supply with consequent leukocytosis, improved absorption and increased removal of toxins. The temperature is lowered. In a case of erysipelas the temperature which had been 106 F. for a week dropped to 102.4 two hours after the first injection of turpentine; four days later the temperature hovering around 102 F. fell to normal after a second injection, and five days later when it was again 102 F. a third injection caused a return to normal, which persisted.

SUMMARY AND CONCLUSIONS

As a result of our experience with injections of turpentine in the treatment of a large number of skin diseases, we recommend its employment in certain conditions. It may be of real value in the pyogenic infections, especially when there is follicular involvement. In such instances the injections may be given in conjunction with the local application of the roentgen rays. Good results were observed in tinea barbae. Further observations should be made for the abortion of pityriasis rosea. In old ulcers the administration of turpentine was followed by evidence of stimulation and a tendency to healing. Fair results were attained in acne indurata. A dose of from 0.5 to 1 c.c. of a 15 per cent. solution of rectified turpentine in sterile olive oil injected intramuscularly causes no pain and gives the best result. The effect is both local and general. Locally there is apparently cell irritation, while the vital centers in the medulla oblongata are reflexly stimulated.

63 West Seventy-Third Street.

A LICHEN PLANUS ERUPTION AFTER ARSPHENAMIN *

LAWRENCE K. McCAFFERTY, M.D.

NEW YORK

It is a well recognized fact that the administration of arsphenamin may produce definite dermatoses of which the most familiar type is the erythematous eruption, which in some instances develops into an exfoliative dermatitis.

Recently Queyrat, Louis, and Rabut,[1] Kleeberg,[2] Buschke and Freymann,[3] and Keller,[4] have reported cases of arsphenamin dermatitis with lichenoid lesions. The following case is reported because, following treatment by arsphenamin, the patient developed a condition which in its clinical appearance, in the histology of the lesions, and in the course of the disease was indistinguishable from true lichen planus. While the possibility that this was a mere coincidence cannot be excluded, the evidence to be presented favors the assumption that the eruption was caused by arsphenamin.

REPORT OF CASE

History.—A mulatto woman, aged 40, married, was admitted to the outpatient department of the Presbyterian Hospital, June 1, 1921, complaining of a skin eruption on the right forearm. The history was irrelevant except that her present husband had been under treatment for syphilis. The patient gave no history of primary or secondary syphilitic manifestations. She had suffered for six years from the lesion which was present on admission.

Physical examination revealed a gauntlet shaped eruption confined to the right forearm and hand. It extended from the finger tips to the middle of the forearm, on the extensor and flexor surfaces. The eruption was brownish-red and did not disappear on pressure. The veins shone through. It was slightly scaly except on the palm, which showed a marked hyperkeratosis. The upper limit was serpiginous and extended completely around the forearm. The cervical nodes were palpable, the knee and ankle reflexes were hyperactive. The Wassermann test was four plus. The urine was negative.

* From the department of medicine of Columbia University College of Physicians and Surgeons, and the Presbyterian Hospital.

1. Queyrat, Louis, and Rabut: Bull. Soc. franç. de dermat. et syph., 1921. No. 2.

2. Kleeberg, L.: Beitrag zur Klinik der Salvarsan Exanthema. Therap. Halbmonatsh. **35**:370, 1921.

3. Buschke, A., and Freymann, W.: Lichen-ruber-ahnliche Salvarsan Exanthema, Med. Klin. **30**:909, 1921.

4. Keller, Philipp: Lichen planus und lichenoide arsendermatitis. Dermat. Wchnschr. **74**:9 (Jan. 7) 1922.

Histology.—A biopsy from the affected area on the right arm revealed slight hyperkeratosis, and atrophy of the rete with a slight prolongation of the rete pegs. There was a slight cellular infiltration into the epidermis. The papillae and upper cutis were infiltrated with mononuclears, plasma and epithelioid cells. The infiltration was rather sharply demarcated in the upper cutis. The connective tissue of the papillae and upper cutis showed an interstitial and parenchymatous edema. The blood and lymph vessels were moderately dilated and surrounded by a sleevelike infiltration of plasma cells. The diagnosis was tertiary syphilid of the right hand and forearm.

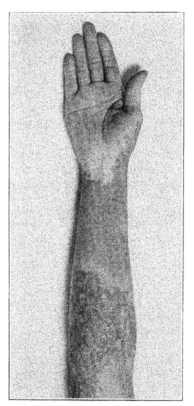

Fig. 1.—Leukoderma of right palm: The skin is normal from middle of forearm to palm. This was the only part of the body unaffected by the lichenoid eruption. It was the former site of the tertiary syphilid.

Treatment and Results.—The patient was given arsphenamin and mercuric salicylate at weekly intervals. She received nine intravenous injections of arsphenamin averaging 0.3 gm. each, and six 1 grain injections of mecuric salicylate intramuscularly. During the antisyphilitic treatment the tertiary syphilid cleared up. The skin of the forearm resumed a normal appearance, but the fingers became leukodermic in places. Within three or four hours after the third and each succeeding arsphenamin injection, the patient complained of a burning sensation in the stomach, and of belching of gas. This indicated arsphenamin intoxication. After the seventh arsphenamin injection, stomatitis, herpes of the lips and vaginitis developed. The mercurial injections were stopped. The ninth and last arsphenamin injection was given, September 1. At this time there were well defined, slightly raised, purplish-red plaques about 1 cm. in diameter, on the left palm and sole. There were a few scattered, lentil-sized, violaceous, ill defined papules on the mesial surfaces of the arms and left axilla.

Second Admission.—As the eruption continued to develop and the patient complained of weakness and malaise, as well as the intense itching, she was admitted to the Presbyterian Hospital, September 8.

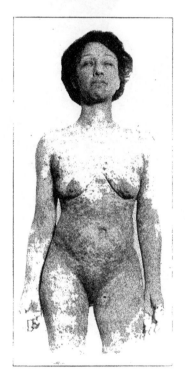

Fig. 2.—Lichenoid eruption: The face. neck and chest are practically clear, although a few lesions appear on the face. The right forearm shows the former site of the tertiary syphilid.

Physical examination disclosed slight lacrimation, inflamed nasal mucosa. and exfoliation of the lips. The tongue and buccal mucosa presented irregular raised grayish areas the size of a pea. The heart and lungs showed no evidence of disease; the liver edge was palpable, but in other respects the abdomen was negative. The systolic blood pressure was 120 mm., the diastolic 70. Blood urea, uric acid, and sugar were within normal limits. The blood count was as follows: erythrocytes, 5,100,000; leukocytes, 8,900; polymorphonuclears, 70 per cent.; small mononuclears, 6 per cent.; large mononuclears, 4 per cent.; eosinophils, 11 per cent. The hemoglobin was 80 per cent. The blood platelets were normal. The urine showed no albumin, no pus, and no casts. Phenolsulphonephthalein excretion was 40 per cent. in two hours and fifteen minutes.

Two days later the eruption faded, but on September 17 it became more severe. The patient then began to improve rapidly, and was discharged, October 8, with a diagnosis of syphilis and lichen planus.

Third Admission.—She was readmitted to the outpatient service, Nov. 7, 1921, complaining of a generalized eruption consisting of shiny, angular papules

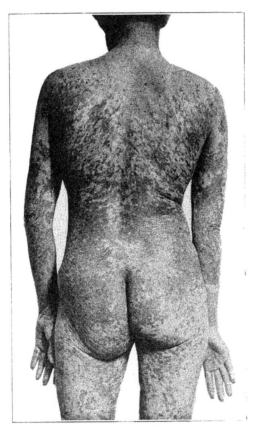

Fig. 3.—Lichenoid eruption. The papules have coalesced in many places, the coffee colored pigmentation is interspersed between many of the papules. The upper back and neck are reasonably clear.

from 3 to 5 mm. in diameter, and from violaceous to deep purple. A few were distinctly umbilicated. These papules were diffusely scattered over the face and neck, the upper portion of the trunk, and the extensor surfaces of the arms. In other areas they became confluent, in some instances forming rings with yellowish-brown centers. Surrounding such patches were areas of yellowish-brown or slate colored pigmentation. The lesions were so numerous on the flexor surfaces of the arms, the axillae, abdomen, lower back, hips and inner surfaces of the thigh that little normal skin remained. On the extensor surfaces of the upper arms and lower legs there was slight follicular keratosis with pigmentation. The areolae of the nipples were deeply pigmented. The palms and soles showed hyperkeratosis. The nails were thickened and had pigmented longitudinal ridges along their entire length. The lower half of the right hand and arm, which was the site of the former syphilitic lesion, was free from lesions. The eyes lacrimated profusely. The entire mucous membrane of the mouth showed scattered minute grayish-white papules. Similar lesions were found in the vagina. The pruritus, which had been a marked symptom in the hospital, had subsided.

Biopsy.—Section of a lichenoid lesion removed while in the hospital revealed a marked hyperkeratosis with a dipping down of the horny layer into the epidermis, forming dells. There was a marked acanthosis with increased granu-

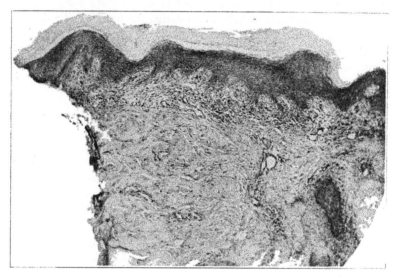

Fig. 4.—Section taken from a papule on the left forearm. Reduced from a photomicrograph × 118.

lar layer, edema, and colloid degeneration of the rete cells. The papillae were widened and edematous. The upper cutis also showed edema, the blood and lymphatic vessels were dilated, and there was a marked cellular infiltration, sharply demarcated from the lower layers.

Under high power the infiltration of the upper cutis and papillae was seen to consist of small mononuclears, larger cells probably of connective tissue origin and melanoblasts, which alone contained pigment granules. The blood and lymphatic vessels of the lower cutis were surrounded by cellular exudate consisting chiefly of mononuclears (Fig. 4).

There was a gradual improvement in her condition, but when last seen, seven months after the first appearance of the lichen planus eruption, she still had a few papules.

There seems little doubt that, had this patient presented the condition just described and given no history of arsphenamin treatment, she would have been regarded as having lichen planus. In view of the fact that the eruption followed treatment, there are three possible interpretations: (1) That it was a mere coincidence. (2) That it was a dermatitis medicamentosa due to arsphenamin. (3) That it was a true lichen planus, in this instance caused by arsphenamin.

Lichen planus, clinically and histologically, is fairly well defined. We have no knowledge of the exact cause, but two hypotheses have been advanced: Pollitzer,[5] Lieberthal,[6] and Hazen[7] believe it is a microbic infection. White,[8] believes that the disease has a neurotic basis. He states that "lichen planus occurs more frequently in educated men and women whose lot in life has been hard." Little,[9] comparing the incidence of lichen planus before and during the war, found a decrease in the latter period, a fact which seems to argue against a neurotic basis. Neither of these hypotheses has any definite proof. Considering the want of knowledge of the cause of lichen planus, this case in which the same syndrome followed arsphenamin intoxication is not without interest.

Previously Reported Cases.—In considering the possibility of arsphenamin causing this eruption, it should be recalled that lichenoid lesions due to arsenicals have been described previously. As far back as 1902, Brooke and Roberts,[10] as well as Barendt,[11] described such lesions occurring in an epidemic of arsenical poisoning from beer. Gans,[12] describing the histology of arsenic melanosis, writes of a case in which the histologic picture was characteristic of lichen planus. This case showed hyperkeratosis, edema of the papillary bodies and a sharply demarcated infiltration of the upper cutis with mononuclears and mast cells. Pigment was scattered through the epidermis, papillae, and upper cutis.

5. Pollitzer, S.: J. Cutan. Dis. **37**:682 (Oct.) 1919.

6. Lieberthal, D.: J. Cutan. Dis. **37**:682 (Oct.) 1919.

7. Hazen, H. H.: Diseases of Skin, St. Louis, The C. V. Mosby Co., 1915, p. 394.

8. White, C. J.: Lichen Planus, J. Cutan. Dis. **37**:671 (Oct.) 1919.

9. Little, E. G.: Lichen Planus, J. Cutan. Dis. **37**:639 (Oct.) 1919.

10. Brooke, H. G., and Roberts, L.: The Action of Arsenic on the Skin as Observed in the Recent Epidemic of Arsenical Beer Poisoning, Brit. J. Dermat. **13**:120 (April) 1901.

11. Barendt, F.: The Skin Lesions Due to the Presence of Arsenic in Beer. Brit. J. Dermat. **13**:148 (April) 1901.

12. Gans, Oscar: Zur Histologie der Arsenmelanose, Beitr. z. path. Anat. u. z. allg. Path. **60**:22, 1914-1915

Since the widespread use of arsphenamin more typical cases have been reported. Queyrat, Louis and Rabut described an eruption on the tongue resembling lichen planus, clinically and histologically, which occurred after the administration of galyl, a drug similar to arsphenamin. The patient also developed an erythema and pigmentation of the body with intense itching.

Kleeberg also reported a case with an eruption on the dorsum of the hands, and lesions of the buccal mucosa resembling lichen planus following a third course of arsphenamin therapy. Buschke and Freymann reported two cases of acute generalized lichenoid eruption occurring during arsphenamin treatment. Their first case had papules on the chest and flexor surfaces of the extremities resembling lichen planus. The entire skin had a silvery, shiny appearance, felt like a nutmeg grater, and resembled lichen planus verrucosus. Histologically the epithelium was slightly changed. The corium was infiltrated with mononuclears and polymorphonuclears, principally in the perivascular spaces. In the second case, the trunk, flexor and extensor surfaces of the extremities were involved, and the face, neck and chest were free. There was a diffuse grayish-brown to coffee colored pigmentation with a varying degree of intensity. The legs presented follicular keratosis with atrophic centers. The histologic picture revealed normal epithelium, a mononuclear infiltration sharply limited to the upper cutis and brownish-black pigment in the papillae. According to the authors, their first case showed a nonspecific inflammation, while their second case resembled lichen planus histologically, but not clinically. At a little later date Buschke and Freymann,[13] reported a third case which resembled lichen planus somewhat. The eruption was not preceded by a dermatitis but by a slight icterus. Shiny red papules were grouped in rings on the sides of the extremities. Some of these papules occurred along linear scratch marks. There were also macules, follicular papules, and pustules. Biopsy revealed only a slight polymorphonuclear infiltration in the cutis under a somewhat acanthotic epidermis. Hoffman[14] described, as a case of lichen planus, an eruption on the body and buccal mucosa, which appeared after the cessation of antisyphilitic treatment. The patient was given arsphenamin again and the lichen planus eruption became more severe. Sections of a typical papule were characteristic of lichen planus. Keller reported a case which, he said, was lichen planus clinically and histologically. His patient had an eruption confined to the face, body and extremities. There was a diffuse

13. Buschke, A., and Freymann, W.: Weiterer Beitrag zu den Lichenruber-ähnlichen Exanthemen nach Salvarsan, Dermat. Wchnschr. **73**:945 (Sept. 10) 1921.

14. Hoffman, E.: Arsenkeratose nach hochgradigen universellen Exanthem durch Sulosozylat, Tr. Bonn. Niederrh. Gesellsch., May 9, 1921.

brownish-red pigmentation with a network of split pea sized reddish-brown shiny papules, and there were characteristic lesions of lichen planus on the buccal mucosa opposite the last molar.   Smith [15] presented a case before the American Dermatological Association in which an exfoliative dermatitis developed following two courses of arsphenamin. In the discussion of this case it was brought out that some lesions strongly resembled lichen planus.   One case of exfoliative arsenical dermatosis with hyperkeratosis reported by Schäfer [16] also presented lesions on the tongue and buccal mucosa which were somewhat like lichen planus.   The chief involvement in this case was on the covered parts of the body, which showed a diffuse pigmentation, but in the pigmented areas lichen like papules were also found.   Similar cases of arsenical melanosis were studied by Gans and by Habermann.[17]

In all of the cases cited, arsenic was considered undoubtedly the cause of the eruption.   In no case was the clinical appearance as close to that of an ordinary lichen planus as in the case reported here. Altogether they form strong evidence for believing that arsenic may produce an eruption simulating this disease.   That the eruption described was caused by arsenic was indicated by slight symptoms of arsenic poisoning during a course of treatment, and also by symptoms which are common in arsenic poisoning and are not associated with ordinary lichen planus: conjunctivitis, stomatitis,[18] and palmar keratosis.   The pigmentation which was pronounced in this case occurs both in true lichen planus and in frank arsenical dermatitis.   In acute generalized lichen planus the papules coalesce and on involuting leave a dark pigmentation which may be confluent.   In the case described, however, there was some pigmentation preceding the appearance of papules. This sequence of events has been observed by Jadassohn [19] in true lichen planus.

SUMMARY

1. This case presented the clinical and histologic picture of lichen planus.

2. The eruption followed shortly after the administration of arsphenamin.

3. Cases of arsenical dermatitis closely simulating lichen planus have previously been described.

4. In the case reported, symptoms and lesions of arsenical poisoning support the belief that arsphenamin caused this eruption.

---

15. Smith, Morton: Arch. Dermat. & Syph. **4**:554 (June) 1921.

16. Schäfer: Einen Fall von exfoliativer Arsendermatitis und Hyperkera-tose, Dermat. Zentralbl. **2**:426, 1921.

17. Habermann, R.: Dermat. Ztschr. **30**:63, 1920.

18. Laurentier, C.: Bull. Soc. franç. de dermat. et syph. **6**:276, 1921.

19. Jadassohn. quoted by Habermann (Footnote 17).

MULTIPLE BENIGN TUMOR-LIKE GROWTHS OF SCHWENINGER AND BUZZI *

S. E. SWEITZER, M.D.

MINNEAPOLIS

Schweninger and Buzzi,[1] in 1891, under the title "Multiple Benign Tumor-Like Growths" described a unique anomaly of the skin.

Crocker [2] gave a very good description of this condition, which we cannot improve on. He wrote: "Clinically, the lesions are soft, round or oval projections, from a lentil to a bean in size, more or less white, with a slight blush or slate color in some of them. Most of them are bladder-like, and can be pressed into the skin by the finger, projecting immediately again like a hernia. The larger ones are flattened and slightly puckered, and harder than the smaller, from which they develop. They undergo spontaneous resolution, and leave only flaccid, loose, foveated scars. They appear very gradually and without sensory symptoms on the trunk, shoulders and thighs and ultimately become numerous, as none disappear entirely, and others keep forming."

Further on, Crocker says: "I have seen very similar lesions associated with fibromata of the ordinary form, when some of them have been absorbed. It is probable that they are the last phase of more than one pathological process."

T. Colcott Fox [3] reported a similar case seen by him, and refers in his article to a case seen by Malcolm Morris and one seen by Van Hoorn. Morris saw the original case of Schweninger and Buzzi and claimed that these three cases were of a similar nature, although no biopsies were made.

Stelwagon,[4] in his book, reported one case which, from his description, seems to belong in this category.

Pusey,[5] in 1917, read a paper on this condition and made a complete report of a case, with microscopic findings. He found a diminution in the elastic fibers.

---

* Read at the Forty-Fifth Annual Meeting of the American Dermatological Association, Washington, D. C., May 2-4, 1922.

1. Schweninger and Buzzi: International Atlas of Rare Skin Diseases, 1891. Part 5, Plate 15.

2. Crocker: Diseases of the Skin, Ed. 3, Philadelphia. P. Blakiston's Son & Co., 1903, p. 702.

3. T. Colcott Fox: Multiple Benign Tumor-Like New Growths of the Skin. Brit. J. Dermat. 4:117-119, 1892.

4. Stelwagon: Diseases of the Skin, Ed. 8, Philadelphia. W. B. Saunders Company, 1916, p. 696.

5. Pusey, W. A.: J. Cutan. Dis. 35:582 (Sept.) 1917.

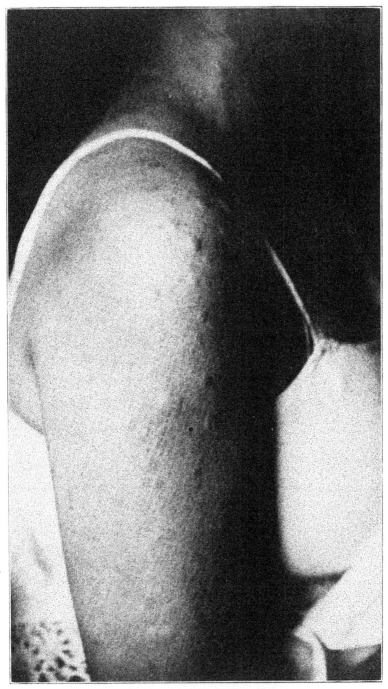

Fig. 1.—Lesions on the right shoulder and arm.

Pringle [6] reported a similar case occurring in a man of 21, showing hard papules, bladder-like tumors and pitted scarring. Pringle maintained that the condition is not a "substansive" disease. A biopsy was not made. Galloway, in discussing Pringle's case, said: "There is no doubt atrophy of the skin, which can be called macular atrophy, but the question is whether this preceding tumor-like appearance of the skin is of the nature of a fibroma, or whether it is some form of degeneration of the white connective tissues, associated with actual atrophy of the elastic tissue, allowing this hernial protrusion, including that of the corium and, to some extent, that of the subcutaneous tissue.

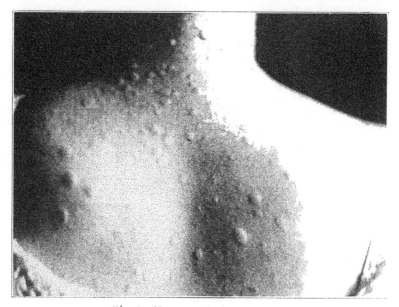

Fig. 2.—Numerous lesions on back.

That it leads on to a condition of atrophy seems perfectly clear, but we agree we have never seen a case of what we call macular atrophy with this excessive amount of tissue, with increase in bulk, so far as the surface is concerned."

Quinn [7] recently presented a somewhat similar case before a meeting of the Chicago Dermatological Society. The discussion brought out the opinion that the lesions were not new growths but a macular atrophy.

Of the nine cases previously reported, all are probably examples of the same condition, except the one mentioned by Crocker, which

6. Pringle: Proc. Roy. Soc. Med. **12**:21, 1919.

7. Quinn: Arch. Dermat. & Syph. **5**:149 (Jan.) 1922.

probably belonged to the fibroma group. Only the original case and the one reported by Pusey have been fully reported.

I am able to report a similar case through the courtesy of Dr. H. E. Michelson. The patient was exhibited before the Minnesota Dermatological Society and was shown to Dr. Ormsby when he visited Minneapolis. The consensus of opinion then was that the case resembled very closely the condition described by Schweninger and Buzzi.

REPORT OF CASE

History.—Mrs. O. C. S., aged 28, a widow, whose family and past history reveal no facts which seem to have any bearing on the dermatologic condition, was a well-nourished and well-developed woman. Her apparent age was no older than her actual age.

The condition present had developed ten years previously, beginning with a single small elevation in the right deltoid region. This elevation was of pea size, hard and bluish-white. It caused her no annoyance, but gradually enlarged to the circumference of a 10-cent piece, and then remained stationary. Insidiously, other similar lesions appeared over the outer surface of the upper arm, the scapular, suprasternal and frontal regions. The patient noticed that the lesions, after being present for some months, retrogressed and became depressed, leaving a wrinkled looking scar.

Examination.—There were numerous small tumor-like projections scattered over the upper anterior and posterior thorax and the arms, and a few on the face and forehead. The lesions varied in size from that of a pea to that of a small cherry. Some were whiter than the normal skin, while others showed a bluish tint, and a few of the lesions had telangiectases over their surfaces. The lesions had the consistency of putty, but there was considerable variation. Some of them were quite soft. The patient stated that the newer lesions were firmer than the older ones. On palpation, many of the lesions could be pushed through a slit-like aperture which admitted the end of the little finger, conveying the impression that the supporting framework had disappeared. The edges of the aperture were smooth and sharply defined. In some locations, the hernia-like lesions had disappeared, leaving the skin over the area thinned and wrinkled in appearance. This scar-like skin was elastic, and when pinched up, seemed to be loosely attached to the underlying tissues. This was evidently the final stage of the disease.

None of the lesions were pedunculated, nor were there any areas of pigmentation or highly pigmented lesions. The surface of all the lesions was smooth, except the wrinkled stage of the older lesions. Sensation was normal, and the location of the lesions seemed in no way to be related to the distribution of the cutaneous nerves. The Wassermann reaction was negative.

Histologic Report.—Three tumors were excised. Two were soft, compressible, old atrophic lesions, while one was an early, firm fibroma-like lesion. The small pieces of tissue excised were hardened in formaldehyd and alcohol in the usual manner, embedded in paraffin and sectioned serially. Hematoxylin-eosin and Weigert's resorcin fuchsin stains were used.

Under hematoxylin-eosin, the epithelium showed marked thinning and complete absence of the rete pegs. There was no hyperkeratosis or parakeratosis;

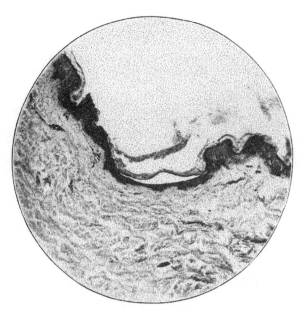

Fig. 3.—Some atrophy of the epidermis and absence of infiltrate in the corium, with hematoxylin-eosin. (Low power.)

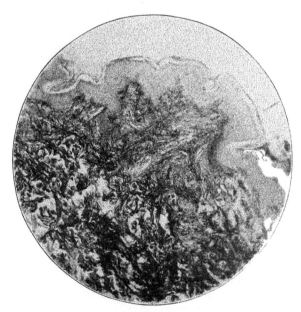

Fig. 4.—New lesion: Elastic fibers present at the periphery of lesion, with Weigert's stain. (Intermediate power.)

nor was there any microscopic evidence of any degenerative processes taking place in the epithelium. There was no infiltration or abscess formation noted in the epithelium.

Examination of the corium revealed: The papillary body projections were lacking. There was no edema, nor destruction of the collagen bundles. Here and there, a few clumps of leukocytes, all of the mononuclear type, were noted. An occasional fibroblast was also seen. There was complete absence of marked infiltration. The sections stained by Weigert's method showed a diminution and atrophy, and in some places complete loss of the elastic fibers, most marked in the upper portion of the center of a clinical lesion. At the periphery of the lesion, the fibers appeared heavier and more numerous.

There were no evidences of new growths. The most marked changes noted were an atrophy of the epidermis and a loss of elastic fibers in the central portion of a clinical lesion.

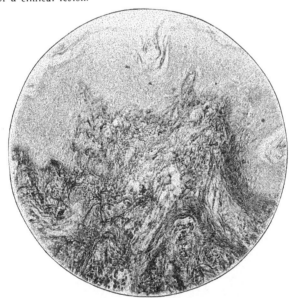

Fig. 5.—Absence of elastic fibers in upper portion of center of lesion, with Weigert's stain. (Low power.)

These findings correspond to those which have been described as occurring in the tumor-like growths of Schweninger and Buzzi, a condition which this case simulated clinically. This case also corresponded closely to a case reported by Pusey.

In endeavoring to classify the case, one must consider two conditions: (1) fibroma molluscum and (2) macular atrophy. Fibroma molluscum may be looked on as a congenital defect or a nevus syndrome which includes pigmented areas, pedunculated tumors, bone changes, with sometimes kyphosis, and, at times, low mentality. These various conditions are not always present, but typical cases often will show them.

Complete absence of pedunculation, pigmented lesions or pigmented areas is strong evidence against fibroma molluscum in this case. Furthermore, sections from a recent lesion did not show the typical structures of fibroma.

Macular atrophy is considered to be due to a loss of elastic tissue. Bag-like pouching is not usually seen in macular atrophy, but has been noted when some concurrent edematous process caused pressure in the surrounding tissues. From Pusey's studies and from a study of our sections, we are convinced that there is an actual atrophy of the elastic fibers, with a subsequent increase of the fibers about the lesions, forming a perceptible slit-like hernial opening through which the tumor-like lesions protrude. Schweninger and Buzzi did not believe that the lesions were new growths, but remarked that the tumor-like lesions were composed of normal elements.

From a survey of the literature and a study of our case, we are convinced that the so-called tumor-like growths of Schweninger and Buzzi should be grouped with the macular atrophies.

CONCLUSIONS

1. This condition should not be regarded as an entity because histologic study reveals that it is a peculiar type of atrophy and not a new growth.

2. We do not believe that this condition is related to fibroma molluscum.

DISCUSSION

Dr. Jay Frank Schamberg, Philadelphia: This paper has cleared up in my mind the diagnosis in a case of my own presented by one of my associates before the Philadelphia Dermatological Association with a condition unlike any I had seen. We were all very much puzzled as to the diagnosis. The patient, a middle-aged woman, had half a dozen or more lesions on the leg that presented a remarkable aspect. At first sight, one would call them large blebs, and only after we had punctured these very distended baggy prominences did we find that they contained no fluid. A small venule ran through soft, wrinkled overlying skin. On pressing this soft growth, the finger went through a small button-hole like opening, through which you could press down the baggy surface. There were other lesions, which had more or less flattened down, presenting a scarred cigaret paper like wrinkling of the skin, but also with this opening at the base. On account of the resemblance to pemphigus, I suggested that we call it atrophoderma pemphigoides.

I never knew the nature of the disease until Dr. Sweitzer read his paper; but now I am sure from the slit-like opening to which he refers, and the very pronounced atrophy of the skin, that it belongs to this group of cases.

Dr. Walter J. Highman, New York: I was particularly interested in Dr. Sweitzer's presentation because I recall seeing the case Dr. Pusey described at the Cincinnati meeting, and, although I had never heard of the condition before, it struck me that the conclusions of Dr. Sweitzer would be tenable. The condition has all of the attributes of atrophies in general, whether primary or secondary. Whether we are dealing with scleroderma or the macular atrophies, or with the cicatricial atrophy or pseudopelade, histologically the same elements are present in the skin, in the disturbance of the elastic tissue. Sometimes, there is a complete disappearance of the collagen, and the crumpling back of the elastic tissue in the vicinity of the lesion; and I feel that this button-hole like sensation imparted to the palpating finger must be really due to the retraction of the elastic tissue. There is a certain vagueness of the tissue when the elastica no longer exists. I think it is only a subvariety of the idiopathic atrophies.

Dr. CHARLES J. WHITE, Boston: We had at the Massachusetts General Hospital a most remarkable case of acrodermatitis atrophicans in which, preceding the atrophy, were the kind of tumors Dr. Sweitzer has described, giving the same baggy sensation. That was as severe a case as I have ever seen, and with this peculiar, progressive symptom which I have seen in but this one instance.

Dr. FRANCIS E. SENEAR, Chicago: I had the opportunity of studying Dr. Pusey's case with him. The peculiar feature in our case was the fact that all of the tumors were present on the lower half of the face and neck. On the body, we found many of the slit-like lesions that Dr. Sweitzer has described. The patient, who was unusually intelligent, had never noticed any of the baggy lesions preceding the macular slit-like lesions, although we felt that they perhaps developed from the baggy tumor. In the light of Dr. Sweitzer's observations, I think perhaps the patient's observation was faulty and that they were the end-result rather than the preliminary lesions.

Dr. SAMUEL E. SWEITZER, Minneapolis (closing): This condition struck us as being a peculiar form of atrophy. In regard to acrodermatitis atrophicans, we frequently find a hard nodule in that disease, but this did not resemble that. There are only the small, tumor-like lesions, and the rest of the skin is normal. The patient presented a few lesions on the face, but they were old lesions and had flattened down and did not photograph well.

The condition apparently began with a small nodule, and we purposely cut out a new nodule as well as an old one to see if we could find any evidence of a tumor growth; but we found only a beginning atrophy in that as well as in the older lesion, so, as nearly as we could find out, the condition began with the small tumors, and eventually the atrophy became sufficiently advanced to make some of the tumors flatten out when the patient was lying down, and on standing, they would puff out.

625 Syndicate Building.

THE PRESENT STATUS OF LEPROSY IN THE HAWAIIAN ISLANDS *

WILLIAM THOMAS CORLETT, M.D., L.R.C.P. (Lond.)

Senior Professor of Dermatology and Syphilology,
Western Reserve University

CLEVELAND

By some, leprosy is supposed to have been introduced into the Hawaiian Islands by the Chinese, many of whom settled there about the middle of the nineteenth century. The reason for this belief rests on the fact that the first name by which the disease as a distinct entity was known in the Islands was *mai pake,* meaning Chinese disease.

Wayson [1] and other leprologists who have lived long on the Islands, as well as others who have recorded earlier observations, do not share this view, but believe that the disease has existed from a more remote period and was probably introduced by sailors or the roving inhabitants of the islands of the South Seas, where from the earliest times it has been endemic. The missionaries who came here in 1820 reported that some of the natives were afflicted with what they called scrofula, "which was not only frequently met with but extremely malignant." [2]

LEPER HOSPITAL AND SETTLEMENT

Soon after the middle of the last century, however, leprosy had made such headway among the native population that in 1865 King Kalakaua called a council to consider means of checking its spread. Segregation of those afflicted and treatment with chaulmoogra oil seemed to offer the most promising means of relief. Accordingly, a hospital for the examination and treatment of persons affected with leprosy was established in November of the same year. It has been in almost continuous existence ever since and is now known as the Kalihi Observation and Detention Hospital. This hospital is situated in the suburbs of Honolulu and consists of a number of small frame buildings pleasantly situated in an inclosure of several acres.

In addition to this hospital, in which it was intended that patients presenting incipient manifestations of the disease and others thought amenable to treatment might be detained, there was established a leper settlement on the island of Molokai, about 80 miles (128 kilometers)

---

* Read at the Forty-Fifth Annual Meeting of the American Dermatological Association, Washington, D. C., May 2-4, 1922.

1. Wayson, J. T.: N. Y. Med. Rec., November, 1904.

2. Report of the board of health to the legislative assembly of 1886.

distant from the island of Oahu and Honolulu, the capital of the island group, known as the Kalaupapa Leper Colony. This is situated on a tongue of land 8 square miles (20 square kilometers) in area, projecting into the sea from the north side of the island of Molokai and walled in by the Kalaupapa, a precipitous mountain range or *pali*, 2,000 feet (600 meters) in height, which affords a natural barrier against escape, as well as complete isolation.

The first consignment of patients arrived at this segregation colony in January, 1866. During the first ten years, 1,587 lepers, who should rightly be called patients, were received.

During this decade, the largest number was received in the year 1873, when 487 lepers were consigned to Molokai; while in 1886 there were only forty-three, this being the smallest number received in any single year during this period. An equal variability in the number of patients domiciled at Molokai at different times is also noted. Thus in 1890 there were 1,213; while in 1886, the end of the first decade, there were only 590.

POLICIES IN DEALING WITH THE DISEASE

This irregularity has continued to the present time, on account of variations in policy in dealing with the disease, which governmental changes have engendered, and bears no relation to the actual number of lepers on the Islands, which, in proportion to the number of inhabitants, has of late slightly decreased.

Mouritz,[3] in his treatise on leprosy in the Hawaiian Islands, speaks thus of this phase of the local situation: "The segregation of lepers has been irregular, spasmodic, and efficient only at certain periods. This is only too plainly evident in the testimony supplied by the yearly number of lepers segregated, as per the following figures, which indicate activity and slackness, alternately; depending in the main on election and non-election years." Then follows the yearly consignments from 1866 to 1899, which varied from 43 to 571 (1888). He continues: "The efforts to stamp out leprosy by segregation have taken on the status of a political football, the party in power being assailed by the outs, who return the attack in kind. Both parties have been offenders, using the care and segregation of lepers as a target or a cudgel, depending on the state of the case. The Hawaiians have the majority of votes, and to placate voters and gain their votes the enforcement of the segregation law has been purposely allowed to lapse temporarily." He then makes a plea for federal control, which has since been partially accomplished.

---

3. Mouritz, A. A. St. M.: The Path of the Destroyer; a History of Leprosy in the Hawaiian Islands, Honolulu, 1916, pp. 165-166.

This shifting policy in dealing with the problem of leprosy, or rather in looking the problem squarely in the face, is also influenced by commercial and social interests. The unwholesome reputation the Hawaiian Islands received in the death of Father Damien in 1889, and the wide publicity it was given, created in the minds of most people a feeling of dread, even of repugnance whenever the Hawaiian Islands were mentioned. This was not warranted by the facts, and to counteract this wrong impression measures tending to the opposite extreme have been from time to time resorted to. This has resulted in the conflicting reports and the consequent uncertainty that exists in the minds of medical men as to the actual status of the leprosy problem in the Hawaiian Islands.

ESTABLISHMENT OF U. S. CONTROL

Soon after the United States took over the Islands as a territory, the Marine Hospital and Public Health Service was asked to take charge of the leper problem. A cooperative plan was devised in which the department of public health works in connection with the local board of health. But the national control of leprosy has not yet accomplished the desired result, that of taking the most efficient measures for controlling the disease.

An attempt was made with, I am told, an expenditure of about $250,000 for buildings and other equipment, including an ice plant and even microscopes, on the island of Molokai. But here again a change in national policy or procedure took place, and the buildings, which have never been occupied, lie rotting, and the other partial equipment remains corroding and unused. In fact, after a lapse of ten or twelve years no benefit has ever accrued from this somewhat ambitious though abortive attempt to study the subject of leprosy and to employ the most efficient means of controlling this widespread disease, which by some is regarded not only as a local, but also as a national, menace.

TREATMENT BY CHAULMOOGRA OIL

The announcement in 1904 that Power [4] and his collaborators in the Welfare Research Laboratory had succeeded in separating certain fatty acids from chaulmoogra oil led many too enthusiastic leprologists to affirm that if the actual cure of leprosy had not been attained its ultimate eradication from the face of the globe was in sight.

Taub further elaborated the separation of the ethyl esters from chaulmoogra oil, and after their extensive use, particularly in Turkey and Egypt, in the treatment of leprosy, the process was patented in the

---

4. Power and Gornall: J. Am. Chem. Soc. **85**:838, 851, 1904. Power and Barrowcliff: ibid. **87**:884, 1905. Barrowcliff and Power: ibid. **91**:557, 1907.

United States in 1910, under the trade name antileprol.[5]   In these letters patent, full and explicit directions are given for the elaboration of the ethyl esters from chaulmoogra oil as used today in the Kalihi Hospital and Station, as well as at the colony of Kalaupapa on the island of Molokai.   The ethyl esters in the form of antileprol were previously used in the Kalihi Hospital at Honolulu by Wayson, between 1910 and 1914,[6] with about the same results as Rogers in India and others were obtaining.

Heretofore, chaulmoogra oil and its derivatives had been given by the mouth. ˙ It was disagreeable to the taste and often its use had to be abandoned on account of the deleterious effect on the patient.   In 1914, Heiser [7] advocated the use of chaulmoogra oil diluted with an equal quantity of camphorated oil, with 4 gm. of resorcin to every 120 c.c. of the mixture.   This was given intramuscularly with encouraging results.

During the World War, letters patent were apparently not considered any more seriously than were other scraps of paper when public necessity required their infraction; consequently Dean,[8] of the University of Hawaii, in 1919, separated the ethyl esters from the crude chaulmoogra oil, as Taub had previously done, and McDonald,[8] and later Wellman, administered them intramuscularly at the Kalihi Hospital.   The enthusiasm with which this treatment was received and entered into seems to have been in inverse ratio to the permanent benefit derived.   Improvement undoubtedly took place in many cases, especially in the early or mild forms of the disease.

PAROLE OF PATIENTS

Although more or less painful, the discomfort was confined to the buttocks, and patients were able to receive more of the active elements of the drug than they had previously been able to receive by way of the mouth, and with less disturbance to their general health.   Consequently, the enthusiasm was not confined to the hospital staff, but was participated in by the afflicted, who saw in this treatment a brighter prospect of being returned to their homes restored to health.   Between July 9, 1919 and March 31, 1921, 140 patients were paroled from the Kalihi Hospital as either cured or no longer a menace to the community at large; thus, a semblance of reality was given to this bright outlook.

5. U. S. Patent No. 957633, May 10, 1910, Washington, D. C.

6. Report of Hawaiian Board of Health, 1912; also personal communication to the author.

7. Heiser, Public Health Reports **29**:2763, No. 42.

8. McDonald, J. T., and Dean, A. L.: The Treatment of Leprosy, Pub. Health Rep. **35**:1959 (Aug. 20) 1920; The Constituents of Chaulmoogra Oil Effective in Leprosy, J. A. M. A. **76**:1471 (May 28) 1921.

During this period, sixty patients were discharged from the leper settlement at Molokai. Of this large number, sixteen have since been returned to the Kalihi Hospital, six have died while on parole, one is known to have escaped from the Islands, and only two have been released from parole as apparently cured, and these prior to the end of the four year period (in which no symptoms of leprosy have appeared, the patient remaining during this time bacteriologically negative) now thought necessary. This still leaves 115 paroled patients from the Kalihi Hospital unaccounted for, as well as those from Molokai.

Two of these paroled patients deserve more than a passing notice. One was a woman of uncertain repute who, on being paroled, entered one of the houses of prostitution in Honolulu, where, after the most intimate exposure of her patrons, who are said to have included soldiers from all parts of the United States, she was finally apprehended as a leper having the disease in its active stage. She is now under treatment at the Kalihi Detention Hospital.

The second patient, also a woman much in the public eye, was discharged from the Kalihi Hospital as cured during the large exodus of 1919, which accompanied the announcement to the world that leprosy was at last completely amenable to treatment. She was exhibited at public gatherings as an example of a cured case of leprosy, and, I am told by eye witnesses, kissed as one "snatched from the jaws of death." This took place during the meeting in Honolulu of the American Press Association and elicited expressions which I will quote from a recent number of what I had considered a conservative weekly publication. "Miss R. B., an Hawaiian woman, had been a leper and was pronounced cured. . . . Miss B., after long treatment at Kalihi, had been among fifty selected to pass across the dark waters of the channels to Molokai—incurable. At the eleventh hour, however, Dr. ——— saw that she was responding to the Dean treatment.[9] The first to be pronounced cured and safe to resume her place among her fellowmen. She is cured."

Again, from a local editorial [10] published during the Press Association meeting:

HONOLULU'S MOLOKAI

The patient who has had leprosy and has been cured may be shy a finger joint, or the tip of an ear, but before God and man he is as clean and free of the disease as a man who has had a carbuncle lanced and has got over it. Hawaii's conquest of leprosy is the greatest achievement of the many of which this land boasts. We not only ask, we urge you to go to Kalihi Hospital today and see this greatest marvel for yourselves, then pass on the word *Hawaii has cured its lepers.*"

In this star case of "cured leprosy," which was given as much publicity as was the life work and death of Father Damien, who, by the

---

9. Names given in original article. Leslie's. July 30, 1921.
10. Pacific Commercial Advertiser. November, 1921.

way, was only one of three priests who have died of leprosy in these islands, the patient was returned to Kalihi Hospital a few months later with the disease under full headway, where I had an opportunity repeatedly to observe the case.

During my stay in the islands, I took occasion to examine a few of the many paroled patients who had either discontinued reporting weekly at the Kalihi Hospital as they are required to do, or had never reported since being released on parole. In one instance, a mother and two children had been paroled. One child, although never having presented any symptoms of leprosy, had been hospitalized with the mother and sister, who were lepers. The mother was now bedridden in her home from active manifestations of the disease, and the affected child also presented macular lesions on the skin, with partial paralysis of one eyelid. One child still remained free from symptoms. Both children were attending school. Neither the mother nor the affected child were reporting at the hospital. Their dwelling was in the center of a large taro plantation which furnishes one of the principal articles of food, poi, of the Islands.

Three other paroled patients who were not reporting at the hospital were following their various vocations, one a flower vendor, one a city employee and one a student. While presenting leprous stigmas, the disease, so far as I could ascertain, was not in an active stage. Whether or not these quiescent or mild forms are a menace to the public health, from our present knowledge of the disease we are unable to say.

SURVEILLANCE OF PERSONS AT LARGE

Koch, during his visit here, it is said, obtained lepra bacilli from the nasal mucosa in some of these apparently inactive cases. Two other persons who were not under surveillance of the board of health came under my observation. One was a teacher in one of the public schools and the other was the elevator boy whom I had the opportunity of repeatedly though somewhat furtively examining throughout my stay. In both, there were visible evidences of implication of the facial and ulnar nerves, with consequent paralysis and atrophy of the levator labii and the adductor pollicis and first dorsal interosseus muscles of the face and hands, respectively.

Granting these were mild or incipient cases of leprosy, with our present lack of exact knowledge as to the mode of transmitting or acquiring the disease, we are unable to say whether or not they are a menace to the public health. Here, it is undoubtedly better to err on the side of safety.

In going through one of the large pineapple canneries in Honolulu, I was impressed with the neatness with which the process was accomplished, and to see the sealed cans finally passing through a steam sterilizer. This, with the wearing of rubber gloves by those who handled the fruit, was especially comforting to me later, on hearing that three employees had previously been afflicted with leprosy. Since which time, all employees of this particular cannery are examined by a member of the board of health once a month.

On the other hand, from what I saw, it is my belief that there are fewer persons at large afflicted with leprosy in the Hawaiian Islands than in most other countries I have seen where the disease prevails to the same extent. This is due, I believe, to the efficient services rendered by Dr. F. E. Trotter, president and officer of the board of health; Dr. James T. Wayson, the leprologist, member of the board of health and former health officer, and Dr. H. E. Hasseltine, of the U. S. Public Health Service, medical officer in charge of the Kalihi Hospital. At the present time, as for the last three years, all cases of leprosy occurring on the Islands are sent to the observation and detention hospital at Honolulu, where they are paroled or detained, as seems best. In mild cases, the patients returning to receive their weekly treatment are permitted to live at home. There are detained at the present time 187 patients. They are comfortably housed in small wooden buildings, with additional structures for schools, cooking and eating.

Since about the middle of 1921, the treatment consists of weekly injections of all the ethyl esters of chaulmoogra oil, the attempt to isolate any particular acid having given less promising results. The medicament is prepared at the chemical laboratory of the University of Hawaii from the crude oil, which is imported from India. From 1 to 6 c.c., varying according to the weight and condition of the patient, are injected into the gluteal muscle. During the last few months, the ethyl esters have been given intravenously to a selected number of patients in 1 c.c. doses, twice or thrice weekly. The ethyl esters in capsule are also given by mouth in some cases. Iodin, which was formerly given in the proportion of 2.5 per cent., is now discontinued.

At Kalaupapa, on the island of Molokai, of the sixty patients paroled during the period between 1919 and 1921, there are recorded eleven relapses, and two who died on parole. The fate of the remaining forty-seven is unknown.

The treatment carried out by Dr. W. J. Goodhue, resident physician at this colony, is said to be that followed at the Kalihi Hospital. The treatment here, however, is not compulsory. Since the leper colony occupies but a small part of the Island of Molokai, and is shut off from the rest of the island, there is apparently an effort to lift the onus of leprosy from Molokai. This, with the almost complete isolation of the colony, has evidently led to the abandonment of Molokai as a haven to which all lepers are sent. No cases of leprosy are admitted to these islands from other parts of the United States.

UNSOLVED PROBLEMS

Since the disease became recognized as a public menace, efforts have been made to ascertain its mode of propagation, the influences which favor such dissemination and the best treatment. Distinguished scientists, among whom may be mentioned Koch and Arning, have studied the disease *in loco,* and still the two major problems, those of dissemination and cure, remain unsolved.

CONCLUSIONS

Leprosy was probably introduced into the Hawaiian Islands from without, some time during the last century. The disease spreads rapidly among the Hawaiians because of their intimate mode of living, together with their *laissez faire* attitude in regard to the disease. With this, complete segregation is difficult of accomplishment.

It is most prevalent during school age. It is most common in the male sex. A specific for leprosy has not yet been fully attained.

If one might be permitted to make a few suggestions on impressions gained from a study extending over only a few weeks they would be:

A more definite plan of procedure should be established. If the changing conditions consequent on our elective form of government are allowed to continue to influence the work, it would seem better that it be assumed by a nonpolitical body, such, for example, as the Rockefeller Foundation could furnish.

If the present system continues, there should be, in addition to Dr. H. E. Hasseltine, the efficient medical officer of the Public Health Service now doing all the work of the Kalihi Hospital, a trained clinician, or at least some one appointed or detailed by the Public Health Service, in place of the more indefinite and heterogenous board of health. Not that there is wanting local ability amply to fill this important position if subjected to a nonpartisan, nonlocalized body.

Then, in addition, there should be sent to this field a research worker of undoubted ability—one of the few who like poets are born and not made—to ascertain, first of all, how the disease is acquired. This, in my opinion, is the first great problem to be solved. Its prevention would then be clear; its treatment is already being elucidated and improved. This position should be untrammeled by local influences, and its incumbent should be given a free hand.

Finally, the ethyl esters of chaulmoogra oil undoubtedly have a beneficial effect on most cases of leprosy; in some, it apparently does harm by aggravating the disease; while in mild or early cases, it apparently, for a time at least, arrests the progress of the disease.

DISCUSSION

Dr. George Henry Fox, New York: I have been greatly interested in the paper of Dr. Corlett. Some twenty-five or thirty years ago it was my privilege to see and treat a large number of cases of leprosy in New York, all of which were imported cases. I remember using Hoang-nan, a Chinese drug, from which I do not remember obtaining great benefit. I remember giving doses of strychnia without any result, but chaulmoogra oil was, in my opinion, then and now a most valuable remedy. Nearly all of the patients that I treated with large or small doses of chaulmoogra oil improved, some of them rapidly. The cutaneous lesions in some cases disappeared rapidly under large doses of the oil. Many of these patients, whether treated with chaulmoogra oil or not, seemed to improve; and I made up my mind that the change of climate in coming to New York was largely responsible for some of the improvement, and I think so now. But that chaulmoogra oil was of value I proved to my own satisfaction then, and I think now that it is the only remedy of great value in this disease. I trust that the ethyl esters will be found to be an improved form of administration, but their precise value does not appear to have been fully determined.

One fact that impressed me strongly was that perhaps no other drug has so many different effects, so much unevenness of action on digestion, as chaulmoogra oil. Some patients could not take more than a few drops without intense nausea, while others could take from 100 to 200 drops daily, and those were the ones that improved most rapidly. One patient under my care in New York for twenty years or more always improved temporarily under chaulmoogra oil, but relapses occurred; so I cannot recommend chaulmoogra oil as a specific or a sure cure. Its varied effect on the stomach in different cases, I cannot explain.

There is one other point in the therapeutics of leprosy that I would like to mention—the psychic treatment. Many lepers are seized by the health authorities and either sent in a box car back to California or elsewhere, or confined in some shanty with food put through a little window on the end of a stick, while the health officer looks at them with a long face and says, "We will do all we can for you, poor fellow, but you have leprosy." No wonder they get worse. If you and I were treated in such a manner, I think we would rapidly deteriorate in health, and perhaps die, whether we had leprosy or not. My opinion is that many of the patients with leprosy if told that it is not an incurable disease will very likely be relieved in mind and benefited physically, if not entirely cured by this encouragement. I think we can accomplish more this way than by the administration of any drug. As I said, I think the change in climate has much to do with improvement. For a long time I believe! that leprosy was not contagious. Perhaps I would not say so now, but I would still claim that a leper in any community is by no means as serious a menace to public health as is a case of mild tuberculosis. I have known of patients with the nodular form living for thirty years before the disease had gone on to a "fatal termination" in spite of what our textbooks used to state; and if these patients were encouraged with the hope of a cure and not scared to death, I think they would all improve, if not recover.

Dr. Harry G. Irvine, Minneapolis: I should like to ask Dr. Corlett whether in his observation in the Islands he saw any children with leprosy. In this regard I should like to relate an interesting experience of my own. We have seen a number of cases in Minneapolis and several in one family starting with a case contracted in Minnesota, so far as we can tell from the history. This woman died with leprosy—I will not say from leprosy—and about a year ago I had an opportunity to examine a daughter, now married and three other children; one was already dead with leprosy. The daughter is just beginning to have thickening of the eyebrows, some loss of hair and three or four nodules. I also examined her husband and two children. At that time there were no signs of the disease in the children, but a few months later her little girl of 3 or 4 years was brought to me for examination. This child then had a peculiar maculopapular eruption, resembling urticaria pigmentosa. It has appeared and disappeared several times, disappearing within a few weeks, and leaving just a little pigmentation. Three months later I saw the child again, and at that time she had three nodules the size of large peas. These were excised and showed all the typical construction of a leprosy nodule. We have never been able to find any bacilli in the nasal secretion or the nodules, but I thought from these findings that the child should be isolated with the mother, at least as a suspect. Both patients were sent to the leprosarium at Carville, La.

Dr. Harry E. Alderson, San Francisco: Dr. Corlett's paper is interesting, and brings up for discussion a subject that is well worth while. Confirming what Dr. George H. Fox said about the beneficial effect of improved hygiene and tonics, I should like to say also that one of the causes of the recent improvement in the matter of the control of lepers in the Islands is the hope that new methods of therapy hold out to the lepers. They feel that there is some chance for them now, and they do not hide away as they formerly did. I have been in Honolulu several times for prolonged visits since 1905 and have been able to observe steady improvement in conditions. An apparent increase in leprosy is believed to have been due to this better cooperation on the part of the natives. More cases are discovered early. On my second visit there I saw a leper who had been hiding away without food, or at least with very little, until he was finally apprehended. When brought into the Kalihi Receiving Station he was in poor physical condition, and the leprosy was correspondingly bad. Under proper feeding, baths, strychnin and arsenic, the physical improvement was remarkable. Such experiences are not uncommon. Similar observations have been made by Dr. George H. Fox.

The last time I was in the Hawaiian Islands I was told that it was much easier to get lepers to report. Perhaps one of the greatest benefits of the new treatment is in the encouragement it offers.

Dr. Corlett spoke of the rather "intimate" life in the Islands. Possibly you might be interested in a few of the details. One good old custom in entertaining guests is to have the entire company occupy one large bed spread on the floor. Perhaps a dozen or more may be accommodated in that way. It is common for entire families and sometimes more than one family, to occupy the same bed. One of the popular native dishes, "poi," is made by pounding out the tara root in a large bowl. I have seen natives laboriously pounding out this food in the hot sun, perspiring over it, and even sneezing in it. The final product is a pasty, starchy raw mass, and it is delicious.

The Hawaiian climate is warm and even, except in the mountains. It is like one huge incubator. At times the humidity is quite pronounced. Conditions for the growth and spread of all kinds of bacterial, insect and vegetable life generally are ideal. In more temperate climates where hygiene conditions are better, of course the spread of leprosy is necessarily much retarded. In tropical and subtropical countries all of the conditions favorable for the spread of bacterial diseases are present.

Dr. A. W. Stillians, Chicago: Chicago has a small colony of lepers, and we have had an opportunity to try the new form of treatment to some extent. From our experience we feel that the ethyl esters have had a much more rapid effect on the cases than either chaulmoogra oil or Sir Leonard Rogers' sodium gynocardate. Our first patient was under treatment for two years and four months before being discharged as clinically well, and is still receiving treatment every week. Our other patients have been sent to Louisiana because our facilities for treatment are not good, in that we cannot allow the patients any freedom in the open air.

Dr. Thomas Casper Gilchrist, Baltimore: I am glad to see that they are not worrying the patients so much. If patients with syphilis and tuberculosis were worried as those with leprosy are, we would not see those patients as we do. I remember one patient that came to Johns Hopkins and another that came in from Virginia; the latter was almost dying from starvation. I wonder if in Biblical times all diseases of the skin were not called leprosy. Josephus refers to 60,000 cases of leprosy at one time; those cases could not have been leprosy. They were probably cases of itch. I wonder whether scabies. because of the idea of its being contagious, was handed down as leprosy before Hansen found the bacillus, and whether the public has its idea of the great contagiousness associated with scabies and that that might be the explanation of the idea.

I had a case two years ago, a bad nodular case of the face and body, in which I began to administer chaulmoogra oil in small doses. The patient stood it pretty well, and I thought I would try radium and the Kromayer lamp on the nodules on his face to see whether they would disappear more rapidly. and use the chaulmoogra oil on the other lesions. I was delighted to see how quickly the lesions on the face disappeared. When the patient came in, sections were taken and one of the nodules was curetted; in the smear we found the lepra bacilli. The chaulmoogra oil in that case improved the condition very much. The effect of that and cheering and feeding him was remarkable.

Dr. E. L. McEwen, Chicago: I wish to refer to two points. The first concerns the relation of newspaper activity to the persecution of lepers. The first leper to remain any length of time in Cook County Hospital was admitted as a patient with tertiary syphilis. A few hours later a correct diagnosis was made, and the man was placed in a room by himself. A turmoil was expected over the situation, but for some reason the matter was scarcely referred to by the newspapers; only one conservative evening sheet carried scare-headlines for one issue. As a result of this newspaper quiet the man stayed in the hospital for six weeks, while his deportation was being arranged. entirely without opposition. Since that time a number of lepers have passed through the hospital without a protest. The second point concerns the beneficial effect of simple tonic and hygienic treatment. The extensive, open lesions of the leper to whom I have referred healed completely with six weeks of good food. rest and tonic medication.

Dr. Harvey P. Towle, Boston: I would like to call particular attention to one point brought out by Dr. Corlett. namely, the influence of the universal public fear of the disease on the treatment of the disease and the handling of lepers. As Dr. Gilchrist has said, the public fear of contagion dates back to Bible times and farther and continues today. The effect is reflected in our laws. The leper is legally torn from his family and segregated with his fellow victims far from men and amid surroundings which, in any other disease would cause an outburst of horror and indignation from the public. As it is now, the public merely sighs with relief when the leper is hurried away—and forgets him. It is our duty to educate the public to more humane treatment. To accomplish this we must seek exact knowledge of how the disease is spread, its incubation period, and other factors. We who treat leprosy know that in this country it is not as contagious as syphilis or tuberculosis. But, unfortunately, we are unable to convince the public. It therefore seems to me that we should methodically and scientifically gather data concerning the propagation and spread of the disease and seek to give them the widest publicity. Once we have induced the public to regard the leper more humanely and to provide for him, at least as well as for the convict, we shall have increased the potency of our therapeutic remedies immeasurably.

Dr. William Thomas Corlett, Cleveland (closing): Little difficulty is usually experienced in finding the bacillus of Hansen in a lepra lesion. A frequent cite of an early invasion is on the ear. If the ear is punctured and a droplet of blood squeezed out and placed on a slide and treated in the usual way for the acid-fast bacilli, numerous groups or clusters are shown if lepra is present. It is more difficult to find them in macular, particularly in the late macular or atrophic, lesions.

In the intravenous administration of the ethyl esters the initial dose at the Kalihi Hospital is 1 c.c., repeated after a few days or according to the reaction. Naturally, all patients do not tolerate well this form of administration.

In some of the instances, notably the one cited by Dr. Morrow, a small blood vessel is entered even when giving the ethyl esters intramuscularly. This, if the quantity is large, is followed by a severe reaction. I am particularly anxious to add a word on the point brought out by Drs Fox, Gilchrist and Towle, namely, the degree of contagiousness of leprosy, and the apparent immunity enjoyed by some who are exposed to the disease. I have on several occasions, in discussing this disease, cited the testimony of the Sister Superior of the leprosarium in Trinidad, who during a period of thirty-five years had not seen a Sister employed as a nurse contract leprosy. I have always interpreted this as an indication that the disease is, under ordinary circumstances, feebly contagious. More recent experience, however, leads me to believe that cleanliness and aloofness are two of the factors which render the nurse more immune to leprosy than others who live more intimately with those afflicted with the disease. Father Damian may be cited as an example. For if the reports of his life while at Molokai be true, he neglected the ordinary precautions of contact and even of cleanliness. I should ascribe about an equal degree of contagiosity to leprosy and tuberculosis; certain factors of environment and racial susceptibility must be recognized in both diseases.

The Hawaiians seem to be particularly prone to leprosy, and to a less extent to tuberculosis—two causes which are acting in the extermination of the native race on these Islands.

Children are especially likely to contract the disease; the records of the Board of Health at Honolulu show that it is largely a disease of school age, and to the intimate life of children at school is attributed the spread of leprosy in Hawaii.

Several members have mentioned the importance of hygiene in the treatment of leprosy, which I believe, next to complete segregation, is one of the important things to bear in mind in controlling the disease.

THE USE OF ULTRAVIOLET LIGHT IN ERYTHEMA INDURATUM *

E. LAWRENCE OLIVER, M.D.

BOSTON

As this paper is based on observations of only five cases of erythema induratum treated with the Kromayer lamp, it seems quite unnecessary to review the literature of the disease or to compare this method of treatment with the results obtained from various other methods of treatment. Neither do I intend to review the literature of the treatment of disease with ultraviolet light in general, for I have found no reports of cases in which the light was used in exactly the same manner in which it was used in this group of cases. General exposure of the body to ultraviolet light, or general exposure of the legs, may prove valuable, but as this paper deals with the effects of the local application of the Kromayer lamp on the individual indurated areas of erythema induratum, the methods are not comparable.

At the outset let me state that I am referring to erythème induré des scrofuleux of Bazin occurring almost exclusively in young women or girls, a disease which I believe should be differentiated from the type occurring in middle-aged women which, according to Whitfield, has nothing to do with tuberculosis, and also from the atypical cases belonging to Darier's sarcoid group.

I believe the five cases here reported all belong in the tuberculous or tuberculid group. All occurred in women under 30. All were in the characteristic situations, the posterior and outer aspects of the lower half of the legs. All of the patients had poor peripheral circulation evidenced by cyanosis or cold feet or both. The one patient with a unilateral case showed evidence of a healed tuberculous gland in the neck, which was, except for its unilateral location, in every respect characteristic of erythema induratum of Bazin.

The treatments were carried out by pressing the quartz glass window of the Kromayer lamp firmly against the indurated areas for from one to two minutes to each area. When the lesions were small the healthy skin outside the area was protected with paper or zinc oxid plaster. The Kromayer lamp was used on a 110 volt direct current and was run at full strength for ten minutes before applying it to the indurated areas.

The following five cases illustrate the probable value of this method in the treatment of erythema induratum of the tuberculous or tuberculid type.

---

* Read at the Forty-Fifth Annual Meeting of the American Dermatological Association, Washington, D. C., May 2-4, 1922.

REPORT OF CASES

CASE 1.—A woman, aged 24, single, well developed and well nourished, who worked in a biscuit factory and was on her feet nearly all day, had had indurated areas in the calves of her legs for two years, somewhat better in summer but never clearing up entirely. She complained of cold feet and occasional swelling of the ankles and legs. She was first seen by me on Oct. 5, 1919. She then had two deep seated indurated areas in the right lower calf and three in the left lower calf. There was no history of tuberculosis and no evidence of tuberculosis elsewhere. There were no ulcerations or scars. The Wassermann reaction was negative. The legs were slightly cyanotic, especially over the indurated areas.

At the first visit one area, 1½ inches (3.81 cm.) in diameter was treated with Kromayer lamp with firm pressure for two minutes. On October 13, she reported that the area treated became blistered the day after treatment; it became hot, red and tender, and the ankle swelled so that she stayed in bed for two days. When seen on October 13, eight days after the first treatment, there was a dried crust covering the area treated; the swelling and pain had subsided, and the induration had entirely disappeared. At this visit the other four areas were treated in the same manner, but for only one minute to each area. One month later the induration had entirely disappeared leaving the skin of these areas purplish bronze, but otherwise normal in appearance.

Two years later, November, 1921, the skin of these areas was still discolored, but she had had no return of the indurations.

CASE 2.—A woman, aged 30, single, weighing 120 pounds (54.4 kg.), whose occupation was housework, had always had cold hands and feet. She was first seen on May 8, 1920. The trouble had been present four years, clearing up every summer but "worse than ever this spring." She complained of getting tired easily and of swelling of the legs toward night, with discomfort rather than pain. There was no history or evidence of tuberculosis elsewhere.

Locally she showed two deep-seated areas of induration about 1 inch (2.54 cm.) in diameter on the outer lower calf of each leg. There were also about a dozen small pea-sized indurations in the calves. The Kromayer lamp was used, the window being pressed against each of the four large lesions, one minute to each. Eighteen days later she came to me again. The burns had hardly troubled her at all, while the indurations had almost entirely disappeared. I did not see her again for a year, when she reported that all the lesions disappeared within six weeks after the treatment, and that she had had no recurrence during the next winter. All the areas treated showed brownish pigmentation, but there was no trace of induration.

CASE 3.—A woman, aged 22, single, a stenographer, had always been well except for trouble in the left eye since early childhood, which was diagnosed as tuberculous keratitis at the Massachusetts Eye and Ear Infirmary. Circulation in the hands and feet had always been poor. The present trouble had existed for six years, becoming somewhat better each summer. At her first visit, April 16, 1921, she showed small and large indurated areas on the calves and outer surfaces of the lower part of the legs. None of the lesions projected appreciably, but all were purplish and deeply indurated on palpation.

The Kromayer lamp was applied to one large induration on the right calf for two minutes. Eight days later this lesion showed a drying crust, but the induration had entirely disappeared. She had had a severe reaction to the light and was in bed for two days after the treatment on account of pain and swelling. On April 24, five more areas were treated for one minute each. On May 7, all areas treated showed complete disappearance of induration. On this date the remaining indurated areas were treated. During the summer the trouble almost entirely disappeared, but the next autumn, on Nov. 21, 1921, she had three new indurated lesions, which were treated in the same manner. On Dec. 21, 1921, she was practically well. There were no palpable lesions, but there was marked pigmentation at the sites of all the old lesions. Since then she had had a few new small indurations which have disappeared, except for pigmentation, after a single treatment with the Kromayer lamp.

CASE 4.—A woman, aged 22, single, a hospital nurse, had always been well except for a tuberculous gland in the neck three years ago. This softened and was opened leaving a scar 2 inches (5 cm.) long on the right side of the neck. She was first seen May 13, 1921. The present trouble began while she was in training one year before. Her general health was excellent.

On the lower portion of the right calf she had two marble-sized deep indurations. The legs were somewhat bluish. On May 13, 1921, one of the areas was treated with the Kromayer lamp, one minute with pressure. Six days later, May 19, 1921, the induration had almost entirely disappeared from the treated lesion, which was covered with a drying crust. On this date the other lesion was treated.

In March, 1922, the patient reported that both lesions had entirely disappeared a month after the last treatment, and that there had been no recurrence.

CASE 5.—A woman, aged 24, married, seen on May 18, 1921, had always been well until the present trouble began, a year before. There was no history or evidence of tuberculosis except tuberculous glands in the neck during childhood. The feet and legs were always cold and bluish. She had received much potassium iodid without benefit. The Wassermann reaction was negative. She had been getting steadily worse during the last six months. She complained of swelling in the legs and ankles toward night.

When examined she had five large deep-seated indurated areas in the calves of the legs. At her first visit, two areas were treated one minute each with pressure. One week later these lesions were covered with drying crusts; the induration had nearly disappeared. The three other lesions were treated for one minute each.

Sept. 15, 1921, she said that she was greatly improved. During the last winter she has been on her feet all day; three new lesions developed which have all responded to treatment, the induration disappearing from each in a week or two after treatment.

CONCLUSION

None of these patients had had ulcerations at any time, so that none of the cases were examples of the severest type of the disease. Furthermore, it is impossible to draw definite conclusions from such a small number of cases. I feel, however, that the uniformity of the results from treatment of the individual lesions in these cases justifies the hope that this method will prove of considerable value in the treatment of this obstinate disease.

DISCUSSION

DR. FRED WISE, New York: The reason I hesitate to discuss the paper is because my experience is limited in the use of the ultraviolet light in this which I am connected, we are accustomed to use the roentgen ray in erythema induratum, with excellent results, so the ultraviolet light has rarely been used. The results in three cases have been very good, but not better than the results from roentgenotherapy.

Dr. A. W. STILLIANS, Chicago: I wish to testify to the value of this method, which was one of the first practical things I learned about ultraviolet light therapy. I think it is a safer method than roentgenotherapy, especially in the hands of those who have not had much experience in roentgenotherapy. According to my experience, it is very easy to cause irritation with the roentgen ray in lesions of the leg.

Dr. E. L. OLIVER, Boston (closing): I offer as a suggestion to those who are using the Kromayer lamp in the treatment of this disease that they press the window of the lamp against the lesions for one minute.

Abstracts from Current Literature

THE SUPERFICIAL REACTION OF RADIUM AS A GUIDE TO DOS-
AGE. WILLIAM S. NEWCOMET, Am. J. Roentgenol. **9**:34, 1922.

The thesis of the paper is that radium effects cannot be measured by
multiplying the time by the quantity of radium, but that larger quantities
produce a relatively greater effect in a less number of milligram hours.

HIGH VOLTAGE X-RAY WORK. W. D. COOLIDGE and W. K. KEARSLEY,
Am. J. Roentgenol. **9**:77, 1922.

A paper devoted to the apparatus for and technic of very high voltage
roentgen-ray currents in therapy.

THE ULTRAVIOLET RAY IN THE TREATMENT OF ROENTGEN-
RAY TELANGIECTASIS. H. H. HAZEN, Am. J. Roentgenol. **9**:101. 1922.

The active ultraviolet lamp, using a compression lens has been found to
cause obliteration of vessels of telangiectasis following the roentgen ray. Two
treatments of from fifteen to twenty minutes in each area have been found
sufficient.

THE RELATION OF TEMPERATURE CHANGES TO ROENTGEN-
RAY SKIN REACTIONS. CHARLES L. MARTIN and GEORGE T. CALDWELL,
Am. J. Roentgenol. **9**:152, 1922.

Observations recently published make it seem likely that the temperature
of the irradiated skin may be a factor in the production of a reaction. Clinical support for this supposition has been had in the observation of patients
who had areas treated in the axillae, in folds of skin in obese patients. beneath
pendulous breasts, and over the buttocks on areas likely to come in contact
with a chair. Areas which were covered by a belt. or heavy dressings or
by ointments, etc., seem to show more intense reactions. Experimental work
on rabbits was done in which areas of the abdomen exposed to heavy doses
of the ray were partially covered with bands of adhesive plaster. The effect
on the skin was that the superficial areas were pulled away with the plaster
on removal about ten days later. This seems to justify the warnings issued
by some roentgenologists that adhesive plaster should not be applied to
irradiated areas. Other experiments seemed to indicate that a covering placed
over an exposed area for a number of days after it had been irradiated
increases the degree of skin reaction obtained. Attempts at cooling the skin
by means of an ice bag for several days after irradiation seem to accentuate
the reaction obtained.

GOODMAN. New York.

GUMMATOUS CERVICAL ADENITIS. W. P. COUES, Boston M. & S. J.
187:65 (July 13) 1922.

A short review of the literature on this subject is given. detailing especially
a case reported by Wile in 1912. An additional case of probable syphilitic
infection of the cervical glands is reported.

LANE. Boston

EPIDERMOPHYTOSIS. A. M. Greenwood, Boston M. & S. J. **187**:176
(Aug. 3) 1922.

This is a good brief account of epidermophytosis. It not only outlines the
clinical characteristics and the more usual types of treatment, but contains
much of interest in regard to laboratory investigation. Considerable detail
is given about the laboratory work, including the choice and examination of
fresh material, with directions in regard to making culture mediums, and the
growth of these organisms.

TUBERCULOUS CHANCRE. J. A. Nixon and A. Rendle Short, Brit. J.
Surg. **10**:44 (July) 1922.

The writers state there is a variety of tuberculosis of the skin which so
closely resembles a primary syphilitic sore that, on the rare occasions when it
occurs, it is likely to be diagnosed as extragenital chancre. Hitherto, if
this lesion has been recognized at all, writers have included it under the
term tuberculosis verrucosa cutis, or verruca necrogenica. Since it is not a
warty type of tuberculosis, however, the observer is not likely to think of
a diagnosis of verruca necrogenica, and the possibility of the lesions being
tuberculosis is overlooked.

Clinically, the lesion appears as a localized indurated papule, resulting
from direct implantation of tubercle bacilli into the skin through a cut or
an abrasion. This papule develops into a small indolent ulcer of cartilaginous
consistency, having an edge that is slightly ramparted and translucent. It is
attended by enlargement of the nearest group of lymphatics. Because of the
induration, the ulcer is mistaken for extragenital chancre, although syphilitic
chancres of the skin are usually not indurated, but assume a raspberry appearance which the tuberculous ulcer never possesses. Sometimes the tuberculous
ulcer may look exceedingly like rodent ulcer, but in the latter case there is
no glandular enlargement.

The writers feel that these tuberculous ulcers are due to inoculation of
tubercle into persons who have a latent tuberculous infection, their tissues thus
becoming intolerant to the presence of the bacilli. The ulcer at the site of
inoculation represents the effort of the tissues to expel the bacilli by local
necrosis.

Several case records are included. Senear, Chicago.

THE NEEDS AND DUTIES OF DERMATOLOGY. Ernest D. Chipman,
J. A. M. A. **79**:419 (Aug. 5) 1922.

The needs of dermatology are defined as: (1) adequate training for those
entering the specialty; (2) more knowledge of the etiology of dermatoses,
and (3) more careful study of the patient from a general medical standpoint.
The duties of the dermatologists of today can be summed up in the word service; service to the patient in the interpretation of the significance of his disease, service to the public in the diffusion of medical knowledge, and service
to the profession in the correlation of the special knowledge of dermatologists
with that of specialists in the other divisions of medicine.

EXPERIENCE WITH CHAULMOOGRA OIL DERIVATIVES IN TREAT-
MENT OF LEPROSY. H. Morrow, E. L. Walker and H. E. Miller,
J. A. M. A. **79**:434 (Aug. 5) 1922.

The authors report their experiences in the treatment of the disease with
the ethyl esters of the fatty acids of chaulmoogra oil. Most of their patients

presented advanced types of the disease. Twenty-one patients were treated; two died, three became worse, five were improved, nine showed no improvement and two absconded. Treatment lasted for from three to eighteen months.

STANDARDIZATION AND PRESERVATION OF COMPLEMENT SERUM FOR THE WASSERMANN TEST. E. H. RUEDIGER, J. A. M. A. **79**:551 (Aug. 12) 1922.

The complement activity of guinea-pig serum can be improved by breeding of animals giving good serums, rejecting those that furnish poor serums and feeding a mixture of raw vegetables to the animals.

The fixability of guinea-pig complement was much better in winter than in summer. Frozen and salted complement serum remained active for several weeks.

A PECULIAR DISCOLORATION OF THE SKIN PROBABLY RESULTING FROM MERCURIAL COMPOUNDS (CALOMEL) IN PROPRIETARY FACE CREAMS. W. H. GOECKERMANN, J. A. M. A. **79**:605 (Aug. 19) 1922.

Two patients presented a peculiar slate colored pigmentation of the face and neck. Each used a face cream containing calomel. Goeckermann concluded from some experiments that the calomel was changed into mercuric oxid and mercury by the alkaline skin secretions of the patient. It is suggested that potassium cyanid in 0.5 to 1 per cent. solution should be used in similar cases.

CONTRIBUTIONS TO THE PHARMACOLOGY AND THERAPEUTICS OF IODIDS. E. D. OSBORNE, J. A. M. A. **79**:615 (Aug. 19) 1922.

The results of two years of study are summarized in this article. There is no striking difference in the rate of elimination of sodium iodid given intravenously as compared with that given by mouth. So far as rectal administration is concerned, it appears that a daily dose of from 2 to 3 gm. by mouth is equivalent to the maximum dose by rectum; thus it would seem that rectal administration of iodids offers no significant advantage. A dose of from 9 to 15 gm. a day by mouth divided into three equal doses is equivalent to 10 gm. in a single dose intravenously. These experiments likewise indicate that iodin given in the form of potassium iodid by mouth forms a sodium protein combination in the serum, while in the form of sodium iodid only traces of iodin enter into combination with the proteins. The question then arises as to the rôle played by the sodium protein combination in the production of iodism. It must be made the subject of further study.

QUARTZ LIGHT THERAPY IN SKIN DISEASES. E. L. OLIVER, J. A. M. A. **79**:625 (Aug. 19) 1922.

Ultraviolet light has been found of special value in ulcers due to poor circulation and in port wine marks. It is of benefit in psoriasis, in localized chronic eczema, in acne vulgaris and in lupus erythematosus. It is curative in some cases of lupus vulgaris.

EXFOLIATIVE DERMATITIS FOLLOWING SILVER ARSPHENAMIN. L. THOMPSON, J. A. M. A. **79**:628 (Aug. 19) 1922.

The patient, who had previously been treated with arsphenamin and had arsphenamin. He reacted with chill, fever and itching followed by a marked erythema and exfoliation. This cleared up in about two months.

WASSERMANN VARIATIONS: A STUDY OF THE SERUMS OF SEVENTY-FIVE PATIENTS BY EIGHT LABORATORIES. L. J. Palmer, J. A. M. A. **79**:724 (Aug. 26) 1922.

Three technics were used by each laboratory: (1) the usual routine test of each laboratory; (2) the routine test, but employing the same antigen, and (3) a common technic using the same reagents. In addition, the Dermatologic Research Institute cooperated, using the new technic of Kolmer.

In the untreated positive cases, the agreement with the clinical evidence was more than 90 per cent., averaging all laboratories, with a range of from 78 to 100 per cent. for individual laboratories. In cases classed as negative, the percentage of agreement varied from 88 to 97 per cent. The author is favorably impressed with the new Kolmer technic.

THE RESULTS IN FOOD ANAPHYLAXIS OBTAINED BY CUTANEOUS AND INTRACUTANEOUS METHODS: THE INFLUENCE OF ARSENICAL PREPARATIONS ON THE ANAPHYLACTIC FOOD REACTIONS. Albert Strickler, J. A. M. A. **79**:808 (Sept. 2) 1922.

There was no material difference in reactions obtained whether the cutaneous or intracutaneous methods were employed. Arsenical preparations whether administered by mouth or intravenously do not appreciably influence the endermic food tests.

SPOROTRICHOSIS. F. W. Cregor, J. A. M. A. **79**:812 (Sept. 2) 1922.

This article contains a discussion of the disease and the report of a typical case. The patient was cured by potassium iodid internally and Lugol's solution locally.

ULCERATING GRANULOMA (GRANULOMA INGUINALE). H. Goodman, J. A. M. A. **79**:815 (Sept. 2) 1922.

The author's experiences with the disease in the tropics and in New York City are recounted. Tartar emetic is a specific, but it must be continued long after the lesions have disappeared to prevent recurrences.

LOCAL BLASTOMYCOSIS: REPORT OF A CASE. M. Haase, E. R. Hall, C. H. Marshall, J. A. M. A. **79**:820 (Sept. 2) 1922.

The patient had a blastomycotic lesion of the cheek for twelve years, which had temporarily healed at times under iodid therapy. He developed an epididymitis, which was culturally proved to be due to blastomyces. The organism had probably spread through the blood stream.

A STUDY OF FOUR HUNDRED AND EIGHTY-FIVE CASES WITH GENITAL LESIONS. J. R. Driver, J. A. M. A. **79**:867 (Sept. 9) 1922.

Syphilis was found 203 times (42 per cent.); chancroids, 177 (36.5 per cent.); ulcerating granuloma, eight; erosive gangrenous balanitis and vulvitis, thirty, and the remainder of the cases were scabetic or herpetic or presented other nonspecific lesions. Of 171 chancres seen, only eight occurred in females.

THE KAHN PRECIPITATION TEST IN THE DIAGNOSIS OF SYPH-
ILIS: A PRELIMINARY STUDY. H. L. Keim and U. J. Wile, J. A.
M. A. **79**:870 (Sept. 9) 1922.

A report is made of the test in comparison with the Wassermann test in
350 cases; approximately half of which were syphilitic clinically.

It was found that the method compares favorably in sensitiveness with the
Wassermann test; over which it has the advantages of simplicity, rapidity, and
reduction of sources of error. The Kahn test is superior to other precipitation
tests in that the precipitate is visible to the naked eye, and there are frequent
spontaneous reactions with strongly positive serums.

Further confirmatory tests, demonstrating parallelism with the Wassermann
reaction, may well lead to the eventual abandonment of the latter in favor of
the simpler precipitation procedure.

STUDIES IN ASYMPTOMATIC NEUROSYPHILIS. IV. THE APPAR-
ENT ROLE OF IMMUNITY IN THE GENESIS OF NEUROSYPH-
ILIS. Albert Keidel, J. A. M. A. **79**:874 (Sept. 9) 1922.

Recent investigations have shown that invasion of the central nervous
system takes place in practically all cases of syphilis. Clinically, however,
it is known that less than 50 per cent. of these patients are neurosyphilitic.
Immunity, treatment and pregnancy are important in the genesis of neuraxial
involvement. Inefficient early treatment increases, efficient early treatment
decreases, the liability to neurosyphilis. The influence of pregnancy is shown
by the fact that the percentage of neurosyphilis in women who have never
been pregnant approximates that of men, while in women who have conceived
the incidence of neurosyphilis is markedly decreased. The formulas of Brown
and Pearce for animal syphilis probably apply to the disease in humans.

FLUMERIN: A NEW MERCURIAL FOR THE INTRAVENOUS TREAT-
MENT OF SYPHILIS; FIRST REPORT OF CHEMICAL, ANIMAL
AND CLINICAL EXPERIMENTS AND RESULTS. E. C. White,
J. H. Hill, J. E. Moore and H. H. Young, J. A. M. A. **79**:877 (Sept. 9) 1922.

Flumerin is a synthetic organic mercurial compound containing about
32.5 per cent. of metallic mercury. After appropriate animal trials, ninety-six
cases of syphilis were treated with it.

The authors do not attempt a comparative estimate of its value but their
clinical impression is that the drug is superior to the soluble mercurial salts
in general use by the intravenous route.

STUDIES OF BACILLUS FUSIFORMIS AND VINCENT'S SPIRO-
CHETE. I. HABITAT AND DISTRIBUTION OF THESE ORGAN-
ISMS IN RELATION TO PUTRID AND GANGRENOUS PROCESSES.
D. J. Davis and Isadore Pilot, J. A. M. A. **79**:944 (Sept. 16) 1922.

There are three chief habitats of these organisms in the human body:
(1) the crypts of the tonsils; (2) the teeth and (3) the smegma. Fusospiro-
chetal organisms are found in great numbers in erosive and gangrenous
balanitis. Proper hygiene of the parts which these organisms normally inhabit
should greatly diminish the incidence of diseases caused by them.

A RING OF CONTACT PRECIPITATION TEST FOR SYPHILIS: A MODIFICATION OF THE KAHN TEST. R. D. Herrold, J. A. M. A. **79**:957 (Sept. 16) 1922.

A proposed modification which has the advantages of simplicity; does not require incubation, and uses very small amounts of material. Comparative tests with the Wassermann reaction and the original Kahn method were satisfactory.

A SIMPLE AID IN THE DIAGNOSIS OF SYPHILIS FROM THE PRIMARY LESION. W. D. Gill, J. A. M. A. **79**:966 (Sept. 16) 1922.

The tip and lowermost part of the barrel of an all glass syringe are removed, thus converting the syringe into a vacuum apparatus. Applied over a chancre, it facilitates withdrawal of serum for dark-field examination.

Michael, Houston, Texas.

NOTES ON A CASE OF TUBULAR LEPROSY TREATED BY INTRA-VENOUS INJECTIONS OF STIBENYL. R. G. Archibald, J. Trop. Med. **24**:277 (Nov. 1) 1921.

A patient with nodular leprosy received six injections of acetyl-p-amino-phenyl sodium stibiate stibenyl in doses of 0.1 gm. to 0.6 gm. during twelve days, followed by a similar course after two weeks of rest. Improvement was noted after the first course, and great benefit after the fourth course.

DHOBIE ITCH PRODUCED BY INOCULATING A CULTURE OF EPI-DERMOPHYTON RUBRUM (CASTELLANI, 1909). Richard de Silva, J. Trop. Med. **24**:303 (Dec. 1) 1921.

This organism was cultured from a case of Dhobie itch, and a typical patch of the disease was produced by inoculation. The organism was recovered and cultured from the experimental lesion. No previous record of disease by inoculation from culture had been reported.

AN EXCEPTIONAL TROPICAL ULCERATION. R. W. Mendelson, J. Trop. Med. **24**:317 (Dec. 15) 1921.

Three cases are reported in which the site of inoculation developed into a small hard painless nodule which later broke down and formed a punched-out ulcer with rounded and elevated edges that tended to become undermined. The surrounding skin was inflamed and tender. Bacteriologic examination was negative for an exciting organism, but careful culturing showed a monilia growth on glucose-agar which completely prevented the growth of ordinary organisms. Ointments tended to allow the ulcer to spread and other applications were of temporary benefit. The ulcers showed a spontaneous cure in two or three months.

NOTE ON THE RECENT EPIDEMIC OF TROPICAL SEPTIC ULCER IN PALESTINE. A. G. Apostolides, J. Trop. Med. **25**:81 (April 1) 1922.

Ulcerations of this type are common to all tropical countries and were found to be clinically identical with the so-called "hospital gangrene." Most of the cases were found to be due to a fusiform bacillus and a spirochete. Ulcers were also produced experimentally by applications of membranes from cases of "ulcero-membranous angina," and the two organisms were found in association in the membrane and also in the ulcers. Infection occurs through a break in the skin and may be spread through the medium of mosquitoes or, possibly, other insects. The incubation period is of two or three days' duration. Beginning as a papule it rapidly enlarges, becomes painful, edematous and gangrenous, with a foul odor. Usually round with undermined edges, it does not penetrate deeply. General symptoms are in proportion to the extent of the gangrene. Many forms of local antiseptic applications have been used with varying success, but the author advocates the intravenous use of neo-arsphenamin and an ointment of 20 per cent. arsphenamin. This method has given excellent results.

FRESHLY DISSOLVED TARTAR EMETIC IN VENEREAL DISEASE. F. G. CAWSTON, J. Trop. Med. **25**:126 (May 15) 1922.

The author believes that tartar emetic produced good results in cases of gonorrhea and chancroids, improvement being noted soon after the treatment was begun. Other methods in many cases were required to finish the treatment. In syphilis also similar results are reported.

JAMIESON. Detroit.

A SURVEY OF THE EFFECT OF VENEREAL DISEASES LEGISLATION IN WESTERN AUSTRALIA FOR A PERIOD OF FIVE YEARS. R. C. EVERITT ATKINSON, Med. J. Australia **1**:65 (Jan. 21) 1922.

From the figures at hand, Atkinson contends that we cannot say whether venereal diseases have been on the increase or not. In the first place, we have no knowledge of the previous prevalence of the disease and, in the second place, we cannot know how much has not come to our knowledge by notification.

Regardless of whether the disease is on the increase or decrease, there is this much in favor of legislative control: the cases are treated earlier and efficaciously, and there is provision for follow-up work and education of the public, and the marriage of diseased persons is prevented.

SYPHILIS IN CHILDREN. H. BOYD GRAHAM. Med. J. Australia **1**:265 (March 11) 1922.

This article deals for the most part with the method of injection of aqueous solution of neo-arsphenamin as performed by the author. The technic consists in the introduction of a concentrated aqueous solution of neo-arsphenamin between the iliotibial tract of the fascia lata, on the sheath of the vastus lateralis. Sixty centigrams of the drug are dissolved in 1 c.c. of sterile distilled water. After careful surgical antisepsis, the needle is inserted at an angle of 60 degrees to the skin. As soon as it is felt that the aponeurosis has been pierced, the solution is injected. The site of injection is then painted with iodin and covered with a strip of gauze. Half an hour later, the gauze is removed and the site of injection is massaged by passing the hand firmly over the site of injection in the direction of the injection. This is repeated two to three times during the ensuing twenty-four hours.

ROUTINE OF A SYPHILIS CLINIC. W. J. BEVERIDGE. Med. J. Australia **1**:382 (April 8) 1922.

Beveridge describes the routine admission and examination of syphilitic
. s in a British expeditionary hospital. He also describes a classification

of venereal sores as adopted by Major White of the British Army. The article also contains interesting statistics of extragenital sores.

POSSIBILITIES OF IRRADIATION IN MALIGNANT DISEASE. L. C. CLENDINNEN, Med. J. Australia 1:456 (April 29) 1922.

This is an interesting and instructive article on the physics and biologic action of the roentgen rays. The article deals also with the new German cross-firing method of treating malignant growths.

GUTIERREZ, Manila.

A HISTOLOGIC STUDY OF CALCIFIED EPITHELIOMA. DUBREUILH and CAZENAVE. Ann. de dermat. et syph. 6:257 (June) 1922.

A summary of seven cases is given, including clinical and histologic findings. It is concluded that we are dealing with an epithelioma whose cells are of a special type, viable only in the very early stages of the process, and soon undergoing necrosis, giant cells later acting as phagocytes. The element of calcification, which has been stressed heretofore, and which is suggested on palpation of the tumor, was found by the authors to be present only in fragmentary form, and its importance diminishes in their estimation.

SYPHILITIC ANGIONEUROTIC AND ANGIONEUROTROPHIC ENDO-CRINIDES. AUDRY and CHATELLIER, Ann. de dermat. et syph. 6:275 (June) 1922.

Raynaud's disease and acrodermatitis chronica atrophicans come under this heading, at least in certain cases, according to the authors, the term 'endocrinide" signifying skin lesions due to endocrine disorders. In addition to the endocrinous element in the causation of these lesions, the authors believe there are also syphilitic changes in the local vessels, and the tumors of acrodermatitis chronica atrophicans are held to be syphilomas. Illustrative cases are cited, including an observation of Fordyce's.

A CASE OF SECONDARY SYPHILITIC PHENOMENA OBSERVED IN A PARETIC. MESTCHERSKY, Ann. de dermat. et syph. 6:269 (June) 1922.

A young man who had contracted syphilis in 1911, and who had received a considerable amount of mercurial treatment and some arsphenamin without a reduction of a strongly positive Wassermann reaction, soon showed signs of paresis, which became more pronounced in 1917 and which increased until his death, in 1919. Early in 1918, he presented patches in the oral mucosa which the author diagnosed as secondary manifestations.

There is a review of the European literature on this subject.

MONILETHRIX. GOLAY, Ann. de dermat. et syph. 6:294, 1922.

The author has made a thorough study of this condition as it appeared in a girl, aged 5 years, in whom it had been present since birth. After reviewing the literature he gives the results of his own investigations, with the following conclusions: The lengths of the enlarged portions of the hairs and of the narrowed parts are not always absolutely identical. The alternation of growth and impediment proceed with a daily rhythm, the former occurring by day, and the latter by night, as the author has clearly shown histologically. Diminution of pigment corresponds with impairment of the growth, and it therefore begins beyond the middle of the enlarged portion, continuing up to the middle of the narrowed part, beyond which point the pigment is more plentiful as the power of growth reappears. For good reasons the author favors a theory of endocrine etiology for the condition, which may simply be an exaggeration of the normal.

AN ERYTHEMATOPAPULAR DERMATITIS IN PLAQUES, OF INTERNAL CAUSATION, DUE TO THE APPLICATION OF A VESICATORY. JEANSELME and BLAMOUTIER, Ann. de dermat. et syph. 6:321 (July) 1922.

A woman, aged 44, presented a symmetrical eruption of papulo-erythematous plaques on the legs, forearms and buttocks, itching and burning, six days after the application of a cantharides plaster to the lumbar region. It disappeared in a week. Eruptions from the systemic effects of cantharides have never been reported, but the authors believe that in this case the possibility of other causative factors can fairly well be excluded.

THE SYPHILITIC SYNDROME OF THE INCISOR BONE. J. NICOLAS, G. MASSIA and D. DUPASQUIER, Ann. de dermat. et syph. 6:323, 1922.

The embryology of the incisor bone is given in detail; it is destined to support the four upper incisor teeth. Syphilis often affects it, congenital syphilis giving rise to dystrophic changes, productive of Hutchinson's teeth and other dental malformations, usually limited to the incisors, and possibly also to harelip. The lesions appearing after birth, due either to congenital or acquired syphilis, are tertiary in character, the resultant tumefaction, ulceration and sinuses involving the anterior palate, the gum and the nose, the frequency being in the order mentioned. Sequestrums may be discharged, but in any case antisyphilitic treatment is to be used first, and surgery only as a matter of last resort, for the removal of lingering sequestrums and the remedy of cosmetic defects. Nineteen cases of tertiary syphilis of this bone are described, three of which were personally observed by the authors.

INTRAVENOUS INJECTIONS OF SODIUM SALICYLATE IN THE TREATMENT OF PSORIASIS. R. LUTEMBACHER. Ann. de dermat. et syph. 6:362, 1922.

In a case of rebellious generalized psoriasis, sodium salicylate was injected daily in the dose of 3 gm. dissolved in 80 c.c. of distilled water. On the eighth day of treatment, the first improvement was noted, and after five weeks the entire eruption had disappeared. A specially purified salicylate was used.

Otto Sachs has reported a similar result (*Wien. klin. Wchnschr.*, April 21, 1921).

THE SPONTANEOUS CURE OF LICHEN PLANUS DURING THE COURSE OF DIPHTHERIA. PAYENNEVILLE and TROTABAS. Ann. de dermat. et syph. 6:364, 1922.

In a young soldier, diphtheria supervened a few days after the onset of a generalized eruption of typical lichen planus, and the eruption rapidly disappeared, leaving no pigmentation.

PSEUDO-ELEPHANTIASTIC CONGENITAL TUMORS OF THE NUCHA. P. Noel, Ann. de dermat. et syph. **6**:366, 1922.

In an African negro soldier, aged 32, there were three cutaneous movable tumors between the nucha and the shoulders, on each side, arranged with exact symmetry. They had been present since infancy.

PRECOCIOUS MALIGNANT SYPHILIS TREATED BY BISMUTH. Tzanck, Bull. Soc. franç. de dermat. et syph. **29**:197, 1922.

At the meeting of Feb. 9, 1922, reported in a recent Bulletin, a patient was presented with a stomatitis which some thought to be due to the medication. However, it subsequently disappeared under continued treatment, and is therefore considered to have been syphilitic.

ROENTGENOGRAM SHOWING PERSISTENCE OF METALLIC DEPOSITS IN GLUTEAL REGION SEVERAL YEARS AFTER INJECTION OF UNKNOWN PRODUCTS (IODIDS OR MERCURY). C. Simon, Bull. Soc. franç. de dermat. et syph. **29**:198, 1922.

There is an illustration clearly showing the presence of aggregated opaque globules.

SERODIAGNOSIS OF SYPHILIS: FLOCCULATION PROCEDURES. Rubinstein (Leredde), Bull. Soc. franç. de dermat. et syph. **29**:201, 1922.

Various procedures, including that devised by Vernes, are reviewed and criticized. Comparative tests were made with 538 serums. The author concludes that the methods of Sachs-Georgi, Meinicke and Dold can be used only in company with the Bordet-Wassermann reaction, for their results are not always specific and their sensibility is insufficient. They cannot be used alone with safety.

PRESENTATION OF A BISMUTH COMPOUND FOR INTRAVENOUS INJECTION: THE FIRST RESULTS. Lacapere and Galliot, Bull. Soc. franç. de dermat. et syph. **29**:210, 1922.

A colloidal bismuth suspension is employed, a series of from twenty to twenty-five injections being given at the rate of three a week. The product is heated on a water-bath and then cooled before being administered. In a series of thirty cases thus treated, excellent results were obtained and the drug was well borne. Stomatitis seems to be far less frequent than with the intramuscular method, possibly because the drug is sooner eliminated when given intravenously. It is recommended for use in cases in which arsphenamin is not tolerated.

NORMAL CEREBROSPINAL FLUID IN A CASE OF PITYRIASIS ROSEA. C. Simon, Bull. Soc. franç. de dermat. et syph. **29**:210, 1922.

These findings, in one case, are presented as a matter of record.

A CASE OF GRANULOMA ANNULARE. Burnier and Rejsek, Bull. Soc. franç. de dermat. et syph. **29**:218, 1922.

The lesions in a girl aged 16 had first appeared three years previously, being located on the forearms and on the dorsum of the left hand. The areas on the forearms, especially, were not suggestive of granuloma annulare so much as of dermatophytosis, but histologic study revealed their nature. Following the biopsies the lesions temporarily disappeared. The patient showed signs of tuberculosis.

A CASE OF LICHEN PLANUS OF THE THORAX PROVOKED BY CUPPING. Burnier, Bull. Soc. franç. de dermat. et syph. **29**:222, 1922.

A man, aged 50, with no history of a previous similar eruption, presented himself with typical annular lichen planus lesions at sites where cupping had been performed. There was a concomitant lichen planus eruption in the oral mucosa.

RESULTS OBTAINED IN SYPHILIS BY AMINO-ARSENO-PHENOL (132). Lepinay, Bull. Soc. franç. de dermat. et syph. **29**:222, 1922.

In a series of thirty-five cases, sixty-eight intravenous and 241 intramuscular injections were given. Intravenously, ten injections were given, at seven day intervals, a total dosage of 2 to 2.5 gm. being reached. By the intramuscular method, the intervals were four or five days, and twelve to fourteen injections were given, making a total of 2.87 to 3.5 gm. of the drug. It is apparently no more toxic than the arsphenamins, and seems quite as effective in treatment. The results from its intramuscular use are said to be fully as rapid as those following intravenous administration, although it is more slowly eliminated thus, and its intramuscular use is tolerated by those who cannot stand intravenous medication.

THE STEPS OF SYPHILIMETRY. Vernes. Travaux et Publications de l'Institute Prophylactique, Paris, Pt. 1: 1, 1922.

The author presents ten of his articles, published since 1913, dealing with the theory and practice of the serologic test which bears his name and which has been so well described by Cornwall in a recent number of the Archives (**5**:433 [April] 1922). The last article, published in the *Presse médicale* for Dec. 3, 1921, after the completion of Cornwall's paper, describes a new and superior method of measurement called "photometrie" whereby the density of the suspension is accurately measured by optical means: this supplants the colorimetric method formerly advocated.

By a thorough perusal of this publication a good working knowledge of this test should be gained. According to the author, it offers a constant reliable gage which is very helpful in controlling treatment, which is thereby rendered more effective; the patient's confidence is stimulated, and the question of permitting marriage is more readily and safely settled.

Parkhurst, Toledo, Ohio.

HISTOPATHOLOGY OF PITYRIASIS VERSICOLOR. P. A. Meineri. Gior. Ital. mal. ven. **63**:755 (June) 1922.

Eight cases of pityriasis versicolor have been histologically studied by the author. The stratum corneum appears thickened and loosely attached to the subjacent stratum lucidum. The microsporum furfur is found only in the stratum corneum and especially in its middle and outer layers. The stratum of Malphigi presents intracellular and intercellular edema and a slight infiltration of leukocytes. In old cases some small microscopic vesicles may be found. There is an increase of pigment in the basal layer. The corium presents a vascular dilatation, numerous proliferating cells, especially around the vessels, and granules of pigment in small groups. The article is illustrated by four photomicrographs.

THREE CASES OF SYPHILITIC REINFECTION. P. MINASSIAN, Gior. Ital. mal. ven. **63**:809 (June) 1922.

This article contains a report of three cases of a second chancre and secondary infection after apparent cure of a first attack of syphilis treated with calomel and arsphenamin.

BISMUTH PREPARATIONS IN THE TREATMENT OF SYPHILIS. A. PASINI, Gior. Ital. mal. ven. **63**:814 (June) 1922.

Pasini has used the tartrobismuthate of potassium and sodium and the citro-bismuthate of sodium. Thirty-one cases of syphilis in its different stages were treated. The injections were given intramuscularly every second day, the amount of the salt being from 0.2 to 0.3 gm. to 1 c.c. of oil. A total of twelve injections comprises a course of treatment, which is followed by a second and sometimes by a third course. After the second or third dose the spirochetes disappear from the chancre and mucous patches. Healing occurs rapidly, but the papular and infiltrated lesions are somewhat slow to respond to the treatment. The Wassermann test remains positive even after several courses of twelve injections. The greatest disadvantage is the sometimes very severe stomatitis which these bismuth preparations produce. The bismuth salts are powerful spirocheticides but are inferior to the arsenicals.

THE TREATMENT OF SYPHILIS WITH BISMUTH SALTS. A. DE BELLA, Gior. Ital. mal. ven. **63**:827 (June) 1922.

The preparation used in the author's eight cases was the tartrobismuthate of potassium and sodium. He reports fairly good clinical results. The Herxheimer reaction occurred in two cases. The Wassermann test remains positive after prolonged treatment. The author concludes that the bismuth salts are useful antisyphilitics but cannot take the place of arsphenamin.

BISMUTH IN THE THERAPY OF SYPHILIS. G. DEFINE, Gior. Ital. mal. ven. **63**:834 (June) 1922.

The tartrobismuthate of sodium and potassium was useful in a case in which arsenic and mercury had failed. There was no improvement in a case of paresis.

SYPHILITIC FEVER. Z. ARMANDO, Riforma med. **38**:697 (July) 1922.

Syphilitic fever may appear during the secondary stage of the disease and is probably a toxic phenomenon. It may occur in the late or tertiary stage, usually in connection with visceral or nervous syphilitic disease. It may be intermittent, continuous or irregular. The author reports a case with localized bronchopneumonia, hypertrophy of the spleen and liver and intermittent fever of malarial type. The Wassermann test was strongly positive. The patient made an uneventful recovery under mercury and arsphenamin.

PROPHYLAXIS OF ARSPHENAMIN ACCIDENTS. A. FONTANA, Riforma med. **38**:699 (July) 1922.

Fontana considers the injection of epinephrin superior to atropin and to the previous injection of a small amount of the arsenical, in the prevention of arsphenamin reactions. He advises thoroughly mixing the blood with the solution in the syringe and injecting very slowly. In cases of malignant syphilis and when there is intolerance to the drug, the previous application of mercury may avoid serious reactions. He considers the Milian sign (arsenical conjunctivitis) of value as indicative of impending trouble if more arsphenamin is used.

MALIGNANT LYMPHOGRANULOMA. G. CASTALDI, Riforma med. **38**: 795 (Aug.) 1922.

Since 1898, when Sternberg described this disease of the hemopoietic system the opinions have been divided as to its etiology; some believing that the condition is due to tuberculosis, while others believe that it is caused by an undetermined virus. The author reports two cases of typical lymphogranulomatosis with Sternberg cells in the glands and the spleen and small granular infiltrations of the liver. No trace of tuberculosis could be found in these cases. Bacteriologic examinations and experimental inoculations in animals were all negative for Koch's bacilli. Castaldi concludes that "the epidemiology, the pathology, the clinical and the experimental pathology are against its tuberculous nature and that malignant lymphogranuloma is a morbid entity with a definite clinical physiognomy."

A CASE OF EARLY SEVERE SYPHILIS. ITALO LEVY, Riforma med. **38**: 800 (Aug.) 1922.

Report is made of a case of serpiginous ulcerations of the face and destruction of the soft palate. The destructive lesions appeared ten months after the chancre. The patient had no specific treatment before.

RECKLINGHAUSEN'S DISEASE. M. ACUÑA and F. BAZAN. Prensa med. Argentina **9**:12 (June) 1922.

Two cases of this disease are reported in children 11 and 12 years of age, respectively. In the first case there was a history of hereditary syphilis, positive Wassermann reaction and symptoms of hypothyroidism. The second patient was mentally defective. The authors think that Recklinghausen's disease may be the result of certain endocrine disturbances.

PARDO-CASTELLO, Havana, Cuba.

A CASE OF PITYRIASIS AMIANTACEA. B. LUDOVICI. Dermat. Wchnschr **74**:153 (Feb. 18) 1922.

A case of this rare and severe form of seborrhea sicca capitis is described, in which, besides the familiar minute scale formation, the shedding of the entire follicular orifice occurs, in such a manner that the latter is taken along as a cuff by the hair in its growth. Some of these cuffs rise as high as 2 mm above the level of the scalp.

REPRESENTATION OF SCHREUS REGARDING THE AUTHOR'S INVESTIGATIONS OF STOMATITIS MERCURIALIS ULCEROSA. J. ALMKVIST, Dermat. Wchnschr. **74**:155 (Feb. 18) 1922.

The author contradicts statements ascribed to him by Dr. H. Schreus, in an article entitled, "A Way to Prevent and Treat Mercurial Stomatitis" (*Dermat. Wchnschr.* **73**:1270, 1921). The bacteria which are causative factors in ulcerative mercurial stomatitis and colitis are not specific micro-organisms, but various putrefactive forms. Their rôle is fulfilled in two ways: first, by a local erosion from hydrogen sulphid, and second, by local resorption, producing together with the mercury in the connective tissue, a connective tissue necrosis. The mercury in the walls of the capillaries is precipitated intracellularly as mercuric sulphid by action of the resorbed hydrogen sulphid. The author recommends disinfection of all bacterial foci in the buccal cavity as the best prophylactic procedure.

TREATMENT AND PREVENTION OF MERCURIAL STOMATITIS. F. HAMMER. Dermat. Wchnschr. **74**:158 (Feb. 18) 1922.

The author recommends from 10 to 20 per cent. of chromic acid applied to the teeth, gums and tonsils with a wooden applicator. Although the treatment is painful, it effectually destroys the putrefactive micro-organisms causing the affection.

MULTIPLE SKIN LESIONS IN FUNCTIONAL ANESTHESIA. E. PICK, Dermat. Wchnschr. **74**:177 (Feb. 25) 1922.

The fact that multiple ulcers occur in nervous and hysterical persons under the aspect of neurotic gangrene, is well recognized; but the question whether the lesions are spontaneously trophoneurotic or artificially produced, is frequently difficult to answer. A case is described occurring in a middle-aged man, who was burned with hot metal on the dorsum of the right hand during routine work in an iron foundry. An ulcer resulted which required three months to heal. Two weeks after the healing was complete, erythematous spots appeared on the forearm. These later became vesicular and ulcerated. There was an accompanying complete anesthesia for touch, pain and temperature of the right arm and hand. This anesthesia and the skin lesions disappeared quickly after slight faradization.

A CASE OF LEUKODERMA IN PITYRIASIS LICHENOIDES CHRONICA. J. ALMKVIST, Dermat. Wchnschr. **74**:201 (March 4) 1922.

Pityriasis lichenoides chronica (Juliusberg). or dermatitis psoriatiformis nodularis (Neisser-Jadassohn), as well as syphilis, psoriasis, and seborrheic eczema. produces leukoderma. A case is described in which the leukodermic spots were generalized and appeared on the sites of the preceding eruption of pityriasis lichenoides chronica.

TECHNIC OF EMPLOYING RADIUM AND MESOTHORIUM IN DERMATOLOGY. W. BRINCKMANN, Dermat. Wchnschr. **74**:204 (March 4) 1922.

The following factors form a basis for technic: The quantity of the radium or mesothorium expressed in milligrams of radium bromid: (1) the extent of surface which is covered by this quantity, (2) the kind and thickness of the filter, (3) the duration of the exposure, and (4) if the first three factors are constant, the last is simply a matter of experience.

A CASE OF UNILATERAL LINEAR PSORIASIS. J. Stangenberg, Dermat. Wchnschr. **74**:210 (March 4) 1922.

The case is described with illustrations, the eruption being segmentally arranged in a manner simulating herpes zoster.

A NEW ELECTRICAL ACCESSORY APPARATUS, "WIGOSTAT TRANSFORMER." T. Benedek, Dermat. Wchnschr. **74**:225 (March 11) 1922.

The apparatus consists of an oxidized wire resistance, rolled on porcelain and polished at its points of contact. Along these, bilaterally arranged, and located in the middle third of the wire, are two sliding springs which may be approximated or separated by means of a spindle with halves of opposite winding. In this manner the length of the resistance wire between the sliding springs may be continually changed. The two springs are connected by metal with two clamps on the outside of the apparatus. In addition the beginning and end of the entire resistance wire lead to two clamps carefully insulated by hard rubber.

THE BILIRUBIN CONTENT OF BLOOD SERUM DURING TREATMENT WITH MERCURY AND ARSPHENAMIN. P. Schneider. Dermat. Wchnschr. **74**:228 (March 11) 1922. (*Continued.*)

After numerous investigations, the author concludes that the bilirubin content is increased in nearly all cases at the beginning of treatment, but that it approaches normal as the treatment progresses.

THE BILIRUBIN CONTENT OF BLOOD SERUM DURING TREATMENT WITH MERCURY AND ARSPHENAMIN. P. Schneider. Dermat. Wchnschr. **74**:250 (March 18) 1922. (*Concluded.*)

Further investigations support the conclusions given in the preceding article. A disturbance of the functions of the liver by the disease or its treatment may account for the augmentation of the serum bilirubin.

COMBINED PRECIPITATION (SIMULTANEOUS SACHS - GEORGI - MEINECKE REACTION). Stern and Evening. Dermat. Wchnschr. **74**: 235 (March 11) 1922.

For the mixture of both extracts distilled water is used as follows (0.5 Sachs-Georgi reaction plus 0.5 Meinecke reaction plus 5.0 distilled water), while the serums are diluted with 2 per cent. sodium chlorid solution. To 0.2 inactivated serum add 0.8 of 2 per cent. sodium chlorid; shake well; add 0.5 cm. of the extract mixture; let it stand for two hours in the water-bath and eighteen hours at room temperature, and read in agglutinoscope.

An examination of 1,500 serums was made. As some Wassermann positive syphilitic serums did not give precipitation, negative precipitation reactions were considered indeterminate.

CUTIS *GYRATA* OF THE FOREHEAD. A. Stuehmer, Dermat. Wchnschr. **74**:249 (March 18) 1922.

The patient, a boy aged 19, had noticed the gradual development of the condition since he had a trauma ten years before. Simultaneously a similar lesion evolved on the occiput. They were asymptomatic. All other findings were normal. There was a deep sagittal furrow between two convolutions on the forehead with symmetrically arranged furrows and convolutions on either side of it. Some of these did not follow the natural lines of wrinkling produced by muscular action.

DERMATITIS FROM SUBSTITUTES FOR TURPENTINE. Galewsky, Dermat. Wchnschr. **74**:273 (March 25) 1922.

Four cases of occupational dermatitis in painters due to the use of substitute products for turpentine are reported. There were no unusual features in the eruptions.

MULTIPLE SOFT WARTS OF THE BUCCAL MUCOSA. E. Stern, Dermat. Wchnschr. **74**:274 (March 25) 1922.

Numerous rounded, pinhead sized soft verrucae were present on the inner surfaces of the lips and in the corners of the mouth of a 14 year old girl. There were no other warts on other parts of the body.

CHANCRE OF THE URETHRA. G. Gjorgjevic, Dermat. Wchnschr. **74**: 276 (March 25) 1922.

Six cases of intra-urethral chancre are presented. Five were in men and one was in a woman. The findings were confirmed by dark-field examination.

THE CAUTERY NEEDLE AS A THERAPEUTIC AND COSMETIC INSTRUMENT. A. Pokorny, Dermat. Wchnschr. **74**:297 (April) 1922.

This instrument is recommended for the treatment of telangiectases, nevus flammeus, angiomas and small pigmented nevi on the face. The author says that keloids do not appear subsequent to this method of treatment.

MY ACTIVATED WASSERMANN METHOD IN *SYPHILIS*. H. Hecht, Dermat. Wchnschr. **74**:300 (April) 1922.

A description of the author's technic and results is presented, using an activated serum.

Andrews, New *York*.

SYPHILITIC ORCHITIS SIMULATING A NEW GROWTH. M. Zeissl, Wien. klin. Wchnschr. **34**:583, 1921.

This is a report of a patient who had been under observation for a number of years. The differential diagnosis of syphilitic involvement of the testicle and new growth is given.

CONSIDERATION OF THE INTRAVENOUS TREATMENT OF PERSISTENT PRURITIC DERMATITIS. Maximilian Strassberg, Wien. klin. Wchnschr. **34**:595, 1921.

In addition to numerous local applications, the author has found the intravenous introduction of autoserum effective. About 100 c.c. of blood are drawn from the vein, allowed to remain at room temperature for three or four hours, and then kept in the icebox for from twelve to twenty hours. The serum is reinjected about twenty-four hours after it had been withdrawn. The injection is repeated at intervals of three or four days. Urticaria, weeping eczema and pruritus senilis have been influenced favorably by this treatment. In addition to autoserum therapy, the use of whole blood has been given a trial In every instance there has been marked relief when this procedure was tried in cases of itchy diseases of the skin. Blood was also withdrawn up to 100 c.c., and replaced with physiologic sodium chlorid solution, but the result was poor. The question of ions in the blood and their effect on the nerves must be considered in this regard.

SECOND INFECTION WITH SYPHILIS WITHIN FIVE YEARS OF THE CURE OF THE FIRST BY STERILISATIO MAGNA. MAXIMILIAN ZEISSL, Wien klin. Wchnschr. **34**:596, 1921.

A student was infected with syphilis in July, 1910. *Spirochaeta pallida* was demonstrated and the Wassermann reaction was positive. He received but one dose of arsphenamin intramuscularly. No secondaries were observed up to July, 1911, despite inspection every other day. The Wassermann reaction was last positive late in 1910. In 1915, the reaction was negative. In January, 1915, after an incubation period of eight weeks, the patient reported with a new infection. *Spirochaeta pallida* was found and the Wassermann reaction was positive. One injection of arsphenamin intramuscularly did not inhibit the secondaries. Despite other treatment, the course of syphilis with this infection was extended.

A NEW METHOD OF INJECTING TUBERCULIN IN WIDESPREAD SKIN TUBERCULOSIS. MAXIMILIAN STRASSBERG, Wien. klin. Wchnschr. **35**:54 (Jan. 19) 1922.

The author uses the dose of O. T. (old tuberculin) to be injected, but dilutes it so as to permit multiple injections locally about the lesions of tuberculosis of the skin. The local reaction of the introduced O. T. has about fifty sites of injection at which to act, and in addition the general reaction need not be different from that of the same dose injected at one place. Of course, only a part of the sum total of reactions can be produced at any one site of injection of the diluted O. T.

IS THERE AN ACTUAL NATURAL RESISTANCE TO SYPHILIS? OBSERVATIONS ON PROSTITUTES. ROBERT BRANDT. Wien. klin. Wchnschr. **35**:223 (March 9) 1922.

A study of a group of· prostitutes for a period of years has shown that. despite every possibility of infection, some of them did not become infected with syphilis until many years of their professional life had elapsed. In the interim, repeated examinations had disclosed no lesions nor serologic evidence of the disease. The women were of the lowest level of professional prostitutes and had undoubtedly been exposed repeatedly to infection.

REMARKS CONCERNING THE CONTRIBUTION OF BUSACCA. ENTITLED, "A NEW INTRACUTANEOUS REACTION IN SKIN TUBERCULOSIS." VJEKOSLAV KUSAN. Wien. klin. Wchnschr. **35**:248 (March 16) 1922.

The use of horse serum for the diagnosis of tuberculosis in human beings is held not to be a reliable test. Such positive reactions as have been reported are conceived to have been due to trauma.

REPLY TO THE REMARKS OF DR. KUSAN. Attilio Busacca, Wien. klin. Wchnschr. **35**:248 (March 16) 1922.

The number of cases on which Kusan bases his conclusions is too small for definite ideas. The factor of traumatism has been properly controlled by injection of warm Ringer's solution in a series of cases taken from Finger's clinic. There were three positive results among forty-one patients with various diseases of the skin. It is interesting that the diagnosis of these three included two cases of lupus vulgaris, and one of lupus erythematosus.

CONTRIBUTION TO THE STUDY OF DERMATITIS OF ARSPHEN-AMIN OR MERCURY OCCURRING DURING THE TREATMENT OF SYPHILIS. Josef Klaar, Wien. klin. Wchnschr. **35**:266, 1922.

In the five-year period of 1916-1921, thirty-four cases of dermatitis due to arsphenamin or mercury have been observed, of which five were brought to the hospital after having treatment elsewhere. There were nineteen patients who had combination mercury and arsphenamin courses; two patients who had had only silver arsphenamin; three patients who had had injections of neo-arsphenamin only; and ten who had had injections of mirion and neo-arsphenamin. The mirion-treated patients, who did not receive arsphenamin, never showed any dermatitis; hence the author absolves this drug from being the cause of the dermatitis. In addition to the classic dermatologic picture, many patients presented edema of the face, loss of weight, hemorrhages, stomatitis, albuminuria, alopecia, enteritis, vulvitis, pyoderma, melanoderma, paronychia, conjunctivitis or pneumonia. The secretion of sweat and sebum is diminished. The loss of hair and nails that may occur is probably due to some disturbance of internal secretion, as evidenced by the occurrence also of disturbances of menstruation.

In individual cases, it is impossible to determine whether the mercury or the arsphenamin has caused the ill-effects.

CONTRIBUTION TO THE STUDY OF ARSPHENAMIN AND MERCURY DERMATITIS OCCURRING DURING THE TREATMENT OF SYPHILIS. Josef Klaar, Wien. klin. Wchnschr. **35**:297, 1922. (*Concluded.*)

A number of cases came to necropsy. In general, it may be said that failure of the heart could be the cause of death. Pneumonia may have been a complication in a youthful individual who died, but he also showed a degenerated heart muscle. Necrotic inflammatory changes in the small and large intestine was present in another case. The mechanism of the dermatitis has not been unfolded by the necropsy studies. The parenchymatous changes of the liver, thought possibly to be of etiologic significance, can just as readily be secondary changes. Patients who have passed through a severe dermatitis may have the Wassermann reaction reversed to negative, and may show no symptoms of syphilis later. The reports of some authors on the favorable influence of fever-exciting injections (milk, typhoid vaccine) are similar in this respect. It is noted that the number of women with dermatitis was about five times greater than the number of men.

EDEMA OF THE TONGUE AFTER MIRION INJECTIONS. N. Nander, Wien. klin. Wchnschr. **35**:296, 1922.

A patient with tabes dorsalis, after numerous courses of mercury and arsphenamin was put on a course of mirion and arsphenamin. After a number of injections of both, his tongue became so edematous that he was unable to talk or eat. The edema did not encroach on the glottis, but did spread to the submaxillary regions. Although the aspect seemed grave enough, within two hours the parts became normal in size, and the edema had disappeared. Although the patient has since received a number of neo-arsphenamin injections, no sign of the edema has returned. It is thought that this swelling was a sign of severe iodism.

EXPERIMENTS WITH SODIUM NUCLEINATE IN THE TREATMENT OF PARESIS WITH MALARIA. Heinrich Kogerer, Wien. klin. Wchnschr. **35**:342, 1922.

In the treatment of paresis at the Vienna Psychiatric Institute with the injection of malarial parasites, one had to determine a cure of the malaria before discharging the patients. After tests of the blood had been negative following treatment of the induced malaria by quinin and neo-arsphenamin, the blood was examined after roentgen irradiation of the spleen. Later, the use of injections of sodium nucleinate, 5 c.c. of a 10 per cent. solution, was found to be more efficacious. In a series of twenty-five patients, three gave positive blood smears after this injection, and continued treatment of the experimental malaria was instituted. It has been shown, too, that experimental malaria is much easier to cure than the malaria ordinarily induced by the bite of the anopheles.

PRACTICAL EXPERIENCE WITH THE SIGNIFICANCE OF THE GUM BENZOIN REACTION ON THE CEREBROSPINAL FLUID. Fritz Mars, Wien. klin. Wchnschr. **35**:417, 1922.

This reaction is to be recommended as it is cheap, easy of preparation and, in a series of cases, has seemed of value in the determination of disease condition. The reaction has been paralleled with the gold sol reaction. The report of this experiment is in course of preparation.

A NEW INTRACUTANEOUS REACTION IN SYPHILIS. Attilia Busacca, Wien. klin. Wchnschr. **35**:523, 1922.

During his experiments with horse serum intracutaneous reactions in tuberculosis, the author made some experiments with gelatin in the same way. A 10 per cent. sterilized solution of gelatin (Merck) was used. In tuberculosis, the positive reaction was present in only 45 per cent. of the cases, a percentage too small to be of use in diagnosis. In syphilis, on the contrary, 71 per cent. of the patients gave a positive reaction with the gelatin, and the patients in the primary stage, sclerosis without exanthem, gave a positive reaction in twenty-seven of twenty-nine instances. The Wassermann reaction was positive in only twenty of this series. In the secondary cases, however, the gelatin reaction was positive in only ninety-five of 149 cases, and the Wassermann reaction was positive in all except nine.

If the horse serum reaction and the gelatin reaction were positive in the same case, the diagnosis of tuberculosis was assured.

The value of the test in early primary syphilis seems to be great, especially in the light of the possibility of abortive treatment. Goodman. New York.

PUNCTURE OF GLANDS AND ITS SIGNIFICANCE IN THE DIAGNOSIS OF SYPHILIS. V. Sedlak, Ceska dermat. **3**:201, 1922.

Puncture of indurated glands resulted in the finding of spirochetes in fifty
... eighteen

out of twenty-one cases in the secondary stage. The puncture seems to be of great diagnostic significance, especially in cases of chancres negative for spirochetes—treated or inaccessible (phimosis)—and while the Wassermann reaction is yet negative. A positive gland puncture may decide the diagnosis in time for abortive treatment.

EXPERIMENTS ON DIFFUSION OF COMPLEMENT. J. Kabelik, Ceska dermat. **3**:211 and 233, 1922.

To study the conditions which influence the diffusion of complement the author superimposed various strengths of complement in the test tubes on thin agar (1 to 0.125 per cent.) to which he added as indicator highly sensitized red corpuscles. His experiments led to the following results: The more concentrated and stronger was the complement, the more sensitized were the corpuscles, the smaller was the number of corpuscles used and the less concentrated was the agar, the greater was the thickness of the hemolyzed · layer. The diffusion of complement was the most rapid at the beginning of the experiment; it became slower rapidly and ceased on the third day by inactivation of complement. Analogous experiments on the diffusion of other substances tend to lead to the opinion that the colloid particles of proteins which carry the complement quality of serum are larger in colloid particles of simple serous proteins.

CUTANEOUS TUBERCULIN REACTIONS IN SKIN TUBERCULOSIS. K. Hubschmann, Ceska dermat. **3**:246, 1922.

The author obtained a positive cutaneous reaction in forty-five cases of various forms of skin tuberculosis (thirty-two of lupus vulgaris). His experiences disagree with the statement of Wolff-Eisner that in lupus a negative reaction is relatively common. Curshmann found more cases giving a positive reaction with bovine tuberculin than with human virus, while Kretschmer's experience was just the reverse. The author did not have a single case giving a positive reaction with one tuberculin and a negative one with the other.

INTRAMUSCULAR INJECTIONS OF NEO-ARSPHENAMIN "GLUCO 914" IN THE TREATMENT OF SYPHILIS. A. Meska, Ceska dermat. · **3**:250, 1922.

This preparation put up by Robert and Carrière, Paris, is recommended for cases in which for some reason or other the intravenous injection cannot be used. The neo-arsphenamin is dissolved in glucose and comes in convenient syringe ampules ready for use. The method is simple and almost painless. Good results of treatment combined with mercury are reported.

PRIMARY CHANCRE OF THE EYELID. Professor Deyl. Ceska dermat. **3**:258, 1922.

A young pregnant woman (five months) presented a painless, cartilaginous, purple-red induration of the right upper eyelid with papulosquamous brownish red lesions on the forehead, falling out of the eyebrows and lashes. The Wassermann reaction was four plus. Genital examination was negative for syphilis. There were no traces of other primary syphilitic lesions on the body. The unusual features of this case are: (1) the lack of a typical primary ulcer—the lesion on the eyelid being without ulceration, and (2) the lack of submental or preauricular adenopathy; there' were a few enlarged posterior cervical glands and one above the clavicle. The findings cleared up in four months under combined treatment. The patient gave birth to a healthy child. The article contains a detailed differential diagnosis, especially the exclusion of tarsitis syphilitica.

EXPERIENCES WITH THE DOLD PRECIPITATION REACTION.
M. DZINBAN, Ceska dermat. **3**:273, 1922.

The author used Dold's original technic in 600 cases and compared the results with those of the Wassermann and Sachs-Georgi reactions. They ran parallel in 92.83 per cent. of cases; in 98.16 per cent. Dold and Sachs-Georgi agreed; Wassermann and Dold reactions agreed in 90 per cent. on early reading and in 93.3 per cent. on late reading of precipitation. To shorten the time of the reaction the author in some cases centrifuged the serum and the antigen, which had been previously incubated from one to two hours. In strongly positive cases the results could be interpreted in five, ten or fifteen minutes. When results were doubtful the author added the complement and the hemolytic system to settle the question, as according to Gaehtgens and Salvioli only specific precipitates hinder hemolysis.

SPINKA, St. Louis.

Society Transactions

URTICARIA PIGMENTOSA. (From the University Clinic.) Presented by
Dr. MICHELSON.

A baby, aged 4 months, for the last two and a half months had shown a
yellowish and brownish-yellow macular eruption located on the trunk and
face. The lesions varied in size from 0.5 to 0.75 cm. in diameter. There was
no scratching, therefore it was concluded that the lesions did not itch. The
baby gained steadily in weight and its general health was perfect. Rubbing
the lesions produced some edema. There was no marked dermographismus.
Biopsy revealed a slight infiltration in the papillary layer. A few mast cells
were noted in the infiltrate, but the infiltrate was not pure mast cells.

MILTOY'S DISEASE. Presented by Dr. MICHELSON.

Miss F., aged 19, born in Minnesota and never out of the state, whose
general health was excellent, said that since birth the left leg had been much
larger than the right. It had never been painful except when injured, and
then it healed slowly. She said that no other member of her family was
afflicted with the same condition. On examination it was noted that the left
leg was 4 inches (10.16 cm.) greater in circumference than the right at the
middle of the calf, and that the swelling was of a doughy character and did
not pit on pressure. The enlargement extended to the groin. There was no
history of febrile attacks or of general disturbance.

CHELITIS GLANDULARIS APOSTEOMATOSA. Presented by DRS.
BUTLER and ODLAND.

A man, aged 74, a retired paint merchant, had had this condition for eight
years. The lower lip was greatly thickened, edematous and everted, and
studded with hemp seed size glistening drops of secretion which had formed
at the orifices of the mucous glands. He gave a history of chronic nasal catarrh.

A CASE FOR DIAGNOSIS (HYPODERMATIC NODULES). (From the
University Clinic.) Presented by Dr. MICHELSON.

Mr. M., a tailor, aged 46, married, who had no children or history of miscarriage in the family, said that he had had a penile sore twenty-five years
ago. There was no history or signs of syphilis. Six months before he
developed two nodules under the skin in the region of the right thigh. They
became painful and after two months discharged pus for several weeks; they
have since healed completely, leaving ordinary scars. The scars did not sug-

gest those which follow gumma. During the last four months several other nodules have developed in the same region. The nodules were apparently deep in the hypoderm and freely movable, and were more easily discerned when the patient was standing erect. They seemed to disappear when he was lying on his side. The periosteum over the trochanter was thickened and rough, but the nodules were not adherent to the bone. Biopsy revealed a chronic, rather diffuse, infiltration of the hypoderm, which was not characteristic of either tuberculosis or syphilis. There was a marked thickening of the blood vessel walls and a profuse polymorphous infiltrate about the vessels and in the pars adiposa. The Wassermann test was negative. The patient was reported for clinical diagnosis of the tumors mentioned.

DISCUSSION

Dr. Ormsby: I worked for some time in London, and during that time we did a great deal of work among tuberculous children. One type of lesion was characterized by a subcutaneous nodule which enlarged, ulcerated and discharged. Then it would heal and a new nodule would form, and the process would be repeated. Before I saw the slide or Dr. Michelson's diagnosis, I had decided that this was a case of scrofuloderma.

In relation to tuberculosis of the hypoderm of Wende, I think that it shows that Wende's case may have been a sarcoid.

Dr. Michelson: Scrofuloderma is a frequent form of tuberculosis of the skin, especially in children. It is often seen in the European clinics. It begins with a deep nodule in the cutis without signs of inflammation, gradually extends into the skin, becomes bluish red, softens and ulcerates. It may originate in glands, bone or the lymphatics of the hypoderm. The nodular tuberculosis as described by Wende is a different condition. In the treatment of tuberculosis of the skin one must take into consideration the type with which we are dealing, whether it is primary or secondary; the prognosis is also guided by the classification.

SCROFULODERMA COLLIQUATIVA. Presented by Dr. Sweitzer.

A. G., a woman, aged 38, single, born in the United States, was seen in April, 1922, with a soft, easily bleeding patch on her right cheek. The patient said that she had had abscess glands in the neck when 16 years old. The present illness started in August, 1921, with the appearance of a small papule on the cheek. The disease spread slowly, and in October, 1921. the patch was the size of a dime. She had been treated with the sun lamp with no apparent benefit. A section taken in April, 1922, showed tuberculosis. Treatment with acid mercuric nitrate was started, and healing has been rapid.

KERATODERMA MACULOSA SYMMETRICA PALMARIS AND PLANTARIS. Presented by Dr. Sweitzer.

M. A., a woman, aged 33, was seen in June, 1922. The patient had numerous small, hard, horny, papular lesions on the palms and soles. The palms were not as extensively involved as the soles; there were numerous small, yellow, horny papules on both heels. Many of the lesions had a small central depression. The condition on the palms and soles had been present since childhood, and the patient's father and one brother were similarly affected.

EPITHELIOMA OF THE CHEEK IN LUPUS ERYTHEMATOSUS SCAR AND ACTIVE LUPUS ERYTHEMATOSUS VISCOIDES OF HANDS. (From the University Clinic and General Hospital Service.) Presented by Dr. MICHELSON.

A man, aged 64, born in Sweden, said that he had had a chronic scaling disease of the skin confined to the scalp and face since he was a young man, that he had received various kinds of treatment, including roentgen-ray and radium treatment, that a growth had developed on the right ear which a physician called cancer and for which he removed the right ear lobe eight years before. During the last year he had developed two elevated hard circumscribed growths on the cheeks within the scar which followed his previous disease. The patient had a typical lupus erythematosus scar of the scalp and face and an active chronic lupus erythematosus on the back of his hands. Two circumscribed hard pearly bordered growths were noted on the right cheek which had developed within the scar, and which had been diagnosed as epithelioma.

CHEILITIS EXFOLIATIVA. Presented by Drs. BUTLER and ODLAND.

A boy, aged 14, presented an eruption on the lower lip of several years' duration. The mucous membranes of the lower lip showed several small, dry areas covered with adherent scales and crusts. At times he had noticed improvement followed by exacerbations.

A CASE FOR DIAGNOSIS. Presented by Drs. BUTLER and ODLAND.

A woman, aged 42, presented extensive mucous membrane lesions of the mouth of four months' duration. She said that the lesions first appeared on the right buccal cavity and rapidly spread to other parts until it involved the inside of the cheeks, the gums, the ventral surfaces and margins of the tongue, the posterior pharynx and fauces. The lesions were grayish white, fairly sharply marginated and raised, giving the appearance of a raised membrane which when detached showed a bleeding surface. Microscopic examination failed to show any mycelia or yeastlike elements. A forty-eight hour old culture showed no growth.

GUMMA FOLLOWING TRAUMA. Presented by Dr. OLSON.

Mrs. W., aged 49 years, showed bilateral gummas at the sites of the patellar bursas. Four months previously she had fallen on the ice. The injury was followed by ecchymoses below both knees. These bruises did not heal but gradually became ulcers. At the time of presentation the patient had received four arsphenamin injections, and the gummas were almost healed.

DYSPITUITARISM WITH HYPERHIDROSIS. Presented by Dr. OLSON.

A boy, aged 14, was first seen eight months ago, when he complained of excessive sweating of the feet. His muscles were well developed and firm. He complained, however, of exhaustion after moderate exertion. He had been unable to take part in such sports as skating. He suffered from severe headaches. The axillary spaces were free from hair, and the pubic hair was feminine in arrangement. Local application of formaldehyd in alcohol and thyroid administered internally had resulted in relief from the hyperhidrosis and improvement in the general condition. The headaches were less frequent and severe, and there was less fatigue after exertion.

RESISTANT THRUSH. Presented by Dr. Olson.

A girl, aged 8 years, was presented at the last annual meeting. The diagnosis had been confirmed by culture. The thrush had not responded to treatment continued over a period of four years. The tongue and mouth showed the white patches of thrush.

LICHEN PLANUS, VERRUCOUS AND ATROPHIC. Presented by Dr. Sweitzer.

R. H., a woman, aged 40, had an eruption which had been present since she had been vaccinated fifteen years before. At first the eruption was general, but after several months it disappeared, with the exception of a few patches on the knees. The left wrist showed typical lichen planus lesions. The right wrist showed a circular lesion resembling a granuloma annulare. On the right tibial region was a round verrucous lesion, and over the region of the knee joint were two irregular atrophic lesions.

PSORIASIS. Presented by Dr. Sweitzer.

M. B., a man, aged 41, presented a verrucous eruption on the thumb and two middle fingers of the left hand and the thumb and third finger of the right hand. The disease had been present for nearly two years, alternately improving and becoming worse. The patient had been treated for eczema of the hands by two physicians. A typical patch of psoriasis was present on the elbows.

DISCUSSION

Dr. Freeman: When I first saw this case I thought it was psoriasis, but I am now inclined to doubt it. I believe that an epidermophyton infection should be considered.

SCROFULODERMA. (From the General Hospital Service.) Presented by Drs. Michelson and Odland.

Mrs. H., a widow, aged 38, who had no children, with a blood Wassermann test repeatedly negative and no history of syphilis, presented herself on account of a rather extensive lesion of the region of the right wrist. She said that two years before she developed a swelling just over the back of the hand, which gradually enlarged and after two months discharged a slight amount of pus. In four weeks this swelling subsided; then another similar swelling developed 4 cm. higher on the wrist. She treated it with hot poultices, but it did not break down. A physician made an incision, and the lesion discharged pus for fifteen weeks. He then burned it with a caustic stick. In March, 1921, new lesions, numbering about five, developed subcutaneously and gradually enlarged until they were the size of a hazelnut. The skin over the nodules was red and slightly painful. The nodules appeared to be adherent to the skin and were closely attached to the underlying tissues. There were no sinuses. Biopsy revealed a deep seated granulomatous structure with typical tubercle formation. Staining for tubercle bacillus was negative. Animal inoculation had been performed, but too recently for report. This condition was apparently scrofuloderma developing in the lymphatics of the hypoderm.

INTERTRIGO INTERDIGITALIS SACCHAROMYCETICA. (From the University Clinic.) Presented by Drs. Michelson and Odland.

A woman, aged 60, had had a disease of the skin between the fingers for the last eight years. It consisted of moist, white lesions located in the interdigital spaces of both hands. The epidermis was accumulated into a mass of undermined, sodden, white, soft débris. It was rather easily removed, and Dr. Odland recovered a saccharomyces from the scrapings, which were easily cultivated. The condition has been refractory to ordinary treatment. The microscope shows finger granules.

NEUROTIC EXCORIATIONS. Presented by Dr. Michelson.

Miss B., aged 76, has for the last four years had lesions on the face, accompanied by an irresistible desire to dig into them. This she had done after retiring. When oozing was produced the desire subsided. There had been no effort to deceive nor any play for sympathy. She simply said that the lesions developed as little bumps and the excoriations were produced and healed by scarring. She showed numerous excoriations and scars on the face and forearms.

IDIOPATHIC MACULAR ATROPHY. Presented by Drs. Butler and Odland.

A woman, aged 21, said that the eruption had been present for three years and that it began as small, slightly reddish spots which, following scaling, became lighter in color. It first involved the neck and shoulders and gradually spread to the upper part of the trunk and lumbar region. When first seen the lesions were atrophic patches, oval in shape, varying in size from that of a split pea to that of a finger-nail. The skin was smooth, thin, wrinkled and white. The lesions appeared to be slightly depressed.

A CASE FOR DIAGNOSIS. Presented by Dr. Armsrong.

J. W., a boy, aged 14, who was first seen April 18, 1921, and at that time presented numerous lesions of a type similar to those now present, gave the following history: He was vaccinated June 30, 1921. This was followed by a rather severe local reaction and the formation of the lesions contiguous to the site of inoculation; afterward the lesions spread to other parts. Until April 18 there had been twenty-seven in all. A Wassermann test had been made before I saw him, and although it was negative, arsphenamin, mercury and sodium iodid had been administered without benefit. Cultures and smears made by me showed staphylococci and streptococci only. The lesions began as raised erythematous plaques from one-half to 1 inch (1.27 to 2.54 cm.) in diameter, which softened and eventually ulcerated, and healed only after a long time. The present lesions were confined mostly to the right tibial region, and the scars of the healed lesions were plainly visible. The boy's general health apparently had not suffered, as he had gained in weight and height during the past nineteen months. Various local treatment had been used. It was the opinion of the presenter that the lesions were those of a staphylococcus infection on a nonresistant skin.

ERYTHEMA FIGURATUM PERSTANS. Presented by Dr. C. D. Freeman.

A man, aged 34, whose physical examination and blood Wassermann test were negative, had always been in good health until about six years ago when he noticed a small dark red lesion about the size of a pea on the left cheek. Other lesions soon appeared and the process gradually spread in the periphery until the upper part of the cheek was practically entirely involved. Two years later a similar eruption appeared on the right cheek. The first lesions appeared on the body two years ago, one over the right scapula, of circinate character. Some of these lesions had disappeared, leaving slight pigmentation, and have again appeared and remained until the present time. There were no subjective symptoms. The lesions on the face had a decided violaceous hue.

ACTINOMYCOSIS. Presented by Dr. H. N. Klein.

A man, aged 35, a farmer, about seven months ago had a sore throat. followed two weeks later by definite swelling of the right cheek and neck which interfered with his breathing. In order to obtain relief he was sent to a surgeon to have the lump incised; after this was done the patient noticed that there was only a slight improvement and that numerous discharging sinuses remained in the region of the neck. Scrapings from the sinuses and growths on glucose agar showed the ray fungus. Under large doses of iodids· and roentgen-ray treatment he showed some improvement. He had been working around infected cattle.

DISCUSSION

Dr. J. H. Stokes commented on the experience of the Section on Dermatology in the treatment of visceral actinomycosis with sodium iodid intravenously. He felt that the intravenous route had no distinctive advantages in such cases, and if there was any reaction, it was unfavorable. He preferred the administration of large doses of potassium iodid by mouth.

In referring to the use of arsphenamin, as suggested by Dr. Ormsby. Dr. Stokes said that three cases under his observation in a series of perhaps ten or twelve had shown strikingly favorable results with arsphenamin, and in one of these cases a permanently satisfactory result was secured without the use of radiotherapeutic measures. In other cases it seemed as if neo-arsphenamin had had either no effect or had hastened the decline of the patient. This was the unpredictable element in the nonspecific use of arsphenamin, to which he had called attention on other occasions.

PALMAR SYPHILID. Presented by Dr. S. W. Sweitzer.

A man, aged 45, married, acquired syphilis in 1906 and took internal treatment for several months. He had had no symptoms since. until April. 1922. when he showed an extensive palmar syphilid. The patient has received six neo-arsphenamin injections and is now being treated with mercury rubs. The lesions have remained unchanged. The Wassermann test is positive.

DISCUSSION

Dr. J. H. Stokes: I note the atrophy over the thenar eminence and the gyrate configurations, which are certainly to some extent suggestive of syphilis On the other hand, palmar syphilids. in my experience. have not 'een as resistant to treatment for the disease as some syphilographers regard them. If a palmar syphilid does not show the beginnings of a definite response after two or three arsphenamin injections, I am inclined to subject the diagnosis to critical revision. In this particular case, the patient had sustained an investigation for syphilis at our hands, with repeated negative Wassermann reactions and a negative spinal fluid. This does not eliminate the disease, and I can very well understand how he might subsequently have had a single positive Wassermann reaction. I can only say that the morphology of the lesion appeals to me as a resistant palmar eczema possibly of occupational origin rather than a syphilid.

D. D. TURNACLIFF, Secretary.

Index to Current Literature

DERMATOLOGY

Anthrax. R. F. Vaccarezza, F. F. Inda and R. Posse. Semana méd. **1**:1013 (June 15) 1922.

Anthrax and Arsphenamin, Human. A. H. Louw and A. Pijper, South African M. Rec. **20**:273 (July 22) 1922.

Anthrax, Neo-Arsphenamin and Anti-Anthrax Serum in. J. Roux, Rev. méd. de la Suisse Rom. **42**:98 (Feb.) 1922.

Anthrax, Treatment of. R. F. Vaccarezza, F. F. Inda and R. Posse. Semana méd. **1**:865 (June 1) 1922.

Argyria After Collargol Treatment. T. Tobler, Schweizer. med. Wchnschr. **52**:774 (Aug. 3) 1922.

Arsphenamin and Human Anthrax. A. H. Louw and A. Pijper, South African M. Rec. **20**:273 (July 22) 1922.

Asthma and Eczema in Infancy and Childhood Controlled by Cutaneous Protein Sensitization Tests, Critical Study of Sixty-One Cases of. H. Herman, Am. J. Dis. Child. **24**:221 (Sept.) 1922.

Bromid Eruption in Nursing Infant, Case of. F. H. Boone, Canad. M. A. J. **12**:570 (Aug.) 1922.

Cancer of Lip. C. M. Hamilton, J. Tennessee M. A. **15**:190 (Aug.) 1922.

Cantharides Blisters for Serologic Tests. Thomas and Arnold, Med. Klin. **18**:899 (July 9) 1922.

Collargol Treatment, Argyria After. T. Tobler, Schweizer. med. Wchnschr. **52**:774 (Aug. 3) 1922.

Cysts, Sebaceous, Treatment of. D. S. Cuneo, Prensa méd. argentina **9**:127 (July 20) 1922.

Dermatitis, Plant. H. N. Ridley, J. Trop. M. **25**:225 (July 15) 1922.

Dermatoses of Present Day Interest. J. W. Miller, Ohio State M. J. **18**:547 (Aug.) 1922.

Dyskeratosis Diffusa Congenita. C. de Lange and J. C. Schippers. Am. J. Dis. Child. **24**:186 (Sept.) 1922.

Eczema and Asthma in Infancy and Childhood Controlled by Cutaneous Protein Sensitization Tests, Critical Study of Sixty-One Cases of. H. Herman. Am. J. Dis. Child. **24**:221 (Sept.) 1922.

Eczema, Diagnosis and Treatment of. B. B. Beeson, Illinois M. J. **42**:140 (Aug.) 1922.

Encephalitis. Herpes Zoster in Epidemic Encephalitis. A. Netter. Bull. et mém. Soc. méd. d. hôp. **46**:1028 (June 30) 1922.

Erysipelas, Quartz Lamp in Treatment of. A. Czepa. Wien. klin. Wchnschr. **35**:564 (June 22) 1922.

Erythema Nodosum. W. Holland, Norsk. Mag. f. Lægevidensk. **83**:626 (Aug.) 1922.

Erythema Nodosum, Epidemic. G. Caussade et al., Bull. et mém. Soc. méd. d. hôp. **46**:1080 (July 7) 1922.

Furuncles, Painless Treatment of. Kritzler, Deutsch. med. Wchnschr. **48**:866 (June 30) 1922.

Herpes Zoster and Vaccine. J. Dumont, Bull. et mém. Soc. méd. d. hôp. **46**:1036 (June 30) 1922.

Herpes Zoster and Varicella. A. Nette, Bull. et mém. Soc. méd. d. hôp. **46**:1004 (June 30) 1922.

Herpes Zoster and Varicella. J. Pignot and H. Durand, Bull. et mém. Soc. méd. d. hôp. **46**:1002 (June 30) 1922.

Herpes Zoster and Varicella. J. Ratea, Bull. et mém. Soc. méd. d. hôp. **46**: 1022 (June 30) 1922.

Herpes Zoster in Children. J. Comby, Bull. et mém. Soc. méd. d. hôp. **46**:992 (June 30) 1922.

Herpes Zoster in Epidemic Encephalitis. A. Netter, Bull. et mém. Soc. méd. d. hôp. **46**:1028 (June 30) 1922.

Herpes Zoster, Present Status of. A. Civatte, Bull. méd. **36**:591 (July 22) 1922.

Hydrargyria: Two Cases. C. Pelfort, Arch. de méd d. enf. **25**:420 (July) 1922.

Impetigo Herpetiformis, Importance of Internal Secretions in Etiology of. F. Walter, Polska Gaz. lek. **1**:425 (May 21) 1922.

Leg, New Variety of Streptothrix Cultivated from Mycetoma of. J. W. Cornwall and H. M. Lafrenais, Indian J. M. Res. **10**:239 (July) 1922.

Leprosy. Treatment of. Oreste Calcagno, Semana méd. **1**:928 (June 8) 1922.

Lip, Cancer of. C. M. Hamilton. J. Tennessee M. A. **15**:190 (Aug.) 1922.

Lupus Erythematosus. L. Lortat-Jacob, Progrès méd. **37**:303 (July 1) 1922.

Lymphogranulomatosis. Inguinal. Gastinel and J. Reilly, Bull. méd. **36**:577 (July 15) 1922.

Madura Foot, Case of. H. W. Dyke and N. M. Macfarlane, South African M. Rec. **20**:270 (July 22) 1922.

Measles, Serotherapy of. O. Jervell, Norsk Mag. f. Lægevidensk. **83**:601 (Aug.) 1922.

Measles, Experimental, Studies on. II. Enanthematous, Exanthematous, Pyrexial and Leukocytic Syndrome Produced in Rabbit by Intravenous Inoculation of Blood from Cases of Human Measles. C. W. Duval and R. D'Aunoy, J. Exper. M. **36**:231 (Aug.) 1922.

Measles, Experimental, Studies on. III. Symptom-Complex in Guinea-Pig and Rabbit Following Intratracheal and Intravenous Injections of Filtered Nasopharyngeal Secretions from Cases of Human Measles. C. W. Duval and R. D'Aunoy, J. Exper. M. **36**:239 (Aug.) 1922.

Measles, Present Status of. P. L. Marie, Presse méd. **30**:711 Aug. 19) 1922.

Mycetoma of Leg, New Variety of Streptothrix Cultivated from. J. W. Cornwall and H. M. Lafrenais, Indian J. M. Res. **10**:239 (July) 1922.

Myiasis, Cutaneous, Caused by Larvae of Sarcophaga Sp., Two Cases of? W. S. Patton, Indian J. M. Res. **10**:60 (July) 1922.

Picric Acid, Disinfection of Skin with. F. Slek, Polska Gaz. lek. **1**:427 (May 21) 1922.

Pigmentation, Xeroderma; Report of an Unusual Case. W. H. Guy, Penn. M. J. **25**:780 (Aug.) 1922.

Plant Dermatitis. H. N. Ridley, J. Trop. M. **25**:225 (July 15) 1922.

Psoriasis. Roentgen Irradiation of Thymus in Psoriasis. Schneider, Wien. klin. Wchnschr. **35**:565 (June 22) 1922.

Rhododendron Poisoning. S. W. Hardikar, J. Pharmacol. & Exper. Therap. **20**:17 (Aug.) 1922.

Roentgen Irradiation of Thymus in Psoriasis. Schneider, Wien. klin. Wchnschr. **35**:565 (June 22) 1922.

Sarcomatosis. Cutaneous, Copper in Treatment of. A. Tomaselli, Riforma med. **38**:631 (July 3) 1922.

Scabies, Variations in Prevalence of. G. Thibierge, Bull de l'Acad. de méd. **88**:52 (July 18) 1922.

Scarlet Fever, Causative Agent in. R. Degkwitz, München. med. Wchnschr. **69**:955 (June 30) 1922.

Skin Diseases of Infancy and Childhood. A. M. H. Gray, Practitioner **109**:67 (July) 1922.

Skin, Disinfection of, with Picric Acid. F. Slek, Polska Gaz. lek. **1**:427 (May 21) 1922.

Skin Eruptions, Hits and Misses in Diagnosis of. C. Pijper, South African M. Rec. **20**:268 (July 22) 1922.

Skin, Lipochrome Sarcoma of. C. Pinedo, Semana méd. **1**:1050 (June 22) 1922.

Smallpox in Monkeys. J. C. Bleyer, München. med. Wchnschr. **69**:1009 (July 7) 1922.

Smallpox, Inoculation with. I. Holmgren, Hygiea **84**:494 (June 30) 1922.

Trichophytosis, Treatment of. C. Maderna, Riforma med. **38**:625 (July 3) 1922.

Tuberculous Dermatitis, Soluble Tuberculous Toxin in Treatment of. C. Felugo, Riforma med. **38**:633 (July 3) 1922.

Vaccine and Herpes Zoster. J. Dumont. Bull. et mém. Soc. méd. d. hôp. **46**: 1036 (June 30) 1922.

Vaccinia of the Eyelids by Homo-Inoculation. J. M. Ball and N. Toomey, J. A. M. A. **79**:935 (Sept. 16) 1922.

Varicella and Herpes Zoster. A. Netter, Bull. et mém. Soc. méd. d. hôp. **46**: 1004 (June 30) 1922.

Varicella and Herpes Zoster. J. Pignot and H. Durand, Bull. et mém. Soc. méd. d. hôp. **46**:1002 (June 30) 1922.

Varicella and Herpes Zoster. J. Rateau. Bull. et mém. Soc. méd. d. hôp. **46**:1022 (June 30) 1922.

Xeroderma Pigmentation; Report of an Unusual Case. W. H. Guy, Penn. M. J. **25**:780 (Aug.) 1922.

SYPHILOLOGY

Anemia, Pernicious, Syphilis Simulating. J. H. Landwehr, Nederlandsch Tijdschr. v. Geneesk. **1**:2529 (June 24) 1922.

Anemia, Syphilitic: Banti's Disease; Case Reports. L. W. Frank, Kentucky M. J. **20**:551 (Aug.) 1922.

Aortitis, Syphilitic, Cause of Sudden Death. L. R. Woodward, Iowa M. J. **12**;319 (Aug.) 1922.

Arsenicals, Eruptions Under. Desaux et al., Presse méd. **30**:668 (Aug. 5) 1922.

Arsphenamin, Intravenous, Spinal Drainage Following. C. B. Craig and L. B. Chaney, J. Nerv. & Ment. Dis. **56**:97 (Aug.) 1922.

Banti's Disease: Syphilitic Anemia; Case Reports. L. W. Frank, Kentucky M. J. **20**:551 (Aug.) 1922.

Bismuth in Treatment of Syphilis. C. Levaditi, Presse méd. **30**:633 (July 26) 1922.

Bismuth in Treatment of Syphilis. Simon and Bralez, Bull. méd. **36**:523 (June 24) 1922.

Bismuth Treatment of Syphilis, Results in. R. Bernhardt, Polska Gaz. lek. **1**:473 (June 4) 1922.

Bladder, Syphilitic Disease of. S. Faragó, Ztschr. f. Urol. chir. **10**:144 (July 12) 1922.

Blood. Studies of Cerebrospinal Fluid and Blood of Syphilitic and Normal Persons; with Special Reference to Immunity Reactions and Colloidal Gold Test on Original and Ultrafiltered Fluids and Serums. C. E. Nixon and K. Naito, Arch. Int. Med. **30**:182 (Aug.) 1922.

Brain Abscess in a Syphilitic, Case of. T. L. Saunders, Laryngoscope **32**:619 (Aug.) 1922.

Central Nervous System, Case of Syphilis of. I. Morgan, M. J. Australia **2**:129 (July 29) 1922.

Cerebrospinal Fluid and Blood of Syphilitic and Normal Persons. Studies of: with Special Reference to Immunity Reactions and Colloidal Gold Test on Original and Ultrafiltered Fluids and Serums. C. E. Nixon and K. Naito, Arch. Int. Med. **30**:182 (Aug.) 1922.

Cerebrospinal Fluid, Colloid Reactions of. G. Laroche, Bull. méd. **36**:530 (June 24) 1922.

Cerebrospinal Fluid of Horses, Precipitation of Colloidal Gold in, with Dourine. F. H. K. Reynolds and H. W. Schoenig, J. Infec. Dis. **31**:59 (July) 1922.

Chloroform Test for Syphilis, Unreliability of. G. Lonero, Riv. crit. di clin. med. **23**:197 (June 15) 1922.

Cirrhosis and Syphilis. M. Villaret, H. Bénard and P. Blum, Médecine **3**:766 (July) 1922.

Colloid Reactions of Cerebrospinal Fluid. G. Laroche, Bull. méd. **36**:530 (June 24) 1922.

Colloidal Benzoin Test in Neurosyphilis. E. Benveniste, Rev. méd. de la Suisse Rom. **42**:353 (June) 1922.

Colloidal Gold, Precipitation of, in Cerebrospinal Fluid of Horses with Dourine. F. H. K. Reynolds and H. W. Schoenig, J. Infec. Dis. **31**:59 (July) 1922.

Colloidal Gold Reaction: Diagnostic Aid of Unquestionable Value. A. G. Kelley, J. M. A. Georgia **11**:310 (Aug.) 1922.

Colloidal Gold Test. Studies of Cerebrospinal Fluid and Blood of Syphilitic and Normal Persons; with Special Reference to Immunity Reactions and Colloidal Gold Test on Original and Ultrafiltered Fluids and Serums. C. E. Nixon and K. Naito, Arch. Int. Med. **30**:182 (Aug.) 1922.

Contact or Ring Precipitation Test for Syphilis: A Modification of the Kahn Test. R. D. Herrold, J. A. M. A. **79**:957 (Sept. 16) 1922.

Diabetes of Syphilitic Origin. F. Rathery and P. Fernet, Bull. méd. **36**:527 (June 24) 1922.

Diabetes, Syphilis in Relation to. C. Pfeiffer, Progrès méd. **37**:381 (Aug. 12) 1922.

Ear. Report of Two Cases of Syphilis of Eighth Nerve and Inner Ear. E. G. Gill, Laryngoscope **32**:634 (Aug.) 1922.

Eyes, Syphilitic Disease of. R. Hessberg, Med. Klin. **18**:954 (July 23) 1922.

Eyes, Treatment of Syphilitic Disease of. H. Boas, Ugesk. f. Læger **84**:757 (June 29) 1922.

Flocculation, Serologic Demonstration of Syphilis by. Sachs, Deutsch. med. Wchnschr. **48**:891 (July 7) 1922.

Glandular Disease of Syphilitic Origin. J. Golay, Rev. méd. de la Suisse Rom. **42**:296 (May) 1922.

Granuloma, Venereal, Case of. C. Morales Macedo, Crón. méd. **39**:201 (June) 1922.

Immunity Reactions. Studies of Cerebrospinal Fluid and Blood of Syphilitic and Normal Persons; with Special Reference to Immunity Reactions and Colloidal Gold Test on Original and Ultrafiltered Fluids and Serums. C. E. Nixon and K. Naito, Arch. Int. Med. **30**:182 (Aug.) 1922.

Metasyphilis, Pathogenesis of. W. Gennerich, München. med. Wchnschr. **69**: 922 (July 23) 1922.

Neosilver-Arsphenamin in Syphilis. Liebner and Rado, Med. Klin. **18**:996 (July 30) 1922.

Nephritis, Early Syphilitic. K. A. Rombach, Nederlandsch Tijdschr. v. Geneesk. **1**:2414 (June 17) 1922.

Nerve, Eighth, and Inner Ear, Report of Two Cases of Syphilis of. E. G. Gill, Laryngoscope **32**:634 (Aug.) 1922.

Nervous System. Early Syphilitic Affections of the Central Nervous System. G. L. Dreyfus, Deutsch. med. Wchnschr. **48**:860 (June 30) 1922.

Nervous System, Syphilis of. N. M. Owensby, J. M. A. Georgia **11**:297 (Aug.) 1922.

Neurosyphilis. H. del Campo, Rev. méd. d. Uruguay **25**:537 (July) 1922.

Neurosyphilis, Colloidal Benzoin Test in. E. Benveniste, Rev. méd. de la Suisse Rom. **42**:353 (June) 1922.

Neurosyphilis, Diagnosis and Treatment of. C. M. Byrnes, Virginia M. J. **49**:269 (Aug.) 1922.

Novarsenobillon, Unusual Local Effect (Skin Eruption) of. M. O'B. Beadon, Lancet **2**:508 (Sept. 2) 1922.

Pachymeningitis, Syphilitic Cervical: Case Report. R. C. Bunting, J. Tennessee M. A. **15**:188 (Aug.) 1922.

Picric Acid, Action of, on Syphilis. Brill and Steusing, Polska Gaz. lek. **1**:423 (May 21) 1922.

Pigmentation in Syphilitic. M. Pinard, Bull. et mém. Soc. méd. d. hôp. **46**: 1009 (June 30) 1922.

Pregnancy. Treatment of Syphilis in Pregnancy in Department of Health in Detroit. W. E. Welz and A. E. Van Nest, Am. J. Obst. & Gynec. **4**:174 (Aug.) 1922.

Ring or Contact Precipitation Test for Syphilis: A Modification of the Kahn Test. R. D. Herrold, J. A. M. A. **79**:957 (Sept. 16) 1922.

Sachs-Georgi Test for Syphilis. H. W. Y. Taylor, China M. J. **36**:344 (July) 1922.

Saprophytism of Causal Agents of Venereal Disease. S. Mazza, S. Sonnenberg and C. Guerra, Prensa méd. argentina **9**:117 (July 20) 1922.

Skin Infections, Syphilis Revealed by. J. May, Rev. méd. d. Uruguay **25**:572 (July) 1922.

Spleen, Enlargement of, in Incipient Syphilis. B. Peiser. Med. Klin. **18**:925 (July 16) 1922.

Stomach. Gastric Ulcer and Syphilis. A. Cade, Médecine **3**:752 (July) 1922.

Stomach, Manifestations of Syphilis in. Bensaude and Rivet, Médecine **3**:747 (July) 1922.

Syphilids, Action of Picric Acid on. Brill and Steusing. Polska Gaz. lek. **1**:423 (May 21) 1922.

Syphilis, Acute, of Central Nervous System, Case of. I. Morgan. M. J. Australia **2**:129 (July 29) 1922.

Syphilis and Cirrhosis. M. Villaret, H. Bénard and P. Blum, Médecine **3**:766 (July) 1922.

Syphilis and Gastric Ulcer. A. Cade, Médecine **3**:752 (July) 1922.

Syphilis. A Ring or Contact Precipitation Test for Syphilis: A Modification of the Kahn Test. R. D. Herrold, J. A. M. A. **79**:957 (Sept. 16) 1922.

Syphilis. A Simple Aid in the Diagnosis of Syphilis from the Primary Lesion. W. D. Gill, J. A. M. A. **79**:966 (Sept. 16) 1922.

Syphilis, Bismuth in Treatment of. C. Levaditi, Presse méd. **30**:633 (July 26) 1922.

Syphilis, Bismuth in Treatment of. Simon and Bralez, Bull. méd. **36**:523 (June 24) 1922.

Syphilis, Congenital, Plan for Intensive Treatment of. H. Schussler, California State J. M. **20**:257 (Aug.) 1922.

Syphilis, Curability of. V. G. Vecki, California State J. M. **20**:274 (Aug.) 1922.

Syphilis in Pregnancy, Treatment of, in Department of Health in Detroit. W. E. Welz and A. E. Van Nest. Am. J. Obst. & Gynec. **4**:174 (Aug.) 1922.

Syphilis in Relation to Diabetes. C. Pfeiffer. Progrès méd. **37**:381 (Aug. 12) 1922.

Syphilis in Stomach, Manifestations of. Bensaude and Rivet. Médecine **3**:747 (July) 1922.

Syphilis, Incipient, Enlargement of Spleen in. B. Peiser. Med. Klin. **18**:925 (July 16) 1922.

Syphilis, Intravenous Use of Mercury Cyanid in Treatment of. M. Q Howard. Colorado M. **19**:184 (Sept.) 1922.

Syphilis, Reinfection with: Two Cases. G. Cornaz. Rev. méd. de la Suisse Rom. **42**:453 (July) 1922.

Syphilis, Relation of, to Diagnosis and Surgery. A. M. Crance, New York State J. M. **22**:357 (Aug.) 1922.

Syphilis, Results in Bismuth Treatment of. R. Bernhardt, Polska Gaz. lek. **1**:473 (June 4) 1922.

Syphilis Revealed by Skin Infections. J. May, Rev. méd. d. Uruguay **25**:572 (July) 1922.

Syphilis, Serodiagnosis of. P. Esch and J. Wieloch, München. med. Wchnschr. **69**:926 (June 23) 1922.

Syphilis, Serologic Demonstration of, by Flocculation. Sachs, Deutsch. med. Wchnschr. **48**:891 (July 7) 1922.

Syphilis Simulating Pernicious Anemia. J. H. Landwehr, Nederlandsch Tijdschr. v. Geneesk. **1**:2529 (June 24) 1922.

Syphilis, Tardy Inherited, in Adults. C. Du Bois, Rev. méd. de la Suisse Rom. **42**:219 (April) 1922.

Syphilis, Tertiary, Diagnosis of. E. E. Butler, Kentucky M. J. **20**:517 (Aug.) 1922.

Syphilis, the Fight Against. L. Bizard and J. Bralez, Bull. méd. **36**:532 (June 24) 1922.

Syphilis, Unreliability of Chloroform Test for. G. Lonero, Riv. crit. di clin. méd. **23**:197 (June 15) 1922.

Syphilis, Wassermann Test Late in. T. E. Hess Thaysen, Ugesk. f. Læger **84**:846 (July 13) 1922.

Venereal Diseases, Bismuth in Treatment of. F. Balzer, Paris méd. **12**:81 (July 22) 1922.

Venereal Disease Cases, Social Investigation and Follow-Up in. G. Bates, Pub. Health J. **13**:362 (Aug.) 1922.

Venereal Diseases, Data for Lectures on. A. Lassueur, Rev. méd. de la Suisse Rom. **42**:171 (March) 1922.

Venereal Disease, Fourth. L. Bory, Progrès méd. **37**:373 (Aug. 12) 1922.

Venereal Disease Program, Some Notes on the Effectiveness of. H. G. Irvine, J. A. M. A. **79**:1121 (Sept. 30) 1922.

Venereal Disease, Saprophytism of Causal Agents of. S. Mazza, S. Sonnenberg and C. Guerra, Prensa méd. argentina **9**:117 (July 20) 1922.

Venereal Granuloma, Case of. C. Morales Macedo, Crón. méd. **39**:201 (June) 1922.

Wassermann Tests Late in Syphilis. T. E. Hess Thaysen, Ugesk. f. Læger **84**:846 (July 13) 1922.

Wassermann Test, Standardization of. L. Bory, Progrès méd. **37**:349 (July 29) 1922.

Wassermann Test, Value of. F. T. Cadham, Canad. M. A. J. **12**:563 (Aug.) 1922.

Archives of Dermatology and Syphilology

VOLUME 6 DECEMBER, 1922 NUMBER 6

THE PREVALENCE OF YAWS (FRAMBESIA TROPICA) IN THE UNITED STATES *

HOWARD FOX, M.D.
NEW YORK

Among the more serious diseases of the tropics, yaws or frambesia tropica is of interest not only because it is striking in appearance, easily communicable and disabling, but also because of its close resemblance in many respects to syphilis. Though often simulating syphilis both clinically and pathologically, it is a much less serious disease, as it does not attack the central nervous system or viscera and is not transmitted by heredity. It is, furthermore, much more easily eradicated by arsphenamin than is syphilis. It is with the object of discussing the prevalence of yaws in the United States and recording a case recently observed in New York that this communication has been written.

REPORT OF CASE

History.—L. C., aged 18 years, unmarried, a full blooded negress, born in Montserrat, British West Indies, applied for treatment at the dermatologic department of the Harlem Hospital, Nov. 30, 1921. Her parents and an only brother, aged 17 years, were living and well. None of her family, to her knowledge, had ever suffered from a similar disease. She did not remember having had any of the diseases of childhood and had been attended only once in her life by a physician, when suffering from cramps incident to menstruation. The menses were established at 13, and since then had been regular.

The patient had lived all her life on the island of Montserrat until July 10. 1921, when she sailed for the United States, arriving in New York, July 22. About two weeks before leaving Montserrat, she had come in contact with two young children who were suffering from sores on the face and hands. On inquiring of the parents as to the nature of these sores, she was told that a physician had said that the children were suffering from yaws. On arriving in New York, she secured work by the day as a housemaid. As far as she was aware, none of the people with whom she came in contact had any disease

---

* Read at the Forty-Fifth Annual Meeting of the American Dermatological Association, Washington, D. C., May 2-4, 1922.

* From the Department of Dermatology and Syphilis of the Harlem Hospital.

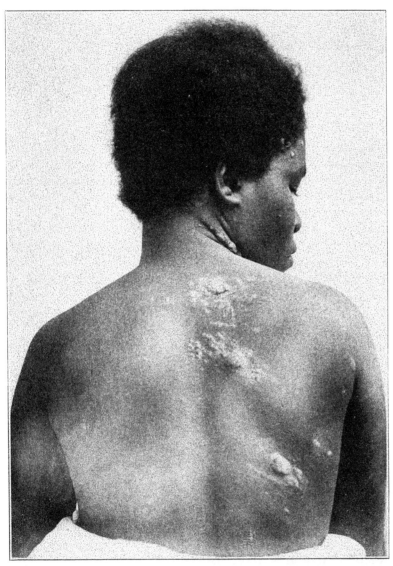

Fig. 1.—Generalized eruption consisting of individual and grouped lesions covered with crusts, some of them suggesting the appearance of a corymbiform syphilid.

of the skin. The patient was certain that she had been entirely free from any eruption until November 10, when she noticed on her right thigh a "pimple" which occasioned considerable itching. It grew larger and in a few days attained its maximum size, that of a 5-cent piece.

Coincident with the first appearance of this lesion, she began to suffer from headache and rheumatic pains in the left shoulder and chest and from sore throat. The pains had continued to the time of treatment. She had not suffered from malaise or fever. About one week after she had first noticed the lesion on the thigh, the rest of the eruption which she now presented made its appearance. Some of these lesions, she stated, lasted only a few days, leaving a scaly surface after their disappearance. She said that she had had sexual intercourse only once in her life, five or six weeks before the appearance of the eruption.

Physical Examination.—Examination revealed that the patient was well nourished and in apparent good health. She weighed 125 pounds (57 kg.) and was 5 feet and 1 inch (1.5 meters) in height. The eruption consisted of about thirty individual and grouped lesions, varying in size from that of a split pea to that of a silver quarter. They were distributed as follows: on the scalp, there were six lesions; on the face and neck seven (the largest being about the size of a 10-cent piece), and on the trunk and arms, twelve, the largest being the size of a quarter. In the midscapular region were two large lesions surrounded by a number of smaller satellites resembling a corymbiform syphilid. The eruption on the lower extremities was confined to a single lesion on the anterior aspect of each thigh and a flattened macerated patch on the sole of the right foot, the macerated appearance being partly due, perhaps, to a poultice which she had applied.

The individual lesions were all painless, and fairly firm to the touch. They gave the appearance of being superficially attached to the skin. Some of them were dry and scaly; others were covered with dirty, yellowish crusts, suggesting an impetigo. All of the lesions, except the dry ones in process of involution, exuded pus on pressure; and, when the crusts were removed, a red, papillomatous, raspberry-like surface was presented. When the lesions were irritated by friction, there was a profuse serous discharge. Under the breast, there was a patch from which the crust had been removed by friction and maceration, giving the appearance of a syphilitic condyloma. The mucous membranes of the mouth and genitalia were entirely free of any eruption. The palms were also unaffected. The eruption did not cause any disagreeable odor. the patient being very cleanly in her habits.

Laboratory Examinations.—Examination by dark-field illumination of the serous discharge revealed large numbers of spirochetes indistinguishable (by the ordinary observer) from *Spirochaeta pallida.* These examinations were made on several occasions by Dr. Howard T. Phillips (a former associate). A Wassermann test by the New York Board of Health was reported negative. December 2, while a similar examination by Dr. Oliver Hillman gave a four plus reaction with both cholesterinized and crude alcoholic antigens.

Animal inoculations were made by Drs. Wade H. Brown and Louise Pearce of the Rockefeller Institute, who reported: "Examination of fluid obtained from several nodules from patient L. C., Dec. 20, 1921, showed an abundance of long and delicate spirochetes of the type *Treponema pertenue.* Inoculations were made from this fluid into the testicles of four normal rabbits. One of the animals inoculated developed a secondary bacterial infection. The others showed practically no immediate reaction. Within three to four weeks, there was a definite inguinal adenitis in all animals, and there was suggestive enlargement and increased tension of the testicles. The adenitis persisted for some time. The testicular condition, however, subsided. At the end of six weeks, transfers were made from lymph nodes of two of the original animals. These animals gave a reaction analogous to those of the first group, but the lesions which developed in the testicles were very slight, consisting chiefly in slight swellings and increased resistance, with some thickening of the tunics.

"Castration of one of these animals performed eleven weeks after inoculation showed slight but definite enlargement of the testicle, diffuse thickening of the tunics and a small nodule situated in the region of the head of the epididymis. There was also well marked adenitis in this animal. Dark-field examination of material showed no spirochetes, but this material was used for a third series of transfers.

"Examination of another animal inoculated with material from lesion of patient showed, at the end of seventeen weeks, a condition which was more characteristic. Both testicles were slightly enlarged, somewhat congested and over the surface of the tunics there were a number of minute granulomatous nodules which were identical in all respects with tunic nodules, which we have frequently observed in the strain of yaws, originally isolated by Dr. Nichols and studied in this laboratory during the last year.

"The mild reaction in the testicles which followed inoculation of comparatively large numbers of actively motile spirochetes associated with slight but definite lymphadenitis, and finally the production of the tunic lesions described, leads us to believe that there is very little doubt that the infection in this case is due to *Treponema pertenue* rather than to *pallidum*."

Histologic Examination.—December 8, a piece of tissue was excised from the chest, under local anesthesia, and the following histologic report was made by Dr. Walter J. Highman:

"Low Power Zeiss, Ocular 4, Objective A. Epidermis is found thrown up in almost verrucous manner and on account of confluence of strands of epidermis inclusions of papillae are established which resemble small islands. Within these, as well as in the corium underlying the epidermis, is an infiltration.

"High Power, Ocular 4, Objective D.D. The infiltration in the islands is found to consist of lymphoid and epithelioid cells in a lacey network of connective tissue fibers, a high degree of edema present and occasional actual minute abscesses. In the corium the infiltration in general has the same character but added thereto are numerous foci consisting almost entirely of plasma cells filling perivascular spaces about the arterioles, which themselves have slightly, if at all, thickened walls and swollen endothelium.

"Comment: The conditions simulated are tuberculosis verrucosa, syphilis, blastomycosis, sporotrichosis and kerion. Tuberculosis verrucosa is excluded by lack of giant cells and the large number of plasma cells. Syphilis can be less readily excluded but gummas practically never show the verrucoid appearance here exhibited and the vascular changes are on the whole not sufficiently profound. The other three conditions are excluded by the relatively small number of true abscesses. By exclusion, diagnosis remains: Yaws."

Diagnosis.—The patient was presented before the Dermatological Section of the New York Academy of Medicine, December 6 by me (in conjunction with

Dr. B. F. Ochs) as a questionable case of frambesiform syphilis.[1] Having had no previous experience with yaws and having had little opportunity to study the case, we did not wish to hazard a diagnosis of this disease. Dr. Herman Goodman, the only one present who had had any personal experience with yaws, made a diagnosis of this disease from the clinical appearance. Dr. Pearce, who had recently seen cases of yaws in Africa, saw the patient a few days later, and unhesitatingly agreed with this diagnosis, on clinical grounds.

Treatment.—The treatment consisted solely of six intravenous injections of neo-arsphenamin, administered during a period of seven weeks, beginning, Dec. 22, 1921. After the fourth injection, the eruption had entirely disappeared, leaving a brownish pigmentation, which had persisted to the time of writing. The dosage of the first two injections was 0.45 gm., and of the succeeding four injections, 0.6 gm. The subjective symptoms, including headache and pain, had entirely disappeared one week after the first treatment. A second Wassermann test made, April 21, 1922, by Dr. Hillman was reported as plus minus.

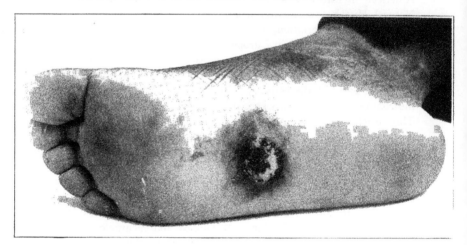

Fig. 2.—Large individual macerated yaw of the sole.

Summary.—The patient, a negress of 18, who came directly to New York from the West Indies (Montserrat) where she had always lived and where she claimed to have been exposed to yaws two weeks before sailing, after nearly four months residence in New York developed a generalized eruption which corresponded with descriptions of yaws and which was so diagnosed by two observers who were familiar with the disease. There was a general adenopathy. There were no lesions of the mucous membranes. Spirochetes were found by dark-field illumination. The Wassermann test was positive, and the eruption cleared up readily under neo-arsphenamin. The histologic diagnosis by exclusion was yaws, and the result of rabbit inoculations strongly favored the same diagnosis. The conclusion would, therefore, seem warranted that the patient was suffering from yaws, and that the infection had been imported from the West Indies (where the disease is common) to New York, where even a single case appears to be a great rarity.

1. Fox, Howard: Arch. Dermat. & Syph. **5**:411 (March) 1922.

THE LITERATURE

The question of the occurrence of yaws in the United States was discussed in 1915 by Edward J. Wood.[2] He attempted briefly to mention every case that had been reported in the United States previous to his publication as he had found "the records of yaws in the literature so few." In addition to recording a case of his own, he was able to find only eight other case reports, one of which concerned a patient observed in Canada. I have also been surprised at the small number of cases recorded in this country and have only been able to find a few additional cases which had not been included by Wood and a few cases subsequently reported.

According to Wood, the first authentic reference to yaws in American literature is to be found in a volume by Brickell on the Natural History of North Carolina, etc., published in 1737. In the course of his description, this early writer says "The Yaws are a disorder not well known in Europe but very common and familiar here. It is like the Lues Venerea having most of the symptoms that attend the Pox, such as Nocturnal pains, Botches, foul Eruptions and Ulcers in several parts of the body.... This distemper was brought hither by the Negroes from Guinea where it is a common distemper among them. This distemper though of a venereal kind, is seldom cured by Mercurials, as I have often experienced." According to Joseph Jones,[3] the first recorded observations on yaws as occurring among the negroes of Louisiana were made by Du Pratz in 1758, in his "History of Louisiana." The author mentions yaws in giving advice to prospective purchasers of negro slaves, saying in the course of his remarks, "You must ask your examining surgeon if he is acquainted with the distemper of the yaws which is the virus of Guinea and incurable by a great many French surgeons though very skillful in the management of European distempers." Roman, is his history of Florida, in 1776 (quoted by Jones) writes " I have seen three or for instances of the disease called body yaws (in the islands) and in Carolina the same distemper. Mercurial medicines are used against it."

Humphreys,[4] in a letter written to Benjamin Rush in 1770, said that among a number of slaves "was a lad about 18 years of age who was a miserable object; from the disorder called the yaws; he was vastly more affected with it than any person I ever saw, before or since; from his head to his feet he was thickly set with those sorts

---

2. Wood, E. J.: The Occurrence of Yaws in the United States, Am. J. Trop. Dis. **2**:431 (Jan.) 1915.

3. Jones, J.: Medical and Surgical Memoirs of Various Diseases, New Orleans **11**:1184, 1887.

4. Humphreys, T.: Minutes of a Case of Yaws, Philadelphia Med. Museum **1**:442, 1805.

of knots or ulcers which that disorder produces when it is in its worst stages."

Van Zandt,[5] in 1831, reported a case of yaws seen in New York. The patient was a negro cook on board a vessel from the West Indies, who stated that previous to sailing he had slept in a bed in which a "negro had died with the yaws." The disease appeared after he arrived in New York. There were febrile symptoms for a few days, followed

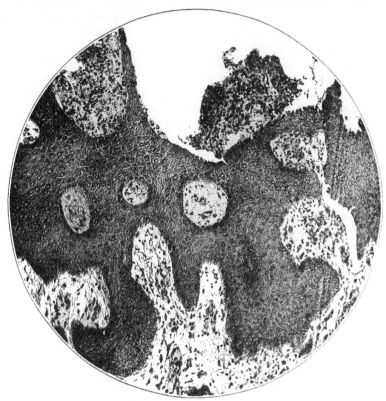

Fig. 3.—General topography of frambesia lesion showing high degree of epidermal hyperplasia (acanthosis) with island-like inclusions of papillae. At the upper left hand corner is an abscess and there is a similar one at the upper right below crust. The distribution of the infiltration is clearly shown. (Low power.)

by an eruption of small pimples not larger than a grain of mustard seed which later became protuberant pustules. One crop of pustules followed another in regular succession. When the patient was nearly convales-

5. Van Zandt, C. A.: Case of Yaws, New York Med. Chirurg. Bull. 2:4 (Nov.) 1831.

cent, there were painful hard swellings of the soles. It is interesting, in view of the present almost miraculous remedy (arsphenamin) for yaws, to read the formulas of seven different prescriptions which the writer had used in treating this patient.

McDowell,[6] in 1858, wrote a short and rather unsatisfactory report entitled "Framboesia or Yaws." The patient was a negro infant of 2 years. He presented an ulcerating, fungoid growth about the anus which was large enough to interfere with defecation. His mother was a native of Africa and was said to have had the "same disease." About three months previously, the child had had fever and "an eruption over most of the body."

Cartwright,[7] in the following year, reported a case of yaws associated with vesicorectovaginal fistula. The patient was a negress in New Orleans. The eruption involved the nates and lower abdomen as far as the umbilicus. "Hard excrescences had formed on the spots occupying the integuments of the labia and through fissures in these excrescences granulated pallulations resembling mulberries had protruded distilling a very fetid ichorous humor. The mama pian or mother yaw was situated near the upper commissure of the right labium majus." There were torturing pains by night, and inguinal swellings which were painful and hard but not suppurating.

Doane,[8] in 1876, wrote a brief and unconvincing report entitled "A case of yaws framboesia or fungoid growth arising from syphilis." The patient was a negress of 35, from Jamaica. The writer stated that she "had a growth (resembling raspberries placed in layers) upon the external and outward portions of the right leg. There was also a small ulcer, undoubtedly syphilitic in its origin. On pressing over the tibia, great pain was caused and upon the back syphilitic papules were seen causing some itching." The writer added that the patient had been seen in consultation with Dr. E. L. Keyes, Sr., "who pronounced the above diagnosis of yaws correct."

Jones,[9] in 1878, reported a case of yaws in New Orleans in a thorough and painstaking manner. His patient was a sailor, born on an island on the coast of Africa. His father was a native of France, his mother of Africa. He stated that he had contracted the disease three months previously, his ship having been visited by natives suffer-

6. McDowell, G.: Framboesia or Yaws, New Orleans M. J. 15:192 (March) 1858.

7. Cartwright, S. A.: Case of Framboesia and Vesico-Recto Vaginal Fistula, New Orleans M. J. 15:512 (July) 1859.

8. Doane, L. G.: A Case of Yaws Framboesia or Fungoid Growth Arising from Syphilis, Pharmacist & Physician 9:6 (Aug.) 1876.

9. Jones, J.: Observations on the African Yaws, etc., in Insular and Continental America, New Orleans M. & S. J. 5:673 (March) 1878.

ing from yaws. During the voyage, he had suffered from severe constitutional symptoms. The eruption first appeared on the face as vesicles, drying to form crusts. It became generalized and was especially severe on the fingers and toes, with swelling and ulceration of the phalanges.

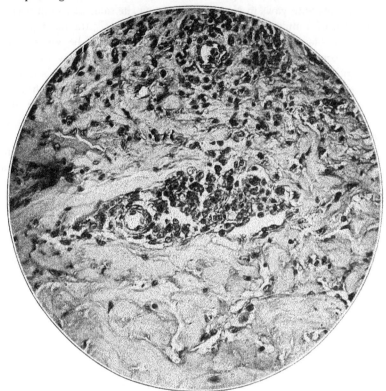

Fig. 4.—Two features of the frambesia lesion stand out in this section: In the center is a transsected arteriole, the perivascular space of which is distended by an infiltration, prevailingly of plasma cells. The vessel itself is but slightly altered, if at all. The independent infiltration above is in vague relation to venules and consists of lymphocytes, a few plasma and epithelioid cells, and a moderate number of fibroblasts. This area, with more vascular changes, would be suggestive of syphilis. (High power.)

McCosh,[10] in 1895, presented a case before the New York Surgical Society as "syphilis cutanea vegetans or framboesia." The report was brief, not mentioning yaws and merely describing a "papillomatous excrescence on the tip of the nose which looks much like a large ras-

10. McCosh, A. J.: Syphilis Cutanea Vegetans or Framboesia. Ann. Surg. **21**:46 (Jan.) 1895.

berry." Microscopic examination revealed simple inflammatory tissue. The patient who was an unmarried woman, about 24 years old, had previously suffered, at different times, from rhinitis and sores on the roof of the mouth, throat and nasal septum.

Matas,[11] in 1896, writing in Dennis' "System of Surgery," spoke of two patients with yaws in New Orleans. One, he said, was an imported case, that of a mulatto from Mauritius, seen in 1877; the other patient was a full blooded negro seen in 1895. "This patient," he wrote, "was a Louisianan by birth and there is no clue in his history by which contagion may be traced. Still we are loath to believe that this disease can originate de novo in the United States." A photograph showing the patient's face, with numerous warty excrescences that were also said to cover the body, certainly seemed to present a condition characteristic of yaws.

McMurran,[12] in 1900, in a communication entitled "Yaws and Smallpox," described the clinical symptoms of the two diseases and followed with a report of a classic case of smallpox, for comparison with the report of a somewhat different condition which he surmised might be yaws. An epitome of this report, which was not very convincing, was as follows: The patient was an unmarried woman of 24, who, on the preceding night, had complained of pains in her back. There was no inflammation of the mucous membranes of the mouth and throat. The temperature was 101 F., pulse 100, respirations 20. The next morning the temperature was 100 F. On the fifth day, there was a vesicular eruption on the forehead and hands and a slight eruption on the breast. At this time, the temperature, pulse and respirations were normal. Her condition continued to improve, with no impairment of health. "The tubercles peeled off and I did not observe any pitting on her face." The patient had never been vaccinated.

In 1910, Nichols and Siler,[13] in separate communications, reported a case of yaws, from both the clinical and pathologic standpoint. The patient was a colored soldier returned from the Philippines, where, according to the writers, his infection had probably occurred. This entailed the rather long incubation period of eighty-six days. The clinical diagnosis was made when the patient was suffering from his second crop of lesions, appearing as typical fungoid papules covered with dirty, yellowish crusts. *Spirochaeta pertenuis* was found by dark-

---

11. Matas, Rudolph, in Dennis' System of Surgery, New York and Philadelphia, Lea Brothers & Company **4:**866, 1896.

12. McMurran, R. L.: Yaws and Smallpox, Virginia M. Semi-Month. **4:**646 (Feb. 9) 1900.

13. Nichols, H. J.: Yaws: with a Demonstration of Infected Tissue. Proc. New York Path. Soc. **10:**1 (Feb. and March) 1910. Siler, J. F.: Report of a Case of Yaws, Mil. Surgeon **27:**306 (Sept.) 1910.

field illumination in the serous exudate. The Wassermann reaction (Noguchi method) was negative. Inoculation of a monkey's eyebrow was positive, the spirochaeta being found and transferred to rabbits testicles, and transmitted through five generations.

White and Tyzzer,[14] in the following year, recorded another imported case of yaws in the person of a Porto Rican sailor. While the eruption was not at all typical of yaws, a probable clinical diagnosis of this disease was made by exclusion. The eruption consisted of "four strange looking, elevated, dry, tumor masses unaccompanied by any signs of local or general inflammation or disturbance." There was also a general and marked glandular enlargement. The Wassermann reaction was negative (Noguchi method). Puncture of a gland showed "a small infrequent spirochaeta which corresponded sufficiently with Castellani's *Spirochaeta pertenuis.*" Inoculation of the eyebrow of a monkey was successful, lesions appearing at sites of inoculation after a period of incubation of sixteen days. Inoculation of the cornea of ten rabbits was unsuccessful. A detailed histologic examination revealed that the epidermis was "markedly acanthotic and hyperkeratotic or moderately parakeratotic." The cutis showed a marked mononuclear infiltration with no giant, epithelioid or plasma cells, the vessels being normal except for moderate dilitation.

Lyle,[15] in 1912, reported a case of "gumma of the liver as a sequel to yaws." The patient was a man, 46 years old, from the West Indies, who gave a history of having yaws thirty-nine years previously. As confirmatory evidence, he stated that at that time he had been isolated, together with two other members of his family, in a "hospital given over to the treatment of yaws." There was no history of syphilis. and a positive Wassermann reaction was obtained only after a provocative injection of arsphenamin. The case was recorded as disproving the relationship between syphilis and yaws as "it has been claimed that an attack of yaws gave an immunity to syphilis."

Wood, in 1915, reported what he considered to be a case of yaws in North Carolina, in an infant whose "parents had always lived in that state and at no time had come in contact with any one from the West Indies or other endemic center of the disease." The importance that this case would assume is unfortunately greatly lessened from the fact that the diagnosis was only made later in retrospect from a study of notes and photographs. There is no mention of any search for spirochetes or of a Wassermann test having been made. The patient was an infant of 5 months who presented a generalized. fungating

14. White, C. J., and Tyzzer, E. E.: A Case of Framboesia. J. Cutan. Dis. **29**:138 (March) 1911.

15. Lyle, H. M. H.: Gumma of the Liver as a Sequel to Yaws. Ann. Surg. **55**:111 (Jan.) 1912.

pustular eruption, part of which was shown by accompanying photographs. The lesions appeared in crops, were autoinoculable and were accompanied by itching and constitutional symptoms. The palms and soles were affected and there was a dactylitis. There was no glandular enlargement. When the patient was seen four years later. there was only a scar on the forehead to indicate the past trouble. According to the mother, all the children in the house had had the disease in milder form.

Davis,[16] in 1916, briefly reported two cases of yaws in a girl of 6 and a brother of 11 years who had apparently acquired the disease during a visit to Porto Rico. The eruption appeared after their return to this country. "The little girl showed one lesion on the lower lip, two in the right popliteal space and one typical cauliflower growth about 3 inches above the right popliteal space and one a few inches below. The boy had a few lesions of the same character on the legs. There was one sister at home who had a very large lesion on the buttock."

Evans,[17] in the following year, reported, in a brief and casual manner, two cases in which the patients were supposedly suffering from some manifestation of yaws contracted in tropical countries. The first patient was a returned missionary, from the South Sea Islands. He gave a history of suffering from frambesia eleven years previously. He presented "callouses or nodules about the size of a grain of wheat on the palmar surface of the index finger and thumb of the left hand. These were itchy and painful. There was also a small elevated spot in the left nostril." The lesions had been present two weeks or less. The second patient was a man who had served in the Philippines during the Spanish-American War. Since then, he had suffered from painful, recurring crops of vesicles and pustules of the soles, causing great pain and difficulty in walking. No spirochetes were found by staining. The eruption disappeared and did not return after one injection of 0.6 gm. arsphenamin.

Stephenson,[18] in 1920, reported fully the case of an American sailor in whom yaws developed while he was stationed at Brest, France. The writer thought the infection probably took place in a barber shop which was patronized by French Colonial troops recently returned from Africa. The patient was transferred to the United States, with the diagnosis of impetigo contagiosa. The eruption consisted of "crusted, circumscribed and pustular foul smelling lesions" of face, scalp and

---

16. Davis, C. N.: *Yaws* (Familial), J. Cutan. Dis. **34**:466 (June) 1916.

17. Evans, E.: *Yaws*: A Clinical Report of Two Cases, Wisconsin M. J. **15**:380 (March) 1917.

18. Stephenson. C. S.: *Yaws*; with Report of a Case which Developed in a Temperate Climate. Mil. Surgeon **47**:344 (Sept.) 1920.

penoscrotal junction. Some were "granulomatous and not unlike a fig in both color and consistence." When the eruption appeared, the patient had been away from Brest more than nine months. On admission to hospital, the diagnosis of frambesiform syphilis was made. The Wassermann reaction was positive. He was taken to the Vanderbilt Clinic, where opinions differed, the majority considering the disease to be syphilis. However, a Brazilian dermatologist was present that day, and he made the unhesitating diagnosis of yaws. Examination of serum from lesions showed spirochetes. Under arsphenamin, the eruption promptly cleared up and in ninety days the patient was returned to duty. The Wassermann reaction was then negative. A histologic examination revealed acanthosis and a plasmoma and marked polymorphonuclear infiltration, with here and there small abscess formation. There was an absence of changes in the vessels and connective tissue, suggestive of syphilis.

Schamberg and Klauder,[19] in 1921, published an elaborate study of a case of yaws in the person of a white American soldier returned from service in France. The eruption involved the palms, soles, scalp, forearms and penis. There were "brownish-yellow crusts which on being detached disclosed a raw surface consisting of red or yellowish fungoid granulations, secreting a thin, slightly purulent secretion." He gave no history of syphilis. Dark-field examination of the skin lesions showed "spirochetes with the morphological characteristics of *Spirochaeta pallida.*" The Wassermann reaction was four plus with several types of antigen. There was a successful inoculation of rabbit testicles, but failure to produce corneal and scrotal lesions in the rabbit by intravenous injection of blood in the acute stage. Several attempts were also made to inoculate a monkey, but without success. The eruption entirely disappeared after a second full dose of neo-arsphenamin. A histologic examination, revealed hyperkeratosis and acanthosis of the epidermal tissue and extensive lymphoid and polymorphonuclear infiltration of the corium, with absence of blood vessel changes. Spirochetes were found in the "leukocytic areas of the apices of the papillae subadjacent to the rete."

FURTHER REFERENCES TO CASES

In the search for further references to cases of yaws in the United Stated, some dermatologic statistics were consulted. In 1914, a report of the committee on statistics of the American Dermatological Association was published by the chairman, Dr. S. Pollitzer.[20] This was

19. Schamberg, J. F., and Klauder, J. V.: Study of a Case of Yaws Contracted by an American Soldier in France, Am. J. Trop. Med. **1**:49 (Jan.) 1921.

20. Pollitzer, S.: Report of the Committee on Statistics of the American Dermatological Association, J. Cutan. Dis. **32**:312 (April) 1914.

a combined report from various clinics scattered over the United States. It covered a period of thirty-four years, from 1877 to 1911 inclusive, and contained a tabulated list of more than 679,376 cases. In this enormous total, there were only twenty-eight cases of yaws. Thinking that even this very small number of cases had been largely observed in some of the southern clinics, I consulted the individual annual reports of previous years and was surprised to learn that none of these cases had been reported from the south. Of the twenty-eight cases, twenty were reported from Boston alone, twelve of these being seen in the year 1878. Of the remainder, three were reported from Chicago, one each from New York and Philadelphia and two from cities not mentioned. The fact that the great majority of these patients were observed in the large seaports strongly suggests that the disease was imported from some foreign country. In the statistical report of the American Dermatological Association from the year 1916, a total of more than 58,000 cases were reported from seventeen different cities, and not a single case of yaws was mentioned.

OPINIONS AS TO PREVALENCE OF THE DISEASE

It is evident from the small number of cases of yaws recorded in our literature and from the statistics here quoted that the disease is either very rare in the United States or that its presence is unrecognized. Yaws could scarcely be prevalent in the northern part of this country, as it is strictly a tropical disease. It seems evident that the comparatively few cases seen in the northern states are imported from elsewhere. That yaws is more prevalent in the South than is generally supposed is the opinion of Wood, who writes "Since studying the condition more fully I am inclined to suspect that we have been overlooking yaws and that among the negroes the disease has occurred in the South frequently and has been counted as syphilis." Continuing, he says that "every negro is assumed by most writers to be guilty of syphilis until he proves his innocence. Can it be," he adds, "that syphilis is being generally confounded with yaws in this manner and can it explain the well-recognized mildness of present day syphilis among the negro? Surely, we see comparatively few cases of tertiary manifestations among the negro in comparison to that seen in the white man." In a similar vein, McMurran writes that "a great many of the cases that have been diagnosed by the members of our profession may not have been smallpox but the disease I shall briefly describe" (referring to yaws).

An opposing view to the ones here quoted was expressed by Matas, in 1896, who wrote "How rare yaws has become in this country is demonstrated by the records of the Charity Hospital in New Orleans which show that only two cases have appeared in its clinics in the last nineteen years. That yaws must be a rarity in the Southern as well as Northern states would seem highly probable to me from the paucity of scientific reports in the South.

In an attempt to obtain further information on this subject, I have recently corresponded with a number of dermatologists in the South. Of the ten correspondents who answered a brief questionnaire, only one, Dr. H. E. Menage of New Orleans, had personally seen a case of yaws in the United States. This was a case observed "years ago at the Charity Hospital," which, he wrote, "we took for yaws," and added "if my memory serves me correctly he was a negro, native born." The others who wrote that they had not encountered the disease in this country were Drs. Marcus Haase (Tennessee) J. B. Shelmire, I. L. McGlasson and E. D. Crutchfield (Texas) J. L. Kirby-Smith (Florida) J. H. Edmonson (Alabama) E. P. McGavock (Virginia) C. O. Abernethy (North Carolina) and J. H. Fox (Mississippi). Of these, Dr. Kirby-Smith had formerly studied the disease in the Philippine Islands. He wrote "I am sure I would recognize yaws when seen in my practice." In answer to the question as to whether yaws was at all prevalent in the United States at present, all answered in the negative except one (Dr. McGavock). All who expressed an opinion regarding the former prevalence of the disease (in slavery times) answered in the negative. In this connection, Dr. Haase wrote "I do not think it was prevalent among the slaves as the negroes were excellently cared for at that time because they were valuable property"; an opinion that coincides with my own regarding some other skin diseases in the negro.

The question of the former prevalence of yaws among the negro slaves imported from Africa, particularly in the seventeenth and eighteenth centuries, is purely a matter of speculation. One thing seems certain, namely, that the disease has never gained a foothold and become endemic to any degree in the United States. From his study of the subject, Jones concludes that "the yaws is an African disease and disappears gradually when introduced upon the North American Continent."

Granted that yaws has not obtained a permanent foothold in the southern states, such an occurrence in the future would seem to be within the range of possibilities on account of the prevalence of the disease in neighboring countries. In his volume on the "Geography of Diseases," Clemow [21] says, in regard to yaws, that the West Indies "form one of the most important centres in the world of this disease." According to this writer, it is especially prevalent in Jamaica, Guadaloupe, Martinique, Trinidad, St. Lucia, Grenada, Antigna and Dominica

---

21. Clemow, F. G.: The Geography of Disease. London. C. J. Clay & Sons. 1903, p. 560.

It appears uncommon in Central America, but is fairly widely distributed in South America. The great prevalence of yaws in Santo Domingo is shown in a recent and most instructive study of 1,046 cases by Moss and Bigelow.[22] During the last two weeks of their stay in the island, the daily number of new and old cases ranged between 100 and 300.

If yaws by some possibility should become endemic in the southern part of the United States, it would not be a great cause for alarm. Though the disease is a most undesirable one, its diagnosis can now be aided by laboratory methods, and its successful treatment by arsphenamin constitutes one of the great triumphs of modern medicine.

CONCLUSIONS

1. Whether yaws was prevalent in the Southern states during the earlier days of slavery appears doubtful. It is a question at all events that can never be settled.

2. Yaws is a rare disease at the present time in the United States, in spite of its great prevalence in certain parts of the West Indies.

3. The majority of the recorded cases have been observed in our northern seaports and have evidently been imported from foreign countries.

4. Yaws would probably never thrive in the northern states as it is purely a tropical disease. With modern laboratory aids to diagnosis, and treatment with arsphenamin, the disease could easily be eradicated if it ever obtained a foothold in the Southern states.

DISCUSSION

Dr. John E. Lane, New Haven: Dr. Fox's reference to the history of yaws in this country reminds me that the Rev. John Clayton, in 1687, referring to Virginia, wrote to Dr. Nehemiah Grew of London as follows: "Among the Indians they have a Distemper which they call *Y*aws, which is nearly related to the French-Pox; which they are said to cure with an Herb that fluxes them. But this I have only by Hear-say." A description of yaws is given in a book attributed to John Tennant, published in Annapolis about 1730, entitled "Every Man His Own Doctor, or the Poor Planter's Physician." The treatment described in this book is rather interesting. A decoction of sumac root, bark of pine and bark of spanish oak was used for purge and emetic, and in addition two pills made of equal parts of deer's dung and turpentine were to be taken at bedtime.

Dr. William Allen Pusey, Chicago: I think Dr. Fox has done a service to us in giving the facts of this matter in America. It is gratifying that yaws has not obtained a foothold here. This is rather difficult for me to understand, because communication between gulf ports and the West Indies has been very intimate since the settlement of the country; the conditions among the negroes in the subtropical districts along the gulf are very like those in the West Indies, and it is very remarkable to my mind that the disease has not

---

22. Moss, W. L., and Bigelow, G. H.: *Y*aws: An Analysis of 1,046 Cases in the Dominican Republic, Bull. Johns Hopkins Hosp. **33**:43 (Feb.) 1922.

obtained a foothold there. This suggests the possibility that there is some other factor in its propagation, which is not included in the ordinary term "tropical climate," because the tropical and other features of the climate of a good part of our gulf border are not unlike those of the West Indies. The only part of Dr. Fox's conclusions that I would be inclined to say is not self-evident is the view that yaws cannot get into this country because it is a tropical disease. I should say rather that the possibility of its communication to this country is exceedingly unlikely, owing to some factor as yet unknown, because it may be some other thing—perhaps the variety of sugar cane or of bananas which these people eat—rather than the climate that is responsible for the disease.

Dr. Charles J. White, Boston: I am sorry to say that I cannot enlighten the association on the great number of cases recorded in Boston. I was entirely unaware of such an occurrence. It was before my day, of course. We cannot account for it in the way of immigration; we do have some inhabitants from the Cape Verde Islands, but, so far as I am aware, they do not have yaws. The man we saw was treated with iodid of potassium and the lesions disappeared very quickly.

Dr. Jay Frank Schamberg, Philadelphia: From the clinical photographs and the histologic pictures shown by Dr. Fox, it is evident that his is a classic case of yaws. The pictures are almost identical with those in the case reported by Dr. Klauder and myself. There are some points of general interest. In the first place. I believe it is beyond the powers of any man to distinguish between *Spirochaeta pallida* and *Spirochaeta pertenuis* under the dark field. But you will find that the field will swarm with spirochetes in yaws; whereas, in the secondary eruption of syphilis, they are sparse. We also found that *Spirochaeta pertenuis* was very difficult to stain with coloring agents that are very quickly taken up by *Spirochaeta pallida*. Another point is the difficulty of perpetuating this infection through successive generations of rabbits. Dr. Klauder succeeded in carrying it through a series of rabbits, but after a time lost it. We sent a strain on to Dr. Nichols of the Army and after a time his strain died out too. It appears to be easier to perpetuate *Spirochaeta pallida* than the spirochete of yaws.

A matter of importance is that, in this disease, we have an infection very strongly resembling syphilis, yielding a strongly positive Wassermann reaction. exhibiting a spirochete difficult to differentiate, and succumbing to the same arsenicals as syphilis. This may readily cause confusion in diagnosing the disease and, by a posteriori reasoning, it may lead to injustice to men enlisted in the Army or Navy. This happened in the case we reported. A soldier in France contracted a disease which was diagnosed as syphilis but which was proved to be yaws. If it had been syphilis, the man would not have been entitled to compensation because the disease would then not have been contracted in the line of duty. I think the diseases are of common origin. But in yaws the spirochete has become attenuated and is readily destroyed. The organisms in yaws appear to be very easily exterminated by a few injections of neo-arsphenamin. They are occasionally found in the spleen. An observation that may shed some light on our obscure comprehension of the significance of a persisting positive Wassermann reaction is this: While there is a very rapid disappearance of the lesions in yaws after one or two injections. the Wassermann reaction does not clear up right away. There is nothing in the literature on this, but in the case studied by us we made tests from week to week. and in spite of the prompt disappearance of the lesions. there was a very slow disappearance of the positive Wassermann reaction.

It was still slightly positive when the patient disappeared from observation. What is the significance of this persisting Wassermann reaction? Does it mean that the arsphenamin treatment killed most of the spirochetes and that those that survived were gradually destroyed by the natural defenses of the body, or does it mean that all were destroyed and that the positive Wassermann reaction was due to the presence of antibodies in the blood? In view of the fact that the statement is commonly made that yaws is cured by one or two injections of one of the arsphenamins, it is urged that the Wassermann reactions in these cases be followed up.

Dr. Charles M. Williams, New York: This case is of interest in connection with the case I presented before the New York Academy of Medicine which was diagnosed syphilid. I think the evidence is correct. The resemblance of yaws to syphilis is exceedingly close; and, if a man is not on the lookout for yaws, the diagnosis is rarely made. Considering how many men treat syphilis and how few think of yaws, there is opportunity for a great leak. There are two points in the diagnosis. The case of Dr. Fox is classic. One special point is the great number of lesions. This is a diagnostic point between yaws and the lesions of syphilis. Very often we think of secondary syphilis as being all over the body, and this is ordinarily the case; but, in my experience, there have been very few lesions in the cases of frambesiform syphilis; whereas, in yaws, there are many. Also, in looking up the literature in my own case, I found that lesions on the scalp and over the forearm are a very common feature in yaws.

Dr. E. L. Oliver, Boston: I should like to say a few words about the case Dr. White reported. I was working under Dr. White at that time, and one of the tests mentioned in the literature of this disease is the lack of sensitiveness of the lesions to acetic acid. In the case reported by Dr. White, I removed the crust covering one of the lesions and then applied 30 per cent. acetic acid, and I found that the lesions were totally insensitive to the acid, although they looked as if they would be very sensitive.

Dr. Marcus Haase, Memphis: It is easy to understand why yaws was not imported to the United States during the time of slavery. The dealers naturally picked the specimens that they brought to the Southern states. These men were placed on the block with nothing more than a strap on, if they were not entirely naked, when they were shown by the auctioneer, and naturally they would not bring one into the country with any such blemishes as yaws would produce.

Dr. Howard Fox, New York (closing): In regard to Dr. Schamberg's remarks concerning the profusion of spirochetes seen by the dark-field illumination, this was apparent when our examinations were made. I do not feel that the average observer could possibly distinguish morphologically between *Spirochaeta pallida* and *Spirochaeta pertenuis*. That the organisms, as Dr. Schamberg mentioned, have been found in the spleen, is true, but they do not seem able to obtain a foothold in this or other internal organs and produce any damage. It does not seem probable that yaws could become endemic in temperate climates. Up to the present time, it has been a strikingly tropical disease, and it has been said that in the tropics it is not encountered at an elevation higher than 800 feet. Dr. Williams' suggestion that many cases are overlooked is perfectly plausible. The disease in the United States must either be rare or unrecognized. It seems unlikely that yaws is really prevalent considering the present large number of well trained dermatologists scattered over different sections of the United States.

114 East Fifty-Fourth Street.

EROSIO INTERDIGITALIS BLASTOMYCETICA *

JAMES HERBERT MITCHELL, M.D.

CHICAGO

Saccharomycetic infections of the skin have long been recognized, but only recently has the subject been given the attention that it merits. Among the earlier studies were those of Gougerot and Goncea,[1] who described saccharomycetic organisms which they had isolated from lesions on the hands and feet. In our [2] paper on ringworm of the extremities, we mentioned the finding of a similar organism which was encountered in three cases. In our later work on mycotic infections of the hands and feet the yeast was grown from time to time, but as we were concerned with *Epidermophyton inguinale* and other related fungi, the yeast was disregarded.

In May, 1917, Fabry [3] described a series of yeast infections of the hand, to which he gave the name *Erosio interdigitalis blastomycetica*. In 1918, Berendsen [4] published an inaugural dissertation on the same subject. In 1918, Fabry [5] published another paper, and in April, 1921, Stickel [6] reported a series of forty-five cases, thirty-eight of which occurred in women. In March, 1922, Greenbaum and Klauder [7] made a valuable contribution to the subject of yeast infection.

The cases described by the German authors are all characterized by the appearance of a benign, superficial, well-defined, red, shiny lesion situated on the web of the finger, usually in the third or fourth interspace. In Stickel's series of cases there were thirty-eight women and only seven men. The disorder was never encountered in children. It is most commonly seen in women who wash clothing or have their hands in water in the course of housework. Soap suds seems particularly to be a causative factor in the production of the disorder or at

---

* Read at the Forty-Fifth Annual Meeting of the American Dermatological Association, Washington, D. C., May 2-4, 1922.

1. Gougerot and Goncea: Bull. Soc. franç. de dermat. et de syph., July, 1914; December, 1915, p. 335.

2. Ormsby, Oliver S., and Mitchell, James Herbert: Ringworm of Hands and Feet, J. A. M. A. **67**:711 (Sept. 2) 1916.

3. Fabry: München. med. Wchnschr., 1917, No. 48, p. 1557.

4. Berendsen: Inaugural Diss., Berlin, 1918.

5. Fabry: Weitere Mitteilungen über Erosio interdigitalis blastomycetica. Dermat. Wchnschr. **66**:321 (May) 1918.

6. Stickel, J.: Dermat. Wchnschr. **72**:257 (April 2) 1921.

7. Greenbaum, S. S., and Klauder, Joseph V.: Yeast Infections of the Skin: Report of Cases and of Studies on the Cutaneous Yeasts. Arch. Dermat. & Syph. **6**:332 (March) 1922.

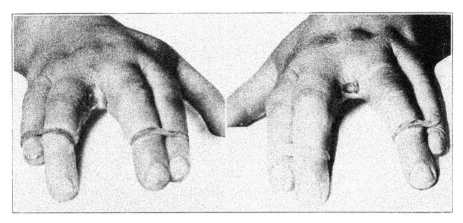

Fig. 1.—Appearance of hands when first seen in August, 1921.

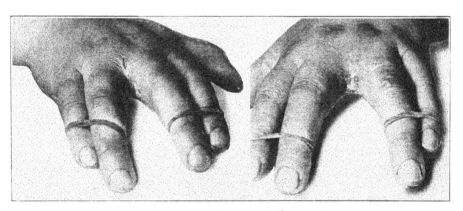

Fig. 2.—Appearance of hands in January, 1922.

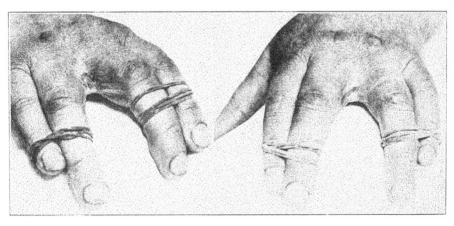

Fig. 3.—Appearance of hands at present time.

least in the continuance of the infection. Neither vesication nor lymphangitis was observed in any of the cases. In only one case did the infection spread over the volar surface.

Examination of the squames with potassium hydroxid in the usual way disclosed double contoured yeastlike spores. Inoculation of the interdigital surfaces with the pure culture of the organism was successful in seven cases. Subcutaneous injection of the organism in white mice caused a formation of abscesses with local alopecia.

Greenbaum and Klauder report, among their other cases, seven cases of the interdigital type yielding pure culture of yeast. The authors made a careful study of the different types of yeast organisms and divide them into four groups. Greenbaum and Klauder also successfully produced a typical lesion by inoculation of the pure culture.

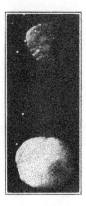

Fig. 4.—Cultures of yeast organism.

My own observations were made in three cases seen in dispensary practice; two of these patients disappeared after the first visit and were lost to view. All three patients were women who were doing heavy housework. The third case has been under constant observation since August 10, 1921, and was demonstrated at the January meeting of the Chicago Dermatological Society.

REPORT OF CASE

History.—The patient was an untidy Jewish woman, 26 years of age, who weighed 300 pounds. She had been married twice, and owing to nonsupport by her second husband, she had been washing clothes for a living. The lesions first appeared six years before on the web of the third interspace on either hand. They had been present constantly since the onset six years before, with only an occasional slight remission. The lesions had remained constantly in the same areas and had shown no tendency to spread either to the dorsal or to the palmar surfaces.

According to the statement of the patient, there was never any vesication before coming under observation, and since August, 1921, there had been no suggestion of vesicle formation. There was a moderate amount of itching and burning which was intensified by having the hands in soapy water.

Examination.—The lesions consisted of well-defined areas of shiny red epidermis surrounded by a collarette of upturned scales. Here and there were small areas of white macerated thin epidermis which could be removed only with a great deal of difficulty and much discomfort to the patient. In cold weather a fissure was occasionally seen in the center of the lesion on the dorsal margins.

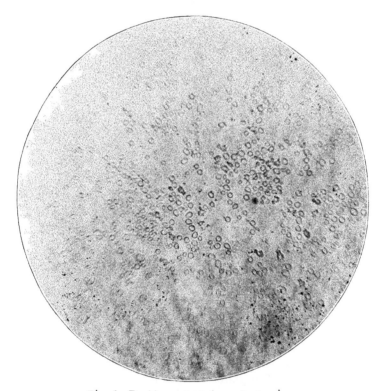

Fig. 5.—Double contoured yeast organism.

At no time had the lesions spread beyond the opposed surfaces of the web of the third and fourth fingers. The feet were free from any suggestion of mycotic infection.

Microscopic Examination.—Examination of the very small pieces of tissue which could be removed with difficulty disclosed double contoured spores which were budding here and there. There were also numerous mycelial threads which appeared to be solid rather than made up of segments, as is the case with *Epidermophyton inguinale.* There were also here and there spores which lacked the double contour and which showed no signs of budding. Plants of the tissue on Sabouraud's proof medium had given rise to creamy, white, shiny colonies of yeast organisms which microscopically were seen to be double contoured and to be budding quite freely. The colonies appeared three to five days after implantation, and when the culture attained a size of about 3 cm. the colony ceased to extend peripherally. Owing to the extreme intractability of the disorder to treatment, no attempts were made to inoculate the organisms on the hand of this or other patients.

Treatment and Course.—The treatment consisted at first in the use of Whitfield ointment in the usual strength. This apparently had no effect and was abandoned. Later chrysarobin in both chloroform solution of gutta percha and petrolatum was used, but likewise without effect.

Radiotherapy was then administered, but despite all the radiotherapy that was deemed safe the lesions persisted apparently unchanged. The treatment tried by Stickel, consisting of the application of a weak tincture of iodin night and morning and the rubbing on four or five times during the day of 20 per cent. salicylic acid powder, was carried out, but this likewise was without effect. As the patient was obliged to wash clothes she had her hands in water constantly. Aid from the United Charities finally enabled her to give up washing for a time, and apparently the discontinuance of laundry work was the only thing that was of any value in the management of the case.

The term erosio interdigitalis blastomycetica is confusing as it leads to the supposition that the causative organism is the well-known blastomyces, with which it has. nothing to do. Substitution of saccharomycetica for blastomycetica would be advisable.

The chronicity of the disorder, the fixed location of the lesion. the absence of vesication, the resistance to therapy and the occurrence of the disorder on the hands of washer-women, make the dermatosis worthy of consideration as an entity.

Whether or not the yeast is the causative organism I am not prepared to say, as I have carried out no inoculative experiments. for the reasons given in the foregoing.

MALIGNANT ENDOTHELIOMAS WITH CUTANEOUS INVOLVEMENT *

A CLINICAL AND HISTOPATHOLOGIC STUDY WITH A REPORT OF THREE CASES

GEORGE J. BUSMAN, M.D., M.S.

Fellow in Dermatology and Syphilology, The Mayo Foundation, and First Assistant, Section on Dermatology and Syphilology, Mayo Clinic.

ROCHESTER, MINN.

The rarity of occurrence, the peculiarities of the clinical course, and the fact that the true nature of the tumor is often concealed because of early surgical or medical interference make a malignant endothelioma peculiarly difficult to distinguish by its clinical characteristics. Because of the difference of opinion regarding the actual existence of endotheliomas, and because of the possibility of serious diagnostic error, illustrated by our own experience, I shall discuss malignant endothelial tumors in the light of three cases which clinically and histopathologically appear to aline themselves with this group.

The variability of the endothelial cell in neoplasms and the ability of endothelium to undergo metaplasia, simulating the epithelial type at one point and the connective tissue type at another, has given rise to confusion in the differential diagnosis of endothelial tumors. The controversy with regard to the actual existence of endothelial tumors and the criteria for diagnosis is, in part, due to the difficulty of obtaining material from the primary focus at a point where the structure still shows that undoubted endothelial cells gave rise to the tumors. Because of the relatively slow onset and low grade of malignancy of tumors from cells lining blood vessels, lymph vessels, lymph spaces, and serous surfaces, the neoplastic change is usually well advanced before a diagnosis is even attempted. The size of the growth at the time of study makes it practically impossible to trace the various cells through their transition stages to the original proliferating endothelium. This point, among others, is illustrated by the first case [1] of my series.

REPORT OF CASES

CASE 1.—*History.*—J. C., a man, aged 34, was first examined at the Clinic, April 10, 1921. He had a large ulcer on the left forearm (Fig. 1). His general

---

* Thesis submitted to the Faculty of the Graduate School of the University of Minnesota in partial fulfilment of the requirements for the degree of Master of Science in Dermatology and Syphilology, April, 1922.

1. This case was presented for diagnosis by the Section on Dermatology and Syphilology of the Mayo Clinic before the joint meeting of the Minnesota, Chicago and St. Louis Dermatological Societies at Rochester, Minn. August, 1921.

health had been good, except for the lesion described, up to the time of his first examination in the Clinic. Thirteen years before he had been kicked on the forearm by a mule, but the arm had not been fractured, and little swelling or soreness had resulted. A few days later, he had noticed a small lump on the forearm about 5 mm. in diameter, which had gradually increased to 1.5 cm. in diameter within a year. He had had practically no pain. In 1914, five years after the onset of the lesion, the nodule, which had grown to be about 2 cm. in diameter but had not broken down, had been surgically removed. The mass had recurred in situ, and a year later, April, 1915, a second operation was performed. An infiltrated mass which extended from 7.5 cm. above the wrist to within 7.5 cm. of the elbow had been removed leaving a large granulating surface which had healed partially. In October, 1915, the lesion had again been explored and cauterized. Following this operation the wound had remained open and had given off a continuous bloody discharge. At no time had there been much pain or tenderness, a remarkable fact in view of the size and nature of the lesion.

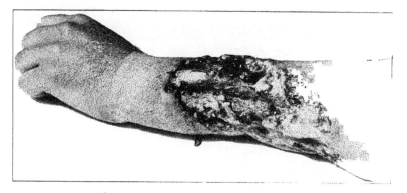

Fig. 1 (Case 1).—Large ulcer on forearm.

From October, 1915, to the date of admission to the Clinic the patient had received intensive local and systemic treatment without benefit. The treatment consisted of six intravenous injections of arsphenamin, twelve intramuscular injections of mercuric salicylate, potassium iodid by mouth, two exposures to radium of two hours each, the number of milligrams not known, violet and roentgen-ray exposures, various antiseptics including a surgical solution of chlorinated soda, continuous wet dressings, and continuous local baths. The patient did not give a history of syphilis, and the blood Wassermann reaction had always been negative.

Examination.—The ulceration extended from 7.5 cm. above the wrist to within 5 cm. of the elbow. The borders were irregular, indurated, undermined, reddish to purple and markedly hemorrhagic. Along the upper margin the border was slightly rolled and "pearly." The arciform configuration suggested a syphilitic lesion. The ulna was exposed, and although there was no evidence of periostitis, the bone was necrosed, the shaft being partially destroyed. The extensors of the thumb and finger were destroyed. The elbow and lower third of the arm were swollen. A mass was palpable in the axilla, and cordlike lines of infiltration extended from the broken down tissue to the elbow flexure. There was also a nodule higher on the brachial lymphatics, with slight diffuse infiltration of the surrounding skin. There was tumid induration of the tissues above the lesion.

In investigating the possibility of syphilis seven Wassermann reactions on the blood following a provocative injection of 0.3 gm. of arsphenamin were made, biopsy was performed, and cultures were taken; the provocative series of reaction was negative, the biopsy demonstrated subepithelial fibrosis with inflammatory changes, and the culture revealed an acid-fast bacillus.

Treatment.—On the hypothesis that the lesion might be an infectious granuloma allied to granuloma inguinale tropicum, the patient was given ten daily injections of from 3 to 10 c.c. of a 10 per cent. solution of tartar emetic. Local wet dressings of a 1:4000 solution of potassium permanganate, were used, and the lesion was exposed three times to rays from an Alpine sun lamp. The lesion became less hemorrhagic, and there was less odor and sloughing. The edges of the ulcer were then painted with a 5 per cent. scarlet-red ointment, and the base with a 10 per cent. solution of balsam of Peru. An aluminum

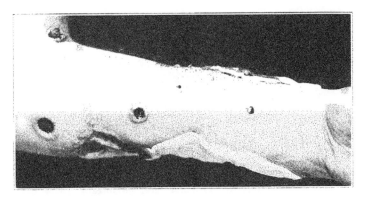

Fig. 2 (Case 1).—New nodules which developed and broke down while the patient was under observation.

acetate wet dressing was used. During the following three weeks an abscess slowly developed in the left axilla. Cultures from aspirated pus showed short-chain streptococci. Three days after drainage a profuse hemorrhage occurred from the axillary wound, and blood transfusion was performed. The lesion on the forearm continued to improve slowly under the local treatment, and July 30 a second biopsy was performed. The sections revealed a vascular, inflammatory, granulomatous tissue, with marked plasma cell infiltration around the vessels, inflammatory muscle tissue, fibroblastic strands and septums, no giant cells, no bacteria and no epithelial change except a moderate degree of acanthosis. The lesion was then regarded as a granuloma of unknown type, and treatment for syphilis was again resorted to. The patient was given six intravenous injections of arsphenamin at weekly intervals in conjunction with twenty intramuscular injections of mercuric succinimid, one-sixth grain (0.01 gm.), without local improvement. Following this treatment radium was used on the nodules in the axilla and upper arm, and the lesion in the forearm was exposed to the roentgen ray. October 15, six months after the patient was first seen in the Clinic, Dr. Stokes suggested the possibility of new light on the diagnosis by the removal of a small new nodule near the older lesion (Fig. 2). This material was examined microscopically by Broders and diagnosed as endothelioma. The importance of obtaining a specimen from an early nodule was demonstrated, for in two previous biopsies on the border of the old ulcer only a vascular structure with inflammatory change (granuloma) was revealed, and there was no evidence of the true character of the original process. After the diagnosis of endothelioma was made, the arm was amputated at the juncture of the middle and lower third of the upper arm. A small nodule from the inner side of the upper third of the arm was excised. The sites of possible metastasis were then repeatedly exposed to the roentgen ray and radium until the patient was dismissed, apparently in good health.

Histology.—The histologic structure of the fresh nodule in this case was, on first examination, rather unusual and complex. The most striking features, when viewed with the low power lens, were an undifferentiated polymorphic cell type of growth, a whorl arrangement of the cells, the formation of elongated cellular

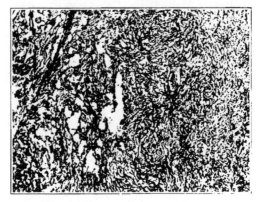

Fig. 3 (Case 1).—Section from a new nodule having the two characteristic structures of the tumor: a solid area with cells arranged in whorls, and an area of more advanced differentiation into vascular structures, × 50.

strands and narrow trabeculae, and the close association of the tumor with blood vessels and the formation of channels which might contain blood cells (Fig. 3). Many of the cell strands or trabeculae, when studied with higher magnification, appeared to be essentially ingrowths from or proliferations of the endothelial lining of the blood vessels and blood spaces. The cellular ingrowths by constant proliferation first formed the solid or whorled masses of cells; then vacuolization of the individual cells in the clumps and solid masses occurred with the formation of loose trabeculated areas and an attempt at differentiation into capillaries and blood spaces. The individual tumor cells were, in general, larger than normal endothelial cells, but they varied enormously in size and shape, having no typical form. Oval, cuboidal, spherical, flattened, and long columnar forms occurred, but the majority were spheroidal. In certain areas, syncytial or branching forms were seen which resembled the true vasoformative type of cell. These cells suggested the true nature of the growth. There were neither characteristic tumor cells nor foreign body giant cells. A constant feature of the tumor was the occurrence of what appeared to be vacuoles in the cytoplasm of practically all cells. These vacuole-like areas which did not take stain, and which apparently did not contain fat, glycogen, hyalin, or colloid material, were of great importance, for by their confluence the lumina of the large characteristic sinuses and channels were formed (Fig. 4). In the solid areas composed of whorls of cells, the vacuoles of the individual cells were small, but they showed evidence of coalescence to form larger spaces (Figs. 5 and 6). In less dense portions of the neoplasm, vacuoles displaced almost the entire cytoplasm of the cells, and by their confluence formed much larger spaces. These parts of the tumor represented, apparently, an attempt at differentiation into vascular structures. This differentiation, however, was incomplete, and these spaces at best represented only rudimentary capillaries and blood spaces. In the walls, the tendency of the cells to exhibit their true nature was easily seen. The cells bordering on these spaces arranged themselves in rows, became elongated, and formed a rudimentary endothelial

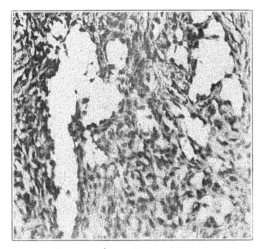

Fig. 4 (Case 1).—Tumor cells form trabeculae; vacuoles in the cytoplasm of individual cells; the coalescence of these vacuoles forms large spaces, × 160.

lining of the spaces. The cells were thicker than normal endothelium, however, and the lining usually consisted of several layers, although in some it might have consisted of a single layer, or might have been absent altogether (Fig. 7). These lining cells also expressed the character of the tumor by the formation of new vacuoles in the cytoplasm. There was a suggestion of further proliferation of the lining with the formation of new cellular ingrowths into the newly formed spaces themselves.

The sinuslike spaces were occasionally filled with erythrocytes which, apparently, had been extravasated, following the rupture of true blood vessels in the vicinity (Fig. 8). There was no evidence of circulation; neither could connection between these spaces and the true circulation be demonstrated. The individual tumor cells had nuclei which were extremely variable in shape and larger than the nuclei of normal endothelial cells. Occasionally multinucleated cells could be found, but no mitotic figures. A delicate intercellular cement could often be distinguished. In certain regions free infiltration into the muscle

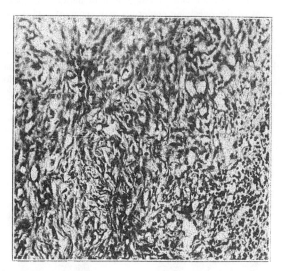

Fig. 5 (Case 1).—Early stages of vacuole formation, × 160.

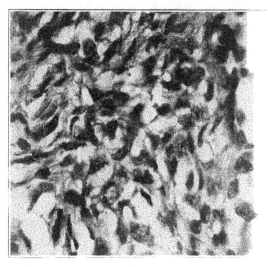

Fig. 6.—Various types of cells with vacuoles in the cytoplasm. × 500.

tissue of the surrounding part was demonstrable, and isolated muscle fibers were surrounded by tumor cells. There was moderate round-cell infiltration. No involvement of the overlying epidermis was apparent. There was, however, moderate acanthosis. Slight plasma-cell infiltration around the vessels occurred even in the early noninflammatory nodule.

CASE 2.—*History.*—C. M., a woman, aged 24, came to the Clinic because of an ulcer on the left heel. At the age of 7, she had had a furuncle over the left Achilles tendon, and later an abscess on the same leg just below the groin. Ten years before, in 1900, a nodule had developed on the inner side of the left heel. In 1906, the nodule had ulcerated and had begun to discharge. Four operations had been performed without benefit, and contracture of the Achilles tendon had resulted. Since 1908, the patient has had severe hemorrhages from the bowels at intervals of about six months.

Examination.—Proctoscopic examination of the lower bowel was negative. A biopsy of the ulcer on the heel was performed, and the diagnosis was sarcoma

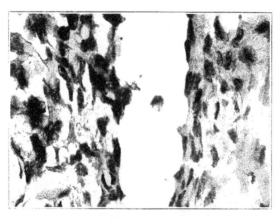

Fig. 7 (Case 1).—Cells bordering the spaces arrange themselves in rows to form an endothelial lining for the space, × 500.

or endothelioma. The lesion was cauterized and packed, but there was recurrence, and a second operation was performed, Nov. 30, 1910. Again, the lesion recurred and was operated on, Jan. 20, 1911. Microscopic examination again revealed malignant growth. A specimen removed, Feb. 23, 1911, presented the pathologic picture of oval-cell sarcoma. March 3, 1911, a new nodule which had developed on the ankle, the ulcer on the foot and the left inguinal glands were removed, and the cautery was used. Specimens from all of these areas presented the same pathologic picture. The patient went home, and Nov. 14, 1912, in reply to an inquiry, said she had recurrent lesions at the former sites, and also five small tumors in various other parts of the body. She did not return for further examination or treatment, and died, May 4, 1913, three years after examination in the Clinic, and thirteen years after the first apperance of the lesion.

Histology.—The histopathologic findings in the lesions from this case varied considerably according to the time and place of removal of the specimens.

Here too a polymorphic-cell, undifferentiated type of growth (Fig. 9), was found. The cells at certain points in the tumor had a whorl arrangement, and at other points were arranged in ropes or cords with the formation of trabeculae. There was no close association with blood vessels. With high magnification, the cell strands and cell masses appeared to have the characteristics of endothelium. The cells in general, however, were larger than ordinary endothelial cells. They varied in shape from spheroidal to cuboidal. Giant cells were not demonstrable. An occasional dividing cell and mitotic figure were seen. The conspicuous and constant feature was the occurrence of vacuoles in the cytoplasm of the cells, which tended to coalesce with the formation of spaces and channels. The cells lining these spaces were flattened, and had taken on the character of true endothelial cells (Fig. 10). Erythrocytes were found in a few of these spaces, but as in Case 1 no connection with the true circulation could be demonstrated. The vacuolization, however, and the attempt at differentiation into vascular structures were much less evident

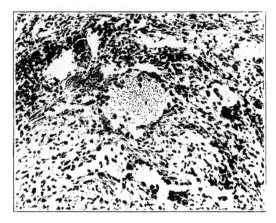

Fig. 8 (Case 1).—Red blood cells in newly formed sinuses. × 100.

than in the former case. The nuclei of the individual cells were large, and extremely variable in size and shape. Only a delicate intercellular substance was present. There was free infiltration into the surrounding tissues. Examination of the overlying epidermis did not reveal a lesion. The tumor merged into surrounding highly vascular granulation tissue (Fig. 11). Specimens from the heel, ankle, and groin exhibited the same characteristics, but in different degrees.

CASE 3.—*History.*—O. W. C., a man, aged 26, one year before had received a slight injury to the hand in cracking a nut. A small growth without pain or soreness had appeared. Ten months later, a glandular enlargement developed on the right side of the neck which grew to be 3.5 cm. in diameter. Examination revealed besides these nodules an enlarged gland in the right axilla. Both nodules were removed surgically.

Histology.—Microscopic examination of both tumors revealed almost identical pictures. The low power lens showed a cavernous type of growth, in parts of which the cells were whorled or solid (Fig. 12). In the cavernous areas the cells were arranged in strands with the formation of trabeculae. The individual cellular elements varied considerably in shape and size, but the occurrence of vacuoles in the cytoplasm was a common feature. It was clearly demonstrated that the larger cavernous spaces were formed by the coalescence of these vacuoles. The cells lining the lumina or spaces were flattened out with the formation of endothelium. The occurrence of the large spaces lined with flattened endothelial cells represented a more advanced attempt of the tumor to differentiate into vascular structures than in Cases 1 and 2 (Fig. 13).

DISCUSSION OF THE HISTOPATHOLOGIC AND CLINICAL PICTURES

In Case 1 six months elapsed, during which time the patient was under observation in the Clinic, before the true character of the tumor was discovered. The distorted picture at the first examination made it

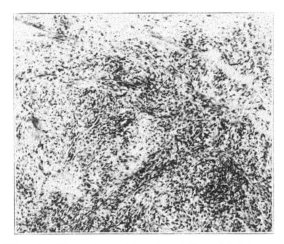

Fig. 9 (Case 2).—The polymorphic cell, undifferentiated type of growth in tumor on the ankle. In certain areas differentiation into sinuses is beginning, × 75.

almost impossible to recognize the character of the growth either by inspection or microscopic study. The history of a tumor of thirteen years' duration without definite metastasis suggested a benign rather than a malignant growth. No evidence of the original character of the lesion remained in the large ulcer. Repeated biopsies on the border of the lesion did not show a tumor of endothelial origin. In its place was a granuloma, probably the product of chronic infection. An imperfectly arciform configuration suggested the possibility of syphilis rather than malignancy. This was considered improbable, however, because of the inability of serologic confirmation, and the failure of the lesion to respond to treatment for syphilis. The distorted clinical picture is explainable on the ground that the lesion had been subjected

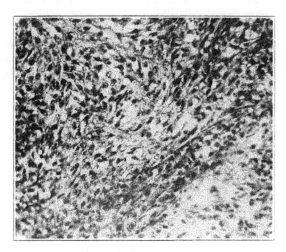

Fig. 10 (Case 2).—Vacuole formation in practically all cells. × 150.

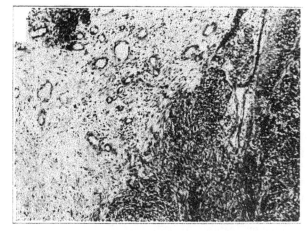

Fig. 11 (Case 2).—Characteristic masses of tumor cells closely associate with surrounding highly vascular granulation tissue. × 75.

to repeated surgical interference and that, to a large extent, secondary pyogenic infection was present, as evidenced by the purulent discharge and the metastatic abscess in the axilla. A culture from the lesion revealed a gram-negative bacillus, probably saprophytic. The response of the lesion, and the improvement in the general health of the patient under local medication, is explained by the fact that the local infectious process was partially controlled. There was no effect, however, on the original neoplastic element, as evidenced by the occurrence of new nodules in the upper and lower arms. In Case 1 the original tumor was almost completely replaced by a secondary condition. In retrospect,

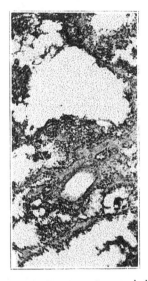

Fig. 12 (Case 3).—Cavernous structure characteristic of this tumor, × 50.

the hemorrhagic character of the tumor, the relatively benign course of the lesion, the good general condition of the patient, the long delayed metastasis, which did not occur until the tumor had reached considerable size, and the appearance of the original lesion at a site of trauma might have led one earlier to suspect malignant endothelial tumor.

Cases 2 and 3 presented clinical pictures in many ways similar to Case 1. Common features of both were the hemorrhagic character of the lesion, the onset following trauma, the relatively benign course of the growth, the late metastasis and the good general health of the patients. Histologically the tumors in the three cases presented essentially the same picture. These three tumors, because of the infiltrative and destructive growth and metastasis, must be regarded as malignant growths. Should they be designated as endotheliomas, even though they reproduce the structure of the hyperplastic endothelial cell?

The inability to obtain an early nodule showing the actual beginning proliferation of the endothelial cells makes it, of course, difficult to demonstrate that cells of undoubted endothelial origin give rise to the cell masses. However, the tumor cells, in general, exhibit so many characteristics of the endothelial cell that it seems justifiable to designate them as such. The undifferentiated, polymorphic-cell type of growth, the appearance within the cells of vacuoles which in turn coalesce to form the rudimentary blood spaces, the syncytial or branch-

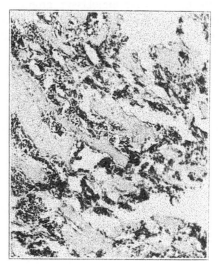

Fig. 13 (Case 3).—Section from metastatic nodule showing the same cavernous structure as the parent tumor, × 75.

ing forms which resemble the true vasoformative type of cells, and the differentiation of the cells lining the newly formed spaces into fairly typical endothelium, are all constant features which suggest endothelial origin. In Case 2 the differentiation into capillaries and spaces was the least complete, and the tumor from its clinical behavior was the most malignant. In Case 1 the differentiation was more advanced and malignancy less marked. The tumor in Case 3, however, showed almost complete differentiation into vascular structures and, to judge from its clinical behavior, was least malignant. It seems evident, then, that the malignancy of the tumor depends, in part, on the degree of differentiation as in other neoplasms, the differentiation in this case being into vascular structures.

THE CLASSIFICATION OF ENDOTHELIAL NEOPLASMS

According to Ziegler,[2] Delafield and Prudden,[3] MacCallum,[4] and others, the classification of tumors depends on whether their growth is typical or atypical, on their morphology and on their histogenesis. Two tumors may be the same morphologically and histogenetically, but one may be benign and the other malignant, depending on whether or not it is a typical or an atypical growth. Carcinoma is an atypical growth of epithelial origin. It is a malignant tumor derived from tissues which have their origin in the ectoblast or entoblast, the only exception being the lining of the genito-urinary tract whose epithelium, as far as the bladder, is of mesoblastic origin, and hence genetically closely related to the extensive mesoblastic group of tissues. In the same way, a sarcoma is an atypical growth of connective tissue origin. It is a malignant tumor of structures which are products of the mesoblast. Carcinoma and sarcoma differ in both their morphology and their histogenesis. Their atypical growth characterizes them as malignant. According to Böhm, Davidoff and Huber,[5] Prentiss,[6] and others, the cells which constitute the endothelium that lines the serous surfaces, including those of the pericardium, pleura, dura and peritoneum, with those of the blood and lymph vessels and lymphatic spaces throughout the body, are modified cells of mesoblastic origin. The endothelial cell belongs to the connective tissue group, and is properly regarded as a modified element of that type of tissue. Endothelial cells resemble, however, those of squamous epithelium in that they are markedly flattened with faintly granular protoplasm, possess flattened, oval or nearly round nuclei, are of polyhedral shape, and are united into a single layer by a small amount of intercellular cement substance; although the borders of the cells may be quite regular or slightly wavy, more often they are serrated. The quantity of intercellular cement substances between endothelial cells is so small and the cell boundary so indistinct that it is necessary to resort to special staining methods in order clearly to bring out their outline. On the other hand, in the connective tissues it is the intercellular substance and not the cells that characterize the tissue, the cellular elements themselves forming

2. Ziegler, E.: General Pathology, Ed. 11, New York, William Wood & Co., 1908. pp. 419, 425.

3. Delafield, F., and Prudden, T. M.: A Text Book of Pathology, Ed. 10, New York, William Wood & Co., 1914.

4. MacCallum, W. G.: A Text-Book of Pathology, Philadelphia, W. B. Saunders Company, 1919, p. 904.

5. Böhm, A. A.; von Davidoff, M., and Huber, G. C.: A Text-Book of Histology, Philadelphia, W. B. Saunders Company, 1900, pp. 84-85.

6. Prentiss, C. W.: A Laboratory Manual and Text-Book of Embryology, Philadelphia, W. B. Saunders Company, 1915, pp. 45, 64.

the less conspicuous portion (Prentiss,[6] Boehm, Davidoff and Huber,[5] Piersol, and others).

An endothelioma, according to the interpretation which is placed on the morphology and histogenesis of the endothelial cell, may be either a tumor of mesoblastic or connective tissue origin (histogenetically a sarcoma), or it may be a tumor composed of cells resembling epithelium (morphologically a carcinoma). The material available in the cases here presented does not permit a decision of this interesting question. The term endothelioma must then stand essentially as a name representing a compromise between the histogenetic and the morphologic views of the classification of tumors. The endothelioma is histogenetically of mesoblastic or connective tissue origin, but morphologically its cellular unit most closely resembles the epithelial cell of ectodermic or entodermic origin which is characteristic of the carcinomas.

THE LITERATURE

There has been much doubt regarding the actual occurrence of endotheliomas. Maurer,[7] in 1879, described two cases of malignant tumors of slow growth composed of ingrowths from the endothelial lining of blood vessels. The tumors exhibited hemorrhagic tendencies and also metastasized. Microscopic examination showed cell masses arranged in whorls and trabeculae which grew by infiltration into and around nerves, ligaments and muscles. Many small round cells with large nuclei were present. The cytoplasm showed a tendency to disintegrate with the formation of vacuoles. By the coalescence of these vacuoles distinct channels and blood spaces were formed, some of which contained erythrocytes. Because of the tendency toward capillary and sinus formation, he called the tumors angiosarcomas. In 1890. Franke [s] described a tumor 11 cm. in diameter, of five years' duration, consisting of tissue and blood spaces lined by endothelial cells in which could be seen what he called hyalin deposits resembling vacuoles. The tumor was formed in the lumen of a vessel from its endothelial lining. He, therefore, suggested the name endothelioma rather than the former name sarcoma. Limacher,[9] in 1898, described a tumor of the thyroid in which there was a distinct attempt at capillary formation. The cells of the tumor appeared to develop from the lining of blood vessels.

7. Maurer, F.: Ein Beitrag zur Kenntniss der Angiosarcome. Arch f. path. Anat. u. Physiol. **77**:346-363. 1879.

8. Franke, F.: Beiträge zur Geschwulstlehre: Endotheliome intravasculare hyalogene der Submaxillargegend, Arch. f. path. Anat. u. Physiol. **121**:465-482. 1890.

9. Limacher, F.: Ueber Blutgefässendotheliome der Struma mit einem Anhang über Knochenmetastasen bei Struma maligna. Arch. f. path. Anat. u. Physiol., suppl., pp. 113-150. 1898.

Krompecher,[10] in the same year said, "Tumors of the testicle of epithelial character (adenoma and adenocarcinoma) seldom have the histogenesis of epithelium." He believes that testicular tumors other than of epithelial origin usually develop from lymphatic endothelium, but occasionally from connective tissue. He asserts that the origin of lymphendotheliomas in the large lymph spaces has been demonstrated to be from endothelium; the origin of those developing from the lymph vessels had not been definitely proved to be from endothelium but evrything suggested endothelial origin. The term endothelioma characterized the tumor histogenetically and angiosarcoma morphologically. His statement that it is difficult to demonstrate that the tumors in blood and lymph vessels are directly of endothelial origin, although their structure strongly suggests it, is entirely in accord with my observation. Harris,[11] in 1893, mentioned a case of primary cylindrical cell endothelioma of the pleura. In 1895, Volkmann [12] in discussing endotheliomas, characterized them as tumors originating from the endothelial lining of blood vessels, lymph vessels and spaces, and pleural and peritoneal serous surfaces. He asserts that the vacuole-like appearance is due to deposits of glycogen in the cytoplasm, as opposed to the idea of former writers on hyalin degeneration. The vacuoles or spaces in the tumor cells in the three cases of my series apparently contained neither hyalin nor glycogen. Barth,[13] in 1896, differentiated endothelial tumors from carcinoma and sarcoma in that they were new growths with the histogenesis of a fibroma or sarcoma and the morphology of endothelial structures. The case he described was that of a tumor composed of minute capillaries and blood spaces. The endothelial cells were thickened and contained large nuclei. Vacuole formation was a common occurrence in the cell cytoplasm. He traced the origin to a definite proliferation of the endothelial cells of lymph vessels and lymph spaces. Borrmann,[14] in 1898, and Marckwald,[15] in 1899, reported cases

10. Krompecher, E.: Ueber die Geschwülste, insbesondere die Endotheliome des Hodens, Arch. f. path. Anat. u. Physiol., suppl. **151**:1-65, 1898.

11. Harris, T.: A Contribution to the Pathology and Clinical Features of Primary Malignant Disease of the Pleura, J. Path. & Bacteriol. **2**:174-189, 1893-1894.

12. Volkmann, R.: Ueber endotheliale Geschwülste, zugleich ein Beitrag zu den Speicheldrüsen- und Gaumentumoren, Deutsch. Ztschr. f. Chir. **41**:1-180, 1895.

13. Barth, T.: Ein Fall von Lymphagiosarkom des Mundbodens und Bemerkungen über die sogenennten Endothelgeschwülste, Beitr. z. path. Anat. u. z. allg. Path. **19**:462-496, 1896.

14. Borrmann: Ein Blutgefässendotheliom, mit besonderer Berücksichtigung seines Wachstums, Arch. f. path. Anat. u. Physiol., suppl. **151**:151-194, 1898.

15· Marckwald: Ein Fall von multiplem, intravasculärem Endotheliom in den gesammten Knochen des Skelets (Myelom, Angiosarcom), Arch f. path. Anat. u. Physiol. **141**:128-152, 1895.

of endotheliomas of the scrotum and bone. The latter does not say that he was able to demonstrate their origin from endothelium, but their structures suggested such origin.

From 1900 to 1905, opinions differed with regard to the occurrence of endotheliomas, and the definite identity of this group. Wolters,[16] in 1900, reported the case of a patient with nodules of endothelial structure on the chest. Warthin,[17] in 1901, reported a case of a tumor of the parotid which consisted of an overgrowth of the endothelial cells of the lymph spaces, lymph vessels and capillaries. The spindle-shaped cells were directly traceable to endothelium through all their transition stages. Colmers,[18] in 1902, described a nodule in the penis with metastasis in the lymph glands, lungs and pericardium. Histologically, a proliferation from the endothelial cells lining the cavernous spaces of the penis had occurred. Burkhardt,[19] in the same year, said, "Histogenetically one cannot differentiate sarcoma from endothelioma," and he suggested that the term endothelioma be dropped. He believes that if a tumor morphologically resembles endothelioma it should be called a sarcoma-endothelioma. He says that tumors of the same histogenesis may differ in morphology, and that the morphology does not determine the type of the original cell. According to Burkhardt, sarcomas are derived from the various cells which form connective tissue. In the purest and least modified type of sarcoma, the spindle-cell type, there is a definite participation of the endothelium of the lymph spaces. In such tumors the predominating type of cell and the endothelial cells respond to the same stimulus, but in a different degree.

Lazarus-Barlow,[20] in 1903, in discussing the status of endotheliomas held that the term includes a class of tumors which, ontogenetically, belongs to the class of sarcoma, and yet, so far as histologic character is concerned, bears a close resemblance to carcinomas. He says that these tumors are composed of cells having the characteristics of endothelium, and as a result they must originate in structures in which these

16. Wolters. M.: Haemangioendotheliome tuberosum multiplex und Haemangiosarcoma cutis, Arch. f. Dermat. u. Syph. **53**:269-312, 1900.

17. Warthin, A. S.: A Case of Endothelioma of the Lachrymal Gland (Myxo-Chondro-Endothelioma Cylindromatodes), with an Analysis of Previously Reported Cases of Lachrymal Gland Tumors. Arch. Ophth. **30**:601-620, 1901.

18. Colmers, F.: Ueber Sarkome und Endotheliome des Penis: im Anschluss an die Beobachtung eines Blutgefässendothelioms der Corpora cavernosa. Beitr. z. path. Anat. u. z. allg. Path. **34**:295-330, 1903.

19. Burkhardt. L.: Sarkome und Endotheliome nach ihrem pathologisch-anatomischen und klinischen Verhalten. Beitr. z. klin. Chir. **36**:1-122, 1902.

20. Lazarus-Barlow, W. S.: The Elements of Pathological Anatomy and Histology for Students. London, J. and A. Churchill, 1903.

elements are present. Coenen,[21] in 1905, described lesions on the scalp similar to those reported by Wolters. Wood,[22] in the same year, reported a case of endothelial tumor of the testicle with metastasis in the kidney, liver and lung. He believes that endotheliomas are directly related to sarcomas.

Lazarus-Barlow,[23] in 1906 and 1907, expressed the belief that the supposed phylogenetic origin of these tumors, combined with the method of arrangement of normal endothelium, should lead one to expect that endotheliomas would show great structural variation ranging between that presented by a typical spheroidal-cell carcinoma on the one hand to that of a typical sarcoma on the other. He contended that the group of endotheliomas in man must be enlarged to include certain growths of the breast, cervix and so forth, which heretofore had been considered carcinomas. He maintained, further, that the variations in certain growths in the human uterus and certain mouse tumors are explicable on the theory that such growths are endotheliomas.

Zeit,[24] in 1908, asserted that tumors which cannot, from a pure histogenic and morphologic point of view, be classified as either epithelial or connective tissue tumors should be called endothelial tumors. He explained their polymorphous structure on the supposition that the mesoderm comes from both the ectoderm and entoderm. Tumors of mesodermal origin, then, might have epithelial characteristics by reversion to their double embryonal anlages, or again might resemble connective tissue growths from mesoderm as such. Zeit described the clinical picture of endothelioma as differing from that of either carcinoma or sarcoma.

Ziegler,[2] in 1908, said that we should consider the endothelioma as a special form of sarcoma, and that endotheliomas in general often so closely resemble sarcomas that they cannot be distinguished from them. He says, "It is by no means determined that endothelial cells of lymph spaces and vessels do not take part in the formation of sarcomas." Delafield and Prudden,[3] in 1914, said that the stroma of an endothelioma may become sarcomatous. In 1908, 1909 and 1910,

21. Coenen: Ueber Endotheliome, Deutsch. med. Wchnschr. **31**:1131-1132, 1905.

22. Wood, E. J.: Report of a Case of Metastatic Endothelioma, Am. J. M. Sc. **130**:642-643, 1905.

23. Lazarus-Barlow, W. S.: The Histological Diagnosis of Endotheliomata, Arch. Middlesex Hosp. **7**:79-87, 1906; Glasgow M. J. **68**:265-274, 1907; The Relations of Endothelioma to Other Forms of New Growth, Proc. Roy. Soc. Med., Path. Sect. **1**:167-172, 1908.

24. Zeit, F. R.: Morphologic and Histogenetic Characteristics of Endothelial Tumors, J. A. M. A. **46**:567-576, 1906.

respectively, Hansemann,[25] Minne,[26] and Lofaro [27] described tumors of endothelial origin occurring in the skin. These tumors presented malignant characteristics, and the histology was that of endothelioma. Börst,[28] in 1913, reported similar tumors of the pleura, peritoneum, dura and skin, and designated those occurring in the pleura and peritoneum as mesotheliomas.

A gradual change in the trend of opinion and a decline in the opposition to the concept of endothelioma has occurred during the last five years. Matheny,[29] Fraser,[30] Schöppler,[31] Kron,[32] Pernet [33] and Kettle [34] reported cases of tumors, the structure of which characterized them as tumors of endothelial origin. Common features of all were the polymorphic-cell type of growth, the whorl arrangement of the cells, the formation of elongated cell strands and narrow trabeculae, and the formation of vacuoles which coalesce to form sinuses and channels which contain blood. These authors define endotheliomas as tumors of mesodermal origin, the cells of which tend to differentiate into flat endothelial cells such as form the intima of blood and lymph vessels, and the inner surface of certain cavities or spaces such as the pleura, peritoneum and the arachnoid and subdural lymph spaces. They are characterized as hemangio-endotheliomas if the tumors arise from cells lining blood vessels, and as lymphangio-endotheliomas if they arise from cells lining lymph or serous spaces. The tumors are also classified into perivascular, endovascular and peri-endovascular, depending on whether the original cells are in the perithelium, the endothelium or both.

ORIGIN OF THE TUMOR

A history of trauma was reported in thirteen (48 per cent.) of the cases. In general, the clinical course in cases reported in the

25. Hansemann, D.: Ueber "Endotheliome," Deutsch. med. Wchnschr. **22**: 52-53, 1896.

26. Minne: Endotheliomes endolymphatiques flexiformes primitifs et secondaires de la peau, J. med. de Bruxelles **14**:226-231, 1909.

27. Lofaro, P.; Endotheliom auf einem dermoidalen Mutternaevus, Deutsch. Ztschr. f. Chir. **106**:537-557, 1910.

28. Börst, M.: Quoted by Schöppler (Footnote 31).

29. Matheny, A. R., and Wallgren, A. B.: Report of Two Cases of Sarco-Endothelioma (Plexiform Angiosarcoma), Penn. M. J. **21**:143-145, 1917-1918.

30. Fraser, J.: The Hemangioma Group of Endothelioblastomata, Brit. J. Surg. **7**:335-342, 1919-1920.

31. Schöppler, H.: Ueber ein Endotheliome sarcomatodes, Centralbl. f. alls. Path. u. path. Anat. **30**:323-329, 1919-1920.

32. Kren: Ein echtes Haemangioendotheliom, Wien. klin. Wchnschr. **30**:28, 1917.

33. Pernet, G.: Case of Multiple Infective Lymphangio-Endothelioma, Proc. Roy. Soc. Med., Dermat. Sect. **13**:17-21, 1920.

34. Kettle, E. H.: Tumours Arising from Endothelium, Proc. Roy. Soc. Med. Path. Sect. **11**:19-34, 1918.

literature, as in my own, is that of a tumor of slow growth, developing at the site of former trauma. The lesions do not produce metastasis until late, when the tumor has reached considerable size. The tumors in all reported cases exhibit a marked tendency to bleed. A similar tendency was evident in my cases. The late metastasis is in marked contrast to that in carcinoma. The results of early excision with thorough removal are good, and the outlook apparently is much better than following removal of either carcinoma or sarcoma.

TABULATION OF TWENTY-SEVEN REPORTED CASES

Sex	Cases	Per Cent.
Males	20	74.7
Females	5	18.5
Sex not given	2	7.4
Age		
1 to 5 years	1	3.7
21 to 30 years	3	11.1
31 to 40 years	5	18.5
41 to 50 years	11	40.7
51 to 60 years	4	14.8
Age not given	3	11.1
*Location of Initial Lesion**		
Lower extremities	6	22.2
Upper extremities	4	14.8
Skin (location not given)	4	14.8
Thorax (pleura)	3	11.1
Chest	1	3.7
Head	1	3.7
Bone	1	3.7
Lacrimal gland	1	3.7
Penis	1	3.7
Testicle	1	3.7
Scrotum	1	3.7
Location not given	2	7.4
Average Duration of Lesion		
Less than one year	1	3.7
1 to 2 years	4	14.8
3 to 4 years	1	3.7
4 to 5 years	4	14.8
5 to 6 years	2	7.4
6 to 7 years	1	3.7
7 to 8 years	3	11.1
8 to 10 years	2	7.4
10 to 13 years	2	7.4
13 to 14 years	1	3.7
15 years	1	3.6
Duration not given	5	18.5

* Metastasis occurred in twenty-four (89 per cent. of the cases.

Various opinions are offered in the literature with regard to the etiology of endothelial tumors. Frazer expressed the belief that they are congenital in origin, supposedly developing from "rests" in the early formation of the vascular system. This point, however, is quite as unsettled as in other cases of malignant tumors. The development of the tumor takes place by endothelial cell proliferation with the formation of embryonic blood vessels. Further development may vary in different ones. A tumor of this type may undergo arrest, or, while retaining its capillary characteristics, it may grow by infiltration into and between the surrounding tissues; it may change from a capillary to a cavernous structure, or it may become compact and solid. In the latter, the endothelial cells form masses and whorls without capillary formation. This type probably is the malignant endothelial tumor which gives rise to metastasis.

Kettle has shown, by cutting entire nodules in serial section, that there is no physiologic connection between the blood spaces of the tumor and the vessels of the host. Small capillaries of the stroma rupture as a result of infiltration of their walls, and hemorrhage occurs into the surrounding tissues, forming cisterns, as it were, from which blood oozes into the vacuoles of the tumor. There is no true circulation of blood in the growth. As Kettle remarks, the condition is comparable to that in the early weeks of the development of the ovum where, as a result of rupture of the maternal capillaries, blood is extravasated into the choriodecidual spaces, and reaches the vacuolated spaces of the trophosphere. For this reason, hemorrhage is a common incident in the development of these tumors. The blood-containing spaces in the malignant endotheliomas merely represent an attempt on the part of the tumor cells to perform their normal function. The spaces result from a degenerative process which has its counterpart in the physiology of the normal angioblast, although it is quite uncontrolled in the malignant cell.

The degree of malignancy of endotheliomas, as in carcinoma and sarcoma, depends first, not on the morphology, histology or type of the original cell, but on the number and behavior of the individual cells. The higher the degree of differentiation, the lower the malignancy; the richer the tumor is in cells and the more independent of intercellular substance, the more malignant it is. The location of the lesion is important. The literature bears out the fact that. if the tumor is situated in a highly vascular area, or one rich in lymphatics. metastasis occurs more readily.

SUMMARY

1. Three cases are reported of tumors whose cellular elements present the histologic characteristics of endothelial cells.

2. The clinical course of the lesions in general is that of tumors of slow growth, often developing at sites of trauma. Metastasis does not appear until late, when the tumor has reached considerable size. The tumors in all cases exhibit a marked hemorrhagic tendency.

3. Clinically the lesions must be distinguished from syphilis. carcinoma, sarcoma, sporotrichosis and the infectious granulomas. The hemorrhagic character of the tumor. the relatively benign course of the lesion, the long delayed metastasis, and the good general condition

of the patient are features which should lead one to suspect malignant endothelial tumor. A final diagnosis, however, is practically impossible without histopathologic study.

4. Because of the variability in arrangement of endothelial cells, the ability of the cells to undergo metaplasia, the distortion of the original picture by secondary factors, such as infection, and the difficulty of tracing the tumor cells through their transition stages to preexisting endothelium, the earliest lesions obtainable should be employed in the histopathologic study.

5. The histologic structure of the tumors is that of an undifferentiated polymorphic-cell type of growth presenting a whorl arrangement of the cells with the formation of elongated strands and narrow trabeculae. There is definite evidence of an attempt to differentiate into vascular structures. A constant feature is the occurrence of vacuoles in the cytoplasm of practically all cells. These vacuoles coalesce with the resultant formation of large spaces. The cells bordering on these spaces arrange themselves in rows, become elongated, and form an endothelial lining of the space. There is a close association of the tumor with blood vessels. Capillary and sinus-like channels are formed which may contain blood, but have no apparent connection with the circulation of the host.

6. According to the interpretation which is placed on the morphology and histogenesis of the endothelial cell, the tumor may be regarded either as a structure of mesoblastic or connective tissue origin, histogenetically a sarcoma, or it may be regarded as a tumor composed of cells resembling epithelium, and hence, morphologically carcinoma.

7. The term endothelioma, as applied to my cases, represents a compromise between the histogenetic and the morphologic views of the classification of tumors.

8. Treatment consists of radical surgical removal of the original process followed by roentgen-ray or radium application to the site of the original lesion and to all probable areas of metastasis.

9 A gradual change in current opinion and a decline in the opposition to the conception of endothelioma as a type of neoplasm have occurred during the past five years. The three cases which I have described help to substantiate the belief that malignant endothelioma is an actual pathologic entity.

MELANOBLASTOMA OF THE NAIL-BED
(MELANOTIC WHITLOW)

ARTHUR E. HERTZLER, M.D.

HALSTEAD, KAN.

DEFINITION

Under this head may be described a malignant disease of the nail-bed marked by the formation of nodules of neoplastic tissue about the border and beneath the nails. The growth is characterized by the formation of melanin and a tendency to spread by way of the lymphatics. Hutchinson called this condition melanotic whitlow, a designation obviously inapt in the more advanced cases. I have adopted the term "melanoblastoma," in harmony with the teachings of Mallory, in order to emphasize the fact that, genetically, they are different both from the sarcomas and carcinomas.

INCIDENCE

The condition is rare, though obviously not so rare as the literature would indicate. The reported cases do not much exceed twenty. It has been my privilege to treat two of these patents, and, since American literature is all but devoid of case reports, a presentation of my cases, together with a general summary of the recorded cases, will be presented here. The case histories resemble each other so closely that a detailed account of each is uninteresting. Since, however, the literature is not readily accessible, the principal papers heretofore published will be presented in abstract.

REPORT OF AUTHOR'S CASES

CASE 1.—A widow, aged 64, a year and a half previously, as a result of a slight injury, had an ulceration beginning along the outer border of the left thumb nail. It was treated with iodin and salves without result. In a year, the greater part of the nail-bed had become involved, and the nail was removed. The pain had never been severe, but it was a constant annoyance. The pain became severe after prolonged use of the thumb.

When she came under my care, the nail was absent and the nail-bed was occupied by a blue-black granular area (Fig. 1, A). To the touch, the nodules were firm and did not tend to bleed. About the border of the granular area was a border of darkly pigmented tissue. About the relatively unchanged skin small deeply colored areas could be seen through the epidermal covering. There was no involvement of the neighboring lymphatic glands.

The thumb was amputated. It is now two years since the amputation, and the patient still is free from evidence of recurrence.

CASE 2.—A woman, aged 54, four years previously, first noticed a black spot under the left thumb nail near its base. The spot was then about the size of a black-headed pin, and looked like a blood blister following a bruise, but there had been no injury and it was not painful. About three months later, the center of the nail became white, dry and scaly and stripped off very easily. In a few months, this central strip of nail had completely separated itself, leaving a strip of healthy nail on either side with a hard, dry surface beneath. There was no soreness, but the area was sensitive to slight injury. The condition remained the same a year and a half. At this time, the remaining portions of the nail became dry and separated. The original black spot did not change until six months ago, when it began to spread and grew up like a wart. It now became sensitive. The patient attributed this to the innumerable slight injuries it received while she was nursing a sick daughter. She tried many kinds of salves and it was burned out a number of times by a physician. Following this the previously healthy skin at the base became brown. Five weeks previously, she had consulted another doctor. He sent her to a dermatologist who applied radium. The condition grew rapidly worse under this treatment and became excessively sensitive.

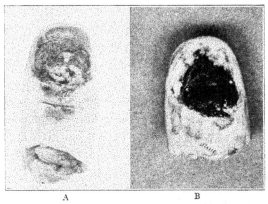

A   B

Fig. 1.—*A*, the nail-bed is covered with dry granulations. The surrounding skin is well preserved. At the base of the nail-bed, the tumorous masses are approaching the skin surface from beneath. *B*, the nail-bed is covered with a granular mass in which hemorrhages have taken place. The surrounding skin is in part exfoliated, exposing the developing tumor masses beneath. Above the nail-bed, the tumor masses are still covered with unchanged skin, but they are well distinguished by their color.

When the patient came to see me the nail-bed had a granular surface covered with recently coagulated blood (Fig. 1, B). The granules appeared to have some hemorrhage into their substance. The whole surface was blue-black. The skin surrounding this area was hard, dry and yellowish white. Near the border of the lesion, small brownish black spots shimmered through. The lesion was very sensitive to the slightest touch. The lymph channels and lymph nodes were not involved.

An amputation at the midphalangeal joint was made. Healing took place without reaction.

This patient was operated on only two months ago, hence a recurrence for some time is not to be expected.

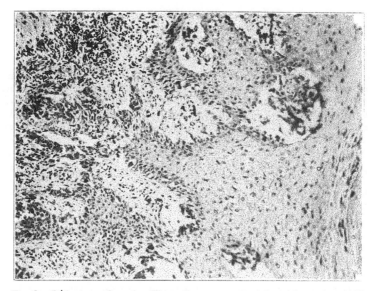

Fig. 2.—Slide from Case 1: The cell masses extend down from the papillary layer of the skin. The farther they advance the more elongated they become. Distributed among and within these cells are abundant pigment granules.

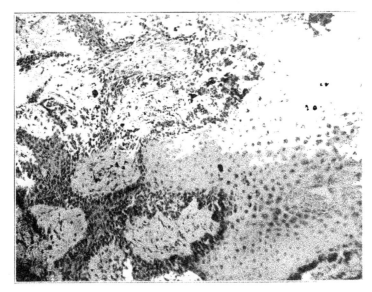

Fig. 3.—Slide from Case 2: The histologic findings are parallel with those in the preceding case.

Following are the only clearly typical cases that could be found in a somewhat extended search of the literature.

CASES IN THE LITERATURE

CASE 3 (Boyer[1]).—A man, aged 57, presented a tumor the size of an egg on the little finger of his left hand. The tumor developed thirty years before as a little black line about the finger nail. This remained stationary for twenty-eight years. During the last two years, the line had become inflamed and extended in breadth and was painful. It became nodular as the size increased. The finger was amputated.

CASE 4 (Demargnay and Monod[2]).—A woman, aged 59, had a tumor occupying the thumb of her left hand by covering the second and part of the first phalanx. It was dark and bled easily. It began as an excrescence near the nailbed. It had been removed some months previously and the base cauterized. It reappeared and hard masses appeared in the axilla, and an indurated cord could be felt along the arm. The slide showed large cells containing nuclei and nucleoli.

CASE 5 (Annendale[3]).—The patient, aged 56, fifteen months before, had observed a small red ulcer, formed beside the nail of the right index finger. The nail was removed, but the lesion spread. A fungus mass formed, extending to the palmar surface. There was a fine line of demarcation between the denuded and the normal tissue. A strip of skin separated the dorsal from the palmar nodules. After amputation, the dorsal part was found to be pigmented, the palmar pigment free. The slide showed cells of all forms.

CASE 6 (Nieberg[4]).—A man, aged 51, a year and a half before, suffered an injury to the ungual phalanx of his left thumb. A granular area appeared along the nail border, which was frequently cauterized and finally removed. This failing to cure, amputation was performed. Metastases in the axilla followed, these lesions containing pigmented cells. Necropsy showed extensions of the nodules along the vessels to the aorta and vena cava.

CASE 7 (Willett[5]).—A woman, aged 80, had a more or less spherical growth springing from and surrounding the ungual phalanx of the thumb. The surface was nodular and uneven, the skin ulcerated. The nail still embedded in the growth was pushed upward from its bed. The lesion appeared strictly limited to last phalanx, which was involved so that the remains of the bone could not be made out. Amputation was performed. The growth consisted, microscopically, of irregular masses of deeply stained nucleated cells. The cells appeared to be epithelial, similar to those forming a healthy nail. They did not grow from the surface. Their arrangement recalled the structure of rodent ulcer. There were no cell nests. Three years later, there was a mass in the axilla.

CASE 8 (Sacin and Keser[6]).—A man, aged 62, developed the lesion six years before entering the hospital, following a small lacerated wound. An ulcer was

---

1. Boyer: Gaz. méd. de Paris, 1854, p. 212.

2. Demargnay and Monod: Gaz. d. hôp., 1855, p. 415.

3. Annendale: The Malformations; Diseases and Injuries of the Fingers and Toes and Their Surgical Treatment, Edinburgh, 1865, p. 167.

4. Nieberg: Diss. Würzburg, 1882, p. 27.

5. Willett: Tr. Path. Soc., London **46**:152, 1895.

6. Sacin and Keser: Jahresb. ü. d. chir. Abt. d. Spit. in Basel, 1885, p. 114.

formed which secreted abundantly, covering the second and third phalanges of the fourth finger, elongated, with an irregular surface showing pigmented areas. The cervical and axillary glands were enlarged. Amputation was performed. The end-results are not stated.

CASE 9 (Hallé[7]).—A man, aged 46, presented an affection of the thumb which had existed seven years. The nail became deformed, shriveled up and cracked, and finally came off completely. The area of the nail became red and thickened. An incision was made into it, but only blood escaped. The wound did not heal, and the tumor advanced. Curettage and cauterization with a hot iron was performed, followed by a recurrence. A granular surface, dark red, with some dark spots sharply defined from the surrounding pale skin, developed. Amputation of the thumb was performed and two glands were removed between the biceps and the brachial artery.

The tumor was firm and black on section and sharply limited. The skin was destroyed over the surface. The glands removed from the arm were ovoid and definitely encapsulated. The section showed pigment. The slide showed large fusicellular alveolar sarcoma, more or less pigmented.

CASE 10 (Hutchinson[8]).—A man, middle-aged, presented a thickened nail along one edge of which was a black line which looked as if it had been touched with lunar caustic. Amputation was performed. Eight or ten years later, the disease recurred, involving the axillary glands.

CASE .11 (Hutchinson[9]).—A middle-aged man presented a tumor which had been growing on his thumb for several years. The growth was as large as a walnut. It was ulcerated over the whole surface, but showed no tendency to slough or become fetid. Just under the overhanging border of the unswollen skin was a narrow coal black margin.

CASE 12 (Lediard[10]).—A woman, aged 40, had a small melanotic tumor growing from the side of the nail of the index finger. The growth was painless for two years. The nail was torn off, the growth clipped off and the phalanx scraped. The finger was amputated two days later, after examination of the tumor had been made. The growth was three quarters of an inch (1.8 cm.) long, one-half inch (1.2 cm.) broad and three quarters of an inch deep. The patient died two years later of numerous melanotic tumors, distributed over the body.

CASE 13 (Faguet[11]).—A woman, aged 63, two years before, ran a splinter under the medial border of the left ring finger. The splinter was not removed and a phlegmonous inflammation developed. The splinter was finally expelled. but left a fistulous tract and a tumefied area. Later, a black nodule the size of the head of a pin developed near the fistulous opening. This spread, finally covering the entire nail-bed.

When examined by the author, the entire phalanx had been completely destroyed. The surface of the extremity of the finger was covered with a black, granular, ulcerating surface. The consistency was hard, particularly at the base. Three or four glands the size of a little nut were discovered in the axilla.

7. Hallé: Bull. de la Soc. Anat. de Paris 58:436, 1883.
8. Hutchinson: Am. J. M. Sc. 91:470, 1886.
9. Hutchinson: Tr. Path. Soc., London 36:468, 1885.
10. Lediard: Tr. Path. Soc., London 39:307, 1888.
11. Faguet: Arch. clin. de Bordeaux, 1894, No. 18, p. 448.

At operation, seven glands, black on section, were found in the axilla. Metacarpophalangal amputation of the finger was performed. The section of the tumor was mottled black and brown, with lighter areas. The slide showed small round cells, separated from one another by small bundles of connective tissue. Other areas show definite epithelial structure, without intercellular connective tissue, but with elongated cells.

CASE 14 (Coley, W. B.[12]).—A man, aged 37, seven years before observation, had bruised his thumb. Several years later, he bruised it again. It soon became painful, and five months later discoloration about the nail appeared. It was examined by L. L. McArthur, who called the lesion melanotic sarcoma of the round cell type. Amputation was performed, and a few months later shot-like nodules appeared in the skin of the wrist. Soon similar tumors occurred in various parts of the body. The patient was treated with toxins, and improvement followed, but soon large tumors appeared, and the patient died.

CASE 15 (Trimble, Wm. B.[13]).—A woman, aged 39, two months before had run a splinter under the thumb nail. Suppuration followed, and a growth the size of a walnut developed. The palmar surface of the skin remained unaffected. The tumor was a fungus mass which overlapped the healthy skin. Amputation was performed.

CASE 16 (Trimble, Wm. B.[13]).—A man, aged 45, whose nail, six months before observation, split slightly, and later came off entirely, noticed small pigmented spots in the nail bed. When first examined, the thumb showed a large fungus mass 2 by 3 inches (5 by 7.5 cm.) involving the whole distal phalanx. Amputation was performed.

Specific treatment was given in each case for a month, without result.

CASE 17 (Murphy, J. B.[14]).—A man, aged 56, six years before, noticed a slight serous discharge with reddening and irritation under the tip of the nail of the right middle finger. The finger was amputated three years later.

Five weeks later, enlarged epitrochlear and axillary nodes were removed. Two years after this, a node the size of a coconut appeared in the axilla. This was removed.

Murphy assumed that the tumor arose from the irritation of a "wart."

PATHOLOGY

Both of my cases represented a relatively early stage of the disease. They both presented the characteristic black border about the lesion. The lesion was granulomatous and looked out through a relatively unchanged skin. In some situations, small black points could be seen shimmering through the skin. This is well shown just about the nail-bed in Figure 1. The important point in the gross appearance is the fact that the growth seems independent of the skin, growing from beneath and displacing it.

The slides from my cases resemble each other so closely that the same description applies to both. Just beneath the epithelial layer, the

---

12. Reported in discussing a paper by Galloway on pathologic pigmentation preceding malignancies.

13. Trimble: Am. Med. **5**:788, 1903.

14. Murphy: Murphy's Clinics **14**:663, 1915.

tumor cells extend in more or less fringelike arrangement (Figs. 2 and 3). These projections seem to be direct continuations of the epithelial layer. The projections extend downward with little tendency to nest formation. The cells tend to become elongated and the nuclei pronouncedly ovoid. The continuation from the epithelial cells is only apparent. Because of the subsequent development and the clinical course, we are warranted in assuming that it is the chromatophore cells that form the starting point of these tumors.

PATHOGENESIS

The genesis of pigmented tumors has been much discussed. Ribbert is of the opinion that they are derived from the chromatophores. These cells lie beneath the epidermis, particularly along the blood vessels. Gibson and I [15] made a study of the pigmented tumors of the lower extremity. We showed that the clinical course of all pigmented tumors was strikingly similar, though the histologic structure may vary markedly. In Figure 16 of our paper, the histologic picture resembles the slides from the cases herein reported. Other slides, as Figures 15 and 17, show, respectively, an alveolar and a spindle form arrangement. We pointed out that, notwithstanding the variation in the histologic appearance of the physical characters of the tumor on the slides, the clinical course is the same. The tendency is to local recurrence, particularly spreading to the neighboring lymph glands or along the lymphatics.

Exactly the same thing is observed in the tumors of the nail-bed of the fingers. Local recurrence and lymph gland metastases are reported in all cases in which the course has been followed long enough. The histologic diagnosis of the reported cases has shown a great variation, carcinoma, sarcoma and sarcocarcinoma. In all these pictures, the clinical course is the same. It seems fair to assume that when the course is so markedly similar, the underlying conditions must be the same.

The clinical course and the histologic picture resemble the like lesion of the lower extremity. I believe the term "melanotic whitlow" should give place to the more accurate term "melanoblastomas of the nail-bed."

DIAGNOSIS

The appearance of a slowly developing granular area about the nail-bed, showing a pigmented border is characteristic of the disease. When the nail has been lost at the time that the examination is made, the history of onset and the deep pigmented areas beneath the otherwise unchanged skin leave no doubt as to the nature of the disease.

---

15. Hertzler and Gibson: Ann. Surg., July, 1914, p. 80.

PROGNOSIS AND TREATMENT

Apparently, all patients so afflicted sooner or later die of the disease. Some have remained free as long as ten years.

From what we know of like lesions in the lower extremities, there is reason to hope that early diagnosis and prompt amputation may produce a cure. Roentgen ray and radium, in these as in all melanotic disease, are worse than useless.[16]

16. In addition to the references already given, the following will be found of interest:

Galloway: Brit. M. J. **2**:873, 1897.

Wheeler: Proc. Path. Soc., Dublin. 1880-1881, N. S. 9, p. 171.

THE KOLMER MODIFICATION OF THE WASSERMANN REACTION

A REPORT OF ITS TRIAL IN A SERIES OF ONE THOUSAND AND FOURTEEN SERUMS [*]

ROBERT A. KILDUFFE, A.M., M.D.

Director, Laboratories, Pittsburgh Hospital and McKeesport Hospital;
Bacteriologist, City of McKeesport

PITTSBURGH

There are few laboratory procedures in common use which have aroused greater interest in the recent past or have been subjected to more intensive and extensive investigation than the complement-fixation reaction as applied to the serologic diagnosis of syphilis, or, as it is commonly known, the Wassermann reaction.

Both investigation and discussion have centered on two points: its reliability and the exact significance to be placed on the results obtained, and matters of technic as affecting the delicacy and reliability of the test. It is to be regretted that these two important phases of the question have not infrequently been discussed and investigated as separate entities rather than as intimately related factors of a most complicated and intricate problem.

It is impossible artificially to assign to this reaction a predominant value in any set stage of syphilis. If an arbitrary division is to be made, it seems fair to conclude that its value as a means of diagnosis can hardly be overestimated, as it is on the early diagnosis and the prompt initiation of treatment that the greatest hopes of ultimate success are firmly founded; on the other hand, without a reliable criterion by which to determine when treatment can be discontinued with any degree of safety, the management of syphilis and the avoidance of late and often intractable complications, while a "consummation devoutly to be wished," presents a problem of the utmost difficulty.

It is true, of course, that absolute dependence as to the absence of syphilitic infection, or an exact degree of safety and confidence as to a sufficiency of treatment cannot—and should not—be determined by the results of a single Wassermann test, and this fact is well known and admitted. Nevertheless, in the present state of our knowledge, it can be safely said that the Wassermann reaction constitutes the most constant single symptom of the disease, even though at times too great a reliance has been placed on the findings of a single examination.

---

[*] From the Laboratories of the Pittsburgh Hospital.

While much has been added to our knowledge concerning the reaction, much still remains to be elucidated. In spite of prolonged and extensive investigations by various workers, the true nature and mechanism of the production of the substance producing the reaction is still unknown.

Many factors concerned with the proper conduct and interpretation of the test have been brought to light, however, and on one phase of the question both serologist and clinician are in thorough accord: the vital necessity for the development of a standard technic which, exclusive of its value per se, will permit of a comparative analysis of the results of the test as conducted by workers of every community, which will form a reliable basis for diagnosis and an equally reliable criterion of the effects of treatment. The importance of this need has long been recognized and often proclaimed and the efforts of many investigators, therefore, have been directed toward this end with the resultant proposal of several "standard" methods.

The solution of the problem presents many difficulties arising both from the inherent complexities of the subject per se and as a natural concomitant to the personal preferences of individual workers, each of whom, using a method satisfactory to himself and tried in the fires of his experience, is naturally reluctant to abandon or modify it in favor of another. As a result, most of the proposed "standard" methods represent the personal preference of individuals fortified by prolonged experience.

It becomes obvious, therefore, that the evolution of any method having a legitimate claim to be adopted as a standard must follow directly on a careful, keen, unbiased and minute analysis of every possible phase and factor entering into the reaction. The technic must arise from and be based on the results of such studies and must present a logical basis for the modifications it involves, and must be subjected to fair, impartial and extensive investigation to determine whether or not the results indicated by the premises on which it is founded can be substantiated in the light of practical experience.

Such a study has recently been concluded by Kolmer and his associates, as a result of which Kolmer[1] has presented for trial a technic based on a careful study and analysis of the results of their work.

Through the courtesy of Dr. Kolmer the details of this proposed new method were made available to these laboratories some time in

---

1. Kolmer, J. A., and Associates: Studies in the Standardization of the Wassermann Reaction, a series of thirty-two papers published in the Am. J. Syph., 1919-1921. Kolmer, J. A.: New Complement-Fixation Test for Syphilis Based on the Results of Studies in the Standardization of Technic, Am. J. Syphilis **6**:82 (June) 1922.

advance of their publication, and I shall present the results of a trial of the method in a series of 1,014 cases tested by parallel methods.

Any technic offering itself as a standard method to supercede and push aside all others must, of necessity, be subjected to careful, extensive and analytic study before its unquestioning acceptance can be advocated; the results of this comparatively small series are of interest only as indicating, to some extent, the degree of usefulness of the method under ordinary routine conditions, and as acting as a possible stimulus to its comparative trial and the resultant accumulation of more voluminous statistics by others.

As has been noted in the foregoing, if the importance of the Wassermann reaction in the management of syphilis can be arbitrarily subjected to gradation, there is some justice for the contention that it is at least of great importance as affecting the matter of diagnosis. So far-reaching are the consequences, to the patient, his family and his associates, of either a false positive or a missed diagnosis, and so great has oftentimes been the unwarranted confidence placed in the results of isolated tests that the development of a technic the results of which may be looked on with a high degree of confidence is a matter the importance of which cannot be overestimated. Of no less importance is it that the method should prove equally delicate and reliable as a criterion for the estimation of the efficiency of treatment.

So far as can be at present ascertained, certain generalities seem justified: (1) In the present state of our knowledge concerning the complement-fixation reaction it does not seem likely that this method of examination presents a possibility of infallible diagnosis, nor that it— or any other method—because of factors inherent in the disease itself. can be depended on to detect unerringly the presence of syphilitic reagin at any and all stages of the disease. (2) The substance or substances now, for want of definite knowledge, grouped under the term "reagin," are not produced in constant mathematical proportion in various stages of the disease. (3) Because of these two facts, absolute reliance must not be placed on the results of a single Wassermann reaction, which should not be made the basis for dogmatic diagnostic or prognostic assertions. (4) No matter what the technic the results of the test must always be approximated with and interpreted in terms of all the other findings in the case at hand.

The problem as it presented itself in the investigation herewith reported was, therefore, to determine, as far as possible, the degree of delicacy to be imputed to the technic on trial and the degree to which reliance could be placed on the findings obtained with it, without any attempt to discuss the premises on which the modification is based. as these have been amply and thoroughly covered in the investigations of which this modification is the sequel.

Owing to the inability of the laboratory to regulate the type and character of the case tested, it was not possible to collect a large number of any one kind; indeed, this was not attempted as it was felt that greater interest might arise from a consideration of the results of the examination of unselected serums. The serums tested, therefore, were examined just as they came from the following sources:

1. Specimens taken as a routine in the wards of the Pittsburgh Hospital, the majority being taken for informative purposes with or without a possibility of syphilitic infection.

2. Specimens sent to the laboratory for diagnosis or as a control of syphilitic treatment.

3. Specimens from "Morals Court" cases forwarded by Dr. A. H. Eggers, to whom acknowledgement is due for his aid in securing "follow-up" data concerning them.

These last cases comprised those of many known prostitutes, the determination of whose infectivity was a matter of great interest, those of many known syphilitic persons, and many cases at various stages of treatment.

Ordinarily the Wassermann reaction is made in these laboratories on every day but Monday, Thursday and Sunday. The Kolmer method was performed on Tuesday and Friday.

While the majority of the serums were tested within twenty-four hours of their reception, many, such as those received on Tuesday afternoons, for example, were held over until the following Friday so that the Kolmer method might be used. Hospital specimens, as a rule, were examined within twelve to twenty-four hours of their collection. "Outside" specimens and those from Dr. Eggers were sometimes not received until from twenty-four to forty-eight hours after collection; they were occasionally hemolyzed in varying degree, and were subsequently, of necessity, held in the laboratory for a further period before being tested by the Kolmer method.

This was not looked on as a disadvantage but rather as approximating the conditions obtaining in laboratories in general, especially those receiving specimens from a wide area, and represents the conditions confronting any method proposed for standard or general adoption.

All serums of this series were tested by two technics; one, the routine method used in this laboratory, hereafter referred to as "routine"; the other, the Kolmer method, hereafter called "Kolmer."

In all instances complement, sheep cells, amboceptor, salt solution and inactivation period were identical in both methods.

All serums were separated from the clot as soon as received, except hospital serums, which were allowed to stand for some hours, placed in sterile, stoppered tubes, and kept at a temperature of from 4 to 6 C. until examined by both methods.

On Tuesdays and Fridays both tests were made, one immediately after the other; on the intervening days the routine method was performed, the Kolmer test of the same serums being made on the subsequent Tuesday or Friday as the case might be.

TECHNIC OF ROUTINE METHOD

Serums: These were inactivated for fifteen minutes at 56 C. and used in doses of 0.1 c.c. No attempt was made to test for or remove the natural antisheep hemolysin.

Salt Solution: An 0.85 per cent. solution was freshly prepared by diluting a stock 8.5 per cent. solution of dried chemically pure sodium chlorid 1 : 10 with sterile distilled water.

Complement: Preserved complement was used throughout in order to permit the use of the same complement in both methods. The pooled serum of four guinea-pigs was preserved both by the Rhamy method (the addition of one and one-half parts of 10 per cent. sodium acetate in physiologic sodium chlorid solution to each cubic centimeter), or by the addition of 0.3 gm. of dried sodium chlorid to each cubic centimeter of serum as advised by Kolmer. The treated complement was then kept frozen.

The former method of preservation was used in approximately three-fourths of the series, and the latter in the remainder.

Complement titration in 1 : 10 dilution was performed immediately before the main test, using a constant dose of 0.1 c.c. of amboceptor and 0.5 c.c. of a 2.5 per cent. suspension of sheep cells with water-bath incubation for one hour at 38 C. At the end of this time the unit of complement was read as the smallest amount giving complete hemolysis and twice this amount, or two units, used in the main test.

Amboceptor: Antisheep amboceptor was preserved by the addition of equal parts of chemically pure glycerin in ampule of 1 c.c. amounts. each ampule, therefore, containing 0.5 c.c. of serum. The contents of one ampule were transferred to a sterile, glass-stoppered bottle and diluted according to titer with sterile 0.85 per cent. salt solution so that 0.1 c.c. gave satisfactory hemolysis with a complement dose of 0.5 c.c. of 1 : 10 dilution, approximately 2 per cent. of 5 per cent. phenol in physiologic sodium chlorid solution added to prevent contamination, and the stock bottle was used until the supply was exhausted. The amboceptor throughout the series came from the same lot.

Sheep Cells: These were secured by bleeding the sheep (four animals bled in rotation to avoid producing undue fragility of the corpuscles) the day previous to the test in 10 per cent. sodium citrate in physiologic sodium chlorid solution; the cells were then washed four times the same day in physiologic sodium chlorid solution and twice more on the morning of the test, the supernatant fluid crystal being clear, as a rule, in the last three washings. The final mass of washed cells was made up in 2.5 per cent. suspension in physiologic sodium chlorid solution.

Glassware: This was utilized for Wassermann purposes only and sterilized by dry heat for one hour at 160 C. All solutions, suspensions, etc., were made in sterilized tubes or flasks.

Antigens: A triple battery was used, consisting of the following:

1. Cholesterinized extract of human heart: an alcoholic extract of human heart muscle containing 0.4 per cent. cholesterin and used diluted 1:20 with 0.85 per cent. salt solution.

2. Acetone-insoluble lipoids of the human heart, diluted 1:10 with 0.85 per cent. salt solution.

3. Alcoholic extract of syphilitic (fetal) liver, diluted 1:10 with 0.85 per cent. salt solution.

All dilutions were freshly made as needed. All antigens were retitrated at monthly intervals and used in doses of not less than five times the antigenic unit, which amount was always from ten to twenty times less than the anticomplementary unit. The hemolytic unit was determined at the time of the original titration but not thereafter, and no extract was used until it had been run with tried antigens in not less than fifty to 100 tests to determine the constancy with which it reacted.

The Test: Four tubes were used for each serum, the first three for the various antigens, the last being the serum control. During the incubation of the complement titration, which was first set up, the test racks were prepared, serums numbered, requisitions and laboratory numbers checked, etc., and the antigen dilutions prepared. The antigen was then placed in the tubes, followed by the serum dose. An interval of from fifteen to twenty minutes then generally occurred before the complement titration could be read. The proper dose of 1:10 complement was then added, and the racks incubated for one hour at from 2 to 5 C. in an ice-water bath, according to the method of Duke.[2]

After the primary incubation period the racks were placed in the 38 C. bath for a few minutes (not more than five), and the hemolytic system added. Secondary incubation was at 38 C. in the water-bath, readings being made when the antigen and serum controls were hemolyzed.

Controls:

1. Corpuscle and salt solution control: 0.5 c.c. of cell suspension plus 2 c.c. salt solution; no hemolysis.

2. Amboceptor Control: Amboceptor dose plus dose of cells plus 2 c.c. salt solution; no hemolysis.

---

2. Duke, W. W.: Ice Water-Bath in Complement Fixation for the Wassermann Reaction—a Shortened Technic, J. Lab. & Clin. Med. **6**:392 (April) 1921.

3. Complement Control: Dose of complement plus cell suspension plus 2 c.c. of salt solution; no hemolysis.

4. Antigen Control: Dose of complement plus dose of antigen plus salt solution plus hemolytic system after primary incubation; complete hemolysis.

5. Serum Control: One-tenth c.c. of serum tested plus dose of complement plus salt solution plus hemolytic system after primary incubation; complete hemolysis.

6. Positive Control: One-tenth c.c. of a mixture of several known positive serums; no hemolysis.

7. Negative Control: One-tenth c.c. of a mixture of several known negative serums; complete hemolysis.

Readings: These were made separately for each antigen on a $+ + + +$, $+ + +$, $+ +$, $+$ basis.

The degree of fixation given by each antigen was noted separately, all three forming the complete report.

In accordance with observations recorded elsewhere,[3] a serum was considered positive if reacting to the cholesterinized antigen in $+ 2$ degree, even if the other antigens were negative.

The technic outlined in the foregoing, with the exception of the primary incubation in the ice-water bath, represents that which I used over a period of years and on the basis of results obtained and an analysis of records, is believed to be reasonably delicate and satisfactory, so much so as to form an acceptable balance by which to weigh the results obtained with the Kolmer modification and to present a fairly strict standard for comparison.

TECHNIC OF THE KOLMER MODIFICATION

The technic used was exactly as outlined in the original paper except that, in the last several hundred tests, the serum dilutions were rendered less abrupt from Tube 2 onward.

The serum dilutions as originally devised were as follows: 0.1, 0.02, 0.004, 0.002, and 0.001 c.c. With this range a large number of $+4000$ results (classed as moderately positive) were obtained, and it became obvious that the drop from 0.02 to 0.004 c.c. was too abrupt. A similar conclusion was reached and recorded by Kolmer,[4] and a change to the following dilutions advocated: 0.1, 0.05, 0.25, 0.005, and 0.0025 c.c. Following this change in the range of dilutions an increase in the flexibility of the readings was noted, and this series of serum dilutions appears to be in every way satisfactory.

---

3. Kilduffe, R. A.: Concerning the Specificity of Cholesterinized Antigens in the Serologic Diagnosis of Syphilis, Arch. Dermat. & Syph. **3**:598 (May) 1921.

4. Kolmer, J. A.: Quantitative Fixation Test in Syphilis, Am. J. Syphilis, to be published.

Before proceeding to an analysis of the results obtained in the series it seems timely here to take note of some general factors concerned with the test as weighing for or against its permanent adoption.

It is not a technic to be readily acquired or grasped by the tyro—but then the tyro should not be permitted to sit in judgment on any question so gravid with important and far-reaching sequelae as the serologic diagnosis of syphilis or the serologic determination, so far as it can be determined, of the efficiency of treatment and the wisdom of the dismissal of a patient from observation.

To the experienced serologist, well grounded and at home in the intricacies of the subject, it presents absolutely no difficulty, and especially since the adoption of the new range of serum dilutions, the large series of tubes required for any considerable number of tests can be set up and filled with remarkable rapidity and certainty. By the accustomed eye no difficulty will be experienced in reading the results with a marked degree of accuracy; until experience is acquired, or in case of doubt, there is always a most ingenious and accurate reading scale for comparison.

From the standpoint of technical difficulty the new technic presents none that is insurmountable or even difficult to overcome, and extreme facility in its performance is rapidly and easily acquired.

The disadvantage of the added time necessitated before a report can be made, owing to the long incubation period, is more than counterbalanced by the greater delicacy of the test, as will hereafter be discussed; and the factors of expense, time and trouble in the preparation of the reagents and the conduct of the test can be disregarded.

The use of preserved complement decidedly lessens the expense of this item, and the new antigen used in the method [5] is so far in advance of any with which I am familiar as to render the expense of its preparation negligible. Indeed, the use of dried heart muscle powder which can be kept indefinitely, and the marked stability of the extract, together with the fact that it is very slightly anticomplementary and antigenic in dilutions as high as 1:2400, make it probably even a smaller item of expense than the continued maintenance of a supply of various extracts, which may require the preparation of several extracts before one which is entirely satisfactory is found.

If this new method had resulted in nothing more than this new antigen, a decided advance in technic would have been made.

Even at the expense of forestalling the analysis of the results obtained, some mention must be made of the clarity, distinctness and definite character of the readings. One is at once impressed with the

5. Kolmer, J. A.: A Superior Antigen for Complement Fixation Tests in Syphilis (a Cholesterinized and Lecithinized Alcoholic Extract of Heart Muscle), Am. J. Syphilis **6**:74 (June) 1922.

graphic and definite character of the results and soon acquires a sense of elation in the flexibility of the readings and the distinct separation into degrees of positiveness; where, before, between two plus four serums there is not a pin to choose, now there are definite. distinct and clearly outlined differences in the strength of the reaction graphically illustrating the intensity of the reaction to infection or a hitherto indistinguishable effect of treatment.

This feature alone constitutes no slight advance and advantage in the interpretation of the serologic index to the response to infection or the effect of treatment.

The readings are made on the basis of the degree of reaction in each serum dilution using a $+ + + +$, $+ + +$, $+ +$, $+$, 0 scale; the reaction is, therefore, a strictly quantitative test, which, it is admitted, forms the sine qua non of any method satisfactory for general adoption.

The readings are recorded as follows: Each figure represents the degree of fixation obtained with the respective serum dilution. When familiarity with the technic is obtained, by the clinician as well as the serologist, the reaction can easily be grasped by the fixation figures—to call them such for convenience—which may be set down much like the figures for a colloidal gold test.

Very Strongly Positive: Fixation *in any degree* in the first four or all five tubes, that is, with 0.005 c.c. of serum or less, for example. 44310, 44441, 34210.

Strongly Positive: Fixation in any degree in the first three tubes or in 0.025 c.c. of serum, for example, 44000, 34400, 41100.

Moderately Positive: Fixation in any degree in the first two tubes or in 0.05 c.c. of serum, for example, 44000, 34000, 13000.

Weakly Positive: Fixation in any degree in the first tube only or in 0.1 c.c. of serum, for example, 40000, 30000, 10000.

Negative: No fixation in any tube of the series, for example, 00000.

As noted by Kolmer in his original communication and confirmed in this series, occasionally there will be, with a positive serum, a lesser degree of fixation in the first tube containing 0.1 c.c. of serum than in the other tubes containing lesser amounts of serum, as, for example, 34100.

The natural inclination is to ascribe this phenomenon to the presence of antisheep amboceptors naturally present in the serum, but this supposition is untenable, as the phenomenon occurs with hemolysin-free serum. It is possible that there are other serum constituents which interfere with the union of antigen and syphilitic reagin, or that, in some way yet to be explained, the phenomenon is analogous to that seen in the proagglutinoid zone of macroscopic agglutination tests. This occurrence, however, is infrequent, and presents no difficulty in making the readings as the strength of the reaction is gaged by the *smallest quantity* of serum capable of giving fixation. As pointed out by Kolmer, it presents, however, an important possible source of error in technics in which doses of 0.1 or 0.2 c.c. of serum only are used.

Tables 1 and 2 give the gross results of the series with both methods. It will be noted that, first of all, there were fewer anticomplementary results with the Kolmer modification and that a larger number of positive results were obtained. Expressed in percentage, 1.5 per cent. more positives were obtained by the Kolmer modification than by the routine method.

AUTHOR'S SERIES

TABLE 1.—General Results with Routine Method
in Author's Experiments

Plus 4, all antigens...	150
Cholesterin plus	93
Total plus, 243 or 2.39 per cent.	
Anticomplementary	36
Negative	735
Total number of cases examined...................................	1,014

TABLE 2.—General Results with Kolmer Standard Technic
in Author's Experiments

Very strongly positive..	82
Strongly positive	37
Moderately positive *	126
Weakly positive	68
Total positive, 313 or 3.8 per cent.	
Anticomplementary	22
Negative	679
Total number of cases examined...................................	1,014

* The large number of moderately positive cases is in part accounted for by the fact that in the serum doses originally used the dilution between Tubes 2 and 3 was too abrupt; after the change in dilution, the number of moderately positive results was decreased in favor of an increase in the number of strongly and very strongly positive cases.

TABLE 3.—Results with Serums Anticomplementary by the
Routine Technic

Anticomplementary by both methods..................................	3
Negative with Kolmer technic...	26
Positive by Kolmer technic..	7
	36

Granting the validity of the additional positive reactions, the apparent gain in delicacy is not overwhelming, and were the analysis of the results to stop here, an entirely false idea would be obtained of the delicacy, reliability and flexibility of the new technic, factors only evident on a closer and more detailed scrutiny.

In Table 3 the results with serums anticomplementary to the routine method are grouped. Despite the fact that many of the serums were tested by the Kolmer modification when older than when tested by the routine method, a decided decrease in the number of anticomplementary reactions is noted, and in a large proportion of the serums definite positive and negative readings could be made by the Kolmer method.

This is a factor of importance and value as obviating in many instances the necessity for the collection of a second specimen, often a matter of grave inconvenience and annoyance to both patient and clinician.

In Table 4 several points of decided interest are at once evident.

By the routine method of sixty-six such cases, forty-three or 65 per cent. were negative and twenty-three or 34 per cent. were positive

TABLE 4.—SERUMS FROM PATIENTS WITH SYPHILIS UNDER TREATMENT

Number	Routine	Kolmer	Number	Routine	Kolmer
3142	0	44000	617	0	00000
3264	0	44000	619	C 4	44400
3294	Plus 4	44440	109	0	00000
3425	C 4 A 4	44000	5173	0	44100
3482	0	40000	5285	0	44400
3769	C 4	44000	5347	0	40000
3883	C 4	44440	5481	0	40000
4192	0	44440	511	0	40000
4236	0	44440	6076	0	44100
4371	0	44440	536	0	10000
4709	0	44000	6584	0	44000
4862	0	44000	6076	0	44100
4885	0	00000	6786	0	44000
McK. 454	0	00000	6841	0	40000
McK. 458	0	44400	7309	0	44400
McK. 462	0	44000	7383	0	44440
McK. 480	Plus 4	00000	7407	0	44310
McK. 498	0	44000	607	0	44441
5590	0	44000	7533	0	44400
5684	0	44000	609	0	4441
5823	0	44000	173	0	10000
5917	Plus 4	44440	5639	Plus 4	00000
McK. 532	0	44000	513	C 4	00000
McK. 539	0	44600	7261	Plus 4	40000
6289	0	00000	3424	C 4	00000
6350	Plus 4	44400	4500	C 4	00000
6820	0	00000	4809	C 4	44000
6948	C 4 A 4	44000	4802	C 4	44100
7213	0	40000	5007	C 4	44000
7379	Plus 4	44440	513	C 4	00000
7380	0	40000	6348	C 4	Ac
7384	0	00000	7562	C 4	00000
7403	Plus 4	44440	7450	C 4	00000

in varying degree, many being cholesterin positive only. By the Kolmer modification, however, fifty or 70 per cent. were positive in varying degree, fifteen or 23 per cent. negative, and one anticomplementary.

In the positive cases the graphic character of the readings forming a definite index to the degree to which response had been elicited by the treatment, and presenting a possible basis for the estimation of the degree to which it should be further pursued, is obvious.

It is to be noted that of the known cases of syphilis, two (480 and 5639) plus four to all antigens with the routine method, were negative to the Kolmer modification; and six (7450, 7562, 513, 4500, 3420, and 513) cholesterin-plus by the routine method, were also negative to the Kolmer modification.

Disregarding, for the moment, any question as to the validity of the cholesterin-plus reactions, this gives a total of eight cases of known syphilis in which, by the Kolmer modification, negative reactions were obtained which probably did not represent the absence of syphilitic reagin.

This is in accordance with the known fact that syphilitic reagin may, at times, present a selective action in regard to antigens and is illustrative of the fallacy of relying on a single negative Wassermann reaction as a criterion for dogmatic assertions. Bearing in mind the work of Thaysen,[6] who demonstrated, in known syphilitic persons, a wide range of varying reactions from plus to minus or dubious occurring without explanation, with fluctuations in the same case from time to time, it is another illustration of the necessity for repeated observations and emphasizes the fact that the reacting substance in syphilis is not pro-

TABLE 5.—DISEASES OTHER THAN SYPHILIS

Disease	Routine	Kolmer
Pneumonia.......	Plus 4*	00000
Pneumonia..	0	00000
Pneumonia..	Plus 4	00000
Enlarged thyroid and aortitis.......................	0	00000
Pneumonia...	0	00000
Uremia..	Ac*	00000
Cancer, stomach...................................	0	00000
Sudden deafness..................................	0	00000
Diabetes...	0	00000
Diabetes.,..	0	00000
Pneumonia...	0	00000
Tuberculosis..	0	00000
Rheumatism..	0	00000
Nephritis...	C 2*	00000
Nephritis...	0	00C00
Diabetes...	0	00000
Pneumonia...	0	00000

* Plus 4, all antigens; C plus, cholesternized antigen only; Ac, anticomplementary.

duced in mathematical proportion, may vary from time to time, and may show a selective preference for various antigens.

It demonstrates anew the unlikelihood of devising a complement-fixation technic which will be infallible at all times.

A study of Table 4 shows at a glance the extreme delicacy of the new technic, its flexibility and its decided advantage as a means of regulating and estimating the efficiency of treatment.

By this method far fewer negatives will be obtained, but when obtained they will be of far greater value. As a result, treatment when checked by this method will be likely to be more prolonged and more adequate and the ultimate results more gratifying.

In Table 5 are shown the results in conditions other than syphilis. A large number of hospital serums were, naturally, from a variety of

6. Thaysen, T. E. H.: Spontaneous Variations in the Wassermann Reaction, Acta med. Scandinav. **55**:281 (June 17) 1921.

conditions other than syphilis, but only those are noted in which false positives are known to be occasionally obtained by methods in ordinary use.

It will be seen that the Kolmer modification gave consistently negative results, a further enhancement of the value of the method and an added point in its favor.

In Table 6 are grouped the results of tests on the blood from twenty-three umbilical cords. One was cholesterin-plus by the routine method, the mother and father being Wassermann negative by the same technic. By the Kolmer method the same serum was negative. The blood from three cords was positive to the Kolmer modification, in only one of which was clinical or other corroborative evidence obtainable.

TABLE 6.—RESULTS OF TESTS OF BLOOD FROM TWENTY-THREE UMBILICAL CORDS

Number	Routine	Kolmer	Remarks
3922	C 4	00000	Mother and father negative by both methods; no history
4342	0	00000	
5721	0	44000	No history; mother and father not tested
6077	0	00000	
6157	0	00000	
6226	0	Ac	
6247	0	011000	No history; mother and father not tested
6290	0	00000	
6413	0	00000	
6468	0	00000	
6555	0	00000	
6789	0	00000	
6971	0	00000	
7102	0	00000	
7213	0	00000	
7235	0	40000	History positive: mother treated with neo-arsphenamin and mercury; child apparently healthy
7384	0	00000	
7397	0	00000	
7469	0	00000	
7490	0	00000	
7597	0	00000	
7619	0	00000	
7688	0	00000	

As has been recorded elsewhere,[7] the reliability and usefulness of the Wassermann reaction as conducted on the cord blood as an indication of syphilitic infection has been the subject of some discussion. The composite data of various investigators has shown that the results of the Wassermann reaction in pregnancy must be interpreted with great care, and that the cord blood is especially prone to give fallacious results when tested by methods in common use. In view of the fact, however, that the cord blood specimen is the most easily obtained, and that, except under the most ideal conditions, when it is possible to examine the mother and father as well as the child, this method of

7. Kilduffe, R. A.: The Clinical Evaluation of the Wassermann Reaction. Arch Dermat. & Syph. **6**:147 (Aug.) 1922. The Wassermann Reaction in Its Relation to Prenatal and Congenital Syphilis. Am. I. Med. Sc., to be published.

investigation will always be used to a greater or less degree, it is of decided interest to note the results of the Kolmer modification in even this small series.

The number of specimens is, of course, too small to allow any conclusions, but the results obtained indicate at least the advisability of an extensive trial of the method in obstetric cases which, in all probability, will give results tending to further enhance the value of the method and present added testimony to its general usefulness.

In view of the fact that, in the present series in toto, evidence tending to substantiate a positive finding was obtained in a high propor-

TABLE 7.—Results of Spinal Fluid Examinations

Number	Routine	Kolmer	Remarks
3101	Plus 4	44000	History positive; diabetes; fluid bloody
3168	0	00000	Recurring iritis; blood negattive
3297	C 4	40000	History negative; colloidal gold negative; cells 6
3293	C 4	40000	History negative; colloidal gold 1000000000
3794	Plus 4	44444	History positive; cells 64; colloidal gold 2342341000
3374	0	00000	History positive; cells 6; colloidal gold 1000000000
3393	0	00000	History and colloidal gold negative
3525	0	00000	History and other findings negative
3747	0	00000	History and other findings negative
4062	C 4	44100	Bloody; history negative
4139	0	00000	History negative; colloidal gold negative: cells 6
5582	Plus 4	44444	History positive; blood plus 4; colloidal gold 3222211000; cells 40
5658	0	00000	History negative; cells 19; colloidal gold 1210000000
5659	0	00000	Cells 8; encephalitis; colloidal gold negative
6271	Plus 4	44444	History positive; cells 40; colloidal gold 322221100
6282	0	00000	Cells 19; colloidal gold 121000000; history negative
6435	0	44400	Bloody; no history; symptoms relieved by mercurial treatment
6922	Plus 4	44444	History of chancre 25 years previously; cells 6; colloidal gold 1210000000; gumma (?) abdomen; relieved by antisyphilitic treatment; blood negative
6764	0	44444	History positive; cells 28; colloidal gold 2333430000
6944	Plus 4	44441	History positive; cells 128; colloidal gold 5555554300
7011	0	00000	Cells 10; colloidal gold negative; puerperal sepsis
7030	0	00000	Encephalitis; cells 16; colloidal gold negative
7032	0	00000	Cells 16; colloidal gold 1100000000; gives history of having had three chancres (?)
7450	C 4	00000	Sells 104; colloidal gold 4155555000; chancre 10 years previously
7597	0	00000	Cells 16; colloidal gold 3345544540; history negative; symptoms suggestive of cerebrospinal syphilis
5917	Plus 4	444100	Colloidal gold 555432110; history positive; chancre 15 years previously

tion of cases, the results obtained with these few cord bloods are, at least, of highly suggestive value.

In Table 7 are shown the results of spinal fluid examinations. Most of these fluids were examined because of known or suspected syphilis and a high proportion of positive results was looked for, an expectation amply verified.

With the routine method ten of twenty-five fluids, or 40 per cent., gave a positive reaction in varying degree. There were, however, two cases (6435, 6764) positive to the Kolmer modification but negative to the routine method, in one of which the only finding suggestive of syphilis was a prompt symptomatic response to mercurial treatment, the other (6764), presenting a positive history and classical cytologic and colloidal gold findings.

One case (7450) with suggestive cytologic and colloidal gold findings and a positive history was negative to the Kolmer modification and positive to the routine test. This is in conformity with findings already referred to and their possible explanation.

The final balance shows twelve or 48 per cent. positive by the Kolmer modification, a gain of 8 per cent.

It will be noted that the phenomenon of stronger reactions in Tube 2 containing a lesser amount of fluid than in Tube 1 did not occur in this small series of spinal fluids and, further, that the strength and degree of fixation could be definitely and graphically set down.

Of some interest are the results in a small series of cases tested when the primary lesion was in its early stage, as shown in Table 8.

In these cases the Kolmer modification picked up the reagin as early as in three and four days, when the routine method was still negative. In other instances, when a cholesterin-positive was obtained

TABLE 8.—Results of Tests in Early Lesions

Age of Lesion	Routine	Kolmer
4 days	0	44100
7 days	C 4	40000
7 days	C 4	44000
5 days	C 4	44120
10 days	C 4 A 2	44440
3 days	0	10000

with the routine method, a distinct variation in the reaction to infection was vividly shown by the Kolmer modification.

In Table 9 are a group of cases of decided interest: serums negative with the routine method but positive by the Kolmer modification. Of 111 such cases, one was a spinal fluid from a known case of syphilis, two were cord bloods without history of syphilis, tests of the mother and father direct not being obtainable; in forty-nine there was definite knowledge of syphilitic infection, many being cases under treatment; and fifty-one were specimens obtained from prostitutes in whom syphilis is a not remote possibility.

In the total series of 1,014 serums, therefore, approximately 10 per cent. additional positives were obtained by the Kolmer modification, in 50 per cent. of which definite evidence of syphilis was obtainable with strong presumptive evidence as to the correctness of the findings in the remaining 50 per cent.—results which speak for themselves.

In view of the strong efforts being made at present toward the control and eradication of venereal infections by health departments, it is of striking significance to note that here were fifty-one prostitutes

TABLE 9.—Cases Negative with Routine Technic
But Positive with Kolmer

Number	Routine	Kolmer	Remarks
3007	0	44000	Prostitute
3142	0	44000	Prostitute; syphilis 5 years previously
3165	0	44420	Prostitute; no history
3264	0	44000	Prostitute; history positive; spinal Wassermann plus 4
3482	0	40000	Syphilis, under treatment
3552	0	44200	Prostitute; no history
3883	0	44440	Syphilis, under treatment
4073	0	11000	Syphilis, under treatment
4192	0	44444	Syphilis, under treatment
4105	0	44400	Prostitute; no record
4217	0	01120	Prostitute; no record
4335	0	01100	Syphilis, under treatment
4236	0	44440	Syphilis, under treatment
4253	0	44400	Syphilis, under treatment
4342	0	44000	Cord blood; no history
4501	0	44000	Prostitute; no record
4709	0	41000	Syphilis, under treatment
4798	0	44400	Prostitute; no history
4799	0	44400	Wife is prostitute and has syphilis
4868	0	44400	Prostitute; has had previous Wassermanns (4), all negative to routine technic; no history or lesions
545	0	10000	Syphilis, under treatment
5073	0	44000	Alopecia; adenopathy; sore throat; gonorrhea
5079	0	44000	Cohabits with previous patient; no history; prostitute
487	0	44400	Syphilis, under treatment
462	0	44000	Syphilis, under treatment
463	0	44000	Syphilis, under treatment
5143	0	44100	Prostitute; gonorrhea; no history of syphilis
5172	0	44000	Had prevous plus 4 test by routine technic; prostitute
5173	0	44100	Prostitute; treated syphilis; 10 neo-arsphenamin
5174	0	44000	Runaway; lives with prostitute under quarantine for syphilis
5234	0	44400	Prostitute
5235	0	44400	Syphilis, under treatment
5236	0	44000	Syphilis, under treatment
5347	0	40000	Syphilis, under treatment
5479	0	44000	Prostitute; no hstory
5481	0	40000	Syphilis, under treatment
5313	0	40000	Syphilis, under treatment
5513	0	40000	Prostitute; husband has plus 4 spinal fluid
5522	0	40000	Has been treated for syphilis
498	0	44000	Syphilis, under treatment
5590	0	44000	No record
5593	0	44000	Prostitute; no record
5595	0	40000	No history
5600	0	44000	No history; prostitute
5601	0	44000	Prostitute; no history
5603	0	44000	Amateur prostitute; no history
5515	0	44000	Prostitute; no history
5683	0	44000	Prostitute; no history
5691	0	41000	Prostitute; no history
5745	0	42000	Prostitute; no history
5782	0	43000	Prostitute; no history
5807	0	43000	Prostitute; no history
5823	0	44000	Syphilis, under treatment
511	0	40000	Syphilis, under treatment
6075	0	12000	Prostitute; no history
6076	0	44100	Syphilis, under treatment
532	0	44100	Syphilis, under treatment
536	0	10000	Syphilis, under treatment
539	0	22000	Syphilis, under treatment
6467	0	10000	No history
6505	0	44000	Prostitute; no history
5511	0	44400	Prostitute; no record
6513	0	44000	Prostitute; no history
6519	0	44000	Prostitute; no record
6520	0	41000	Prostitute; no history
6521	0	41000	Prostitute; no history
6522	0	42000	Prostitute; no history
6526	0	41000	Prostitute; no history
6529	0	41000	Prostitute; no history
6531	0	42000	Prostitute; no history
6556	0	44000	No history
6581	0	44200	Prostitute; no history
6583	0	44400	Prostitute; no history
6584	0	44000	Syphilis, under treatment

TABLE 9.—Cases Negative with Routine Technic But Positive with Kolmer—(*Continued*)

Number	Routine	Kolmer	Remarks
6588	0	44000	No history
6624	0	04400	Prostitute; no history
6649	0	04400	Prostitute; no history
6651	0	40000	Prostitute; no history
6694	0	40000	Prostitute; syphilis
6435	0	44440	Spinal fluid syphilis
6732	0	41000	Prostitute; no history
6736	0	44000	Prostitute; no history
6738	0	04200	Prostitute; no history
6741	0	44820	Prostitute; no history
6786	0	44000	Syphilis, under treatment
6841	0	40000	Syphilis, under treatment
6858	0	02000	Prostitute; no history
7023	0	442100	Prostitute; no history
7035	0	44431	Prostitute; no history
7052	0	44410	Prostitute; no history
7074	0	44100	Prostitute; no history
7127	0	44000	Prostitute; no history
7213	0	40000	Cord blood; syphilis, under treatment
7217	0	40000	Prostitute; no history
7249	0	44440	General adenopathy; prostitute
7251	0	43210	General adenopathy; four miscarriages
7259	0	44440	Prostitute; no history
7309	0	44400	Neurosyphilis
7311	0	44000	Prostitute; no history
7332	0	44000	Prostitute; no history
7333	0	42000	Prostitute; no history
7380	0	40000	Syphilis, under treatment
7383	0	44400	Syphilis, under treatment
7407	0	44311	Syphilis, under treatment
607	0	44410	Syphilis, under treatment
7533	0	44440	Syphilis, under treatment
609	0	444100	Syphilis, under treatment
7723	0	44444	General adenopathy; knee reflexes absent; no history
1	0	12110	Cord blood: no history
173	0	10000	Syphilis, under treatment
194	0	44100	Syphilis, under treatment

all released from quarantine on the basis of a negative Wassermann test by a technic comparable to those in common use, many of whom, if not all, it is highly reasonable to suppose were infected with syphilis. Further comment seems unnecessary except to say that if the Kolmer modification were adopted by municipal laboratories charged with the study and control of venereal diseases, a much larger proportion of this element of the population will be held in quarantine and under control than is now the case.

Of no less interest are the thirty-one serums grouped in Table 10 —all positive to the routine method and negative by the Kolmer modification.

In fourteen of these there was a definite history of syphilis; one serum was from a case of pneumonia in the febrile stage, in which non-specific fixation of complement is known occasionally to occur, and the remainder are cholesterin positive serums in which a history of syphilis was not obtained.

These findings again demonstrate the fallacy of relying on a single negative reaction by any technic yet devised as infallible evidence of the absence of syphilitic infection at any time in any given stage of the disease, and also demonstrate the relative infrequency with which such false negatives occur with the Kolmer modification.

Table 11 shows results by the Kolmer modification with ninety-one cholesterin-plus serums. In sixty-four, or 70 per cent., both tests agreed, and of these sixty-four cases, forty-three were known to be syphilitic, many being cases of persons under treatment; in ten no data was obtainable, and eleven were prostitutes in whom the possibility of syphilis cannot be overlooked.

The high percentage of agreement between the two methods is of interest as affecting the question of the reliability of cholesterin-plus findings, a factor of interest because the new antigen used in the

TABLE 10.—CASES POSITIVE BY ROUTINE TECHNIC BUT NEGATIVE
BY KOLMER MODIFICATION

Number	Routine	Kolmer	Remarks
2050	C 2	00000	No history
2051	Plus 4	00000	Known syphilitic; dark field positive
3041	C 2	00000	No history of syphilis
2088	C 4	00000	No history of syphilis
3238	C 4	00000	Syphilis, under treatment
3297	C 4	00000	Spinal fluid: cells 6; colloidal gold negative; no history
3349	C 4	00000	No record
3356	Plus 4	00000	Primary lesion present
3403	C 4	00000	Nasal lesion clearing up under antisyphilitic treatment; roentgenogram suggestive of syphilis; history negative
3686	C 4	00000	Prostitute; has had previous plus 4
4046	C 4	00000	Syphilis, under treatment
447	C 4	00000	Syphilis, under treatment
4441	C 4	00000	Syphilis, under treatment
4483	Plus 4	00000	Pneumonia; febrile stage
4579	C 4	00000	Prostitute; syphilis, under treatment
4580	C 4	00000	No history
480	C 4	00000	Syphilis, under treatment
5439	Plus 4	00000	Prostitute; now has annular syphilid; three previous tests plus 4; under treatment
5438	C 4	00000	Prostitute; no record
5735	C 4	00000	No record
5838	C 2	00000	Enlarged thyroid and aortitis; no history
513	C 4	00000	Syphilis, under treatment
523	Plus 4	00000	Syphilis
524	C 4	00000	No record
6597	C 4	00000	Prostitute; no history
7148	C 4	00000	Wife has syphilis
7562	C 4	00000	Syphilis, under treatment
7450	C 4	00000	Spinal fluid from cerebrospinal syphilis; cells 10?; colloidal gold 445555530; chancre ten years before
619	C 4	00000	Syphilis, under treatment
49	C 4	00000	Lives with prostitute
104	C 2	00000	No record

Kolmer modification is a cholesterinized antigen, albeit reinforced by the addition of the acetone-insoluble lipoids incorporated in it, and if the standard Wassermann test of the future is to rely on such antigens, it behooves serologists, in general, to come to some agreement as to the reliability of cholesterin-plus reactions in general.

This matter of the specificity of cholesterin-plus reactions has been discussed in a previous communication [3] and the results obtained with the Kolmer modification are in no small measure confirmatory of the conclusions then formulated.

TABLE 11.—Cholesterin-Plus Serums

Number	Routine	Kolmer	Remarks
2050	C 2	00000	No record
2052	C 2	44210	No record
2072	C 4	00000	Prostitute; treated syphilis
3041	C 2	00000	No record
2088	C 4	00000	Interstitial keratitis; no history
3136	C 4	44000	Treated syphilis
3140	C 4	44000	Prostitute; lost
1514	C 4	41000	Prostitute; lost
3201	C 4	42000	Wife is prostitute and has syphilis
3238	C 4	00000	Syphilis, under treatment
3297	C 4	00000	Treated syphilis
McK. 3	C 4	34000	Treated syphilis
8349	C 4	00000	Prostitute; lost
3362	C 4	20000	Treated syphilis
3403	C 4	00000	Prostitute; lost
3411	C 4	41100	Treated syphilis
3424	C 4	342000	Syphilis, under treatment
3550	C 4	44000	No record
3571	C 4	40000	Prostitute; lost
3579	C 4	44000	Treated syphilis
3723	C 4	40000	Syphilis, under treatment
3764	C 4	40000	Cerebrospinal syphilis; spinal fluid plus 4 all antigens
3769	C 4	41000	Syphilis, treated
3820	C 4	44000	Prostitute; no record
3899	C 4	44400	Treated syphilis
3922	C 4	44000	Cord blood; mother and father negative to routine method
4046	C 4	00000	No record
4047	C 4	00000	No record
4062	C 4	44100	Spinal fluid, neurosyphilis
4083	C 4	40000	Treated syphilis
4089	C 4	40000	Treated syphilis
4309	C 4	44400	Prostitute; no record
4341	C 4	44000	Syphilis, under treatment
4441	C 4	00000	No record
4500	C 4	44000	Syphilis, under treatment
4515	C 4	44000	No record
4550	C 4	44000	No record
4579	C 4	00000	Syphilis, under treatment
4580	C 4	00000	No history of syphilis
4734	C 4	44400	Neurosyphilis; spinal fluid plus 4 all antigens
4760	C 4	44400	Syphilis, under treatment
4809	C 4	44000	Treated syphilis
4862	C 4	44100	Syphilis, under treatment
4866	C 4	44110	Syphilis, under treatment
4867	C 4	44440	Syphilis, under treatment
4850	C 4	40000	No record
4888	C 4	40000	Prostitute; lost
4906	C 4	40000	Syphilis, under treatmentt
4927	C 4	41000	No record
4932	C 4	40000	Syphilis, under treatment
4935	C 4	40000	Prostitute; no history
5007	C 4	44000	Syphilis, under treatment
5171	C 4	44000	Prostitute; no history
5291	C 4	31000	Syphilis, under treatment
5348	C 4	44440	Adenopathy; husband has syphilis
5458	C 4	00000	Prostitute; no history
5516	C 4	44000	No record
5519	C 4	40000	Neurosyphilis; spinal fluid positive
5962	C 4	44000	Treated syphilis
5742	C 4	44444	Primary lesion still present
5753	C 4	00000	No record; arrested in raid
5814	C 2	44000	No history; lancinating leg pains
5838	C 2	00000	Enlarged thyroid; aortitis
513	C 4	00000	Treated syphilis
522	C 4	40000	Treated syphilis
524	C 4	00000	Treated syphilis
5966	C 4	44000	Chancre three weeks old
6161	C 2	01000	Chancre seven days old
6348	C 4	Ac	Treated syphilis
6349	C 4	Ac	Prostitute; no record
6597	C 4	00000	Prostitute; no record
6740	C 4	44000	Syphilis, under treatment
6785	C 4	44000	Treated syphilis
6948	C 4	44000	Syphilis, under treatment
6931	C 2	44000	Spinal fluid; cells 28; colloidal gold 33334400; no history
7126	C 4	44400	Syphilis, under treatment
7148	C 4	44400	Treated syphilis
7279	C 4	44430	Prostitute; lost

TABLE 11.—Cholesterin-Plus Serums—(*Continued*)

Number	Routine	Kolmer	Remarks
7280	C 4	44400	Treated syphilis
7381	C 4	44440	Syphilis, under treatment
7562	C 4	00000	Syphilis, under treatment
7450	C 4	00000	Cerebrospinal syphilis; cells 104; colloidal gold 4455555310; chancre ten years previously
7693	C 4	11000	Chancre four weeks ago
619	C 4	44400	Provocative; suggestive history
623	C 4	34430	No record
49	C 4	00000	No history of syphilis
52	C 4	44410	Syphilis, under treatment
104	C 2	00000	No record; prostitute
110	C 4	44400	Prostitute; no history

SUMMARY AND CONCLUSIONS

The results of tests on 1,014 serums examined in parallel series by a routine method of complement-fixation and by the Kolmer modification of the Wassermann reaction are recorded and the findings tabulated and discussed.

As a result of the study the following conclusions seem warranted:

1. There are no disadvantages militating against the adoption of the Kolmer modification as a standard method of complement-fixation in the serologic diagnosis of syphilis.

2. The method presents the following advantages in favor of its adoption, as compared to methods in common use:

(*a*) It possesses greater delicacy.

(*b*) It presents a greater flexibility and elasticity.

(*c*) Strictly quantitative readings are easily made.

(*d*) Nonspecific fixations were not obtained in this series and are, apparently, extremely rare, if they occur at all.

(*e*) It is equally well adapted to the control of treatment as to the diagnosis of syphilis.

3. The new antigen used in the method is superior in every way to any hitherto devised.

4. As a means of determining the efficiency of treatment the method is far superior to any with which I am familiar, giving fewer negative reactions than by the usual methods, and thus ensuring more protracted and adequate treatment.

5. As far as is indicated by the evidence at hand, a positive reaction by this method constitutes extremely good presumptive evidence as to the presence of syphilitic reagin.

6. The method is not infallible and occasionally fails to detect syphilitic reagin in known cases of syphilis, in this respect being similar to all other technics, *except that such false negative reactions occur with much less frequency.*

7. Absolute reliance as to the absence of syphilitic reagin at a given time cannot be placed on the results of a single negative reaction by any method of complement-fixation yet devised.

8. In early primary syphilis the Kolmer modification gives earlier and stronger results than routine methods.

9. The results with this method are in close agreement with the clinical findings in a high percentage of cases.

10. It is a strictly quantitative method and as such better adapted to the study of treated syphilis.

11. It appears to be eminently worthy to supercede and supplant the methods now in common use.

12. It presents by far the most acceptable technic yet proposed for adoption as a standard method and as such should be subjected to extensive, exhaustive and impartial trial and study.

THE SPECIFICITY OF CHOLESTERINIZED ANTIGENS IN THE SEROLOGIC DIAGNOSIS OF SYPHILIS

SECOND COMMUNICATION *

ROBERT A. KILDUFFE, A.M., M.D.

Director, Laboratories, Pittsburgh Hospital and McKeesport Hospital;
Serologist, Providence Hospital

PITTSBURGH

In a previous communication concerned with this subject,[1] attention was directed to the importance of this question and its thorough investigation was urged.

There are few laboratories in which cholesterinized antigens do not play some part in the serologic diagnosis of syphilis, either forming a part of a multiple antigen battery or even constituting the sole standard by which the positiveness of the reaction is to be gaged.

As noted elsewhere,[2] the problem is one well worthy of, and even compelling, the attention of both serologist and clinician, for its satisfactory solution depends not on either alone but on the combined efforts of both.

It is worthy of comment, and a hopeful augury, to note the gradual eradication, in the discussion of syphilis, as of other conditions, of the tendency to discuss the laboratory and the clinical angles of the problem as more or less separate entities; for the effect of such an attitude can only be stultifying and obstructive. Only when the mutual dependence of clinician and serologist is recognized and emphasized can either attain their supreme effectiveness in the attack on this or any other of the multitude of problems confronting the earnest student of today.

In syphilis, the problem can be divided into two great sections: its diagnosis and its treatment.

The importance of the first is obvious; of no less importance is the question of treatment: how long should it be continued; when may it safely be discontinued?

To all of these, the question of the specificity of cholesterinized antigens is intimately related.

It is, perhaps, rather generally admitted that the treatment of syphilis should be persisted in until a negative reaction is consistently obtained with a cholesterinized extract; it is, therefore, rather with the

---

* From the Laboratories of the Pittsburgh Hospital.

1. Kilduffe, R. A.: Concerning the Specificity of Cholesterinized Antigens in the Serologic Diagnosis of Syphilis, Arch. Dermat. & Syph. **3**:598 (May) 1921.

2. Kilduffe, R. A.: Footnote 1. The Clinical Evaluation of the Wassermann Reaction, Arch. Dermat. & Syph. **6**:147 (Aug.) 1922.

discussion of the interpretation of cholesterin plus reaction from the standpoint of diagnosis that this communication is particularly concerned.

CORRELATION OF CLINICAL AND SEROLOGIC FINDINGS

What is to be the attitude of the clinician and serologist when confronted with such a reaction, in the absence of a positive or suspicious history or of easily discernible clinical findings?

Certain general premises previously laid down [2] may be repeated here:

1. If cholesterinized antigens are to be regarded as frequently prone to give nonspecific or false reactions, then, without question, to make a Wassermann test with these as the sole antigens is a dangerous procedure and one which should not be countenanced by either clinician or serologist.

This is a proposition which it seems difficult to deny; and yet this is the situation which obtains in numerous institutions and laboratories of standing both here and abroad, and this was the technic relied on by the laboratories of both the British and the American expeditionary forces in the World War.

It is inevitable and can be admitted without question that some of the reactions reported must have been weakly positive. Where is the borderline between the specificity and nonspecificity of such reactions? What degree of fixation to cholesterinized antigens is specific and what nonspecific? How is this determined? What are the data on which reliance on such reactions is obtained?

These are all pertinent queries, of interest to patient, clinician and serologist alike, of sufficient importance to demand a concerted attempt at a satisfactory answer.

2. In the unknown case tested for diagnosis, a cholesterinized plus reaction should form the basis of an exhaustive clinical, historical and laboratory study, fortified by repeated serologic blood and possibly spinal fluid examinations. Under such circumstances, corroboratory evidence will be obtained in a large percentage of cases.

3. To pass over a cholesterin plus reaction, in the absence of fixation with other antigens, as generally nonspecific and of no moment is an attitude certainly not justified by the data available.

It is unfortunate that, in the matter of diagnosis in the doubtful case, the clinician and the serologist are still some distance apart. The opinion of the serologist as to the interpretation of his examination is too infrequently sought, and still more infrequently is he in possession of sufficient clinical as well as laboratory data on which to formulate such an opinion.

The division of physicians into clinicians and pathologists should be merely an arbitrary one, denoting the particular phases of medicine in which each has a compelling interest. The ability and skill of the clinician is best founded on a broad knowledge of the pathology of the conditions he essays to treat; the pathologist finds his greatest usefulness when he regards and interprets his findings in the light of their clinical application; neither can work in separate fields or do good work in the same field if they elect to remain apart and solitary.

It is impossible for either to make of himself a Robinson Crusoe; inevitably, he will find on his solitary strand the footprints of the other.

It is unfortunate that the clinician is too often content to leave in abeyance the question of the competence of the serologist to whom he refers his examinations; and too often is he satisfied with a negative or positive report from the laboratory, while remaining in abysmal ignorance of the identity of the worker or the reliability of his technic. And far too often is the result of a single Wassermann report deemed sufficient basis for definite diagnostic and prognostic assertions.

Many of the reports thus accepted without cavil are based on reactions to cholesterinized antigens alone and, if this is the case, the clinician should be so informed, and he should be possessed of data on which to formulate a conclusion.

VARIATIONS IN TECHNIC

The question of cholesterinized antigens cannot be evaded by the adoption of a standardized technic, a consummation devoutly to be wished.

So far, but two worthy of note have been proposed, one by Hinton,[3] in which three antigens are used: two different cholesterinized extracts of human heart and one cholesterinized extract of guinea-pig heart— thus relying entirely on cholesterinized antigens. With this method, I have had no experience.

Kolmer[4] has recently published a technic based on an extensive and long-continued series of studies, which has been tested in these laboratories in a series of 1,014 cases, a report of which is to be published.

In this method, which is a strictly quantitative one, but one antigen is used, a polytropic cholesterinized extract of beef heart to which is added the acetone-insoluble lipoids of the same extract. A careful trial of this method has shown a remarkable degree of delicacy, specificity and agreement with the clinical findings, and the technic seems eminently worthy for adoption as a standard.

3. Hinton, W. A.: A Standardized Technic for Performing the Wassermann Reaction, Am. J. Syphilis **4**:598 (Oct.) 1920.

4. Kolmer, J. A.: A New Complement-Fixation Test in Syphilis Based upon the Results of Studies in the Standardization of Technic, Am. J. Syphilis **6**:1 (Jan.) 1922.

It seems apparent that the standardized technic of the future will certainly involve the use of cholesterinized antigens, and some conclusion as to their reliability must, therefore, be agreed on.

This can only be attained by the careful collection and analysis of statistics concerned with cholesterin plus reactions, and by the cooperation of clinician and serologist. All such cases should be carefully investigated as to the presence or absence of clinical signs, the history and the results of further serologic tests.

STUDY OF CASES REACTING TO CHOLESTERIN ANTIGENS

In the present communication, such a study of 159 cases reacting to cholesterin antigens has been attempted.

The cases were collected from those in which reactions occurred in routine Wassermann tests made in these laboratories during the past year (May, 1921, to May, 1922), and were not selected in any way.

Whenever a cholesterin plus reaction occurred, an effort was made to secure all the history and clinical data possible and, if possible, further specimens for examination.

In many of these cases of persons held by the morals court, specimens were secured through Dr. A. H. Eggers, county medical inspector of Allegheny County, Pa., to whom acknowledgment is due for historical data and subsequent specimens. In not a few of these cases, the subsequent serologic examinations were made in other laboratories, using various modifications of technic. The remainder of the series were cases from the wards of the Pittsburgh Hospital and from patients sent to the laboratory for examination.

The technic of the Wassermann reaction as employed in this series has been detailed elsewhere.[5] In brief, it consisted in the employment of a triple antigen battery (cholesterinized extract of human heart, acetone-insoluble lipoids of human heart, and alcoholic extract of syphilitic fetal liver), with two units of titrated complement and fixation in the cold water bath at from 2 to 4 C.

The accompanying table presents the cases and the results obtained in detail.

Including repeat tests, a total of 213 Wassermann tests were made.

It will be noted that, of 159 cholesterin plus reactions, a history of syphilis or clinical evidence of syphilitic infection was obtained in eighty, or approximately 50 per cent.

These cases, on investigation, were found to be either cases of known syphilis under treatment, cases with a history of syphilis

---

5. Kilduffe, R. A.: The Kolmer Modification of the Wassermann Reaction: A Report of Its Trial in a Series of 1,014 Cases. Arch. Dermat. & Syph., this issue, p. 709.

Case	Wasser-mann	Comment	Other Tests
1	C 4 *	Treated syphilis	Two negative
2	C 4	Prostitute; lost	None
3	C 4	Treated syphilis	None
4	C 4	Cohabits with prostitute; no history	One negative
5	C 4	Prostitute; no history	C 4; C 4 A 3 †
6	C 4	Treated syphilis	Plus 4 ‡
7	C 4	Prostitute; no history	C 4 A 1
8	C 4	Prostitute; no history	None
9	C 4	Prostitute; no history	None
10	C 4	Treated syphilis	C 4
11	C 4	Prostitute; no history	Two negative
12	C 4	Treated syphilis	None
13	C 4	Treated syphilis	None
14	C 4	Prostitute; no history	None
15	C 4	Prostitute; no history	C 3; C 4; negative
16	C 4	Treated syphilis	None
17	C 4	Wife has syphilis; plus 4 Wassermann reaction	Negative
18	C 4	Prostitute; no history	Negative
19	C 4	Prostitute; treated	None
20	C 4	Prostitute; treated	Two negative
21	C 4	Prostitute; treated	Two negative
22	C 4	Treated syphilis	Negative
23	C 4	Treated syphilis	Negative
24	C 4	Prostitute; lost	None
25	C 4	Prostitute	Plus 4
26	C 4	Lesions present	None
27	C 4	Husband infected	None
28	C 4	Prostitute	Plus 4
29	C 4	Prostitute, treated syphilis	None
30	C 4	Prostitute; no history	Plus 4
31	C 4	Treated syphilis	None
32	C 4	Prostitute; no history	None
33	C 4	Prostitute; treated syphilis	Two negative
34	C 4	Treated syphilis	Negative
35	C 4	Cohabits with prostitute	Spinal fluid plus 4
36	C 4	Treated syphilis	C 4
37	C 4	Prostitute; lost	None
38	C 4	Prostitute; lost	None
39	C 4	Prostitute; lost	None
40	C 4	Prostitute; no history	Negative
41	C 4	Treated syphilis	None
42	C 4	Prostitute; lost	Anticomplementary
43	C 4	Prostitute; lost	None
44	C 4	Visible lesions; treated	None
45	C 4	Prostitute; lost	None
46	C 4	Prostitute; lost	None
47	C 4	Prostitute; lost	None
48	C 4	Treated syphilis	C 4
49	C 4	Prostitute; lost	None
50	C 4	Prostitute; lost	None
51	C 4	Prostitute; lost	None
52	C 4	Treated syphilis	C 4 A 4; C 4
53	C 4	Glandular involvement; lost	None
54	C 4	Treated syphilis	None
55	C 4	Prostitute; lost	None
56	C 4	Prostitute	C 4 A 4; C 4; C 4
57	C 4	Treated syphilis	None
58	C 4	Treated syphilis	None
59	C 4	Prostitute; no history	Plus 4; plus 4
60	C 4	Secondary infection	None
61	C 4	Treated syphilis	None
62	C 4	Prostitute; lost	None
63	C 4	Treated syphilis	Plus 4
64	C 4	Prostitute; no history	Plus 4
65	C 4	Prostitute; lost	None
66	C 4	No history	Plus 4; negative; negative
67	C 4	Prostitute; lost	None
68	C 4	Treated syphilis	None
69	C 4	Chancre present	None
70	C 4	No history	None
71	C 4	Cohabits with prostitute	Plus 4
72	C 4	Prostitute; lost	None
73	C 4	Known syphilis	Died
74	C 4	Prostitute; no history	C 4; C 4; spinal fluid plus 4
75	C 4	Prostitute; no history	"Delayed negative"
76	C 4	Prostitute; no history	None
77	C 4	Treated syphilis	None
78	C 4	Prostitute; no history	None
79	C 4	Syphilis under treatment	Lost
80	C 4	Prostitute; lost	None
81	C 4	Prostitute; treated syphilis	Plus 4

Case	Wasser-mann	Comment	Other Tests
82	C 4	Prostitute...	Spinal fluid plus 2
83	C 4	Treated syphilis	C 3 A 2
84	C 4	Treated four years ago	None
85	C 4	No history	None
86	C 4	No history	None
87	C 4	No history	None
88	C 4	No history	None
89	C 4	Known syphilis; son has congenital syphilis with plus 4 Wassermann reaction	None
90	C 4	Chancre one month ago	None; lost
91	C 4	Prostitute; lost	None
92	C 4	Prostitute; lost	None
93	C 4	Treated syphilis	C 3; C 4
94	C 4	Prostitute; no history	Plus 4
95	C 4	Treated syphilis	"Positive"
96	C 4	Treated syphilis	None
97	C 4	Prostitute; lost	None
98	C 4	Prostitute; treated	Negative
99	C 4	Wife had syphilis	None
100	C 4	Treated syphilis	None
101	C 4	Treated syphilis	C 4 A 4
102	C 4	Prostitute; lost	None
103	C 4	Chancre one month ago	None; lost
104	C 4	Treated syphilis	None
105	C 4	Treated syphilis	None
106	C 4	Prostitute; lost	None
107	C 4	Prostitute; no history	Plus 4
108	C 4	Prostitute; lost	None
109	C 4	Chancre present	Lost; none
110	C 4	Prostitute; no history	None
111	C 4	History doubtful	None
112	C 4	Treated syphilis	None
113	C 4	Treated syphilis	None
114	C 4	Treated syphilis	None
115	C 4	Treated syphilis	None
116	C 4	Treated syphilis	None
117	C 4	Treated syphilis	None
118	C 4	Treated syphilis	None
119	C 4	Treated syphilis	None
120	C 4	Treated syphilis	None
121	C 4	Treated syphilis	None
122	C 4	No history	None
123	C 4	No history	None
124	C 4	No history	None
125	C 4	No history	None
126	C 4	No history	None
127	C 4	No history	None
128	C 4	No history	None
129	C 4	No history	None
130	C 4	No history	None
131	C 4	No history	None
132	C 4	No history	None
133	C 4	No history	None
134	C 4	No history	None
135	C 4	No history	None
136	C 4	Prostitute; no history	None
137	C 4	Prostitute; no history	None
138	C 4	Lesions present	None
139	C 4	Lesions present	None
140	C 4	Treated syphilis	None
141	C 4	Treated syphilis	None
142	C 4	Treated syphilis	None
143	C 4	Treated syphilis	None
144	C 4	Treated syphilis	None
145	C 4	Treated syphilis	None
146	C 4	Treated syphilis	None
147	C 4	Treated syphilis	None
148	C 4	Treated syphilis	None
149	C 4	Treated syphilis	None
150	C 4	Treated syphilis	None
151	C 4	Treated syphilis	None
152	C 4	Treated syphilis	None
153	C 4	Treated syphilis	None
154	C 4	Treated syphilis	None
155	C 4	Treated syphilis	None
156	C 4	Treated syphilis	None
157	C 4	Treated syphilis	None
158	C 4	Treated syphilis	None
159	C 4	No record	None

* Plus 4 to cholesterinized antigen only.
† C 4 A 4: Plus 4 to cholesterinized antigen and to acetone-insoluble lipoids.
‡ Plus 4: Plus 4 to all antigens.

previously treated, or cases in which early or late clinical manifestations of syphilis were demonstrable.

In seven cases, a suggestive history ("cohabits with prostitute," "lives with infected prostitute," "husband or wife has syphilis," etc.) was elicited, thus providing presumptive evidence of syphilitic infection. Including these, there is a total of eighty-seven, or 54.7 per cent., in which syphilis could be proved or its possibility not denied.

There were fifty serums from admitted professional prostitutes who, naturally, gave a negative history or concerning whom, for one reason or another, no data could be had; many of these were examined but once, and it is debatable how many could have been proved infected if more exhaustive examinations could have been obtained.

In this connection, it is interesting to note that, of a total of ninety-one professional prostitutes examined, twenty-five, or 26 per cent., were definitely shown to be syphilitic.

In twenty-one cases of the series, no data of any kind were obtainable nor was a repetition of the test possible.

It is, of course, realized that this series is too small to permit of exhaustive deductions or analysis, and it is obvious that, for evident reasons, it was not possible to conduct an extended or thorough investigation in any one case. Nevertheless, even this incomplete survey is sufficient to indicate that, in more than 50 per cent. of the persons examined, a cholesterin plus reaction could be shown to be indicative of the presence of syphilitic reagin in the blood. If such reactions are to be looked on as meaningless and of no value, then eighty syphilitic persons would have been overlooked or prematurely discharged from treatment, not a few being professional prostitutes and thus a source of continual danger to the community.

The problem seems an important one and well worthy of extended investigation.

The salient features may be thus briefly expressed:

1. Cholesterinized antigens form a permanent factor in the serologic diagnosis of syphilis.

2. It seems highly probable that the standard Wassermann technic of the future will depend in no small measure on the results of tests against such antigens.

3. Under ordinary circumstances, nonspecific reactions with normal serums are certainly much more infrequent than has generally been supposed, and with a carefully titrated, checked and controlled antigen are rare.

4. Nonspecific fixation by cholesterinized antigens with normal serums (in the absence of lobar pneumonia in the febrile stage, pregnancy, leprosy and yaws), in 100 per cent. or four plus degree, is very rare and infrequent.

5. The cavalier refusal to grant any significance to cholesterin plus reactions in general is an unjustifiable attitude, not supported by available data.

VALUE OF REACTIONS

If a cholesterin plus reaction, in the presence of an early chancre, is a true indication of the presence of syphilitic reagin, what is the status of the same reaction when the presence of the chancre is not known? If treatment cannot be safely discontinued in the persistent presence of a cholesterin plus reaction, what is to be done when the syphilitic person denies or presents no obvious signs of previous infection or treatment?

It would seem of the highest importance for both clinician and serologist to evolve a concerted opinion as to the general reliability and specificity of these reactions and to determine the exact degree of dependability to be assigned to them.

It is not for the clinician alone to determine. Too often he is not sufficiently familiar with, or, what is worse, not sufficiently interested in, matters of technic to bestir himself in an endeavor to ascertain the competence of his serologist or the dependability of his technic.

Nor is it a problem for the serologist alone; if he is concerned only with the serum and his pipets and test tubes, his information and his avenues of investigation are limited to and imprisoned within the walls of his laboratory.

It is a problem necessitating both clinical and laboratory investigations, not as separate but as united forces; investigation by clinicians sufficiently familiar with the theory and mechanism of the methods of investigation they employ, and by serologists in sufficiently close contact with the clinical sides of their work, to properly evaluate their findings.

When confronted with the borderline case, it is only when both are met on the neutral ground of consultation that results of value will be obtained.

Ponderous arguments as to whose shall be the prerogative and glory of the diagnosis are of little moment. Syphilis—or any other condition —cannot be segregated into widely separated zones of diagnosis and clinical findings; the clinician must be sufficiently a pathologist to apply properly the studies of the laboratory; the pathologist must be sufficiently a clinician to properly interpret the results of his investigations. and both must cooperate to properly correlate and evaluate the results of their combined investigations.

CONCLUSIONS

1. Cholesterin plus reactions cannot be safely disregarded as generally nonspecific.

2. The problem of the specificity of cholesterinized antigens should be exhaustively investigated.

3. The occurrence of a cholesterin plus reaction constitutes strongly presumptive evidence of the presence of syphilitic reagin and necessitates a further and an exhaustive examination—clinical, historical and laboratory.

EXPERIENCE WITH THE KOLMER QUANTITATIVE COMPLEMENT FIXATION TEST FOR SYPHILIS *

LESTER J. PALMER, M.D., AND W. E. GIBB, B.S.

SEATTLE

The new quantitative technic for complement fixation in syphilis, as recently published by Dr. John A. Kolmer,[1] has been employed by us since November, 1921, in the examination of 362 specimens of serum from 329 patients. The Dermatologic Research Institute of Philadelphia examined 100 of these serums in collaboration with this laboratory, employing both their old method and the new Kolmer technic. The serums of these 100 patients were drawn for both laboratories at the same sitting. These serums were all from patients who have been thoroughly studied clinically. In many of them, the diagnosis has been proved in the surgery or at necropsy, and in only a few has there been clinical uncertainty as to the condition present.

The 362 serums may be grouped as follows: positive Wassermann reaction, positive clinically, 136; negative Wassermann, negative clinically, 181; positive Wassermann, negative clinically, fifteen; negative Wassermann, positive clinically, two; syphilitic patients under treatment, with previously strongly positive Wassermann reactions which are now negative, three; and unclassified serums in which the Wassermann reactions were variable on different days, fifteen, all of which were from five patients.

Throughout this series, the usual good technical care was exercised and all serums were examined in our laboratory by the same technician. The new technic was exactly adhered to in every detail. The old method (A) as employed in this laboratory consists of a water-bath fixation technic, employing 0.5 c.c. of a titrated 0.4 cholesterinized human heart antigen, two units of titrated antisheep amboceptor, 0.5 c.c. of a 1:10 dilution of guinea-pig complement, 0.5 c.c. of a 1:20 suspension of sheep cells and 0.2 c.c. of desensitized patient's serum, with a sharply adjusted hemolytic system. This we considered in our hands a sensitive technic. An acetone insoluble antigen with otherwise the same reagents was employed as a control (B). A second control consisted of a 0.2 cholesterolized lecithinized beef heart antigen, pre-

* From the Virginia Mason Hospital Laboratory.

1. Kolmer, J. A.: Studies in the Standardization of the Wassermann Reaction; a New Complement Fixation Test for Syphilis Based upon the Results of Studies in the Standardization of Technique, Am. J. Syphilis 6:82 (Jan.) 1922.

pared according to the method of Kolmer,[2] with a primary short icebox incubation of four hours (C). The old method, as applied at the Dermatologic Research Institute, employs three antigens, a cholesterinized, an alcoholic syphilitic liver, and an acetone insoluble lipoid.

An analysis of the results of this study leads us to the following conclusion: The new Kolmer quantitative technic has greater sensitivity than our old methods.

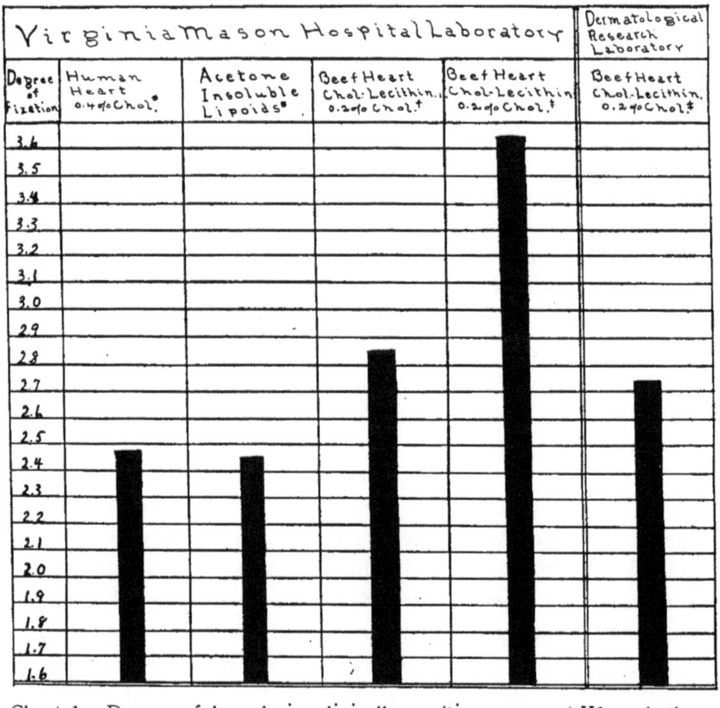

Virginia Mason Hospital Laboratory				Dermatological Research Laboratory
Degree of Fixation	Human Heart 0.4% Chol.*	Acetone Insoluble Lipoids*	Beef Heart Chol-Lecithin. 0.2% Chol.†	Beef Heart Chol-Lecithin 0.2% Chol.†	Beef Heart Chol-Lecithin. 0.2% Chol.‡
3.6					
3.5					
3.4					
3.3					
3.2					
3.1					
3.0					
2.9					
2.8					
2.7					
2.6					
2.5					
2.4					
2.3					
2.2					
2.1					
2.0					
1.9					
1.8					
1.7					
1.6					

Chart 1.—Degree of hemolysis, clinically positive cases. * Water-bath, one-half hour. † Icebox incubation four hours. ‡ Kolmer quantitative icebox incubation, eighteen hours.

The results with the new technic agreed with the clinical evidence in the clinically positive cases in 97 per cent. in our laboratory and 81 per cent. in Philadelphia. Our old technics agreed in 92 and 83 per cent., respectively. Even the short icebox method agreed in only 93 per cent. The percentages with the old technics are comparatively

---

2. Kolmer, J. A.: Studies in Standardization of the Wassermann Reaction; a Superior Antigen for Complement Fixation Tests in Syphilis (A Cholesterolized Lecithinized Alcoholic Extract of Heart Muscle). Am. J. Syphilis 6:74 (Jan.) 1922.

higher because one plus reactions, which are usually considered questionable, are counted as positives, while none of these weak reactions occurred with the new technic. The average degree of hemolysis with the new technic in our laboratory, in this group of the cases, was plus 3.6 and in Philadelphia was plus 2.7. We believe that this low degree of hemolysis obtained in Philadelphia was due to the fact that from eight to fourteen days were consumed on the average in shipment

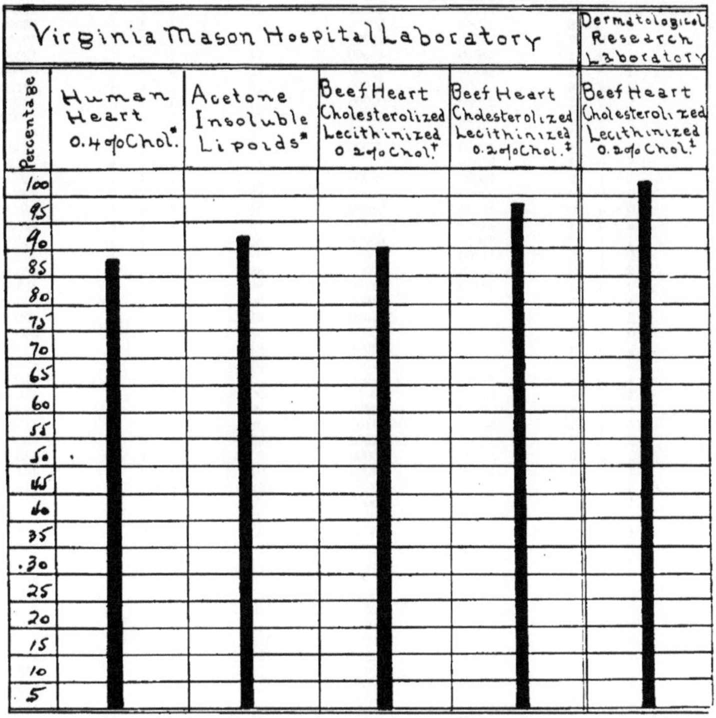

Percentage	Virginia Mason Hospital Laboratory				Dermatological Research Laboratory
	Human Heart 0.4%Chol.*	Acetone Insoluble Lipoids*	Beef Heart Cholesterolized Lecithinized 0.2%Chol.†	Beef Heart Cholesterolized Lecithinized 0.2%Chol.‡	Beef Heart Cholesterolized Lecithinized 0.2% Chol.‡
100					
95					
90					
85					
80					
75					
70					
65					
60					
55					
50					
45					
40					
35					
30					
25					
20					
15					
10					
5					

Chart 2.—Percentage agreement with clinical evidence, clinically negative cases. * Water-bath, one-half hour. † Icebox incubation, four hours. ‡ Kolmer quantitative icebox incubation, eighteen hours.

and that many of the serums were deteriorated or showed a weakening of reagin. The average degree of hemolysis with our old technic was plus 2.5 (A) and plus 2.4 (B) respectively, and only plus 2.8 (C) with the short icebox method. It is evident, therefore, that employing the new Kolmer cholesterolized lecithinized antigen, in a short icebox technic, does not give the same high degree of sensitivity as does the new Kolmer quantitative method. Criticism of the new technic, based on any modification of the Kolmer method, is, in our opinion, not dependable. For instance, shortening the primary icebox incubation

TABLE 1.—CLINICALLY POSITIVE REACTIONS UNDER OLD AND NEW TECHNIC

	Clinically Positive Reactions								
	Virginia Mason Hospital			Kolmer,		Virginia Mason Hospital			
Case	Old			New	New	Case	Old			New
1	4	4	4	44200	44100	69	1	2	3	42100
2	4	4	4	43100	43000	70	4	4	4	42000
3	3	4	3	32100	43000	71	0	0	0	32100
4	3	2	3	42200	30000	72	4	4	4	33000
5	0	0	2	43200	20000	73	1	0	1	40000
6	4	4	4	44000	44000	74	1	2	2	12000
7	1	2	2	44330	42000	75	4	4	4	04000
8	4	4	4	44300	41000	76	4	4	4	44433
9	2	1	3	21000	00000	77	1	2	3	43200
10	3	3	3	33100	40000	78	2	2	3	44000
11	2	2	3	44310	40000	79	4	4	4	44430
12	4	4	4	44210	30000	80	2	2	2	43000
13	1	0	2	32000		81	4	4	4	44430
14	1	1	2	21000	32000	82	4	4	4	44000
15	0	0	0	00000	42000	83	1	2	2	30000
16	0	0	0	20000	44000	84	4	4	4	44000
17	4	4	4	44000		85	4	4	4	44000
18	1	1	2	33000	00000	86	3	3	3	44300
19	2	1	3	41000	00000	87	4	4	4	44300
20	2	3	3	44320	44000	88	0	0	0	22000
21	4	4	4	44430	44100	89	1	2	2	32000
22	1	3	3	44320	44000	90	2	2	2	32000
23	2	4	4	44333	44000	91	....			30000
24	0	0	0	44200	00000	92	1	1	1	30000
25	3	3	4	43300	43000	93	1	1	1	22000
26	3	2	4	43000	44000	94	2	3	3	42100
27	4	4	4	44200	44000	95	2	2	2	41000
28	4	4	4	44320	A C	96	2	3	2	41000
29	4	4	4	43100	44000	97	4	4	4	44300
30	4	4	4	44330	44200	98	2	2	2	42000
31	2	2	3	42000	44000	99	4	4	4	43000
32	2	3	3	33000	00000	100	1	1	2	42000
33	4	4	4	44100	44000	101	3	2	3	44400
34	4	4	4	44332	10000	102	4	4	4	44442
35	1	1	2	43200	00000	103	3	2	3	44800
36	2	2	3	40000		104	1	2	3	43000
37	1	0	2	31000	00000	105	3	3	4	44300
38	3	2	4	44200	44000	106	0	2	2	33000
39	4	4	4	44100	44000	107	2	2	3	31000
40	2	2	3	42000	42000	108	1	0	2	31100
41	3	2	3	43000	10000	109	2	2	3	43100
42	3	3	3	43000	42000	110	4	4	4	44200
43	4	4	4	43100	44000	111	1	0	2	41000
44	2	1	3	43000	41000	112	1	1	2	42000
45	2	2	2	42000	42000	113	4	4	4	44200
46	1	0	2	31000	42000	114	1	1	1	41000
47	1	1	1	44000	43000	115	3	3	4	44300
48	4	4	4	44200	44000	116	2	3	2	44400
49	3	2	4	44000	44000	117	1	1	1	43000
50	....			41000	44000	118	2	2	3	31000
51	4	4	4	44430	44100	119	2	2	3	41000
52	4	4	4	44300	00000	120	2	1	2	41000
53	3	3	4	43000	A C	121	4	4	4	43000
54	3	2	3	44300	20000	122	4	4	4	44300
55	1	0	2	44000	44000	123	1	0	1	02000
56	1	1	1	40000	00000	124	2	1	3	03000
57	0	0	0	20000	00000	125	0	0	0	31000
58	4	4	4	44210		126	2	2	3	43200
59	0	0	0	44000		127	2	1	2	44300
60	2	1	2	44200		128	0	0	0	32000
61	2	2	2	43200		129	0	0	0	31000
62	4	4	4	44430		130	4	4	4	44300
63	4	4	4	44300		131	3	3	4	44300
64	4	4	4	44000		132	4	4	4	44300
65	4	4	4	44000		133	4	4	4	44300
66	4	4	4	44320		134	2	2	3	44420
67	4	4	4	44320		135	3	3	3	30000
68	1	2	2	44300		136	4	4	4	43000

to less than twelve hours in the Kolmer technic has proved to be less sensitive than our old technic (C), which employed a cholesterinized antigen and a four-hour icebox primary fixation. The new technic gave stronger reactions in fifty-three of the 136 positive Wassermann and clinically positive cases, while in only three cases was the reaction weaker than with the old technic. More important is the fact that the new technic gave a diagnostically positive reaction in nine of the 136 clinically positive cases in which the old technics gave a negative.

The new Kolmer technic has greater specificity than our old methods.

The results with the new technic agreed with the clinical evidence in the clinically negative cases in 94 per cent. in our laboratory and in 97 per cent. in Philadelphia. Our old technics agreed in 83 per cent. (A) and 87 per cent. (B), respectively, and the short icebox method (C) agreed in 85 per cent. If a false positive does occur with the new technic, the degree of hemolysis is greater than with the old technics.

TABLE 2.—CLINICALLY NEGATIVE, WASSERMANN POSITIVE REACTIONS
WITH OLD AND NEW TECHNIC

Clinically Negative Wassermann Positive Reactions								
	Virginia Mason Hospital			Kolmer,		Virginia Mason Hospital		
Case	Old			New	Case	Old			New
1	0	0	0	30000		9	1	2	1	31000
2	0	0	0	43000	00000	10	1	0	1	02000
3	0	0	0	44300		11	2	1	3	03000
4	0	0	0	00000	04210	12	0	0	0	31000
5	1	1	2	43000		13	0	0	0	22000
6	0	0	0	30000		14	0	0	0	41000
7	1	1	2	40000		15	0	0	0	41000
8	1	0	2	23310						

In ten cases with no clinical evidence of syphilis, positive reactions were obtained with the new technic. However, it could not be proved by history or examination that these were not cases of latent syphilis. All the patients had given previous variable Wassermann reactions, and in three of the ten cases in which the serums were checked on different days, the reactions were consistently positive. However, it is possible that some of these reactions were false positives, and they have been considered as such. In compiling the foregoing percentages, there is no more evidence for than against this fact.

In five of the 329 patients, the reactions obtained with their serums, were not consistent on different days, using the new technic. In one case of gastric ulcer, with a positive history of syphilis, and some treatment, a 20000 reaction was obtained; and, two weeks later, a negative. In a second case, with negative clinical findings and no syphilitic history, a 44300 reaction was obtained, followed by two negative reactions about ten days apart. In a third case, with a diagnosis of duodenal ulcer and no findings or history of syphilis, a 44300 reaction was obtained in the same run as the second case, followed by two negative reactions about ten days apart. In a fourth case, that of a colored woman in whom the diagnosis was fibroid uterus and who gave a questionable history of syphilis, a 44000 reaction was obtained, followed a week later by a negative reaction, which was followed, in turn, a week later, by a 44300 reaction. In a fifth case, with no diagnosis other than nervous exhaustion and no history or clinical evidence of syphilis, a 04300 reaction was obtained, followed by a negative reaction a week later. In the first and fourth of these cases, the negatives are considered by us to be false, and in the other three cases, the positives are considered to be false, the opinions being based on careful clinical consideration.

TABLE 3.—WASSERMANN VARIABLE REACTIONS WITH OLD AND NEW TECHNIC

	Wassermann Variable Reactions						
	Virginia Mason Hospital			Kolmer,		Virginia Mason Hospital	
Case	Old		New	New	Case	Old		New
1	4 2 4	20000	41000	3	1 1 2	00000
1	0 0 0	00000		4	0 0 0	44000
2	4 4 4	44300		4	0 0 0	00000
2	0 0 0	. 00000	00000	4	1 1 2	44300
2	1 1 1	00000		5	1 1 2	04300
3	1 1 2	44300		5	0 0 0	00000
3	0 0 0	00000	00000			

The new technic gives in our laboratory a much lower percentage of anticomplementary reactions than the old technics. Only 40 per cent. as many of the 362 serums were anticomplementary with the new technic as with our old technics.

There was total disagreement as to positive or negative reactions in 13 per cent. of the 100 serums examined, both in our laboratory and at Philadelphia. This is high because of changes taking place in the serums during shipment.

The quantitative phase of the new technic is very valuable. The gradation of hemolysis in the five tubes indicates the quantity of reagin present in the serum being examined. Although this is of some value from a diagnostic standpoint, it is of greater importance in cases under treatment. Here it indicates the effect of treatment and acts as an indicator for further therapy.

Certain advantages which stand out prominently in opposition to any criticism that might be made of the new technic have been brought to our attention during the use of it. It is true that the new technic requires more time, and the reports will be somewhat delayed as compared with the old methods, but we believe that this is justified by the greater accuracy of the results obtained. This increased accuracy should not be sacrificed for a little saving of time and labor. The reason that the sensitivity of our old method rates so high is that, in compiling the percentages, one plus reactions were considered positive in the group of clinically positive cases. In a large number of cases, serums giving one, two or three plus positive reactions with the old technic gave a four plus with the new method. Clearcut and easily read reactions are always obtained. Not over five one or two plus reactions have been obtained with the new technic. As emphasized by the author, it has been our experience that in adjusting the hemolytic system, it is important to use the second tube showing complete hemolysis as the unit of complement instead of the first tube, as is commonly done in methods not employing icebox fixation.

CONCLUSICNS

The new Kolmer quantitative complement fixation test for syphilis differs from our old methods as follows:

1. It shows greater sensitivity.
2. It shows greater specifity.
3. It gives fewer anticomplementary reactions.
4. It is more economical.
5. It requires somewhat more time and labor.
6. The reactions are sharper and more easily read.
7. It has the added value of a quantitative phase.

STUDIES IN THE CHEMOTHERAPY OF FUNGUS INFECTIONS

I. THE FUNGISTATIC AND FUNGICIDAL ACTIVITY OF VARIOUS DYES AND MEDICAMENTS *

JAY FRANK SCHAMBERG, M.D.

AND

JOHN A. KOLMER, M.D.

PHILADELPHIA

The new science of chemotherapy, which has achieved brilliant success in the attack on certain spirochetal infections, offers a fertile field for research in connection with other parasites. It is possible to produce new chemical compounds which will possess affinities for cocci, bacilli, fungi, etc. In order to pursue fruitful research along these lines, it is desirable that the parasiticide properties of old and known medicaments be investigated and classified.

Modern medicine employs the experimental method in the development of new remedies for infectious diseases in contrast with the empiric method that characterized the prelaboratory period in medicine. There are two lines of approach in investigative work of this character. One is chemically to modify a drug or compound of clinical value in a certain infection and test the various modifications until an enhanced parasiticidal value is obtained. Starting with atoxyl, which possessed trypanocidal power and a perceptible influence in syphilis, Ehrlich and his associates, after a brilliant research, ultimately elaborated arsphenamin.

In conjunction with Dr. Raiziss, we have shown that an organic mercurial compound—sodiumoxymercury orthonitrophenolate— is from five to seven times more inhibitive to the growths of various cocci than mercuric chlorid. Another mercury compound with which we have been experimenting has a strong affinity for bacilli.

The most desirable method of determining affinities is first to employ the compound in the test tube against cultures of various microorganisms. However, as the results in vitro constitute no convincing evidence of the power of a drug in vivo, it is necessary to infect susceptible animals with various parasites and then inject into each animal the compound under investigation.

In dealing with parasites, such as fungi, which attack merely the skin and its appendages, intravenous or constitutional medication appears to be superfluous.

---

* From the Dermatological Research Institute.

As far as we have been able to determine, no chemotherapeutic research has hitherto been carried out in connection with infections caused by pathologic molds or fungi. The remedies which are in use for ringworm, tinea versicolor and favus have come into employment as a result of empiricism. The thought has occurred to us that laboratory studies of the fungicidal properties of different medicaments would shed light on the chemical affinity of these drugs for different fungi and might lead to the elaboration of compounds superior to those which we already possess.

Two different methods were carried out—one which we have termed the fungistatic test, and the other a fungicidal test. In the former, cultures of certain fungi were planted on mediums containing various strengths of the medicaments to be tested; the results indicated the *restraining* or *inhibitory* power of the compounds. In the fungicidal tests, the strength or amounts of various medicaments necessary to *kill* cultures was determined. The character of this latter test meets more closely the conditions which are present in human infections, as each case of ringworm or favus represents a culture on or in the skin or its appendages.

We have tested twenty-one chemical compounds or drugs and nine dyestuffs. The compounds investigated were iodin, iodoform, phenol, betanaphthol, mercuric chlorid, sodium oxymercury orthonitrophenolate (mercurophen), ammoniated mercury, mercuric salicylate, calomel, salicylic acid, sodium salicylate, benzoic acid, sodium benzoate, resorcin, sulphur, sodium thiosulphate (hyposulphite), sodium hydroxid, chrysarobin, neorobin, arsphenamin and neo-arsphenamin.

In the fungistatic test, three parasites were employed, two types of ringworm fungus, *Trichophyton rosaceum* and *Microsporon audouini*, and *Achorion schoenleinii*, the parasite of favus.

TECHNIC OF FUNGISTATIC TESTS

In these experiments, our purpose was to determine approximately the highest dilutions of various dyes and medicaments incorporated in a solid culture medium capable of inhibiting the growth of three pathogenic molds: *Trichophyton rosaceum, Microsporon audouini, Achorion schoenleinii.*

With the exception of crystal violet, all of the dyes were prepared by Grübler. Each dye and medicament was prepared in a 1 : 100 solution or suspension in sterile distilled water, and higher dilutions were prepared in series of sterile test tubes in amounts of 1 c.c. Numerous controls were included in each set in which sterile water was placed.

To each tube was added 4 c.c. of Sabouraud's maltose medium titrated to 1 per cent. acid to phenolphthalein, melted and cooled to 40 C. The agar and solution or suspension of dye or medicament were mixed, slanted, and allowed to harden. These tubes were then seeded with the respective cultures. As a general rule, each dye and medicament was tested in twenty-four dilutions with each of the three cultures; and each experiment was repeated twice, and the majority three times, in order properly to check the results. After seeding, the tubes were kept at room temperature. The results were read at weekly intervals, but those given in the tables represent the final readings made on the sixth to eighth week of each experiment.

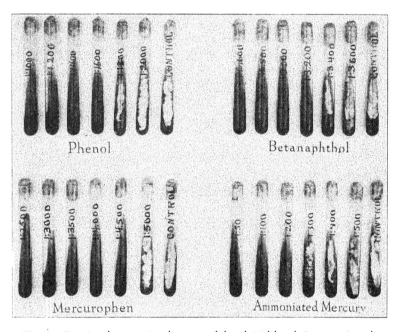

Fig. 1.—Fungistatic test, showing restraining inhibiting influence of various medicaments and stains on Trichophyton rosaceum.

As is true of bacteriostatic (antiseptic) tests, the highest values are found during the first week or ten days in these experiments; but during prolonged incubation the restraining activities of the higher dilutions of the substances being tested are lost until a period is reached when the results remain stationary, thus disclosing the fungistatic activity.

Table 1 gives the restraining power of the different drugs against these three fungi. It will be observed that against *Trichophyton rosaceum,* iodin exerted an infinitely greater inhibition than any other compound; next in order, but far behind, came mercurophen, mercuric chlorid and betanaphthol.

Against the *Microsporon audouini,* mercurophen stood first, closely followed by iodin, with mercuric chlorid and betanaphthol next. With *Achorion schoenleinii* as the test parasite, mercurophen exhibited a marked superiority over iodin, which came second, with mercuric chlorid third.

Reading down the list, one is somewhat astonished to note the low inhibiting power of certain medicaments which have acquired reputations as remedies of value against ringworm. Reference will be made later to this observation.

TABLE 1.—THE FUNGISTATIC ACTIVITY OF VARIOUS MEDICAMENTS

Medicament	Highest Fungistatic Dilutions for		
	T. rosaceum	M. audouini	A. schöenleinii
Iodin..........................	1:100,000*	1:10,000†	1:15,000‡
Iodoform......................	1:400	1:400	1:300
Phenol.........................	1:1600	1:1600	1:1200
Betanaphthol..................	1:3200	1:3000	1:1600
Mercurophen..................	1:4500	1:12.000	1:47.000
Mercuric chlorid..............	1:4000	1:5000	1:6000
Ammoniated mercury..........	1:200	1:300	1:1600
Mercuric salicylate...........	1:200	1:600	1:800
Mild mercurous chlorid.......	1:100	1:400	1:300
Salicylic acid.................	1:50	1:100	1:150
Sodium salicylate.............	Not in 1:20	1:25	1:200
Benzoic acid..................	1:40	1:200	1:200
Sodium benzoate..............	1:20	1:25	1:25
Resorcin.......................	1:200	1:300	1:1600
Precipitated sulphur..........	Not in 1:10	Not in 1:10	Not in 1:10
Sodium thiosulphate..........	Not in 1:20	1:300	1:300
Sodium hydroxid..............	1:1000	1:750	1:3000
Chrysarobin...................	Not in 1:10	Not in 1:10	Not in 1:10
Neorobin.....................	Not in 1:10	Not in 1:10	1:10
Arsphenamin (acid solution)...	1:100	1:160	1:400
Arsphenamin (alkaline solution)..	1:50	1:150	1:200
Neo-arsphenamin..............	1:20	1:100	1:75

* 1:2000 of a 2 per cent. solution (2 gm. iodin crystals; 5 gm. potassium iodid and 100 c.c. water) = 1:100,000 of pure iodin.
† 1:200 of a 2 per cent. solution = 1:10,000 of pure iodin.
‡ 1:300 of a 2 per cent. solution = 1:15,000 of pure iodin.

Studies of the fungistatic power of various dyestuffs are shown in Table 2. It is here seen that brilliant green decisively transcends all the other laboratory stains in restraining the growth of molds. Only against the parasite of favus is it equaled by crystal violet. All of the remaining dyes are infinitely inferior.

TABLE 2.—THE FUNGISTATIC ACTIVITY OF DYES

Dyes	Highest Fungistatic Dilutions for		
	T. rosaceum	M. audouini	A. schöenleinii
Brilliant green....................	1:16,000	>1:47,000	<1:47,000
Crystal violet....................	1:500	1:6000	<1:2500
Methylene blue...................	1:200	1:300	1:800
Methyl green.....................	1:200	1:800	1:900
Gentian violet............	1:200	1:200	1:150
Fuchsin..........................	1:200	1:100	1:20
Eosin.,..........................	1:20	1:10	1:200
Safranin.........................	Not in 1:200	1:200	1:200
Bismarck brown..................	1:200	1:150	1:200

TECHNIC OF FUNGICIDAL TESTS

As has already been intimated, more importance is to be attached to the fungicidal tests, because these denote the comparative destructive influence of medicaments on the growths of fungi.

In these experiments, our purpose was to determine approximately the highest dilutions of various dyes and medicaments capable of killing the cultures of the fungi, employed in fifteen minutes, one hour, three hours and twenty-four hours.

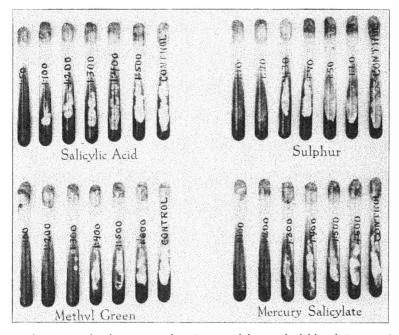

Fig. 2.—Fungistatic test, showing the restraining or inhibiting influence of various medicaments and stains on Trichophyton rosaceum.

Cultures of the respective fungi were removed from Sabouraud's maltose medium with sterile saline solution and shaken mechanically with glass beads for several hours, until a homogeneous suspension was secured corresponding in density to Tube 5 of the McFarland nephelometer.

Solutions of the dyes and medicaments were prepared with distilled water. Equal parts (0.5 c.c.) of varying dilutions and suspension of culture were mixed and kept at 20 C. At intervals of fifteen minutes, one hour, three and twenty-four hours, a portion of each mixture was cultured by transferring several loopfuls to slants of Sabouraud's maltose medium. Controls were included in each experiment in which sterile saline solution was employed. These cultures were kept at room temperature for from three to four weeks, and the results read. These are recorded in Tables 3, 4 and 5.

One would expect that stronger concentration of the compounds would be necessary to kill fungi than to prevent their growth; the investigations prove this assumption to be correct. In the fungicidal tests, brilliant green falls from its high estate and is supplanted by crystal violet. All of the dyestuffs, however, are markedly inferior to the other medicaments.

TABLE 3.—FUNGICIDAL ACTIVITY FOR TRICHOPHYTON ROSACEUM

	Exposure			
	15 Minutes	1 Hour	3 Hours	24 Hours
Brilliant green..............	1:25	1:80	1:200	1:200
Crystal violet..............	1:25	1:50	1:50	1:200
Gentian violet..............	Not in 1:25	1:25	1:50	1:50
Iodin......................	1:5000*	1:5000	1:7500†	1:10,000‡
Phenol.....................	1:25	1:25	1:50	1:150
Betanaphthol..............	1:25	1:25	1:50	1:100
Mercuric chlorid..........	1:10,000	1:10,000	1:10,000	1:15,000
Mercurophen..............	1:10,000	1:10,000	1:10,000	1:15,000
Sodium hydroxid..........	Not in 1:15	1:15	1:25	1:25

* 1:100 of a 2 per cent. solution.
† 1:150 of a 2 per cent. solution.
‡ 1:200 of a 2 per cent. solution.

Against *trichophyton rosaceum,* mercurophen is slightly superior to mercuric chlorid, with iodin third. Phenol and betanaphthol are far inferior. The same sequence holds true for *Microsporon audouinii* and for the parasite of favus (*A. schoenleinii*).

TABLE 4.—FUNGICIDAL ACTIVITY FOR MICROSPORON AUDOUINI

	Exposure			
	15 Minutes	1 Hour	3 Hours	24 Hours
Brilliant green..............	1:100	1:200	1:500	1:500
Crystal violet..............	1:1000	1:1000	1:2000	1:2000
Gentian violet..............	1:25	1:50	1:100	1:200
Iodin......................	1:500	1:1000	1:2000	1:7000
Phenol.....................	1:100	1:100	1:100	1:200
Betanaphthol..............	1:50	1:50	1:100	1:100
Mercuric chlorid..........	1:2000	1:5000	1:10,000	1:15,000
Mercurophen..............	1:5000	1:10,000	1:10,000	1:20,000
Sodium hydroxid..........	Not in 1:25	Not in 1:25	Not in 1:25	Not in 1:25

BACTERICIDAL ACTIVITY OF COMPOUNDS TESTED

Five of the most favorable compounds, mercurophen, mercuric chlorid, crystal violet, iodin and brilliant green, were tested for their destructive power on *Staphylococcus albus.* Their sequence here indicates the order of their efficacy.

It is here observed that while the mercurials come first, crystal violet has a stronger bactericidal effect than iodin, which has been much used as a skin disinfectant in surgery. It should be noted, however, that the iodin in these tests was used in aqueous solution in order to avoid confusion of interpretation from the effect of alcohol. The tincture of iodin might well be more germicidal as such, and moreover the alcohol would doubtless facilitate penetration into the upper layers of the skin.

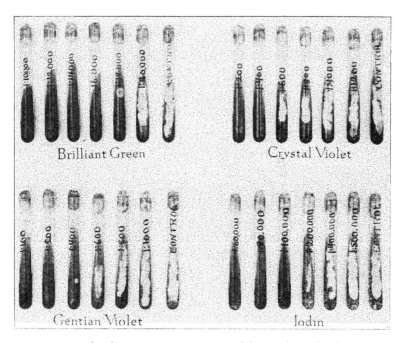

Fig. 3.—Fungistatic test, showing 'the restraining or inhibiting influence of various medicaments and stains on Trichophyton rosaceum.

The superiority of crystal violet over other stains in killing the staphylococcus is of interest in connection with the studies of Farley[1] on gentian violet. Farley incorporated gentian violet in maltose agar for the purpose of restraining the growth of gram-positive bacteria and thus aiding the isolation in pure culture of molds from the skin and hair. He found that 1 : 500,000 dilution would restrain the growth of those bacteria; while 1 : 250,000 did not inhibit the growth of molds.

1. Farley, D. L.: The Use of Gentian Violet as a Restrainer in the Isolation of Pathogenic Molds, Arch. Dermat. & Syph. **2**:459 (Oct.) 1920.

Our investigations indicate that very much stronger concentrations could be used without inhibiting mold growth.[2]

PRACTICAL APPLICATION OF RESULTS

One is somewhat astonished at the relatively poor showing in inhibiting the growth of molds exhibited by salicylic and benzoic acid. These are the essential ingredients in Whitfield's ointment, the favorable effect of which in the treatment of chronic ringworm of the cutaneous surface appears to have strong clinical support.

TABLE 5.—FUNGICIDAL ACTIVITY FOR ACHORION SCHOENLEINII

	Exposure			
	15 Minutes	1 Hour	3 Hours	24 Hours
Brilliant green	1:100	1:100	1:500	1:500
Crystal violet	1:1000	1:1000	1:1000	1:2000
Gentian violet	1:25	1:50	1:100	1:150
Iodin	1:2000	1:4000	1:5000	1:5000
Phenol	1:100	1:100	1:200	1:500
Betanaphthol	1:50	1:50	1:50	1:100
Mercuric chlorid	1:2000	1:5000	1:10,000	1:15,000
Mercurophen	1:2000	1:5000	1:15,000	1:20,000
Sodium hydroxid	1:25	1:100	1:1000	1:1000

TABLE 6.—BACTERICIDAL ACTIVITY FOR STAPHYLOCOCCUS ALBUS

	Exposure			
	15 Minutes	1 Hour	3 Hours	24 Hours
Brilliant green	1:500	1:500	1:600	1:800
Crystal violet	1:1000	1:1000	1:1500	1:3000
Iodin	1:100	1:100	1:100	1:200
Mercuric chlorid	1:1600	1:1600	1:1800	1:3200
Mercurophen	1:1600	1:2000	1:2000	1:4000

It is possible that the beneficial effects of this ointment may be due to the exfoliative effect of salicylic acid rather than to its fungicidal influence.

The laboratory studies herewith reported cannot subvert, and are not designed to controvert, established clinical judgments. They are merely test tube experiments, which must be subjected in due course to clinical trial. They may be regarded as establishing leads to clinical experimentation. The ultimate results may be disappointing, or they may be gratifying. It may, furthermore, prove desirable to subject the most favorable compounds to chemical alteration with the view of enhancing their value. We have had a brief but favorable experience

2. We would suggest that crystal violet be used instead of gentian violet. as crystal violet is a pure substance, whereas gentian violet is an impure compound of variable composition containing crystal violet, methyl violet and perhaps other substances.

with one compound in the treatment of tinea cruris; but the number of cases treated is not sufficiently extensive to warrant a definite statement at this time.

CONCLUSIONS

1. We have endeavored by a fungistatic (restraining) test and a fungicidal (killing) test to determine the affinities of various commonly employed medicaments and of certain laboratory stains for three different pathogenic molds.

2. We have found selective affinities of certain of the medicaments and dyes for the molds as well as for bacteria.

3. At the present time, the use of these tests appears to be an aid in the isolation of molds and bacteria in pure culture.

4. Iodin transcends all other medicaments in restraining the growth of certain molds, but in aqueous solution it is inferior to certain other drugs in killing them.

5. Sodium oxymercury orthonitrophenolate (mercurophen) is superior as a fungicide, in the test tube, to mercuric chlorid and to iodin, and far superior to the other medicaments tested.

6. Among the dyestuffs, brilliant green was the best restrainer of growth, but crystal violet proved distinctly superior as a fungicide. All of the dyes, however, were inferior to the mercurial preparations.

7. These experiments should not be interpreted in such a manner as to subvert established clinical judgments. The findings, however, should stimulate clinical experimentation.

DISCUSSION

DR. CHARLES M. WILLIAMS, New York: We are very much indebted to Dr. Schamberg for this work on the germicidal action of drugs in the skin and for the conservatism with which he has interpreted the results. We shall be thankful to find a reliable drug. It seems that neither benzoic acid nor salicylic acid has any effect on mycotic organisms; and yet there is no question that mild cases are cured by applications of Whitfield's ointment. The exfoliation is probably the most important factor. I think the irritation is a very good thing. This means increased blood supply and a greater power of bringing about a resistance to the organism itself, as we know that kerion is cured by the very acuteness of its own inflammatory reaction.

The work with iodin was interesting; but in practice I have found that iodin is not so useful as we would expect. The boy I mentioned as having tinea on the toes had been applying iodin for some weeks, and I never found more organisms than in that case. There is no way that we can account for the cure by salicylate or benzoic acid, or the roentgen ray, except by their influencing the reaction of the patient.

DR. HARVEY P. TOWLE, Boston: The important thing in Dr. Schamberg's paper, it seems to me, is that, whereas we have been relying on one drug for the cure of all fungus diseases, it is here illustrated that we must select the one that has the most effect on the various types as shown by laboratory experiments:

That is well illustrated in his tables, which I think, bear out our clinical results. Unquestionably, the laboratory conclusions will be modified greatly, because we are dealing, in the clinic, with living tissue; whereas, Dr. Schamberg, as he pointed out, is dealing, in the laboratory, with the inert substances. That is a tremendous factor; but if we learn to pick out a given remedy in a given case with a direct etiologic factor, we shall have made great advance.

Dr. SAMUEL E. SWEITZER, Minneapolis: I should like to ask what diluent Dr. Schamberg used, particularly in iodin. It is possible that, if alcohol was used, it might have had some effect. I should also like to ask if, in his future studies, he will take up the question of potassium permanganate. This will frequently bring about a rapid disappearance of the vesicles.

Dr. WALTER J. HIGHMAN, New York: In 1908, Professor Jadassohn set me to work on a task similar to the research Dr. Schamberg and his co-workers have undertaken less crudely. One of the things he was anxious to determine was whether the vehicles in which parasiticides were used affected their activity. It was brought out that aqueous and alcoholic solutions were more effective; that the incorporation of any medicament in oil or cream diminished its effect two to five fold. In Dr. Schamberg's work, so far as the clinical domain is concerned, it will be necessary, I think, to take into consideration the effect on the parasite of the excipient that is employed in using the medicament clinically. This is only a practical point, perhaps, but it will have to receive consideration.

For the rest, I was amazed at the mathematical accuracy with which the various strains of organisms employed by Dr. Schamberg responded or did not respond to the various medicaments tested, and it is gratifying to see this particular branch of parasitology removed from the field which Sabouraud so long ago exhausted.

Dr. HARRY E. ALDERSON, San Francisco: I should like to ask Dr. Schamberg about the effect of some of these drugs applied in powders. I have recently had the pharmacist make up some crayons containing salicylic acid and benzoic acid with starch and magnesium carbonate. I have used these in a few cases of tinea cruris with good effect. These crayons are not so hard that they irritate the skin and not so soft that they crumble; but they leave an adhesive powder on the skin without much rubbing being necessary.

Dr. WILLIAM ALLEN PUSEY, Chicago: I am obliged to Dr. Schamberg for these definite facts and am willing to let their application take care of themselves. I think this would be borne in mind. We are not looking for the interpretation, but first for facts. I think Dr. Schamberg has used to excellent advantage the opportunities he has for such investigation, and I sincerely hope he will give us more reports of the same sort. This is a stimulating appetizer, but not a full meal, and we shall expect more.

Dr. JAY FRANK SCHAMBERG, Philadelphia: I think the members have fully understood that this paper is more or less a preliminary communication and merely a report of laboratory data. It gives us certain leads for clinical experimentation and for further work.

In reply to the query as to whether iodin was used in alcoholic solution, I would answer in the negative. It was used in an aqueous menstruum. I have no doubt that alcohol would penetrate more readily; but we wished to avoid complications in formulating our deductions. If you have a thickened skin in which the fungus is embedded, it is necessary to reach the fungus before you can kill it. As Dr. Highman has stated, the incorporation of medicaments in unguents would doubtless lessen their effect.

Whether powders will be more effective remains for investigation; we have felt that the experimental work done will give us certain lines of approach.

After all, we must be careful not to interpret laboratory data too sweepingly in their application to clinical ends, because results in vitro are commonly very different from results in vivo. We will have to follow our test tube results with experimental work on the animal infected with the parasites in question in order to demonstrate their practical value. Mercuric chlorid, while it shows up very well in these tables, even in a solution of 1 : 10,000, tends to necrotize tissue cells; so it may be that another drug which we have used will be more advantageous because it does not work material harm on living tissue, but confines its action more to the bacteria.

INOCULATION, AUTOINOCULATION AND COMPLEMENT FIXATION TESTS IN POMPHOLYX (TILBURY FOX) *

SIGMUND S. GREENBAUM, M.D.

Assistant Professor of Dermatology, University of Pennsylvania,
Graduate School of Medicine; Senior Dermatologist
to Mount Sinai Hospital

PHILADELPHIA

In 1919, Darier[1] published an article on the vesicular and the vesicopustular eruptions on the hands and feet. In this article, he found mycelia, on microscopic examination, in the majority of those conditions corresponding to the classic description of pompholyx. His conclusions were that, after excluding eruptions of dermatitides due to plants, trauma, trades and the streptostaphylococci (dematitis venenata; dermatitis traumatica; occupational dermatitis, and infectious eczematoid dermatitis), most cases of pompholyx (80 per cent.) were of mycotic nature.

The opinion expressed by Darier in 1919 created widespread interest. This opinion has not, however, been generally accepted up to the present time by independent observers, because of the general failure to demonstrate mold fungi in the typical lesions of pompholyx. As a matter of fact, Darier, in a most recent expression of opinion,[2] stated that he found parasitic mycelia in 80 per cent. of those cases presenting the clinical aspect of pompholyx. This latter opinion places the question in a totally different light; one in which many dermatologists concur.

Sabouraud,[3] whose work with the ringworm fungi is well known, is of the opinion that pompholyx is not of mycotic origin, though there are pompholyx-like lesions that are; that labeling a disease as of mycotic origin because of the microscopic findings alone is insufficient, for the reason that occasional fragments of mycelium of the penicilium may be found living as saprophytes on the skin; thirdly, that cultures are necessary as additional evidence. In a previous communication,[4] we amply confirmed Sabouraud's contentions that the higher fungi,

* From the Dermatological Research Institute.

1. Darier, J.: Lancet **2**:578 (Sept. 27) 1919.

2. Darier, J.: Presse méd.. July, 1922, No. 52. p. 560.

3. Sabouraud: Bull. Soc. franç. de dermat. et syph., 1921, No. 9, p. 441.

4. Greenbaum. S. S. and Klauder, J. V.: Yeast Infections of the Skin. Arch. Dermat. & Syph. **5**:332-344 (March) 1922.

aside from the fission and the budding fungi, may be found on the normal skin, but that under certain conditions they may develop pathogenic properties.

Koch's laws are too well-known to necessitate description here, but they have not as yet been fulfilled in a way to place pompholyx definitely with the mycoses. Darier's studies were entirely microscopic and positive; Sabouraud's studies were both microscopic and cultural, but entirely negative. Sabouraud's studies have been confirmed, not only be me, but by many others. With the opinions of these two eminent dermatologists diametrically opposed, it was thought that perhaps the problem could be approached from other angles; namely, inoculation, autoinoculation and serologic studies.

The importance of having a clear understanding of the condition under discussion cannot be exaggerated, since all dermatologists are not in accord in considering pompholyx a clinical entity. As a matter of fact, it is not always easy to say that such and such a condition of the hands, feet or both is, for example, a trade dermatitis, a streptococcic dermatitis or a dermatitis venenata. All of us are well aware of the fact that more than one factor (bacterium, exotoxin, endotoxin) may lie behind the development of lesions clinically exactly alike. The reason for this is not far to seek, since we know that the skin can react to any irritant in but a few ways; whereas the number of irritants are far more numerous. If the important fact is recognized that clinical lesions with a varied etiology may not differ, it then becomes evident that other means besides clinical, bacteriologic and cultural measures are necessary to differentiate these etiologic factors.

TYPE OF CASE STUDIED

For the sake of clearness, a brief description of the type of case selected for this study follows:

True pompholyx (cheiropompholyx of Hutchinson, dyshidrosis of Tilbury Fox) is characterized by the development of vesicles and bullae on the hands and feet and, notably, the palms, lateral surfaces of the fingers and soles. This acute, generally symmetrical inflammatory disease is further characterized by the development of its manifestations in crops, its tendency to recur and, as regards a single attack, its limited duration. The vesicles, at first small and deepseated, increase in size, may and often do become purulent, coalesce and later undergo resorption. As a rule, spontaneous rupture does not occur, but accidental rupture of the larger ones is usual. It is to be remembered that all grades of the affection occur, from a few superficial or deep lesions to those involving the entire palm, dorsum of hands and the soles. In order to be absolutely certain that we were dealing with the affection under consideration, only those cases in which the diagnosis was certain, with well-marked lesions and a history of previous attacks, were included in this study. Abortive cases, such as those in which there were but a few vesicles on the lateral surfaces of the fingers, were not included. The cases selected for this study came from private practice, from the Polyclinic Hospital dispensary of Dr. Jay F. Schamberg and from my own dispensary at the Mount Sinai Hospital.

INOCULATION TESTS

The surfaces of vesicles with clear contents were swabbed with alcohol and punctured with a capillary pipet. Sufficient fluid for the tests was thus obtained, and kept in sterile test tubes. The greater vulnerability of children to ringworm infection was recognized and volunteers were consequently used for the experiments. In control experiments, volunteers whom I had previously inoculated with trichophytons and microsporons, from their own scalp lesions, and with cultures from the laboratory, generally developed ringworm of the parts inoculated (glabrous skin) within from seven to ten days. It might be here noted that this autoinoculation test in ringworm of the scalp is quite simple and of value not only as an aid to the diagnosis of tinea capitis, but also as a method of determining the presence or absence of cure. The diagnostic lesion is easily eradicated. The volunteers used for the experiments in this study (five in number) were inoculated with a mixture of fluids obtained from different cases of pompholyx and were kept under observation three weeks.

The tests were uniformly negative.

AUTOINOCULATION TESTS

All the patients used for the complement fixation tests underwent an autoinoculation test. The vesicles generally selected were those in which the contents had not become purulent. When this was not possible, purulent contents were used. The surface was swabbed with alcohol, the vesicle punctured with a sterile capillary pipet and the material thus obtained rubbed into a superficially scarified area on the skin, over the deltoid muscle and in the inguinal region, the site of predilection of the epidermophyton. All the tests, following a three-week period of observation, were negative.

COMPLEMENT FIXATION STUDIES [5]

Kolmer [6] showed that, with a polyvalent antigen of *Microsporon audouini*, complement fixation occurred in 78 per cent. of persons suffer-

5. The complement fixation tests were performed by Miss Anna Rule, following the new standardized technic of Dr. John A. Kolmer.

6. Kolmer, J. A., and Strickler, Albert: Complement Fixation in Parasitic Skin Diseases. J. A. M. A. **44**:800-804 (March 6) 1915.

ing with ringworm of the scalp and that the antigens, not only of the microspora but of an achorion as well, were specific in that they did not fix complement with the serums of syphilitic patients or patients suffering with scabies, acne vulgaris, eczema and impetigo. That study seems to indicate that in superficial ringworm infection there is a concomitant development of "ringworm reagin." It was felt, therefore, that if pompholyx is really of ringworm origin, the depth of the lesions would presumably be associated with the development of complement fixing bodies in the blood.

As a result of certain recent studies in the immunologic relationships of the ringworm fungi,[7] it was determined that the fungi, in certain instances, were so closely related that an antigen of some of them was of sufficient value to determine the presence of ringworm reagin produced in rabbits by the injection of many of the others. In the complement fixation tests in this study (twenty subjects), several such antigens were used independently. The antigens used were made from cultures of *Tricophyton niveum-radians, Tricophyton violaceum* and *Achorion gypseum.* Complement remained unfixed in every case tested.

CONCLUSIONS

1. Pompholyx is a clinical entity whose cause remains unknown. When well defined, ringworm as the etiologic factor can be clinically excluded.

2. There are poorly defined or aborted cases of pompholyx whose differentiation from the pompholyx-like lesions of ringworm require microscopic and cultural examinations. Autoinoculation, as a diagnostic test, is of value, but great care in the collection of the material to be used is advised, as severe scarring· from secondary coccic infection may occur.

3. There are pompholyx-like eruptions having a mycotic origin.

1714 Pine Street.

---

7. Paper to appear shortly.

A CONTRIBUTION TO THE TREATMENT OF PHYTOSIS OF THE FEET *

MILLER B. HUTCHINS, M.D.

ATLANTA, GA.

As the term epidermophytosis seemed about to supplant the ancient titles (White, the author, and others), workers demonstrated that the tricophytons are the majority of the offenders, with others of the higher fungi (Wende-Collins) capable of producing disease. The term tinea, defined worm, was employed as far back as 1829 and has continued to cover several different dermatologic conditions. Tricophytosis, for years, and epidermophytosis, of late, bade fair to break the reign of tinea, but now we must coin a new name. Taenia means tapeworm; tinea, any worm.

While investigators seem not to have complied with Koch's law, the presence of these fungi, with resistance and recurrence of disease induced, as well as the usual sources and methods of infection, leaves little doubt of their pathogenicity. As to the distribution of this class of disease, it is at least universal, almost pandemic, among men; and for the simplest of reasons. Casual reference to "toe trouble" or "foot trouble" in conversation anywhere is more than likely to arouse interest, though it is a natural condition. Cases in children as young as 7 are in my records, an evidence of parental carelessness. I have never seen a very old person with the disease. There is a Y. M. C. A. building here, the shower baths of which are open to all members, whether resident or not. Even before the war, this disease was prevalent. During the war, lay over soldiers often used these baths. The disease has been so common of late that I have heard it referred to as the "M. A. disease." Public baths and showers, the more menacing, even golf club showers, are the leading sources of infection. Socks and stockings may actually bring the disease from the laundry, or reinfect the owner if, as Mitchell suggests, the organisms survive laundering.[1] There is some evidence to support the belief that the

---

* A clinical paper, based on private cases.

1. Many housewives wash socks and stockings at home without boiling. Washerwomen do not boil them. The head of a large laundry states that these articles, of the same colors, are put in meshed bags and run through the mangle, with little heat, the cleansing chemical probably being sodium carbonate. They are then placed on hollow, metal forms, steam-heated to 180 or 200 F., the drying process requiring from two and one-half to four minutes. I am now instructing patients to have hosiery boiled at home for at least fifteen minutes.

fungi may be water-borne, as in a case supposedly contracted from a Georgia stream and another through a laceration of the bare sole of a young woman at a bathing beach near Detroit, though the latter infection could have come from a preceding infection of the foot. The family tub and towels, and the exchanging of footwear, provide other sources of infection.

The disease, while easily transinoculated by the patients' hands, or auto-inoculable, is very rarely directly contagious. A curious illustration of variations in personal local immunity is the frequency of involvement of one foot alone, this condition often persisting for months, even indefinitely. Such local persistence with frequent recurrences is also strong evidence of dormancy and periodic growth of retained organisms, rather than of positive reinfection in loco.

These fungi are known to have survived from five to nine months in a dry envelop, but the ultimate longevity of some of them is yet to be determined. They may rival the Egyptian wheat which germinated after reposing for 2,000 years in a tomb. Mitchell has shown viability of certain phyton forms after boiling in potassium hydroxid solution.

That the organisms may lie dormant during cool or cold weather, either in contaminated articles of apparel or actually in the epidermis, in spite of normal desquamation, is well established. Recurrence of disease in practically the same areas occupied during the preceding summer and the depth from which lesions may arise, as on the plantar surfaces, at least favors the probability of epidermal hibernation. Even in Atlanta, where we average less than one freeze a week in winter and the temperature may get up to 60 F. or higher, many cases give no trouble but reappear as the average daytime temperature reaches 70 F. I see very few of the phytoses in winter, but very many in summer. Yet there are cases even in Boston and Detroit that are unchecked by cold weather, and they are also seen in Atlanta.

Whether being in heated homes, cars and offices, with a minimum of exposure to cold, or whether the variety of organism is responsible for these exceptions, we have no positive knowledge. That warmth and moisture, not necessarily hyperhidrosis, do encourage growth of these fungi is known. In this connection, it is a curious fact that we rarely see phytic infection of the feet in cases of bromidroses.

The depth to which the phytons penetrate, as in plantar regions and the fourth interspace, as well as in callosities, constitutes the primary reason for persistent recurrences and difficulty of cure. Extracorporeal destruction of germs or fungi and destruction in vivo are vastly different propositions. Dry air and sunlight may kill tubercle bacilli, drying suppress gonococci, soap destroy *Spirochetae pallidae* and radiation disintegrate cancer cells, but for cure every organism or cell must yield. When contact is established, as in vitro, such accomplishment may be easy. In the tissues, we must get at the cause or depend on the natural resistant forces of the body cells, reinforced if possible. Schamberg's weak iodin destroys the fungi in vitro, and tincture of iodin is practically useless as applied by patients to these foot conditions. Ruggles' tincture of iodin 1, spirits of camphor 7, did well until his patient went on a six weeks' vacation and left off treatment, with the usual relapse.

Ripened or developed lesions yield rather readily to almost any good dermatologic treatment, most of which are more or less germicidal, though not by far so rapidly as a simple dermatitis. Hidden organisms delay recovery, just as they, with now and then a reinfection, prevent permanent cure. After getting relief, the majority of patients disappear.

TREATMENT

In order to effect a cure, it is imperative that we rid the patient of all harbored fungi, and, in doing this, endeavor to adapt remedies to the destruction of organisms present in articles worn. Whitfield's principles of treatment must be followed in one particular at least, and to extremes. These cases require constant desquamating and exfoliating; in other words, persistent and intensive peeling. This is best accomplished with salicylic acid, combinations of methods to be mentioned later activating its effect. Benzoic acid is probably almost inert as a fungicide, as shown by Schamberg.

Pus cases, secondary coccic infections, have needed but a single remedy to clear them up in from twenty-four to forty-eight hours, whether there be a few pustules or the greater part of the plantar surface is undermined. Small lesions are broken up and the larger buttonholed in such manner as to prevent reclosure and yet leave sufficient epidermis for protection of tender surfaces until new can form. The official ointment of ammoniated mercury, in half or full strength, is specific. A few pus conditions may be too inflammatory, or, more likely, the lesions may have been stained with tincture of iodin, the latter condition contraindicating mercury. A mild boric ointment is satisfactory as a beginning in these cases.

Ointments are heavily applied, with cotton to retain them, and changed at least twice in twenty-four hours. Because of their messiness, doubtful utility and injury to footwear, I do not employ ointments in the nonpyodermic cases, save at night in conditions tending to become very dry.

Stains and dyes have been avoided because of their character as well as doubt of their ability to reach or affect the phytons. Treatment has been limited largely to powders and to mechanical procedures.

It may be stated with positiveness that the majority of cases of phytosis must be treated after the war cry of the Tank Corps, very few yielding definite results under gentle management. Soap, water and scrubbing (Williams) must be employed, not only for cleanliness but also to get rid of as much dead epithelium and as many fungi as possible. Vesicles are broken up, bullae and large subepidermic lakes torn to pieces or buttonholed, as in the pus conditions, and shreds are cut or peeled away in all cases. Plantar callosities are cleansed with soap and water or gasoline and covered with salicylic acid, roofed over with narrow overlapping strips of adhesive plaster—wide sections do not fit—and this dressing renewed as often as it loosens. As the seminecrosed, broken-up, rubber-like epidermis begins to separate, it is removed. The salicylic acid may also be employed on interspace accumulations, particularly the wide fourth. At the same time, salicylic acid is used in all powders, 1:8, or stronger, often alone, on the feet and in socks.

The gamut has been run with everything from a little boric acid even through ground-up hexamethylenamin and, occasionally, thymol iodid or calomel, to sulphur. Salicylic acid in the socks produces definite exfoliation of thick epidermis, as of plantar surfaces, and desquamation alone of lateral and dorsal areas, partly through greater contact from drifting down in the former instance, but also because the thickened epidermis is farther from its blood supply, and so less vital. It not only opens their lair, but possibly has some destructive action on the organisms; spores, as always, being perhaps the hardest to kill.

Proof that going into the treatment of the phytoses is entering a maze in which we wander rather vainly seeking a definite objective exists in the many remedies tried and abandoned or employed with scant success.

If formaldehyd vapor from an open bottle in the laboratory "killed all the ringworm cultures," why could the liquid or vapor not act in phytosis? Vapor was used under a rubber cap, in scalp cases. The disease required its usual time for cure. There is no practical way of applying vapor to foot cases, and any percentage of the liquid is too irritating and of slight penetration.

Hexamethylenamin grossly pulverized was put in socks, shoes and slippers, with the hope of getting some free formaldehyd. The soles were tanned and thickened, but vesicles and small bullae continued to appear even in the leathery tissue. Leather insoles were ruined by the drug. Benzin, or gasoline, applied to perfect sheaths of little black bugs on new shoots of grapevines killed both the bugs and a foot or two of new vine. Applied to broken vesicular points on the toes, it intensely aggravated the itching. Saturating the socks with it in the hope of sterilizing the feet and foot coverings had no apparent effect.

Surgical solutions were not considered worthy of trial and germicidal ointments, even the pus destructive ointment of ammoniated mercury, has been of doubtful utility in the phytoses. Any effect from the roentgen rays was simply due to cell reaction, and transitory. On several occasions, new erythematovesicular patches were treated by momentary freezing with ethyl chlorid, in the hope that refrigeration might hasten recovery. Carbon dioxid snow would have been cheaper, but the treatment was applied in the patient's room. Results of this brief freezing were uncertain.

In desperation, a physician even applied: Oleate of mercury and olive oil, four parts each, and sulphuric ether, sixty parts (mixed), an instantly effective remedy for pediculosis pubis and their ova. Even this mixture had practically no effect, except to ruin the shoes.

Powder prescriptions have always had talcum as the vehicle, since it is insoluble and keeps dry.

Powders have run from the ancient: salicylic acid and boric acid one part each, pulverized zinc oxid from four to eight parts, and pulverized talcum to make thirty parts (mixed) ; on through: salicylic acid, from two to four parts, benzoic acid, four parts, and pulverized talcum to make thirty parts (mixed) ; and salicylic acid, two parts, calomel, four parts, and pulverized talcum to make thirty parts (mixed).

Even pulverized alum has been added to some of these prescriptions for its drying effect ; and, finally : salicylic acid and precipitated sulphur, fifteen parts each (mixed).

He rubbed as frequently as possible on the hands of a patient who could treat them but little during the day ; applying at night : salicylic acid and precipitated sulphur, four parts of each, and zinc oxid ointment to make thirty parts (mixed), on all affected parts. The patient has done well.

A paste of sulphur and lard hastened recovery in one case Whitfield's ointment, stronger than the original, is still employed in some cases at night, and occasionally, the ammoniated ointment or petrolatum.

It will be seen from the foregoing that salicylic acid is depended on as the sheet anchor in all prescriptions.

There has been no opportunity to evaluate results from soaking the feet at night in hot water, salt water or ice water, or from washing them with gasoline, the majority of patients having been unwilling to fight the disease to a finish.

In the light of later experience, and through study of old case records. I am inclined to believe that pompholyx is not a distinct disease, as we get these exact lesions, "sago-grains" and all, in the phytoses.

REPORT OF CASES

Case 1.—J. W. C., aged 23, first seen, May 25, 1892. had six weeks before developed deep bullae and some excoriations on the left toes and foot. When examined, there were several ulcers, with pus and blood, and anterior plantar, flat bullae and denudations. Much of the pus was green. "Antiseptic" salves and powders were employed, and some "mixed treatment" was given, on a dubious history. The foot was well in fifteen days.

November 2: Pompholyx which had developed in the sole of left foot as a group of deep vesicles was drying up.

April 6. 1893: The patient had another attack of pompholyx, with deep-seated, shot-like vesicular lesions.

June 2: New vesicles developed. The patient had been using:

		Gm. or C.c.	
℞	Resorcin	1 4	gr. xx
	Zinc oxid	4	ʒ i
	Pulverized talcum...................q. s. ad	30	ʒ i

July 14: Bullae developed beneath the first and second interspaces of both feet. Asiatic pills were prescribed, and for local application:

		Gm. or C.c.	
℞	Resorcin (pulverized)	1 4	gr. xx
	Salicylic acid	1	gr. xv
	Talcum (pulverized) ad	30	ʒ i

There was hyperidrosis pedum. The eruption was better in two weeks.

March 7, 1894: A prescription for treating seborrhea of the scalp was given the patient. No complaint was made of the feet.

May 10: On both soles, especially beneath the arches, there were pin-head to nail-head diameter vesicles and bullae, and note was made of the "same old trouble." A 1:60 potassium bichromate solution was ordered as a wash and a bidaily dressing:

		Gm. or C.c.	
℞	Salicylic acid	2	ʒ ss
	Resorcin	2	ʒ ss
	Magnesium carbonate	4	ʒ i
	Olive oil.................q. s.	30	ʒ i

May 12: The old lesions were improved. and there were a few new ones. The patient died within the following year. His was a typical case of phytosis, the summer type.

Case 2.—Mrs. H. T., aged 29, first seen May 8. 1912, had pompholyx of the hands and feet, first noted in the spring of 1910, and again in the spring of the present year. On the palms, the fingers over the nail roots and on the toes, there were vesicles and erythematosquamous sequelae. On the soles and sides of the feet, there were bullae up to quarter of a dollar in size. Lesions were ordered broken up and boric acid and salicylic acid, one part each, zinc oxid (pulverized). eight parts, and talcum (pulverized) to make thirty parts was ordered kept on in white stockings and gloves.

The lesions began to dry, but new and painful flat bullae appeared, and new vesicles on the palms and fingers. Treatment, as for dermatitis or eczema. continued through prolonged dry, scaly and occasional vesicular periods, until August 28 when the affected areas showed but slight redness and scaling. All were healed, September 25.

May 7, 1921: The patient had had only one or two slight recurrences. At present, a vesicular to thick scaly itchy patch was present on the dorsum of one finger, and a small disk in the right submaxillary area. The latter soon healed, with simple treatment; the finger was resistant. Recurrence on the finger and a patch on one sole developed in September, and treatment was continued, still without recognition of the possibility of phyton infection, and certainly no treatment was given for this condition. The patient, who was hypersensitive, had plant dermatitis meanwhile, the last outbreak, on the forearms and hand, following gathering garden peas, in May, 1922, at which time the old dermatoses had long since disappeared.

CASE 3.—A medical student, from the country, had had trouble with his feet, summer and winter, for more than a year. When first seen, the anterior half of the plantar epidermis of the left foot was undermined with pus, and there was the usual condition of the toes. The pus was rapidly eliminated with ointment of ammoniated mercury. A large callus beneath the anterior arch was gradually removed with salicylic acid and adhesive plaster. Dermatitis of the toes was reduced by the salicylic acid, calomel and talcum powder; but the use of salicylic acid alone for the whole foot and peeling the sole to infantile thinness really accomplished the cure. This case was fought from fall to spring and definitely cured. The feet were always damp, partly for the reason that he wore overshoes in bad weather and kept them on indoors.

CASE 4.—A college professor, seen recently in May, when the daily temperature was running above 80 F., had had the condition for six summers, always affecting the external three toes of the right foot. It was never present in cold weather and had never been conveyed elsewhere, though the patient was most careless in handling the condition. Clinically, it was a perfect type of phytosis.

CASE 5.—This case is biographic of the disease as affecting the feet of a medical man with whom my relations were not exceeded by those of the Beaumont-St. Martin partnership. In 1918, he contracted the condition in quarters at a base hospital. This erythematosquamous dermatitis of lateral surfaces of the toes and interspaces, with fine fissuring of the latter, was attributed to the shower bath which was so strongly chlorinated that it irritated the eyes. The condition disappeared in cold weather.

In 1919, in Atlanta, there was recurrence with the advent of warm weather, vesicles now appearing about the toes. Diagnosis was made and careless stepping on a boarding house bath rug incriminated. All kinds of treatment and experiments were carried out; however, the salicylic and benzoic powders with talc were employed mostly, as well as occasional trials of most unusual procedures. The lesions disappeared by the time of frost, though the patient was rarely and briefly exposed to cold.

1920: The condition reappeared with the steadily warm days, it now involving also the anterior sole, from vesicles to small bullae. The slippers used in army were worn at home winter and summer. Summer socks, the same used even thus far in 1922, and an old pair of canvas shoes were worn during the hot weather, far into the summer of 1921. The disease had always appeared before these shoes were put on and even with new shoes. Slippers, socks and shoes got practically as much treatment as the feet.

1921: The toes had never been as uniformly affected as in the first year or two. Now the vesicles and deep bullae appeared as far back as the mid-sole, and two or three of the toes were showing small patches of vesicles dorsolaterally, especially near the nails. Vesicles were broken up and salicylic acid rubbed into all new areas or lesions. Gasoline was tried again in spite of its former bad effect on broken points, the socks being saturated with it and slippers or shoes put on. Later, ethyl chlorid freezing was practiced on all new outbreaks, and this season finished with the salicylic-sulphur-talc powder.

There was never hyperhidrosis, though there was a slight dampness of the socks winter and summer. Salicylic acid beneath adhesive plaster on a new patch caused a violent outbreak of vesicles beneath the plaster, peripherally to the salicylic acid application.

In April, 1922, there were a few days on which the temperature rose above 70 F. My impression is that the same socks, some pairs of which had been worn for several summers, cotton or mercerized, bluish-gray, were resumed about this time. Promptly, a large pea-sized bulla appeared beneath the center of the right heel, and a dime-sized patch of vesicles developed on the inner side of the arch of the same foot. All lesions were broken and rubbed with salicylic acid, sometimes the salicylic-sulphur mixture, and for the following weeks the inside of the socks were heavily dusted with salicylic acid, four parts, precipitated sulphur, eight parts, and talcum (pulverized) to make thirty parts (mixed). There was no night treatment. The bullae never itched but they were painful. There was intense itching of the primarily vesicular patches, just as this year, long after there was nothing but a little redness and scaling. At the end of May, there had been no new lesions; the site of the bulla peeled off, and the little patch was pink, thinly desquamative and a bit itchy. Many days in May and June, 1922, the thermometer rose as high as from 82 to 85 F. and the humidity was excessive. Use of the powder was continued and the left foot, thus far, has escaped and the right foot has shown no further lesions.[2] The sulphur accentuates the peeling effect of the salicylic, much of the latter being synthetic and probably weak locally.

We are not prepared thus early to believe that the final chapter in this biography can be written. The same lot of socks, washed by a colored woman, is being worn; the shoes were new in the winter. There is a pair of oxfords of last summer yet to be tested, though personally I would be satisfied to let well enough alone.[3]

This patient will never step on any bath floor and has the greatest repugnance for shower baths—the cement floors of all of which we believe infected.

SUMMARY AND CONCLUSIONS

It is admitted that the term phytosis, an amputated extremity of more definitely descriptive names, is a makeshift. Epidermophytons appearing now in the minority in the tricophyton group, we cannot properly continue epidermophytosis as descriptive. If the term tinea, used since 1829, means worm, it is as bad as many other misnomers. As it is impossible to make a laboratory diagnosis in every case, we must employ the loose term phytosis as a convenient designation.

---

2. The oxfords were later worn through a period of hot June weather, the temperature going as high as 93 F. The powder was never omitted.

3. Post seu propter hoc, within forty-eight hours after putting on a pair of socks not worn since last summer a single pruritic vesicle appeared above the outer edge of right heel. Severe treatment produced terminal peeling on the fifth day.

This disease group has few if any individually distinctive clinical features pointing to the type of fungus, even as the multitude of dermatitides venenatae may result from as many kinds of irritant as there are cases.

The disease is less contagious than infectious through an intermediary, as witness the frequency of unilateral cases and common sources of acquirement. Cases reported from practically every part of the world almost demonstrate pandemicity.

Commonest foci of infection are public baths, especially showers, and family contamination of rugs and floors and perhaps towels. Reinfection occurs from shoes, slippers and socks, even after laundering, or from laundry transference. The duration of viability of the fungi is from many months to an indefinite period, even in dry air. The majority of cases seems to indicate cold weather dormancy of organisms, even if the daily temperature reaches 60 F.

There is some preponderance of evidence that the fungi live as saprophytes in the epidermis all winter, down-growth preventing their removal by normal desquamation, though reinfection from footwear also occurs.

We encounter the same difficulty in treatment that is common in other infective conditions, such as tuberculosis, syphilis and gonorrhea; and, as in the case of inaccessible cancer cells, destruction in vitro and in vivo is hence vastly different. It is essential that desquamation and exfoliation be constantly induced. Salicylic acid is the best agent for this purpose. Aside from the use of an ointment of ammoniated mercury in secondary pus cases, where it is specific, greasy applications, particularly in the daytime, are not only uncomfortable but ruinous to shoes. Dyes, from tincture of iodin through the list, are disagreeable and of doubtful efficacy.

All vesicles must be broken up, all bullae or lakes buttonholed, loose epidermis removed, soap and water freely used and salicylic acid, from 12 to 100 per cent., employed, as a peeling agent. Powders in socks, shoes and slippers have constituted regular treatment, whether salicylic-sulphur or talcum powder, this at present seeming the more effective, salicylic and sulphur equal parts, or, occasionally the salicylic alone. Salicylic acid beneath air tight adhesive is used for the removal of callosities.

If greasy applications are needed at night, Whitfield's ointment, or a salicylic-sulphur ointment or simple petrolatum is used. Ointment of ammoniated mercury seems ineffective against these fungi. Cases extending over years are reported.

631 Candler Building.

COMPARATIVE STUDY OF THE KAHN AND WASSERMANN REACTIONS FOR SYPHILIS *

SOBEI IDE, M.D., AND GEORGE J. SMITH

ANN ARBOR, MICH.

Recently Kahn [1] proposed a precipitation reaction for syphilis for which he claims a high degree of sensitiveness and specificity, combined with simplicity and ease in manipulation. These claims led us to investigate this reaction, and this paper will present a preliminary report of our findings. The Wassermann test was carried out with a sheep-cell system and guinea-pig complement. Two antigens were used on each case. One an absolute alcohol extract of human heart muscle, reinforced with 0.4 per cent. cholesterin, and the other acetone insoluble lipoids with cholesterin, proposed by Kolmer.[2] The fixation period was from sixteen to eighteen hours in the icebox.

RESULTS OF REACTIONS

Wassermann Reaction		Kahn Reaction
296	+ + + +	250
25	+ + +	35
28	+ +	64
349....Total of more than	+ + positive	349
11	+	11
36	±	63
396	+ and ± included	423
1,769	—	1,742
2,165	Grand Total	2,165

The serums were obtained from unselected cases from this hospital, the University Hospital and various state asylums of Michigan. The serums were separated from the clots by centrifugation and were used, as a rule, within twenty-four hours after reaching the laboratory.

Altogether, 2,165 serums were examined with the Kahn and Wassermann reactions. As indicated in the accompanying table, the results of the reactions are identical when more than two plus positives are counted.

---

* From the Laboratory of the State Psychopathic Hospital, University of Michigan.

1. Kahn, R. L.: Simpler Quantitative Precipitation Reaction for Syphilis, Arch. Dermat. & Syph. 5:570 (May) 1922; ibid. 5:734 (June) 1922.

2. Kolmer, J. A.: Am. J. Syphilis 6:74 (Jan.) 1922.

CONCLUSION

The value of the Kahn precipitation reaction is almost as great as that of the Wassermann reaction on the blood serum. This reaction is now being performed as a check on the Wassermann reaction on all serums sent to this laboratory for examination. The relative ease with which this reaction can be carried out leads us to believe that it will attain wide usefulness in many laboratories. A point particularly in favor of the Kahn reaction is that anticomplementary serums give no difficulty with it. Such serums are either positive or negative, depending in the presence of syphilitic reagin. While this test worked very well on the blood serum, it does not, however, work as well on the spinal fluid as does the Wassermann test. It is believed by the writers on this subject that in the very near future this drawback will be overcome by some worker who will cast light on the matter.

News and Comment

CONGRESS OF FRENCH SPEAKING DERMATOLOGISTS AND SYPHILOLOGISTS

The Congress of French-Speaking Dermatologists and Syphilologists will be held at Strasbourg on the occasion of the celebration of the centennial of Pasteur, July 26 to 28. These are the topics on the program: Desensitization in diseases of the skin, Lavaut (Paris) and Spillmann (Nancy); nevocarcinoma, P. Masson (Strasbourg) and Bruno Bloch (Basel); treatment of primary syphilis, Queyrat (Paris) and Malvoz (Liége); value of various methods of using medicaments in the treatment of syphilis, Milian (Paris) and Bodin (Rennes). Queries with respect to the congress should be addressed to Professor Pautrier, president du bureau d'organisation du congrès, 2 Quai St. Nicolas, Strasbourg.

Abstracts from Current Literature

BACTERIAL ENDOCARDITIS AS A SEQUEL TO SYPHILITIC VALVE DEFECT. Le Roy H. Briggs, Am. J. Med. Sc. **164**:275 (Aug.) 1922.

Although syphilitic endocarditis is quite frequent, bacterial invasion following this condition is rare. Age incidence and changes in the vascularity of the valves are cited as possible factors to account for the infrequency of the two conditions. One case is reported.

Jamieson, Detroit.

THE SIGNS OF FILARIAL DISEASE. B. Blacklock, Am. Trop. M. & Parasitol. **16**:107 (July) 1922.

In 240 cases examined in Sierra Leone no correlation could be established between the "signs of filarial disease" and the occurrence in the blood of *Microfilaria bancrofti.*

Jamieson, Detroit.

THE ELIMINATION OF ARSENIC IN THE URINE OF SYPHILITIC PATIENTS AFTER INTRAVENOUS INJECTION OF ARSPHENAMIN. Charles Weiss and G. W. Raiziss, Arch. Int. Med. **30**:85 (July) 1922.

Three cases of previously treated syphilis were observed following doses of 0.6 gm. arsphenamin. Most of the arsenic passing through the kidneys is eliminated during the first three days, gradually diminishing during the next two weeks, the largest amount being 13.5 per cent. during this period. Following the second and third doses the elimination is greater and varies considerably in different persons and even in the same person at different times under the same conditions. A quantity of arsenic is temporarily retained by the liver, kidneys, spleen, etc., and some is eliminated through the feces.

Jamieson. Detroit.

SOME NOTES ON INDIAN CALLIPHORINAE. PART VI. HOW TO RECOGNIZE THE INDIAN MYIASIS-PRODUCING FLIES AND THEIR LARVAE, TOGETHER WITH SOME NOTES ON HOW TO BREED THEM AND STUDY THEIR HABITS. W. S. Patton. Ind. J. M. Res. **9**:635 (April) 1922.

PART VII. ADDITIONAL CASES OF MYIASIS CAUSED BY THE LARVAE OF CHRYSOMYIA BEZZIANA VILL. TOGETHER WITH SOME NOTES ON THE DIPTERA WHICH CAUSE MYIASIS IN MAN AND ANIMAL. Ibid., p. 654.

The contents of these articles are described by their titles. They are technical and not suited to abstracting.

Protection of sores and destruction of all larvae is recommended as a preventive in all countries in which these flies exist.

NOTES ON SOME INDIAN APHIOCHAETAE. W. S. Pattton, Ind. J. M. Res. **9**:685 (April) 1922.

This is a technical article describing the flies of this species which cause cutaneous and intestinal myiasis in man and animals.

A NOTE ON SOME CULTURAL PHASES OF LEISHMANIA DONOVANI. B. M. Das Gupta, Ind. J. M. Res. **9**:809 (April) 1922.

This is a discussion with regard to the encystment of the Leishman-Donovan bodies and whether unrecognized forms can exist in the tissues of its vertebrate **host.**

GATÉ-PAPACOSTAS REACTION IN LEPROSY. D. A. Turkhud and C. R. Avari, Ind. J. M. Res. **9**:850 (April) 1922.

One hundred and sixteen cases of leprosy tested by the formol-gel test all gave a positive reaction. This is regarded by the writers as a valuable serologic test in the diagnosis of leprosy.

Jamieson, Detroit.

STUDIES IN ASYMPTOMATIC NEUROSYPHILIS. II. THE CLASSIFICATION, TREATMENT AND PROGNOSIS OF EARLY ASYMPTOMATIC NEUROSYPHILIS. J. E. Moore, Johns Hopkins Bull. **33**:231 (July) 1922.

The author classifies neurosyphilis appearing within a year or less from the date of infection thus: (1) acute syphilitic meningitis; (2) precocious vascular neurosyphilis; (3) neurorecurrence; (4) neurosyphilis manifested by mild symptoms or slight physical signs, not of themselves diagnostic of central nervous system damage (headache, neurologic pains, etc.), and (5) asymptomatic neurosyphilis.

Moore disregards the first three groups, for reasons mentioned in his article, and confines himself to Groups 4 and 5, under the name of early asymptomatic neurosyphilis. The paper is based on 352 cases of primary or secondary syphilis of less than one year's duration. Ninety-four of the 352 patients developed early neurosyphilis, and of this number 76.6 per cent. fell into the asymptomatic group.

The author places the asymptomatic cases in three groups, the grouping being based on the type of spinal fluid, and, in part, on the response of the various types to treatment. He believes that the central nervous system is invaded in most cases in the first year unless the disease is influenced by treatment. Whether the organisms produce clinical neurosyphilis depends on the defense mechanism of the host. It is interesting to note that early asymptomatic neurosyphilis is more common in the white race than in the black, but it is the same in men and women of both races.

Prolonged regular antisyphilitic treatment intravenously will have a favorable result in Groups 1 and 2, but Group 3 responds only to intraspinous medication. The author's statistics do not support the theory of a neurotropic strain.

That the spinal fluid abnormalities of early asymptomatic neurosyphilis are signs of actual anatomic damage to the nervous system is no doubt true. The author believes that Group 1 may pass on to Groups 2 and 3 if left untreated; and he therefore strongly urges a diagnostic lumbar puncture at the end of the first or second courses; if negative, to be repeated at the close of the treatment.

McCafferty, New York.

A REVIEW OF THE CLINICAL SIGNIFICANCE OF THE WASSER-MANN REACTION. A. STRICKLER, J. A. M. A. **78**:962 (April 1) 1922.

This article gives a general summary of the present knowledge concerning the clinical value of the Wassermann reaction. The author stresses the injustice done patients by subjecting them to specific treatment on the strength of a weakly positive reaction, unsupported by clinical evidence of the disease.

REPORT OF A CASE OF NASAL HERPES DUE TO INGESTION OF PHENOLPHTHALEIN. J. ROSENBLOOM, J. A. M. A. **78**:967 (April 1) 1922.

Recurrent herpes of the nasal region was due to the occasional use of a proprietary pill containing phenolphthalein. Even one-half grain of the drug provoked the eruption.

SOME NOTES ON THE EFFECTIVENESS OF THE VENEREAL DISEASE PROGRAM. H. F. IRVINE, J. A. M. A. **79**:1121 (Sept. 30) 1922.

The reporting of veneral disease by number, and not by name, appears to secure better cooperation from physicians. The spending of large sums of money for quarantine and rehabilitation of prostitutes is condemned. Prostitution is handled best by legal means.

SYPHILIS OF THE MOUTH: COMMON TENDENCY OF THE MOUTH AND SKIN TO THE SAME PATHOLOGIC PROCESSES. W. A. PUSEY, J. A. M. A. **79**:1285 (Oct. 14) 1922.

This is an exposition of the clinical characteristics of syphilis of the mouth with pertinent comments from the author's experience. Despite the general impression to the contrary, Pusey emphasizes his opinion that leuoplakia due to syphilis is much less frequent than leukoplakia of nonspecific origin.

MICHAEL, Houston, Texas.

BISMUTH IN SYPHILIS. C. LEVADITI, Press méd. **30**:632 (July) 1922.

Levaditi discusses in detail the action of tartrobismuth of sodium and potassium in syphilis, from its discovery in 1889 by Balzer to the present time. From a therapeutic point of view, it compares favorably with the best preparations of arsphenamin. Its action is as quick and thorough as that of arsphenamin in all forms of syphilis, whether they be cutaneous, visceral or nervous. The action on the Wassermann test is similar to that of arsphenamin except that the blood which may be positive at the end of a regular course may become negative a short time after the cessation of administration of tartrobismuth sodium and potassium.

It is given in 2 c.c. doses, containing 0.2 gm. of the active substance and injected every three or four days until from 2.2 to 3 gm. are given. An interval of one month is allowed to elapse, and treatment is again given until the Wassermann test becomes negative.

The bismuth is found in all the organs, including the nervous tissue, and is eliminated in the usual ways. Its elimination is begun in twenty hours after an injection, and continues for twenty-five days after the last treatment. There are no contraindications when it is given properly. The compound may be given as a prophylactic, with good results. The author considers it the equivalent of arsphenamin and believes that the patient does not become immune to its action. The good effects of the bismuth continue long after the cessation of treatment.

McCafferty, New York.

PENICILLUM GLAUCUM AS THE ETIOLOGIC AGENT OF ULCER OF THE LEG. U. Rebaudi and G. B. Podesta, Gior. ital. d. mal. ven. **63:** 871 (Aug.) 1922.

Penicillum glaucum was isolated and cultivated from two ulcers of the leg in a middle-aged woman. The complement-fixation test made with the spores of the fungus was strongly positive. The authors call attention to the pathogenic properties of fungi and make a plea to the medical profession for their consideration as etiologic agents of disease.

TREATMENT OF TINEA BARBAE WITH INTRAVENOUS INJECTIONS OF GRAM'S SOLUTION. F. Ronchese, Gior. ital. d. mal. ven. **63:**918 (Aug.) 1922.

Five cases of tinea barbae were treated with Gram's solution. The amount injected varied from 1 to 5 c.c. diluted in 5 c.c. of water, the injections being made every other day. One case showed some improvement, but the other four did not present any change and were finally successfully treated with the roentgen ray. The injections are well tolerated, but there was a local reaction, the vein becoming hard and thrombotic.

Pardo-Castello, Havana, Cuba.

THERAPEUTIC RESEARCHES WITH PERCUTANEOUS ELECTROLYSIS. K. Wirz, Dermat. Wchnschr. **74:**321 (April 8) 1922.

After experimentation, the author found that epinephrin, iontophoretically introduced into the skin, caused a diffuse, intensive and lasting anemia which is useful in small cosmetic operations. Epinephrin, so administered, also favorably influences localized eczema. Ichthyol applied to parasitic sycosis in this manner causes more rapid and certain improvement than any other methods of treatment, including treatment with the roentgen rays. In tricophytosis, iodid of potassium so given causes rapid improvement. In lupus and scrofula these were of little value.

ACID-FAST BACILLI IN ACNE CONGLOBATA. E. Pick, Dermat. Wchnschr. **74:**345 (April 15) 1922.

A case of this disease is reported in which acid-fast bacilli, morphologically characteristic of tubercle bacilli, were observed on animal inoculation and cultural tests. These were conclusively proved to be nonpathogenic saprophytes, and not *B. tuberculosis.*

A NEW TECHNIC FOR INTRAMUSCULAR MERCURY INJECTION. B. Pontoppidon, Dermat. Wchnschr. **74:**348 (April 15) 1922.

Instead of an oil suspension, greater accuracy and sterility is obtained by the use of pellets of cocoa butter containing mild mercurous chlorid (calomel), rod-shaped, with a diameter of a few millimeters, so that they fit into an ordinary 1 c.c. syringe, which is warmed prior to injection.

COLLOIDAL BENZOIN REACTION ON THE SPINAL FLUID. F. Mras, Dermat. Wchnschr. **74**:369 (April 22) 1922.

After extensive researches on the spinal fluids of syphilitic and non-syphilitic persons, the author advocates the value of the colloidal benzoin reaction and says that there is a second precipitation zone, similar to that described by Kafka in the Mastix reaction, which is of value in the diagnosis of menigitic involvement.

A CASE OF RAZOR CHANCRE. H. Helle, Dermat. Wchnschr. **74**:376 (April 22) 1922.

The appearance of a chancre on the site of a cut on the chin received in shaving is described. When observed the patient also had a secondary exanthem and a four plus Wassermann.

SYPHILIS OF THE VEGETATIVE NERVOUS SYSTEM. E. Sklarz, Dermat. Wchnschr. **74**:393 (April 29) 1922.

In the past, little attention has been given this subject. The following subjects are discussed:

The temporary arrhythmias of the heart in syphilitic persons, the appearance of exanthems due to the disease or to the treatment, the Herxheimer reaction. the anaphylactic manifestations subsequent to arsphenamin injections and their relief by sympatheticotropic remedies, syphilis of the suprarenals, alopecia and leukoderma, decubitus and malperforans in neurosyphilitic persons, herpes zoster, the vomiting and hypo-acidity, and the obstipation and incontinence in tabetic patients, their impotence and crises, the occasional appearance of Graefe's and Stelwagon's phenomena without struma, and disturbances of the glands of internal secretion, an instance of which are the anomalies of dental development in persons with congenital syphilis.

THE VALUE OF THE DACTYLOSCOPE IN CRIMINOLOGY. F. Dehnow, Dermat. Wchnschr. **74**:398 (April 29) 1922.

The dactyloscope is an instrument devised for the observation of the papillary line. In no two fingers is this line the same. Observations of it, to supplement finger prints, have proved of value in the identification of various persons.

Andrews, New York.

Book Reviews

ATLAS DER SYPHILIS. By Leo v. Zumbusch. Leipzig, F. C. W. Vogel, 1922.

A recent importation, von Zumbusch's Atlas should have great vogue in this and other countries. The Atlas consists of thirty-one plates portraying sixty-three phases and features of syphilis, as ordinarily encountered, rather than the bizarre and rare manifestations. The choice of subjects is unusually good. The text is short, and is printed with each picture. Indeed, one without any knowledge of German may review the Atlas with profit. One cannot say too much regarding the faithfulness of reproduction of the lesions of syphilis.

LEHRBUCH DER HAARKRANKHEITEN. By Max Joseph. Leipzig: Barth, 1921.

The second edition of this manual of the care and treatment of diseases of the hair has been condensed a little, yet all that is new and has been confirmed has been added. There are twenty-five illustrations in the text, and more than 100 prescriptions. An addenda carries a list of ninety-eight prescriptions for alopecia, hair dyes, hair oils, hair tonics, washes, pomades and soaps.

Index to Current Literature

DERMATOLOGY

Acne Vulgaris. Biochemical Studies in Diseases of Skin. O. L. Levin and M. Kahn, Am. J. M. Sc. **164**:379 (Sept.) 1922.

Alopecia and Its Treatment. L. K. McCafferty, New York M. J. & Med. Rec. **116**:369 (Oct. 4) 1922.

Alopecia Areata, Familial, and Strabismus: Family Group of Cases. J. G. Tomkinson, Brit. M. J. **2**:505 (Sept. 16) 1922.

Anemia, Pernicious, Melanodermia in. M. Mosse, Med. Klin. **18**:1085 (Aug. 13) 1922.

Anthrax. R. F. Vaccarezza et al., Semana méd. **1**:1081 (June 29) 1922.

Cancer of Mouth. J. C. Bloodgood, Northwest Med. **21**:280 (Sept.) 1922.

Cancer of Skin, Roentgen-Ray Treatment of. G. Miescher, Schweizer. med. Wchnschr. **52**:791 (Aug. 10) 1922.

Cancer of Tongue: Pitfalls in Diagnosis and Treatment. W. S. Bainbridge, J. A. M. A. **79**:1480 (Oct. 28) 1922.

Carbuncle, Treatment of. A. U. Williams, J. Arkansas M. Soc. **19**:68 (Sept.) 1922.

Dermatitis Artefacta. G. H. Lancashire, Brit. M. J. **2**:504 (Sept. 16) 1922.

Dermatitis, Occupational. W. J. O'Donovan, Brit. M. J. **2**:499 (Sept. 16) 1922.

Dermatology and Nervous System. G. H. Hyslop, New York M. J. & Med. Rec. **116**:402 (Oct. 4) 1922.

Dermatoses, Occupation. R. Ruedemann, Jr., Ohio State M. J. **18**:618 (Sept.) 1922.

Dermatoses, Precancerous. W. J. Highman, New York M. J. & Med. Rec. **116**:367 (Oct. 4) 1922.

Dystrophia Adiposogenitalis, Pityriasis Rubra Pilaris Associated with. P. E. Bechet, New York M. J. & Med. Rec. **116**:372 (Oct. 4) 1922.

Epithelioma, Retrogression of. M. Helmann, Semana méd. **1**:1111 (June 29) 1922.

Erysipelas, Experimental. Studies in Streptococcus Infection and Immunity. F. P. Gay and B. Rhodes, J. Infect. Dis. **31**:101 (Aug.) 1922.

Erythema Nodosum and Tuberculosis. A. Wallgren, Acta Pediatrica **2**:85 (July 31) 1922.

Erythema Nodosum Plus Phlebitis. C. Achard and J. Rouillard. Bull. et mém. Soc. méd. d. hôp. **46**:1113 (July 21) 1922.

Erythrodermia Desquamativa (Leiner). B. Hackel, Monatschr. f. Kinderh. **23**:197 (May) 1922.

Exanthems in Typhoid Fever in Children. J. Kisters, Monatschr. f. Kinderh. **23**:193 (May) 1922.

Granuloma Inguinale. H. L. Claassen, Ohio State M. J. **18**:685 (Oct.) 1922.

Granuloma Inguinale and Other Granulomas and Granulating Ulcers, Tartar Emetic in Treatment of. K. M. Lynch, South. M. J. **15**:688 (Sept.) 1922.

Herpes, Etiology of. K. Edel, Nederlandsch Tijdschr. v. Geneesk. **2**:263 (July 15) 1922.

Keratitis Punctata, Leprous, Case of. M. J. Levitt, New York M. J. & Med. Rec. **116**:376 (Oct. 4) 1922.

Leishmaniosis, Cutaneous, Two Cases of. H. Fox, New York M. J. & Med. Rec. **116**:365 (Oct. 4) 1922.

Leprosy, Prophylaxis of. I. Vernet, Brazil-med. **2**:61 (July 29) 1922.

Leukoplakia Buccalis. H. H. Hazen and F. J. Eichenlaub. J. A. M. A. **79**:1487 (Oct. 28) 1922.

Measles, Diazo Reaction in. N. Malmberg. Acta Pediatrica **2**:101 (July 31) 1922.

Measles, Inhibition of the Gruber-Widal Reaction by. W. Forche, Deutsch. med. Wchnschr. **48**:1010 (July 28) 1922.

Melanodermia, Case of. Enriquez et al., Bull. et mém. Soc. méd. d. hôp. **46**: 1149 (July 21) 1922.

Melanodermia in Pernicious Anemia. M. Moses, Med. Klin. **18**:1085 (Aug. 13) 1922.

Mouth, Cancer of. J. C. Bloodgood, Northwest Med. **21**:280 (Sept.) 1922.

Myiasis, Cutaneous, Cases of Larvae of Wohlfahrtia Vigil (Walker). E. M. Walker, J. Parasitology **9**:1 (Sept.) 1922.

Nervous System and Dermatology. G. H. Hyslop, New York M. J. & Med. Rec. **116**:402 (Oct. 4) 1922.

Oils, Cutting, Causing Skin Lesions, Bacteriologic Study of. R. C. Rosenberger, New York M. J. & Med. Rec. **116**:377 (Oct. 4) 1922.

Phlebitis. Erythema Nodosum Plus Phlebitis. C. Achard and J. Rouillard, Bull. et mém. Soc. méd. d. hôp. **46**:1113 (July 21) 1922.

Pityriasis Rubra Pilaris Associated with Dystrophia Adiposogenitalis. P. E. Bechet, New York M. J. & Med. Rec. **116**:372 (Oct. 4) 1922.

Pox, Sheep, Studies on. M. Tsurumi, T. Toyoda and T. Inouye, Japan Med. World **2**:221 (Aug.) 1922.

Psychosis. Diffuse Scleroderma with Concurrent Psychosis. C. F. Read, J. Nerv. & Ment. Dis. **56**:313 (Oct.) 1922.

Purpura Fulminans Complicating Scarlet Fever. N. T. Johnston, Nebraska M. J. **7**:284 (Aug.) 1922.

Rhinoscleroma. H. Goodman, New York M. J. & Med. Rec. **116**:391 (Oct. 4) 1922.

Roentgen Rays in Diseases of Skin. E. W. Reed, Brit. M. J. **2**:559 (Sept. 23) 1922.

Roentgen-Ray Treatment of Tinea Tonsurans. J. G. Graham. Brit. M. J. **2**: 563 (Sept. 23) 1922

Roentgen Ray, Value of, in Skin Diseases. M. V. Leof, New York M. J. & Med. Rec. **116**:379 (Oct. 4) 1922.

Scarlet Fever, Purpura Fulminans Complicating. N. T. Johnston, Nebraska M. J. **7**:284 (Aug.) 1922.

Scleroderma, Diffuse, with Concurrent Psychosis. C. F. Read, J. Nerv. & Ment. Dis. **56**:313 (Oct.) 1922.

Skin, Biochemical Studies in Disease of. II. Acne Vulgaris. O. L. Levin and M. Kahn, Am. J. M. Sc. **164**:379 (Sept.) 1922.

Skin. Cases of Cutaneous Myiasis: Larvae of Wohlfahrtia Vigil (Walker). E. M. Walker, J. Parasitology **9**:1 (Sept.) 1922.

Skin Diseases, Value of Roentgen Ray in. M. V. Leof, New York M. J. & Med. Rec. **116**:379 (Oct. 4) 1922.

Skin Eruptions, Hits and Misses in Diagnosis of. C. Pijper, M. J. South Africa **17**:248 (July) 1922.

Skin, Frog's, Electromotor Reaction of. K. Hashida, J. Biochemistry **1**:21 (Jan.) 1922.

Skin Lesions, Bacteriologic Study of Cutting Oils Causing. R. C. Rosenberger, New York M. J. & Med. Rec. **116**:377 (Oct. 4) 1922.

Skin Lesions in Smallpox, Bacteriology of. L. E. Hines, J. Infect. Dis. **31**:89 (Aug.) 1922.

Skin, Roentgen Rays in Diseases of. E. W. Reed, Brit. M. J. **2**:559 (Sept. 23) 1922.

Skin, Roentgen-Ray Treatment of Cancer of. G. Miescher, Schweizer. med. Wchnschr. **52**:791 (Aug. 10) 1922.

Smallpox. Bacteriology of Skin Lesions in. L. E. Hines, J. Infect. Dis. **31**: 89 (Aug.) 1922.

Smallpox, Paul's Rabbit Eye Test for. J. M. Gomes, Brazil-med. **2**:35 (July 15) 1922.

Sore, Oriental, Two Cases of (Cutaneous Leishmaniosis). H. Fox, New York M. J. & Med. Rec. **116**:365 (Oct. 4) 1922.

Sporotrichosis, Case of. C. M. Grigsby and R. H. Moore, South M. J. **15:** 684 (Sept.) 1922.

Sporotrichosis, Report of Five Cases of. E. A. Watson, Nebraska M. J. **7:** 282 (Aug.) 1922.

Strabismus and Familial Alopecia Areata: Family Group of Cases. J. G. Tomkinson, Brit. M. J. **2:**505 (Sept. 16) 1922.

Tar Cancer, Experimental. H. T. Deelman, Nederlandsch Tijdschr. v. Geneesk. **2:**334 (July 22) 1922.

Tinea Tonsurans, Roentgen-Ray Treatment of. J. G. Graham, Brit. M. J. **2:**563 (Sept. 23) 1922.

Tongue, Cancer of; Pitfalls in Diagnosis and Treatment. W. S. Bainbridge, J. A. M. A. **79:**1480 (Oct. 28) 1922.

Tuberculosis and Erythema Nodosum. A. Wallgren, Acta Pediatrica **2:**85 (July 31) 1922.

Tuberculosis Plus Inherited Syphilis in Children. J. Cassel, Med. Klin. **18:** 1048 (Aug. 13) 1922.

Tuberculosis, Syphilis and the Teeth. C. D'Alise, Pediatria **30:**823 (Sept. 1) 1922.

Typhoid Fever, Exanthems in, in Children. J. Kisters, Monatschr. f. Kinderh. **23:**193 (May) 1922.

"Ulcus Tropicum" in North Palestine, Observations on. K. C. Sen, Indian M. Gaz. **57:**286 (Aug.) 1922.

SYPHILOLOGY

Achondroplasia in Infant with Syphilitic Parent. G. Milio, Pediatria **30:**775 (Aug. 15) 1922.

Arsenical Preparations. New Bismuth and Arsenical Preparations for Treating Syphilis. Pomaret, Brazil-med. **2:**76 (Aug. 5) 1922.

Arsphenamin and Mercury, Contribution to Action of, on Treponema Pallidum. D. C. Lee, Am. J. Syphilis **6:**546 (July) 1922.

Arsphenamin and Neo-Arsphenamin, Influence of, on Epinephrin Content of Suprarenals. B. Lucke, J. A. Kolmer and G. P. McCouch, J. Pharmacol. & Exper. Therap. **20:**153 (Sept.) 1922.

Arsphenamin By-Effects. H. Mouradian. Paris méd. **12:**172 (Aug. 19) 1922.

Arsphenamin Derivative Suitable for Subcutaneous Administration. C. Voegtlin. H. Dyer and J. W. Thompson, Am. J. Syphilis **6:**526 (July) 1922.

Arsphenamin in Children, Distribution and Excretion of Arsenic After Intravenous Administration of. S. W. Clausen and P. C. Jeans, Am. J. Syphilis **6:**556 (July) 1922.

Arsphenamin, Jaundice Under. W. Wechselmann and H. Wreschner. Med. Klin. **18:**1080 (Aug. 13) 1922.

Arsphenamin. Possible Excitive Effects of Arsphenamin on Tabes. Paresis and Syphilis of the Brain in Secondary Syphilis. K. Wagner. Wien. klin. Wchnschr. **35:**673 (Aug. 3) 1922.

Arsphenamin—Some Factors Which Influence Its Colloidal Properties. A. E. Sherndal, J. Lab. & Clin. M. **7:**723 (Sept.) 1922.

Arthropathies in Syphilitic Infants. G. L. Hallez. Médecine **3:**852 (Aug.) 1922.

Bismuth and Arsenical Preparations, New, for Treating Syphilis. Pomaret. Brazil-med. **2:**76 (Aug. 5) 1922.

Brain. Possible Excitive Effects of Arsphenamin on Tabes. Paresis and Syphilis of the Brain in Secondary Syphilis. K. Wagner. Wien. klin. Wchnschr. **35:**673 (Aug. 3) 1922.

Chancre, Extragenital. W. J. Young. Am. J. Syphilis **6:**392 (July) 1922.

Chancre, Penile, with Ringworm; Report of Case. F. J. Eichenlaub. J. A. M. A. **79:**1518 (Oct. 28) 1922.

Colon, Syphilis of. J. P. Keith, South. M. J. **15:**709 (Sept.) 1922.

Complement Fixation Test in Syphilis. Quantitative. J. A. Kolmer. Am. J. Syphilis **6:**496 (July) 1922.

Complement Fixation Tests in Syphilis, Study of Factors Influencing Amount of Antigen to Employ in. J. A. Kolmer, Am. J. Syphilis **6**:481 (July) 1922.

Ear. Two Cases of Syphilis of Eighth Nerve and Inner Ear. E. G. Gill, Virginia M. Month. **49**:337 (Sept.) 1922.

Extremities. Trophic Disturbances of Lower Extremities in Relation to Syphilis. S. J. Sinkoe, J. M. A. Georgia **11**:352 (Sept.) 1922.

Heart. Treatment of Syphilitic Liver and Heart: Therapeutic Paradox. U. J. Wile, Am. J. M. Sc. **164**:415 (Sept.) 1922.

Hecht-Weinberg-Gradwohl Test: Studies on Serodiagnosis of Syphilis. L. W. Famulener and J. A. W. Hewitt, J. Infect Dis. **31**:285 (Sept.) 1922.

Jarisch-Herxheimer Reaction; Unusual Reaction Following Antisyphilitic Treatment. H. A. R. Kreutzmann, Am. J. Syphilis **6**:539 (July) 1922.

Jaundice Under Arsphenamin. W. Wechselmann and H. Wreschner, Med. Klin. **18**:1080 (Aug. 13) 1922.

Liver and Heart, Syphilitic, Treatment of: Therapeutic Paradox. U. J. Wile, Am. J. M. Sc. **164**:415 (Sept.) 1922.

Liver, Fatal Syphilis of, in *Y*oung Prostitute. K. Bierring, Ugesk. f. Læger **84**:969 (Aug. 3) 1922.

Liver, Syphilitic Disease of. F. Viola, Policlinico **29**:1040 (Aug. 7) 1922.

Lung. Syphilis of; Report of Case. A. T. Hawthorne, Virginia M. Month. **49**:345 (Sept.) 1922.

Mercurosal. Report Following Use of Mercurosal in Treatment of One Hundred and Fifty Cases of Syphilis. W. E. Keane and J. G. Slaugenhaupt, J. Urol. **7**:197 (Sept.) 1922.

Mercury and Arsphenamin, Contribution to Action of, on Treponema Pallidum. D. C. Lee, Am. J. Syphilis **6**:546 (July) 1922.

Metasyphilis, Combined Treatment of. T. Brunner, Schweizer. med. Wchnschr. **52**:812 (Aug. 17) 1922.

Metrorrhagia and Syphilis. Dalché, Progrès méd. **37**:364 (Aug. 5) 1922.

Mouth, Syphilis of: Common Tendency of the Mouth and Skin to the Same Pathologic Processes. W. A. Pusey, J. A. M. A. **79**:1285 (Oct. 14) 1922.

Neo-Arsphenamin, Death Fifty-Five Hours After Intravenous Administration of. J. H. Schrup, Am. J. Syphilis **6**:544 (July) 1922.

Neo-Arsphenamin. Influence of Arsphenamin and Neo-Arsphenamin on Epinephrin Content of Suprarenals. B. Lucke, J. A. Kolmer and G. P. McCouch, J. Pharmacol. & Exper. Therap. **20**:153 (Sept.) 1922.

Nerve. Two Cases of Syphilis of Eighth Nerve and Inner Ear. E. G. Gill, Virginia M. Month. **49**:337 (Sept.) 1922.

Neurosyphilis, Fatal. H. Vøhtz, Ugesk. f. Læger **84**:1012 (Aug. 10) 1922.

Ophthalmia, Sympathetic, Arsphenamin in. P. Satanowsky, Semana méd. **2**:34 (June 29) 1922.

Paralysis, General, and Tabes Dorsalis, Pathogenesis and Treatment of. L. B. Alford, Am. J. Syphilis **6**:410 (July) 1922.

Paresis. Effects of Antisyphilitic Therapy as Indicated by Histologic Study of Cerebral Cortex in Cases of General Paresis. H. C. Solomon and A. E. Taft, Arch. Neurol. & Psychiat. **8**:341 (Oct.) 1922.

Pipet Washer and Wassermann Test Tube. C. E. Swanbeck, J. Lab. & Clin. Med. **7**:754 (Sept.) 1922.

Radioactive Baths and Wassermann Reaction. Mittenzwey, Wien. klin. Wchnschr. **35**:657 (July 27) 1922.

Reaction, Unusual, Following Antisyphilitic Treatment; Jarisch-Herxheimer Reaction. H. A. R. Kreutzmann, Am. J. Syphilis **6**:539 (July) 1922.

Ringworm, Penile Chancre with: Report of Case. F. J. Eichenlaub, J. A. M. A. **79**:1518 (Oct. 28) 1922.

Sachs-Georgi and Wassermann Reactions in Diagnosis of Syphilis, Relative Value of. C. F. Craig and W. C. Williams. J. A. M. A. **79**:1597 (Nov. 4) 1922.

Stomach. Syphilitic Gastric Ulcer. A. Cade and Morenas, Arch. d. mal. de l'app. digestif. **12**:109 (March) 1922.

Teeth, Syphilis and Tuberculosis. C. D'Alise, Pediatria **30**:823 (Sept. 1) 1922.
Treponema Pallidum, Contribution to Action of Arsphenamin and Mercury on. D. C. Lee, Am. J. Syphilis **6**:546 (July) 1922.
Venereal Disease Control in Army of France, Insistent Campaign for. A. N. Tasker, Mil. Surgeon **51**:240 (Sept.) 1922.
Wassermann Reaction and Radioactive Baths. Mittenzwey, Wien. klin. Wchnschr. **35**:657 (July 27) 1922.
Wassermann Reaction from Clinical Standpoint. L. M. Otero, An. de la Fac. de Med. **7**:131 (May) 1922.
Wassermann Reaction from Clinician's Point of View. C. J. Broeman, Am. J. Syphilis **6**:499 (July) 1922.
Wassermann Reaction, Interpretation of. W. A. Murray, South Africa M. Rec. **20**:306 (Aug. 26) 1922.
Wassermann Reactions. Relative Value of Sachs-Georgi and Wassermann Reactions in Diagnosis of Syphilis. C. F. Craig and W. C. Williams, J. A. M. A. **79**:1597 (Nov. 4) 1922.
Wassermann Reaction, Studies in Standardization of. Study of Factors Influencing Titration of Antigen. J. A. Kolmer and M. E. Trist, Am. J. Syphilis **6**:461 (July) 1922.
Wassermann Test, Interpretation of. H. K. Detweiler, Pub. Health J. **13**:395 (Sept.) 1922.
Wassermann Test Tube and Pipet Washer. C. E. Swanbeck, J. Lab. & Clin. Med. **7**:754 (Sept.) 1922.

INDEX TO VOLUME 6

The star (*) preceding the page number indicates an original article in THE ARCHIVES. Book Reviews, Obituaries and Society Transactions are indexed under these headings in their alphabetical order under the letters B, O and S, respectively.

PAGE

Lightning Source UK Ltd.
Milton Keynes UK
UKHW010322120219
337137UK00004B/370/P

9 780260 850010